D1606727

Manual of Research Techniques in Cardiovascular Medicine

Dedication

To my dear wife, Fahti, for her support and being my companion and best friend. And to my children, Mariam and Ali.
Hossein Ardehali

I dedicate this book to all those who have seen that the complexity of life is infinite and that life itself is a miracle.
Roberto Bolli

To Tina, my love, for all of her love and support, to our son Luke for teaching us the meaning of true joy, and to my parents, Dominic and Louise, who gave me the compass that has guided me throughout my life.
Douglas Losordo

Manual of Research Techniques in Cardiovascular Medicine

Edited by

Hossein Ardehali MD, PhD, FAHA
Associate Professor of Medicine, Molecular Pharmacology and Biological Chemistry
Feinberg Cardiovascular Research Institute
Northwestern University Feinberg School of Medicine
Chicago, IL
USA

Roberto Bolli MD
Professor of Medicine
Chief, Division of Cardiovascular Medicine
Director, Institute of Molecular Cardiology
University of Louisville
Louisville, KY
USA

Douglas W. Losordo MD
Vice President
New Therapeutic Development
Baxter Healthcare Corporation
Deerfield, IL
USA

Section Editors

Sanjiv J. Shah
Marina Bayeva
Amy Rines
Andy Wasserstrom

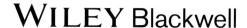

Library of Congress Cataloging-in-Publication Data
Manual of research techniques in cardiovascular medicine / edited by Hossein Ardehali, Roberto Bolli, Douglas W. Losordo; section editors, Sanjiv Shah, Marina Bayeva, Amy Rines, Andy Wasserstrom.
    p. ; cm.
  Includes bibliographical references and index.
  ISBN 978-0-470-67269-3 (cloth) – ISBN 978-1-118-49513-1 (epub) – ISBN 978-1-118-49514-8 –
ISBN 978-1-118-49515-5 – ISBN 978-1-118-49516-2 (epdf)
    I. Ardehali, Hossein, editor of compilation. II. Losordo, Douglas, editor of compilation. III. Bolli, Roberto, editor of compilation. IV. Shah, Sanjiv, editor of compilation. V. Bayeva, Marina, editor of compilation. VI. Rines, Amy, editor of compilation. VII. Wasserstrom, Andy, editor of compilation.
    [DNLM: 1. Cardiovascular Diseases. 2. Cardiology–methods. 3. Models, Cardiovascular. 4. Research Design.
WG 120]
    RC681
    616.1'2–dc23
                    2013017936

A catalogue record for this book is available from the British Library.

Cover image: Background image – Fotolia #42280909 © luchshen. Foreground image – Fotolia #44655249 © CLIPAREA.com
Cover design by Andrew Magee Design Ltd

Set in 9.25/12 pt Minion by Toppan Best-set Premedia Limited
Printed and bound in Malaysia by Vivar Printing Sdn Bhd

1 2014

Contents

Part 3 Manipulation of the Heart and Vessels *in Vivo* and *ex Vivo*

Part 4 Small Animal Imaging

Part 5 Metabolism, Mitochondria, and Cell Death

Part 6 Manipulation of Gene Expression *in Vitro* and *in Vivo*

List of Contributors

E. Dale Abel MB, BS, DPhil
Professor of Medicine and Biochemistry
John B Stokes III, Chair in Diabetes Research
Fraternal Order of Eagles Diabetes Research Center
Division of Endocrinology and Metabolism
Roy J. and Lucille A. Carver College of Medicine
University of Iowa, Iowa City, IA
USA

Abhinav Agarwal PhD
Post Doctoral Scholar
Institute of Molecular Cardiology
Diabetes and Obesity Center
University of Louisville
Louisville, KY
USA

Molly Ahrens PhD
Postdoctoral Associate
Northwestern University Feinberg School of
Medicine;
Lurie Children's Hospital of Chicago Research
Center
Chicago, IL
USA

Gary L. Aistrup PhD
Research Assistant Professor
Department of Medicine (Cardiology)
Feinberg Cardiovascular Research Institute
Northwestern University Feinberg School of
Medicine
Chicago, IL
USA

Hossein Ardehali MD, PhD, FAHA
Associate Professor of Medicine, Molecular
Pharmacology and Biological Chemistry
Feinberg Cardiovascular Research Institute
Northwestern University Feinberg School of Medicine
Chicago, IL
USA

Takayuki Asahara MD, PhD
Professor of Regenerative Medicine Science
Science Division of Basic Clinical Science
Tokai University School of Medicine
Shimokasuya, Isehara
Kanagawa;
Group Leader of Vascular Regeneration Research
Group
Institute of Biomedical Research and Innovation
Kobe, Hyogo
Japan

Christopher P. Baines PhD
Assistant Professor of Biomedical Sciences
Dalton Cardiovascular Research Center
Department of Biomedical Sciences
Department of Medical Pharmacology and
Physiology
University of Missouri
Columbia, MO
USA

Marina Bayeva PhD
Research Associate
Feinberg Cardiovascular Research Institute
Northwestern University Feinberg School of
Medicine
Chicago, IL
USA

Darrell D. Belke PhD
Assistant Professor
Roger Jackson Centre for Health and Wellness
University of Calgary
Calgary, AB
Canada

Donald M. Bers PhD
Silva Chair for Cardiovascular Research
Distinguished Professor and Chair
Department of Pharmacology
University of California, Davis
Davis, CA
USA

Lauren Beussink-Nelson MHS, RDCS
Division of Cardiology, Department of Medicine
Feinberg Cardiovascular Research Institute
Northwestern University Feinberg School of
Medicine
Chicago, IL
USA

Roberto Bolli MD
Professor of Medicine
Chief, Division of Cardiovascular Medicine
Director, Institute of Molecular Cardiology
University of Louisville
Louisville, KY
USA

Donato Cappetta PhD
Research Fellow
Departments of Anesthesia and Medicine
Division of Cardiovascular Medicine
Brigham and Women's Hospital
Harvard Medical School
Boston, MA
USA

Lin Chang MD, PhD
Research Investigator
Department of Internal Medicine
Cardiovascular Center
University of Michigan Medical Center
Ann Arbor, MI
USA

Y. Eugene Chen MD, PhD
Frederick Huetwell Professor of Cardiovascular
Medicine
Departments of Internal Medicine and Cardiac
Surgery
Cardiovascular Center
University of Michigan Medical Center
Ann Arbor, MI
USA

Guangming Cheng MD, PhD
Research Associate
Cardiovascular Research Institute
University of Kansas Medical Center
Kansas City, KS
USA

Daniela Čiháková, MD, PhD
Assistant Professor
Director, Immune Disorders Laboratory
Johns Hopkins University
Baltimore, MD
USA

Hugh Clements-Jewery PhD
Associate Professor of Physiology
West Virginia School of Osteopathic Medicine
Lewisburg, WV
USA

John P. Cooke, MD, PhD
Professor of Medicine and Associate Director
Division of Cardiovascular Medicine
Stanford Cardiovascular Institute
Stanford University School of Medicine
Stanford, CA
USA

Joseph W. Covington MS
Research Associate
Feinberg Cardiovascular Research Institute
Northwestern University Feinberg School of
Medicine
Chicago, IL
USA

Michael J. Curtis PhD, FHEA, FBPharmS
Reader in Pharmacology
Cardiovascular Division
Kings College London
London
UK

Joseph P. Daniels BA
Division of Cardiology
Department of Medicine
Duke University
Durham, NC
USA

Robert S. Danziger MD, FACC
Associate Professor of Medicine, Physiology, and
Pharmacology
University of Illinois at Chicago
Chicago, IL
USA

Jose S. Da Silva PhD
Associate Scientist
Interdisciplinary Stem Cell Institute
Miller School of Medicine
University of Miami
Miami, FL
USA

Arash Davani MD
Postdoctoral Fellow, Cardiovascular Research
Institute
University of Kansas Medical Center
Kansas City, KS
USA

Buddhadeb Dawn MD
Professor of Medicine
Director, Division of Cardiovascular Diseases
Director, Cardiovascular Research Institute
Vice Chairman, Department of Medicine
University of Kansas Medical Center
Kansas City, KS
USA

Angela C. deAlmeida MS
Research Associate
Department of Medicine/Cardiovascular Disease
University of Alabama at Birmingham
Birmingham, AL
USA

Sebastian Diecke PhD
Post Doctoral Associate
Department of Medicine and Radiology
Stanford University School of Medicine
Palo Alto, CA
USA

Igor R. Efimov PhD
Lucy & Stanley Lopata Distinguished Professor
Department of Biomedical Engineering
Washington University
St. Louis, MO
USA

Harold K. Elias MD
Postdoctoral Fellow, Cardiovascular Research
Institute
University of Kansas Medical Center
Kansas City, KS
USA

Anees Fatima PhD
Postdoctoral Research Associate
Feinberg Cardiovascular Research Institute
Northwestern University Feinberg School of
Medicine
Chicago, IL
USA

João Ferreira-Martins MD, PhD
Research Fellow
Departments of Anesthesia and Medicine and
Division of Cardiovascular Medicine
Brigham and Women's Hospital
Harvard Medical School
Boston, MA
USA

A. Martin Gerdes PhD
Professor and Chairman
Department of Biomedical Sciences
New York Institute of Technology
College of Osteopathic Medicine
Old Westbury, NY
USA

Asish K. Ghosh PhD
Associate Professor – Research investigator
Feinberg Cardiovascular Research Institute
Northwestern University Feinberg School of Medicine
Chicago, IL
USA

Kenneth S. Ginsburg PhD
Associate Research Pharmacologist
Department of Pharmacology
University of California
Davis, CA
USA

Magdy Girgis MD
Research Associate, Cardiovascular Research
Institute
University of Kansas Medical Center
Kansas City, KS
USA

Roberta A. Gottlieb MD
Professor of Biology and Director
Donald P. Shiley BioScience Center
San Diego State University
San Diego, CA
USA

Søren Grubb MSc
Danish Arrhythmia Research Centre
Biomedical Institute
University of Copenhagen
Copenhagen
Denmark

Yiru Guo MD, FAHA
Professor of Medicine
Director Murine Research Laboratory
University of Louisville
Louisville, KY
USA

Sarah Gutbrod MSc
Graduate Student
Department of Biomedical Engineering
Washington University
St. Louis, MO
USA

Milton Hamblin PhD
Assistant Professor
Department of Pharmacology
Tulane University School of Medicine
New Orleans, LA
USA

Tariq Hamid PhD
Assistant Professor of Medicine
Division of Cardiovascular Disease
University of Alabama at Birmingham
USA

Joshua M. Hare MD, FACC, FAHA
Louis Lemberg Professor of Medicine
Director of the Interdisciplinary Stem Cell Institute
Interdisciplinary Stem Cell Institute
Miller School of Medicine
University of Miami
Miami, FL
USA

Fatemat Hassan MD
Post-doctoral Researcher
Davis Heart and Lung Research Institute
Division of Cardiovascular Medicine
The Ohio State University
Wexner Medical Center
Columbus, OH
USA

Kyle K. Henderson PhD
Assistant Professor
Department of Physiology
Midwestern University
Downers Grove, IL
USA

Brandon Holtrup BS
Research Associate
Northwestern University Feinberg School of
Medicine;
Lurie Children's Hospital of Chicago Research
Center
Chicago, IL
USA

Ngan F. Huang PhD
Assistant Professor of Cardiothoracic Surgery
Division of Cardiovascular Medicine
Stanford Cardiovascular Institute
Stanford University School of Medicine
Stanford, CA;
Biomedical Engineer
Veterans Affairs Palo Alto Health Care System
Palo Alto, CA
USA

Bruno C. Huber MD
Postdoctoral Fellow
Stanford Cardiovascular Institute
Stanford University School of Medicine
Stanford, CA
USA

Marisa Z. Jackson BA
Graduate Research Assistant
Department of Pathology
Northwestern University Feinberg School of
Medicine
Chicago, IL
USA

José Jalife MD
Cyrus and Jane Farrehi Professor of Cardiovascular
Research
Professor of Internal Medicine
Professor of Molecular and Integrative Physiology
Co-Director, Center for Arrhythmia Research
University of Michigan
Ann Arbor, MI
USA

Jan Kajstura PhD
Associate Professor
Departments of Anesthesia and Medicine
Division of Cardiovascular Medicine
Brigham and Women's Hospital
Harvard Medical School
Boston, MA
USA

James E. Kelly BS
Department of Medicine (Cardiology)
Feinberg Cardiovascular Research Institute
Northwestern University Feinberg School of
Medicine
Chicago, IL
USA

Mahmood Khan PhD
Assistant Professor of Medicine
Davis Heart and Lung Research Institute
The Ohio State University
Wexner Medical Center
Columbus, OH
USA

Gene H. Kim MD
Assistant Professor of Medicine
The University of Chicago Medical Center
Chicago, IL
USA

Raj Kishore PhD
Associate Professor of Medicine
Feinberg Cardiovascular Research Institute
Northwestern University Feinberg School of
Medicine
Chicago, IL
USA

Richard N. Kitsis MD
Professor of Medicine and Cell Biology
Dr. Gerald and Myra Dorros Chair in
Cardiovascular Disease
Director, Wilf Family Cardiovascular Research
Institute
Albert Einstein College of Medicine
Bronx, NY
USA

Stephen C. Kolwicz Jr. PhD
Acting Instructor
Mitochondria and Metabolism Center
University of Washington School of Medicine
Seattle, WA
USA

Klitos Konstantinidis MD
Departments of Medicine and Cell Biology
Wilf Family Cardiovascular Research Institute
Albert Einstein College of Medicine
Bronx, NY
USA

Prasanna Krishnamurthy DVM, PhD
Assistant Professor, Research
Feinberg Cardiovascular Research Institute
Northwestern University Feinberg School of
Medicine
Chicago, IL
USA

Manvinder Kumar BS
Department of Medicine (Cardiology)
Feinberg Cardiovascular Research Institute
Northwestern University Feinberg School of
Medicine
Chicago, IL
USA

Tsutomu Kume PhD
Associate Professor of Medicine
Feinberg Cardiovascular Research Institute
Northwestern University Feinberg School of
Medicine
Chicago, IL
USA

Di Lang MSc
Graduate Student
Department of Biomedical Engineering
Washington University
St. Louis, MO
USA

Roberto M. Lang MD, FASE, FACC, FESC, FAHA, FRCP
Professor of Medicine and Radiology
Past President of the American Society of
Echocardiography
Director Noninvasive Cardiac Imaging Laboratories
Section of Cardiology
Department of Medicine
The University of Chicago Medical Center
Chicago, IL
USA

Jacob Laughner MSc
Graduate Student
Department of Biomedical Engineering
Washington University
St. Louis, MO
USA

Kenneth R. Laurita PhD
Associate Professor of Medicine and Biomedical
Engineering
Heart and Vascular Research Center
Case Western Reserve University
Cleveland, OH
USA

Jerry C. Lee MS
Life Science Research Assistant
Division of Cardiovascular Medicine
Stanford Cardiovascular Institute
Stanford University School of Medicine
Stanford, CA
USA

Qianhong Li MD, PhD, FAHA
Associate Professor of Medicine
Director, Stem Cell and Pathology Core
Director, Biomarker Core of NIH CAESAR
Institute of Molecular Cardiology
University of Louisville
Louisville, KY
USA

Douglas W. Losordo MD
Vice President
New Therapeutic Development
Baxter Healthcare Corporation
Deerfield, IL
USA

Alexander R. Mackie PhD
Post-doctoral Fellow
Feinberg Cardiovascular Research Institute
Northwestern University Feinberg School of
Medicine
Chicago, IL
USA

Raphaël P. Martins MD
Electrophysiology Fellow
University Hospital of Rennes
Rennes
France;
Research Fellow in Basic Electrophysiology
Center for Arrhythmia Research
University of Michigan
Ann Arbor, MI
USA

Haruchika Masuda MD, PhD
Associate Professor of Regenerative Medicine
Science
Science Division of Basic Clinical Science
Tokai University School of Medicine
Isehara, Kanagawa
Japan

Sol Misener AAS, RVT, LATG
Feinberg Cardiovascular Research Institute
Northwestern University Feinberg School of
Medicine
Chicago, IL
USA

Rupak Mukherjee PhD
University of South Carolina School of Medicine
Columbia, SC;
Medical University of South Carolina
Charleston, SC
USA

Carey Nassano-Miller BA
Research Technician
Feinberg Cardiovascular Research Institute
Northwestern University Feinberg School of
Medicine
Chicago, IL
USA

Jeanne M. Nerbonne PhD
Alumni Endowed Professor of Molecular Biology
and Pharmacology
Department of Developmental Biology
Washington University School of Medicine
Saint Louis, MO
USA

Patricia K. Nguyen MD
Instructor
Department of Radiology
Molecular Imaging Program at Stanford
Stanford University School of Medicine
Stanford, CA
USA

Barbara Ogórek PhD
Research Fellow
Departments of Anesthesia and Medicine
Division of Cardiovascular Medicine
Brigham and Women's Hospital
Harvard Medical School
Boston, MA
USA

Alessandro Pingitore MD, PhD
Researcher
Clinical Physiology Institute, CNR
Pisa
Italy

Bradley N. Plummer MS
Research Associate
Heart and Vascular Research Center
Case Western Reserve University
Cleveland, OH
USA

Sumanth D. Prabhu MD
Professor of Medicine
Director, Division of Cardiovascular Disease
University of Alabama at Birmingham
Birmingham, AL
USA

Carrie M. Quinn PhD
Graduate Student
Cardiovascular Research Institute
University of Kansas Medical Center
Kansas City, KS
USA

Md. Abdur Razzaque PhD
Research Associate
Department of Pediatrics
Cincinnati Children's Hospital Medical Center
Cincinnati, OH
USA

Amy K. Rines PhD
Research Assistant
Feinberg Cardiovascular Research Institute
Northwestern University Feinberg School of
Medicine
Chicago, IL
USA

Jeffrey Robbins PhD
Professor of Pediatrics, Executive Co-Director
Department of Pediatrics
Cincinnati Children's Hospital Medical Center
Cincinnati, OH
USA

Eva van Rooij PhD
Senior Director of Biology
miRagen Therapeutics, Inc.
Boulder, CO
USA

Noel R. Rose MD, PhD
Professor of Pathology
Professor of Molecular Microbiology and
Immunology
Director, Johns Hopkins Center for Autoimmune
Disease Research
Johns Hopkins University
Baltimore, MD
USA

Marcello Rota PhD
Assistant Professor
Departments of Anesthesia and Medicine and
Division of Cardiovascular Medicine
Brigham and Women's Hospital
Harvard Medical School
Boston, MA
USA

Sashwati Roy PhD
Associate Professor of Surgery
Director, Laser Capture Molecular Analyses Core
The Ohio State University Wexner Medical Center
Columbus, OH
USA

Rachel Ruckdeschel Smith PhD
Research Scientist
Cedars-Sinai Medical Center, Heart Institute;
Vice President of Research and Development
Capricor, Inc.
Los Angeles, CA
USA

Susmita Sahoo PhD
Research Assistant Professor
Feinberg Cardiovascular Research Institute
Northwestern University Feinberg School of Medicine
Chicago, IL
USA

Fumihiro Sanada MD, PhD
Research Fellow
Departments of Anesthesia and Medicine and
Division of Cardiovascular Medicine
Brigham and Women's Hospital
Harvard Medical School
Boston, MA
USA

Chandan K. Sen PhD
Professor & Vice-Chairman (Research) of Surgery
Associate Dean (Research), College of Medicine
Executive Director, Comprehensive Wound Center
Director, OSU Center for Regenerative Medicine &
Cell-Based Therapies
The Ohio State University Wexner Medical Center
Columbus, OH
USA

Sanjiv J. Shah MD
Associate Professor of Medicine
Division of Cardiology, Department of Medicine
Feinberg Cardiovascular Research Institute
Northwestern University Feinberg School of
Medicine
Chicago, IL
USA

James A. Shuman BS
University of South Carolina School of Medicine
Columbia, SC;
Medical University of South Carolina
Charleston, SC
USA

Hans-Georg Simon PhD
Associate Professor of Pediatrics
Northwestern University Feinberg School of
Medicine;
Lurie Children's Hospital of Chicago Research
Center
Chicago, IL
USA

Neha Singh PhD
Department of Medicine (Cardiology)
Feinberg Cardiovascular Research Institute
Northwestern University Feinberg School of
Medicine
Chicago, IL
USA

Srinivas D. Sithu PhD
Institute of Molecular Cardiology and Diabetes
and Obesity Center
University of Louisville
Louisville, KY
USA

Francis G. Spinale MD, PhD
University of South Carolina School of Medicine
Columbia, SC;
Medical University of South Carolina
Charleston, SC
USA

Sanjay Srivastava PhD FAHA
Professor of Medicine
Institute of Molecular Cardiology and Diabetes
and Obesity
University of Louisville
Louisville, KY
USA

Xian-Liang Tang MD
Associate Professor of Medicine
Institute of Molecular Cardiology
University of Louisville
Louisville, KY
USA

Rong Tian MD, PhD
Professor and Director
Mitochondria and Metabolism Center
University of Washington School of Medicine
Seattle, WA
USA

Warren G. Tourtellotte MD, PhD, FCAP
Associate Professor of Pathology (Neuropathology)
Neurology and Neuroscience
Northwestern University Feinberg School of
Medicine
Chicago, IL
USA

Douglas E. Vaughan MD
Professor of Medicine
Feinberg Cardiovascular Research Institute
Northwestern University Feinberg School of
Medicine
Chicago, IL
USA

Suresh Kumar Verma PhD
Research Assistant Professor
Feinberg Cardiovascular Research Institute
Northwestern University Feinberg School of
Medicine
Chicago, IL
USA

Wei Wang PhD
Staff Scientist
Department of Developmental Biology
Washington University School of Medicine
Saint Louis, MO
USA

J. Andrew Wasserstrom PhD
Jules J. Reingold Research Professor and Associate
Professor of Medicine
Department of Medicine (Cardiology)
Feinberg Cardiovascular Research Institute
Northwestern University Feinberg School of
Medicine
Chicago, IL
USA

Russell S. Whelan PhD
Departments of Medicine and Cell Biology
Wilf Family Cardiovascular Research Institute
Albert Einstein College of Medicine
Bronx, NY
USA

Millicent G. Winner BS
Institute of Molecular Cardiology
and Diabetes and Obesity Center
University of Louisville
Louisville, KY
USA

Matthew J. Wolf MD, PhD
Assistant Professor
Division of Cardiology
Department of Medicine
Duke University
Durham, NC
USA

Joseph C. Wu MD, PhD
Associate Professor
Stanford Cardiovascular Institute
Stanford University School of Medicine
Stanford, CA
USA

Kai-Chien Yang MD, PhD
Postdoctoral Research Associate
Department of Developmental Biology
Washington University School of Medicine
Saint Louis, MO
USA

Yanjuan Yang RN
Research Technician, Cardiovascular Research
Institute
University of Kansas Medical Center
Kansas City, KS
USA

Lei Ye MD, PhD
Assistant Professor of Medicine
Cardiovascular Division
Department of Medicine
University of Minnesota Medical School
Minnesota, MN
USA

Lin Yu PhD
Research Fellow
Division of Cardiology
Department of Medicine
Duke University
Durham, NC
USA

Jianyi Zhang MD, PhD
Professor of Medicine
Cardiovascular Division
Department of Medicine
University of Minnesota Medical School
Minnesota, MN
USA

Sophia Zhang
Cardiovascular Division
Department of Medicine
University of Minnesota Medical School
Minnesota, MN
USA

Preface

Cardiovascular disease remains the number one cause of death in developed countries. Every year, billions of dollars are spent on cardiovascular research, and several laboratories around the world are specialized in conducting experiments related to cardiovascular biology and physiology. Although some aspects of research are common among various fields in medical and biological sciences, cardiovascular researchers utilize an array of techniques and procedures that are unique to their field. Thus, it is important for investigators in this field to have access to a manual that contains protocols on cardiovascular research techniques written by experts, which is currently lacking. Many of us, when we first started our independent career or even when our labs were established and running, have experienced the need for such a resource. It is common for cardiovascular investigators to spend hours looking for the details of a protocol and searching for specific papers where the procedure is used, only to find out that the method is referenced to earlier papers, while those earlier papers refer to yet other papers. It is also common practice for cardiovascular researchers to contact others in the field to get a copy of their protocols when they start a new procedure in their laboratories.

Because of this lack of a centralized manual of common cardiovascular techniques, we decided to put this book together. When we started the process, the three of us acknowledged the difficulties associated with this huge project, and realized that it could be very time consuming. Nevertheless, the need for such a manual was the driving force behind our resolve to get this project completed.

The book is organized into seven different sections: (1) electrophysiology, (2) stem cells, (3) working with heart and vessels *in vivo* and *ex vivo*, (4) small animal imaging, (5) metabolism, mitochondria, and cell death, (6) altering gene expression *in vivo* and *in vitro*, and (7) model systems. We tried to ensure that all of the widely used cardiovascular techniques are covered in this book, and sought the opinion of the leaders in the field to ensure this is the case. The majority of the chapters contain figures and images and some are accompanied by videos that are provided online. We acknowledge that, given the dynamic nature of cardiovascular research, the book will have to be updated in the near future. Thus, we would greatly appreciate any feedback from colleagues.

We would like to thank the section editors, Drs. Andy Wasserstrom, Marina Bayeva, and Amy Rines, for their assistance with the editing of the book. This project would not have been possible without the great contribution of all of the authors. We would like to extend our gratitude to the authors for their excellent contributions to the book and for being on time with their submissions. Finally, we would like to thank our families for being patient with us during the completion of this project.

Hossein Ardehali
Roberto Bolli
Douglas W. Losordo

About the Companion Website

This book is accompanied by a companion website:

www.wiley.com/go/ardehali/cardioresearch

The website includes:
• 7 video clips

Part 1

Electrophysiology

Measurement of calcium transient *ex vivo*

Kenneth R. Laurita and Bradley N. Plummer

Case Western Reserve University, Cleveland, OH, USA

Introduction

Intracellular calcium is a key regulatory signal for cardiomyocyte contraction and has become increasingly recognized as an important mechanism of electrical instability in the heart (arrhythmias) [1]. Measuring intracellular calcium in heart tissue is based on established techniques for measuring intracellular calcium levels in isolated myocytes using fluorescent indicators [2]. However, in tissue preparations additional factors need to be accounted for. Nonetheless, the advantages are: measurements can be performed while cardiomyocytes are in their native setting; it is possible to account for regional heterogeneities of cellular function as they exist normally and in disease conditions; and calcium-mediated arrhythmias can be investigated. The present chapter focuses on measuring intracellular calcium with high temporal and spatial resolution from intact heart preparations.

Preparation and fluorescent indicator loading

Measuring intracellular calcium in heart preparations is most effective when performed *ex vivo*, to provide efficient fluorescent indicator delivery, light excitation and emission collection. Efficient and uniform delivery of the fluorescent indicator is key; accordingly, perfusion in whole hearts (e.g. Langendorff) will provide the best result in this regard. Perfusion of tissue samples (e.g. left ventricular wedge preparations [3], isolated atria [4]) is also possible but careful attention must be paid to the location of the perfusion bed relative to the imaging field of view. Loading of calcium fluorescent indicators by superfusion is difficult in large (i.e. thick-walled) preparations when diffusion to deeper cell layers is limited; however, superfusion of smaller (i.e. thin-walled) preparations, such as the isolated zebrafish heart, is feasible [5].

In general, most calcium-sensitive fluorescent indicators that have been used in isolated myocytes can also be used in *ex vivo* tissue preparations. However, in tissue the cell permanent or acetoxy-methyl (AM) ester form of the fluorescent indicator should be considered. AM indicators, being uncharged and lipophilic, readily penetrate the cell membrane. Once inside the cell, esterases liberate the charged fluorescent indicator by hydrolysis, which is then less likely to cross the cell membrane. Many calcium fluorescent indicators are available in the AM form and can also be used in *ex vivo* preparations, such as Indo-1 [6,7], Rhod-2 [8], Fluo-4 [9], and Fura-2 [5]. The choice of fluorescent indicator depends on several factors, the main being the wavelengths at which peak excitation and emission occur. With some fluorescent indicators, emission (Indo-1) or excitation (Fura-2) occurs at distinct wavelengths depending on whether calcium is bound or not, which can be used to aid calibration (see section Calibration in this chapter). The affinity

Manual of Research Techniques in Cardiovascular Medicine, First Edition. Edited by Hossein Ardehali, Roberto Bolli, and Douglas W. Losordo.
© 2014 John Wiley & Sons, Ltd. Published 2014 by John Wiley & Sons, Ltd.

of the fluorescent indicator for calcium (i.e. K_d) must also be taken into account. Typically, K_d is chosen within the range of expected calcium concentration to enable sufficient sensitivity without saturation. Unlike voltage-sensitive fluorescent indicators, special attention should be given to the concentration of the calcium fluorescent indicator used. If the concentration used is too large (>5 μM) intracellular calcium levels could be unintentionally reduced by the buffering capacity of the indicator.

Several co-agents can be administered with the fluorescent indicator to improve loading and fluorescent measurements *ex vivo*. Pluronic F-127 is a detergent that can aid the dispersion of the lipophilic AM form of fluorescent indicators. In addition, when inside the cell the indicator can be actively removed from the cytosol by anion transporters, which can quickly reduce signal intensity. Probenecid can be used to block this transporter; however, its effects on cellular physiology should also be weighed. Finally, it is very difficult to accurately image fluorescence from contracting heart tissue, thus, inhibiting contraction is essential. It is possible to mechanically restrain the preparation or use ratiometric techniques [10] to reduce some motion artifact, but currently the most common and effective method is to use pharmacological agents that maintain electrical excitation and calcium release yet inhibit mechanical contraction, such as 2,3-butanedione monoxime, cytochalasin-D, and blebbistatin. However, these agents should be used with caution because they can influence calcium regulation and electrophysiological function [11,12].

Optical setup

Shown in Figure 1.1 (Panel A) is an example of an optical mapping system in its simplest configuration to measure intracellular calcium from the Langendorff perfused heart using Indo-1 [7]. One of the advantages of using optical mapping techniques to measure cellular function is that a wide range of preparation size (i.e. field of view) can be accommodated. However, there are several limitations that should be considered. Measuring fluorescence at the level of the whole heart is best achieved using macroscopic objectives (e.g. standard photography lens). In Figure 1.1 (Panel A), two separate camera lenses are optically aligned to face each other in a tandem lens configuration, which significantly improves light collection. Optical magnification is determined by the focal length ratio of the back ("B") lens to the front lens ("F"). For example, an 85-mm front lens with a 105-mm back lens yields a magnification of 1.24×. High numerical aperture lenses are optimized for maximal light collection and are preferred. Macroscopic systems based on standard photography lenses are suitable for imaging fields (i.e. preparations) that range from a few mm (mouse) to a few cm (canine isolated atrial preparations). Larger preparations would require significant demagnification because total detector size is typically not much larger than 1–2 cm. However, standard photography lenses are not optimized for significant demagnification and may produce a fading out of the image at the periphery, known as vignetting. For preparations <1 mm² (e.g. embryonic hearts), a standard fluorescent microscope may be better suited.

Measuring fluorescence *ex vivo* requires a light source for fluorescence excitation, a light detector for fluorescence emission, and a judicious selection of optical filters to optimize light transmission. The light source and optical filters are determined by the fluorescent indicator chosen. For example, shown in Figure 1.1 (Panel A) is UV excitation light (Hg lamp, 365 nm) for Indo-1. In contrast, Fluo-4 is excited with 488 nm light; thus, a quartz tungsten halogen (QTH) lamp that produces light in the visible range will suffice. Light sources with broad output spectra require excitation filters (Ex Filter, Figure 1.1) to pass only wavelengths that maximally excite the fluorescent indicator and do not overlap with the emission wavelength. Filter specifications such as bandwidth, peak transmission, and blocking will all determine the amount of light that excites the fluorescent indicator and will, thus, impact signal fidelity. Modern LED technology can provide an excellent alternative to Hg and QTH light sources given their low cost, low noise, and high power output [13]. Moreover, the wide availability of quasimonochromatic LEDs may obviate the need for an excitation filter.

Light collected from the preparation includes excitation light that reflects off the preparation as well as fluorescence emission. The amount of excitation light is much larger than fluoresced light,

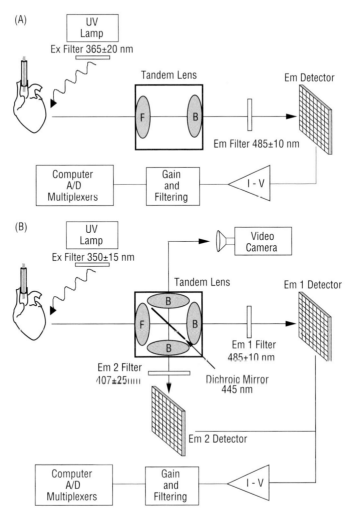

Figure 1.1 System diagram for measuring un-calibrated (A) or calibrated (B) intracellular calcium from intact heart preparations. (A) shows excitation light from an Hg arc lamp directed to the preparation. Fluorescence is collected by a tandem lens assembly consisting of a front (F) and back (B) camera lens. Fluoresced light is allowed to pass through an emission filter (Em Filter) to a detector array (Em Detector). Signals corresponding to each pixel channel are amplified, filtered, and digitized for analysis. (B) shows filtered excitation light (350 nm) from an Hg arc lamp specifically for dual wavelength emission. Fluorescence is collected by a tandem lens assembly consisting of four camera lenses (1 front, 3 back). A dichroic mirror (445 nm) passes fluorescence of longer wavelengths to an emission filter (Em 1 Filter) and detector array (Em 1 Detector) and reflects fluorescence of shorter wavelengths to a second emission filter (Em 2) and detector array (Em 2 Detector). To view the preparation, the dichroic mirror is rotated clockwise by exactly 90° to reflect an image of the preparation to a standard video camera.

requiring the need for an emission filter (Em Filter, Figure 1.1 Panel A) to block excitation light from reaching the detector (Em Detector, Figure 1.1 Panel A). The bandwidth, center wavelength, and maximum transmittance of the emission filter must be taken into account to maximize the amount of fluorescence passed and excitation light blocked.

A variety of detector technologies with sufficient sensitivity and speed (e.g. frame rate) are capable of accurately measuring fluorescence from *ex vivo* preparations. Photomultiplier tubes have sufficient fidelity; however, being a single detector they can only measure fluorescence from multiple sites if the preparation is scanned site by site in a sequential manner with excitation light (e.g. laser) [14]. On the other hand, detector arrays, such as photodiode arrays (PDA), charge-coupled devices (CCD), and complementary metal–oxide–semiconductor (CMOS) sensors can capture fluorescence from hundreds to thousands of sites simultaneously when excitation light illuminates the entire imaging field [15]. These detector arrays are based on similar technology, except for their output format. The PDA output is a parallel stream of voltage signals corresponding to each recording location where each signal needs to be, conditioned (amplified and filtered), multiplexed, and digitized (Figure 1.1). This offers flexibility in signal conditioning and sampling speed in hardware, but with the added cost of a specialized design. CCD and CMOS sensors on the other hand, output a single serial stream of data that is digitized and multiplexed "on chip". This limits signal conditioning to mostly software methods, but offers the advantage of being "plug and play". Currently, the speed and signal fidelity of these arrays are similar; however, CCD and CMOS arrays offer spatial resolutions that can be orders of magnitude higher (more pixels) than PDAs.

Calcium recordings from an intact heart using currently available detectors should not required further signal processing (e.g. filtering) to achieve acceptable signal fidelity (Figure 1.3A). However, in some situations the signal source may be very small (e.g. embryonic hearts, monolayers), which may result in the appearance of excessive noise. Typically, this noise is high frequency and can be filtered out in the time and/or space domain. In the time domain, the signal from each "pixel" can be low-pass filtered in software using standard digital signal processing techniques. In the space domain, signals from neighboring pixels can be averaged together (i.e. binned) in either hardware or software. The choice of filter characteristics for calcium transients may be different than that for action potentials [16]. For example, action potentials have a much faster rise time than calcium transients. However, action potentials are naturally "smoothed" in space due to electrotonic forces (i.e. space constant), but calcium transients are not.

Confocal microscopy can be used to image intracellular calcium from heart tissue [9,17]. The field of view is limited to several cells; however, measured fluorescence only arises from cells within the confocal plane. As such, subcellular events within single cells (calcium sparks, waves) can be resolved, as well as heterogeneities in calcium cycling between neighboring cells. Confocal imaging, however, requires exquisite control of motion, and depth of penetration is very limited depending on the technology used (e.g. single or two photon technology). Finally, the first reported measurements of intracellular calcium *ex vivo* were achieved by attaching a fiber-optic cable to the epicardial surface of a beating rabbit heart [18]. The advantage of such a system is that the fiber-optic cable can be sutured to the heart surface so it can move with the beating heart, thus minimizing motion artifact.

Calibration

Intracellular free calcium concentration and its change during the heartbeat have very important physiological meaning. However, the fluorescence intensity measured can depend on factors unrelated to calcium levels such as the intensity of excitation light, optical transmission, and fluorescent indicator washout. Thus, to quantify intracellular calcium concentration, the fluorescence signal needs to be calibrated to absolute calcium levels. Standard procedures have been developed for isolated cells; however *ex vivo* methods are much more complex due to spatial heterogeneities and limited control of the cellular environment.

A fluorescent indicator that exhibits a dual spectral response or a shifting of excitation wavelength with free calcium concentration is ideal for calibration. For example, fluorescence from Indo-1 will increase with increasing intracellular calcium when measured at ~407 nm but will decrease with increasing calcium when measured at ~485 nm. By calculating the ratio of fluorescence measured at each wavelength it is possible to normalize for factors that influence fluorescence that are unrelated to calcium levels (e.g. excitation light intensity, fluorescent indicator washout). Shown in Figure 1.1 (Panel B) is an example of an optical mapping system designed to measure the fluorescence ratio of Indo-1. This setup is similar to that shown in Panel A, except with several important changes. First, fluorescence emission of Indo-1 at both peak wavelengths is best achieved by ~350 nm excitation.

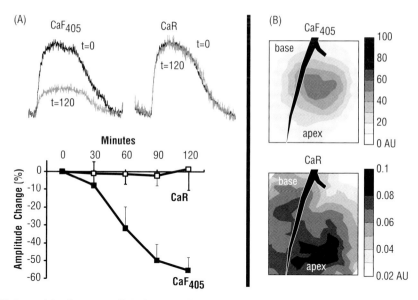

Figure 1.2 (A) shows calcium fluorescence (CaF$_{405}$) and ratio (CaR, background corrected CaF$_{405}$/CaF$_{485}$) transients from the same site over a 2-h period. As demonstrated in the traces (top) and graph (bottom), CaF$_{405}$ significantly decreased, but CaR did not (error bars show SD). (B) shows contour maps of CaF$_{405}$ and CaR amplitude measured across the epicardial surface of the intact heart preparation. CaF$_{405}$ exhibited a circular "bull's-eye" pattern similar to the pattern of excitation light (not shown). In contrast, CaR reflects the physiologic heterogeneity of calcium transient amplitude that is independent of excitation light intensity and heterogeneity.

Measuring fluorescence simultaneously at two separate wavelengths requires two detectors. Therefore, fluorescence emission corresponding to each peak wavelength needs to be split into two light paths. A dichroic mirror placed between the tandem lenses passes light of longer wavelengths (>445 nm) and reflects light of shorter wavelengths. Light directed to each detector is then band-pass filtered to optimally detect emission at each peak wavelength (Em 1 Filter, Em 2 Filter). It is important that both detectors (Em 1 Detector, Em 2 Detector) are in perfect alignment to ensure a one-to-one correspondence (i.e. registration) between the field of view and both detectors. Finally, before the fluorescent indicator is loaded, background fluorescence intensity at each wavelength is measured and then subtracted from all subsequent recordings (i.e. background corrected) after the fluorescent indicator is loaded.

Shown in Figure 1.2 are examples of how the ratio of Indo-1 fluorescence can correct for changes that occur over time due to dye washout (Figure 1.2A) and heterogeneities of excitation light and indicator loading (Figure 1.2B). Calcium transient amplitudes measured *ex vivo* from Indo-1 fluorescence directly (CaF) can significantly decrease by more than 50% over 2 hours. However, the background corrected ratio of Indo-1 fluorescence (CaR) remains unchanged over the same period. Spatial heterogeneities of excitation light and indicator can also significantly influence the calcium transient amplitude measured *ex vivo*. Shown in Figure 1.2B is a contour map of calcium transient amplitude measured across the epicardial surface of the guinea pig heart as measured directly by fluorescence (CaF, top) or the ratio of fluorescence (CaR, bottom). CaF reveals a bull's-eye pattern that mostly depends on the pattern of excitation light directed to the heart. In contrast, CaR reveals a pattern that is dependent on physiological heterogeneities (largest amplitude at apex) that remains the same even if excitation light is reduced or moved to a different position. However, CaR alone cannot account for the nonlinear response of fluorescence to calcium that occurs at concentrations far from K_d (e.g. saturation).

Calibrating the ratio (CaR) to calcium levels *ex vivo* can be performed as it is done in isolated cells using:

$$[Ca^{2+}]_i = K_d S_2 \left\{ \frac{R - Rmin}{Rmax - R} \right\}$$

where R is CaR (as described here) and S_2 is the ratio of fluorescence at the longer peak wavelength (485 nm) measured in absence of calcium (minimum) and in the presence of saturating calcium (maximum). Calibration constants (e.g. K_d) can be borrowed from that used in isolated cells; however, this may not be the same in tissue and there are several factors that complicate the calibration procedure [19]. In addition, R_{min} and R_{max}, the ratios that correspond to maximum and minimum calcium respectively, can be difficult to measure. For example, the reagents that are used to minimize (zero) intracellular calcium (e.g. ionophores) can only be used at the end of an experiment, and these can change the shape of (e.g. shrink) the preparation making it difficult to measure R_{min} at the same recording sites where calcium transients were measured during an experiment. Nevertheless, accurate calibration *ex vivo* is possible [6,7].

Analysis and interpretation

The signal morphology of intracellular calcium (e.g. calcium transient) measured *ex vivo* is similar to that measured from isolated cells *in vitro*. Normally, calcium levels are low at rest (diastole, ~100–200 nM), but several milliseconds after electrical excitation (action potential upstroke) calcium levels quickly increase to levels close to 1000 nM (systole), corresponding to the release of calcium from the sarcoplasmic reticulum (SR) by the ryanodine receptor (RyR). Following systole, calcium levels return to diastolic levels due to, mostly, the uptake of calcium back into the SR by SR calcium ATPase and extrusion of calcium from the cell by the sodium–calcium exchanger. To quantify the rate of calcium removal from the cytosol, the decay phase can be fit to an exponential function, or the duration of the calcium transient can be measured at a predefined amplitude percentage (e.g. duration at

90% amplitude). Unlike calcium measured from single cells *in vitro*, calcium measured *ex vivo* typically originates from an aggregate of cells. Thus, it is possible that if significant heterogeneities exist between cells or single cell events occur (e.g. calcium sparks and waves), the measured response may be significantly different than measured from an individual cell.

One of the advantages of measuring calcium *ex vivo* is that regional heterogeneities can be determined and linked to normal and abnormal physiology. For example, we have previously shown that the decay phase of the calcium transient is significantly slower near the endocardium compared to the epicardium [3]. Shown in Figure 1.3A is an example of calcium transients measured from the endocardium (ENDO) and epicardium (EPI) of the intact canine LV wedge preparation. The decay phase of the calcium transient, when fit to a single exponential, reveals a shorter time constant (135 ms) near the EPI compared to the ENDO (250 ms). These heterogeneities have been linked to the occurrence of cardiac alternans [3] and triggered arrhythmias [20]. In addition, we have also shown in the guinea pig heart that calcium transient amplitude is larger near the apex of the heart compared to the base (Figure 1.2B), which is consistent with a stronger contraction near the apex compared to the base.

Abnormal calcium regulation has become increasingly recognized as an important mechanism of arrhythmia. Accordingly, a very important advantage of measuring calcium *ex vivo* is that calcium-mediated arrhythmias can be fully investigated. For example, arrhythmias can be caused by spontaneous release of calcium from internal stores. Such events are well characterized as calcium sparks and waves in isolated cells [21]. These manifest as a membrane depolarization that, if large enough, can initiate multiple extra beats (extrasystoles) [4,22]. Shown in Figure 1.3B is an example of spontaneous calcium release measured *ex vivo* in a rat heart with myocardial infarction. Immediately following four paced calcium transients, stimulation is halted and activity is measured as spontaneous calcium release (arrows) and full calcium transients (asterisks). Similar studies in canine demonstrate the focal nature

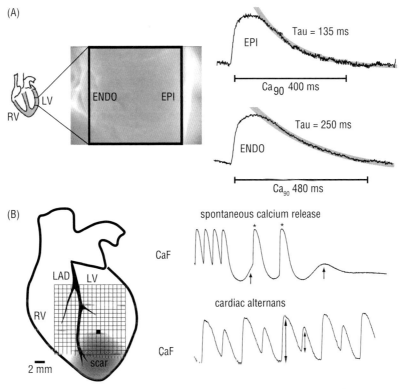

Figure 1.3 (A) shows an image of the LV canine wedge preparation with the mapping field superimposed. Calcium transients (right) reveal that the return of intracellular calcium to diastolic levels is slower at the endocardium (ENDO) compared to the epicardium (EPI), as indicated by the exponential fit (i.e. bold gray line) to the decay phase of the calcium transient and by the calcium transient duration (i.e. CaF_{90}). (B) shows examples of calcium-mediated arrhythmia substrates present in an intact rat heart with myocardial infarction. Calcium transient recordings (CaF) from the mapping field (grid) show spontaneous calcium release (arrows) associated with un-stimulated beats (asterisks), and alternans of calcium transient amplitude (double arrows).

of spontaneous calcium release in tissue [20] (Video clip 1.1). However, CaF recordings and in particular spontaneous calcium release measured *ex vivo* (what we call an m-SCR) must be interpreted with caution. For example, it is not clear if m-SCR activity represents calcium waves and/or calcium sparks. Abnormal calcium regulation has also been linked to reentrant arrhythmias. For example, our laboratory [23] and others [24] have linked calcium transient alternans, a beat-to-beat fluctuation of calcium transient amplitude, to repolarization alternans, an important mechanism of sudden cardiac death [25]. Shown in Figure 1.3B is an example of calcium transient alternans measured *ex vivo* in a rat heart with myocardial infarction. The

arrows indicate alternation in the calcium transient amplitude on a beat-by-beat basis.

Set-by-step procedure

For details of the procedure see Katra *et al.* [7].

1. Optical setup (for Indo-1 AM):
   a. excitation 365 nm, or 350 nm for ratio;
   b. emission 485 nm, or 485 nm + 405 nm with 445 nm dichroic mirror for ratio.
2. Prepare tissue sample and perfuse/ superfuse (e.g. Langendorff).
3. Monitor ECG, and perfusion pressure and flow.
4. Confirm preparation viability and stability (~10 minutes).

5. Position preparation within mapping field and adjust focus.

6. For ratio, record background fluorescence in the absence of calcium indicator. At this point, the preparation position must be maintained (or accurately restored later) for all subsequent recordings.

7. Administer calcium-sensitive dye (~30-45 minutes) prepared in perfusion/ superfusion solution at ~5 μM final concentration, initially dissolved in a 0.5 mL solution of DMSO and Pluronic (Molecular Probes, Inc. Eugene, OR) 20% wt/vol.

8. For ratio, a 20-minute washout period to remove unhydrolyzed dye.

9. Administer mechanical–electrical uncoupler (e.g. blebbistatin) continuously.

10. Confirm pacing electrode placement and threshold strength.

11. Perform experimental protocol.

References

1 Laurita KR, Rosenbaum DS. Mechanisms and potential therapeutic targets for ventricular arrhythmias associated with impaired cardiac calcium cycling. *J Mol Cell Cardiol* 2008; **44**: 31–43.

2 Grynkiewicz G, Poenie M, Tsien RY. A new generation of Ca^{2+} indicators with greatly improved fluorescence properties. *J Biol Chem* 1985; **260**: 3440–3450.

3 Laurita KR, Katra R, Wible B, Wan X, Koo MH. Transmural heterogeneity of calcium handling in canine. *Circ Res* 2003; **92**: 668–675.

4 Chou CC, Nihei M, Zhou S, Tan A, Kawase A, Macias ES, *et al*. Intracellular calcium dynamics and anisotropic reentry in isolated canine pulmonary veins and left atrium. *Circulation* 2005; **111**: 2889–2897.

5 Panakova D, Werdich AA, Macrae CA. Wnt11 patterns a myocardial electrical gradient through regulation of the L-type $Ca^{(2+)}$ channel. *Nature* 2010; **466**(7308): 874–878.

6 Brandes R, Figueredo VM, Camacho SA, Baker AJ, Weiner MW. Quantitation of cytosolic $[Ca^{2+}]$ in whole perfused rat hearts using Indo-1 fluorometry. *Biophys J* 1993; **65**: 1973–1982.

7 Katra RP, Pruvot E, Laurita KR. Intracellular calcium handling heterogeneities in intact guinea pig hearts. *Am J Physiol Heart Circ Physiol* 2004; **286**: H648–656.

8 Del Nido PJ, Glynn P, Buenaventura P, Salama G, Koretsky AP. Fluorescence measurement of calcium transients in perfused rabbit heart using rhod 2. *Am J Physiol* 1998; **274**: H728–741.

9 Aistrup GL, Kelly JE, Kapur S, Kowalczyk M, Sysman-Wolpin I, Kadish AH, *et al*. Pacing-induced heterogeneities in intracellular Ca^{2+} signaling, cardiac alternans, and ventricular arrhythmias in intact rat heart. *Circ Res* 2006; **99**: e65–73.

10 Brandes R, Figueredo VM, Camacho SA, Massie BM, Weiner MW. Suppression of motion artifacts in fluorescence spectroscopy of perfused hearts. *Am J Physiol* 1992; **263**: H972–980.

11 Kettlewell S, Walker NL, Cobbe SM, Burton FL, Smith GL. The electrophysiological and mechanical effects of 2,3-butane-dione monoxime and cytochalasin-D in the Langendorff perfused rabbit heart. *Exp Physiol* 2004; **89**: 163–172.

12 Lou Q, Li W, Efimov IR. The role of dynamic instability and wavelength in arrhythmia maintenance as revealed by panoramic imaging with blebbistatin vs. 2,3-butanedione monoxime. *Am J Physiol Heart Circ Physiol* 2012; **302**: H262–269.

13 Lee P, Bollensdorff C, Quinn TA, Wuskell JP, Loew LM, Kohl P. Single-sensor system for spatially resolved, continuous, and multiparametric optical mapping of cardiac tissue. *Heart Rhythm* 2011; **8**: 1482–1491.

14 Knisley SB. Mapping intracellular calcium in rabbit hearts with fluo3. *Proceedings of the 17th Annual International Conference – IEEE Engineering in Medicine and Biology Society* 1995: 127–129.

15 Salama G, Hwang SM. Simultaneous optical mapping of intracellular free calcium and action potentials from Langendorff perfused hearts. *Curr Protoc Cytom* 2009; Chapter 12: Unit 12 7.

16 Mironov SF, Vetter FJ, Pertsov AM. Fluorescence imaging of cardiac propagation: spectral properties and filtering of optical action potentials. *Am J Physiol Heart Circ Physiol* 2006; **291**: H327–335.

17 Wier WG, ter Keurs HE, Marban E, Gao WD, Balke CW. Ca^{2+} "sparks" and waves in intact ventricular muscle resolved by confocal imaging. *Circ Res* 1997; **81**: 462–469.

18 Lee HC, Smith N, Mohabir R, Clusin WT. Cytosolic calcium transients from the beating mammalian heart. *Proc Natl Acad Sci USA* 1987; **84**: 7793–7797.

19 Brandes R, Figueredo VM, Camacho SA, Baker AJ, Weiner MW. Investigation of factors affecting fluorometric quantitation of cytosolic $[Ca^{2+}]$ in perfused hearts. *Biophys J* 1993; **65**: 983–993.

20 Katra RP, Laurita KR. Cellular mechanism of calcium-mediated triggered activity in the heart. *Circ Res* 2005; **96**: 535–542.

21 Cheng H, Lederer WJ, Cannell MB. Calcium sparks: elementary events underlying excitation-contraction coupling in heart muscle. *Science* 1993; **262**(5134): 740–744.

22 Hoeker GS, Katra RP, Wilson LD, Plummer BN, Laurita KR. Spontaneous calcium release in tissue from the failing canine heart. *Am J Physiol Heart Circ Physiol* 2009; **297**: H1235–1242.

23 Pruvot EJ, Katra RP, Rosenbaum DS, Laurita KR. Role of calcium cycling versus restitution in the mechanism of repolarization alternans. *Circ Res* 2004; **94**: 1083–1090.

24 Goldhaber JI, Xie LH, Duong T, Motter C, Khuu K, Weiss JN. Action potential duration restitution and alternans in rabbit ventricular myocytes: the key role of intracellular calcium cycling. *Circ Res* 2005; **96**: 459–466.

25 Pastore JM, Girouard SD, Laurita KR, Akar FG, Rosenbaum DS. Mechanism linking T-wave alternans to the genesis of cardiac fibrillation. *Circulation* 1999; **99**: 1385–1394.

Confocal imaging of intracellular calcium cycling in isolated cardiac myocytes

Søren Grubb,[1] J. Andrew Wasserstrom,[2] and Gary L. Aistrup[2]

[1] University of Copenhagen, Copenhagen, Denmark
[2] Northwestern University Feinberg School of Medicine, Chicago. IL, USA

Introduction

Intracellular calcium (Ca^{2+}) cycling plays a central role in the cardiomyocyte excitation–contraction (E-C) coupling under both physiological and pathophysiological conditions [1–15]. Briefly, the molecular process of E-C coupling starts with the arrival of an action potential (excitation), which causes the opening of L-type voltage-gated calcium channels (VGCCs) located in the plasmalemma. This current, I_{Ca-L}, underlies the prominent plateau of cardiac action potentials. The resulting Ca^{2+} influx activates calcium-activated Ca channels (or ryanodine receptor channels, RyRs) in the sarcoplasmic reticulum (SR, a specialized intracellular Ca^{2+} store organelle), releasing a larger amount of Ca^{2+} from the SR into the cytoplasm throughout the myocyte – a process referred to as Ca^{2+}-induced Ca^{2+} release (CICR). This released Ca^{2+} then binds to and activates myofilament proteins causing myocyte contraction (*systole*). Relaxation (*diastole*) occurs when sarco-endoplasmic reticulum Ca-ATPase (SERCA) resequesters the released Ca^{2+} in the cytoplasm back into the SR, while the Ca^{2+} that entered via L-type VGCCs is extruded by the Na^+–Ca^{2+} exchanger (NCX). This exchange is in a ratio of $1\,Ca^{2+}:3\,Na^+$ taken in "forward mode", but it can act in "reverse mode" also when intracellular Na^+ is high; and in either case its activity is electrogenic, generating inward or outward current, respectively. The change in $[Ca^{2+}]$ in the cytoplasm during SR Ca^{2+} release and re-uptake is referred to as the intracellular Ca^{2+} transient.

Considerable research has been conducted with isolated cardiomyocytes to study E-C coupling/Ca^{2+} cycling in detail, concerning how it maintains its stability, how its stability is lost and what interventions can be made to correct it if it goes awry. For such studies, a method of rapidly measuring the dynamic changes in intracellular Ca^{2+} concentration is obviously required. This was made possible with improved cardiomyocyte isolation techniques, the development of cell-permeant fluorescent Ca^{2+} indicators and the high temporal and spatial resolution obtainable using confocal microscopy compared to low-resolution information derived from experiments using epifluorescence microscopy. The primary objective of this chapter is to briefly describe a protocol to isolate cardiomyocytes from mammalian heart and then describe in detail how to investigate Ca^{2+} cycling using Ca^{2+}-fluorescence and confocal microscopy.

Manual of Research Techniques in Cardiovascular Medicine, First Edition. Edited by Hossein Ardehali, Roberto Bolli, and Douglas W. Losordo.

Materials and methods

Chamber, electrical stimulation, and superfusate delivery apparatus

For maximal application flexibility, the cell superfusion chamber should be one that exhibits good laminar solution flow, has field stimulation capability, and temperature control. We use a complete system (Cell MicroControls) as illustrated in Figure 2.1. This system includes a three-channel bipolar temperature control unit (TC^2_{bip}) together with a polycarbonate cell chamber (BT-1-TBS) equipped with a paired platinum-wire electric field stimulator (STIM-TB), a solution preheater (HPRE2), and a transparent iridium/ tin oxide (ITO) heater chamber bottom, as well as a temperature-controlled 8-to-1 micromanifold fast-exchange local superfusion apparatus (MPRE8) for rapid drug application. An 8-to-1 solution exchange minimanifold (MP8, Warner Inst.) at the chamber inflow is also useful for effector/ drug preapplication experiments.

Electrical stimulation is provided via paired platinum-wire electric field stimulator electrodes, which are controlled by electrical pulse/ isolated stimulus generator system (e.g. STIM-TB, Cell Microcontrols coupled to a Pulsar 4i, Frederick Haer & Co.; see Figure 2.1), typically utilizing a square-wave pulse of ~150V and ~0.5ms duration with variable frequency, that is 0.5–5Hz, or 2000–200ms basic cycle length (BCL), providing a wide range of physiologically relevant stimulation rates experienced by cardiomyocytes. Note that a greater solution volume requires more field strength; thus,

the chamber solution level must be optimized in order to minimize solution depth in each system. While stimulating, the chamber solution should flow constantly to avoid heavy-metal toxicity due to ionization of the metal stimulation wires.

In order to achieve rapid solution exchange applied directly to individual cardiomyocytes in the chamber without affecting neighboring myocytes, it is recommended to employ a (temperature-controlled) fast-exchange local superfusion apparatus (we use an MPRE8, Cell MicroControls; see Figure 2.1). Changes in flow rate can be minimized by delivering the superfusate via siphoning from the superfusate reservoirs, which ensures a constant superfusate solution column height, and thus constant superfusion rate regardless of reservoir level. Local superfusion, when temperature controlled, also minimizes variations in heating across the chamber bottom. Drawbacks to local superfusion can include: (1) the necessity to coat the chamber bottom with extracellular matrix (ECM) protein to provide for better adhesion of cardiomyocytes to it upon the more prominent superfusion flow (such as ECM, Sigma-Aldrich, which gels almost immediately at 37°C, and so can be quickly reapplied as needed); and (2) the formation of bubbles in the microsuperfusion inflow lines due to solution degassing, particularly when working at 35°C, which can wreak havoc in single-cell experiments. To minimize the latter, use thicker-walled Teflon, polyimide or polyethelene microsuperfusion lines whenever possible; clean the tubing thoroughly with water and alcohol before and after each day of experiments and occasionally

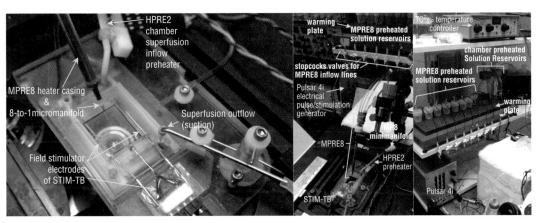

Figure 2.1 Myocyte cell chamber and apparatus.

with nitric acid and/or H_2O_2; and, perhaps most importantly, preheat the solution inflow reservoirs (~5°C above the temperature to be used) to degas the solutions before they enter the microsuperfusion lines. We use polyimide microsuperfusion lines, and preheat the superfusion solutions via a plate warmer (Figure 2.1). While temperature control and fast-exchange local superfusion are not absolutely required, Ca^{2+} cycling in isolated cardiomyocytes is dramatically slowed at room temperature thus limiting the physiological relevance of experiments performed under these conditions, particularly in myocytes from large animals which have longer action potentials than smaller animals, such as in rodents.

Finally, the use of objective heaters is recommended to minimize the objective acting as a "cooling sink" on the heated chamber bottom. Concerning ITO-heated chamber bottoms, we have not found significant potential for an electrical short to the ITO heater when using water immersion objectives, as pure water is a poor electrical conductor. However, care should be taken to electrically insulate the conductor leads at the edges of the ITO heater (liquid heat-shrink or even nail polish works fine) to prevent possible shorting if the actual metal objective housing comes in contact with the edge conductor lead.

Confocal microscope system

While there are different types of confocal micro-copy systems that can be utilized for cellular Ca^{2+} cycling measurements (discussed later, below), the most commonly used presently are laser (raster) scanning confocal microscopes (LSCMs). The LSCM system must be designed to include lasers with lines corresponding to the maximum excitation wave-length for the required fluorescent Ca^{2+} indicators, with dichroic mirrors and long-pass or band-pass filters, enabling the collection of the fluorescence encompassing its maximum emission wavelength as well as those for simultaneous collection of expressed fluorescent reporters or voltage indicators if needed. In addition, appropriate objectives must have optical magnification and resolution sufficient to obtain fluorescent images of the Ca^{2+} cycling phenomena of interest. Objective selection must therefore be based on fluorescence emission wavelength and the objec-tive's numerical aperture (NA) in order to remain in compliance with the equation for minimum

distance resolvable between two points $= \lambda/2 \cdot NA$. In general, an objective capable of higher magnification and resolution is needed for the study of Ca^{2+} sparks versus that for study of Ca^{2+} transients, although additional factors must also be considered, such the spatial field size desired (i.e. whether or not the region of interest encompasses subcellular events or the whole cell).

Another important consideration is that the physiological study of Ca^{2+} cycling in cardiomyocytes typically is best achieved using water immersion objectives in order to maximize the attainable resolution by minimizing the refraction of light entering the objective. That is changes and differences in refractive indices between water (aqueous physiological buffer solution) $\leftrightarrow$ glass (chamber bottom) $\leftrightarrow$ air $\leftrightarrow$ glass (objective lens) are much more than that between water (aqueous physiological buffer solution) $\leftrightarrow$ glass (chamber bottom) $\leftrightarrow$ water (immersion droplet) $\leftrightarrow$ glass (objective lens). The same limitation applies to oil immersion objectives as to air. Also, water immersion objectives are often manufactured with a correction collar to adjust for differences in glass chamber bottom thickness. Without such collars, objectives are generally corrected for a standard 0.17 mm thickness (#1) cover glass. Our system has three water immersion objectives (Zeiss) for acquiring single-cell level images: a LCI Plan–Neofluar 25 × 0.8 (NA), 0–0.17 mm adjustable correction; a C-Apochromat 40 × 1.2, 0.14–0.17 mm adjustable correction; and a C-Apochromat 60 × 1.2, 0.14–0.17 mm adjustable correction. Data acquisition on a confocal microscopy is accomplished via computer interfacing, the specific hardware and software for which varies depending on the system manufacturer (Zeiss, Leica, Olympus etc.; we use a Zeiss LSM 510/Observer Z1 system). The software serves as the user interface in controlling specifically how the confocal image is to be acquired, including choice of fluorophore excitation wavelength (laser lines), laser intensity, emission dichroic and long-pass filters, pinhole adjustments, and the speed and duration of line or image scans. The latter is investigation-dependent since the speed of capture at a desired spatiotemporal resolution depends on the magnitude, brightness, timing and duration of the events (Ca^{2+} sparks, transients, waves, etc.). In general, the more complex the experiments, the more sophisticated the software must be.

Cell loading of fluorescent Ca²⁺ indicators

Non-protein fluorescent Ca^{2+} indicators, all of which are Ca^{2+} chelators based on BAPTA (1,2-bis-(2-aminophenoxy) ethane-N,N,N',N'-tetra acetic acid), differ in Ca^{2+} affinities (ranging from nanomolar to millimolar), and excitation/ emission spectral properties [16,17]. Some indicators have dual excitation or dual emission properties that provide for ratiometric cancellation of variations in cell loading, optics, and instrumentation, thus enabling true quantitative amplitude-dependent measurements of Ca^{2+} and accurate cell-to-cell comparisons [18,19]. Unfortunately, ratiometric Ca^{2+} indicators usually require UV-excitation spectra (thus requiring UV-lasers) and are susceptible to photodegradation and bleaching. Furthermore, ratiometric indicators require LSCM setups that must switch rapidly between multiple excitation or emission wavelengths. The choice of indicator(s) must be established by the investigator, who should not only take into consideration the experimental objectives and whether true or only relative quantification of Ca^{2+} is needed, but also the practical aspects such as available excitation lasers, potential spectral overlap with other fluorescence indicators (such as autofluorescence or fluorescent transgene reporters such enhanced green fluorescent protein (eGFP)) and experiment duration (with respect to bleaching and indicator retention limitations).

Whatever the choice, fluorescent Ca^{2+} indicators are made cell-permeant by masking their carboxylates as acetoxymethyl (AM) esters. Once inside the cell, endogenous intracellular esterases cleave off the esters, trapping the now membrane impermeant fluorescent Ca^{2+} indicator inside the cell. The latter process is referred to as indicator loading, which commonly proceeds via incubating an appropriate dilute aliquot of isolated myocyte suspension in physiological buffer solution (e.g. 500 μL suspension with ~500 cells in normal HEPES-buffered Tyrode's) for 20–30 minutes prior to the start of experiment with a fluorescent Ca^{2+} indicator (usually fluo-4AM or rhod-2AM, Invitrogen) to give a final concentration of ~5 μM (from a 1 mM stock in DMSO). Loading also requires a similar volume of 20% (w:v) pluronic acid in DMSO solution, which aids in dispersing the typically very water-insoluble indicators. As a practical rule of thumb, *use the least amount of indicator/ pluronic acid to allow just sufficiently measurable Ca²⁺ fluorescence as empirically determined*, since high concentrations of indicators can lead to undesirable intracellular organelle compartmentalization (due to overwhelming the endogenous intracellular esterase capacity to expediently cleave the indicator AM esters) or non-negligible intracellular Ca^{2+} buffering due to the Ca^{2+} chelating properties of the indicators.

Of practical note regarding the use of the very commonly used non-ratiometric Ca^{2+} indicators, fluo-3/4/8, we have found that while the intracellular signal-to-noise intensity for these indicators is nominally stable at 25°C, it quickly deteriorates at 37°C, probably due to dye extrusion from the cell via anion exchangers. Probenecid may prevent this, but in our hands it does so minimally and at the expense of an apparent probenecid-mediated decrement in signal-to-noise ratio. However, we have found that the signal-to-noise ratio when using rhod-2 is quite stable at 37°C and is therefore preferable for recordings at physiologically relevant temperatures. We are aware that rhod-2 is often cited to localize to mitochondria but we only see mitochondrial rhod-2 fluorescence when myocytes are overloaded or loaded for an extensive amount of time beyond ~20 minutes.

In addition to the normal loading of fluorophore, it is sometimes desirable to record action potentials or specific currents via sharp electrodes or whole-cell patch clamp simultaneously with Ca^{2+} events. Care must be taken so that patch pipette dialysis does not significantly interfere with Ca^{2+} cycling through the inclusion of EGTA, which buffers intracellular Ca^{2+}. High resistance microelectrodes or nystatin/ amphotericin-perforated patch techniques can be used to avoid disruption of intracellular ion balances that occur with ruptured patch electrodes. If extremely exact subcellular measurements are desired, cardiomyocyte contraction, particularly when the myocytes are not sufficiently adherent to the cell chamber bottom, must be suppressed because contraction can influence measurements via introducing motion artifacts. This can be circumvented by using paralytic agents such a cytocalasin-D [20] and/or blebbistatin [21]. However, cytocalasin-D can alter ion channel function or Ca^{2+} cycling to some degree at higher concentrations [22], and blebbistatin is light (laser) sensitive [23], and thus these limitations must be taken into consideration in LSCM physiological experiments.

Experimental approach

X-t line-scanning is most commonly used to visualize Ca²⁺ cycling, including Ca²⁺ transients, sparks, and waves. The following is a description of line scan imaging in single cardiac myocytes.

1. Myocytes loaded with indicator are placed in the experimental chamber without perfusion or temperature control and allowed to settle and adhere to the chamber bottom (5–10 minutes), at which point perfusion and temperature control are initiated.
2. Using the software interface to scan (2-D) the optical field, a cardiomyocyte is chosen and the focal plane is established at which maximal fluorescence (F) occurs in the cardiomyocyte. This should be done while cells are stimulated, first with visual light to identify contracting myocytes, then with fluorescence confocal imaging to determine which cell(s) are giving the brightest transients.
3. A scan line is placed along the cardiomyocyte where scanning should occur – a line drawn parallel to the short axis of the cardiomyocyte constitutes transverse X-t line scanning (Figure 2.2, top), whereas a line drawn parallel to the long axis of the cardiomyocyte constitutes longitudinal X-t lines scanning (Figure 2.2, bottom).
4. F at each point of the line is acquired for the desired duration of the scan, which entails a serial X-t (F(x) vs. time) line stack that is assembled to give a 2-DF(x)-t image. Ordinarily, a 512-pixel line is scanned at 2 ms/line in order to obtain sufficiently high spatial and temporal resolution of Ca²⁺ cycling events in heart cells. An obvious limitation of the confocal line scan is the spatial restriction of the line, which equals the length of the user-drawn scan line (x) × 1 pixel in "width" (y) × the optical "slice" depth (z).

When designing the experiment, it is essential to consider the cellular location in which the line scan recordings are to be acquired. Transverse line-scan recordings (parallel to the short axis of the myocyte, traversing edge-to-edge; Figure 2.2, top) constitute a shorter scan length, and can therefore have a higher resolution per scan; but at the expense of sampling a smaller portion of cell, and thus fewer Ca²⁺ cycling events are encountered. On the other hand, longitudinal line-scan recordings

(parallel to the long axis of the myocyte, traversing end-to-end; Figure 2.2, bottom) sample a larger portion of cell, and thus encounter more events but at the expense of lower resolution per scan. The orientation of the line may be important in determining the results, as shown in Figure 2.2 (top panels), where a transverse line scan recording in an atrial myocytes exhibits "V-shaped" Ca²⁺ transients in X-t images. Because there are no t-tubules in atrial cells, CICR occurs only at the periphery of atrial myocytes, while the rest of the SR Ca²⁺ release occurs more slowly as a Ca²⁺ wave propagated by activating RyRs in the corbular (non-junctional) SR. The regionally extracted F(x)-t profiles of junctional versus corbular Ca²⁺ transients are depicted below the whole-cell mean transverse line-scan image and show the differences in amplitude and timing of SR Ca²⁺ release between these two regions of atrial myocytes.

In contrast, Ca²⁺ transients are not V-shaped in longitudinal line scan recordings (Figure 2.2, bottom panels), since the spatiotemporal aspects of Ca²⁺ release are relatively equivalent along the entire length of the line scan except, nominally, at the ends. For comparison, Figure 2.3 depicts the same perspectives of transverse versus longitudinal line scanning in ventricular myocytes, which do have extensive t-tubules (note differences between atrial vs. ventricular myocyte X-Y images in Figures 2.2 vs. 2.3). Indeed, Ca²⁺ transients are not V-shaped in the ventricular myocyte transverse recording, and in both ventricular line scans the Ca²⁺ transient is more uniform across either cell axis compared to those in atrial myocytes.

Data analyses

Computer-assisted data analyses of confocal microscopy recordings of Ca²⁺ cycling in cardiomyocytes are, for the most part, performed off-line. Most of the manufacturers of confocal microscopes provide software customized for their microscopes, but these vary widely in sophistication and capabilities, particularly when analyzing X-t time series images. Image J (freeware from NIH) is of great utility for first-pass analyses, including automated Ca²⁺ spark analysis. However, if details of Ca²⁺ transient characteristics (i.e. rise time, decay time, etc.) are needed, most often custom or user-made software (e.g. via MatLab®, MathWorks,

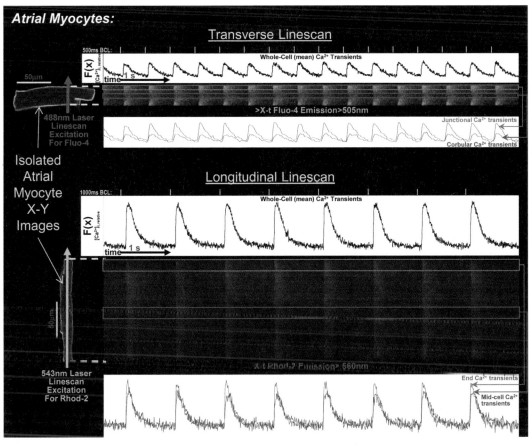

Figure 2.2 LSCM transverse versus longitudinal X-t line scanning in atrial myocytes (yellow tics above mean whole-cell F(x)-t profile represent the electrical stimulus).

Natick, Massachusetts, USA) is employed, which include noise filtering in the analysis. Most parameters of mean $F(x)$-t Ca^{2+} transient profiles of cardiomyocytes can also be obtained using the Clampfit module of P-Clamp® (Molecular Devices, Sunnyvale, California, USA) electrophysiology software (or similar specialty software). Ingenuity is definitely an attribute in efficient and accurate analyses of confocal recordings of Ca^{2+} cycling in isolated cardiomyocytes.

Weaknesses and strengths of the method and alternative approaches

While we have specifically discussed the use of LSCM, as mentioned above, there are two other types of confocal microscope systems that can and have been used to measure Ca^{2+} cycling in cells: (1)

spinning-disk; and (2) programmable array [24]. Laser scanning confocal microscopes offer the greatest degree of confocality, but the raster scanning employed is inherently slow, and so are inadequate for two-dimensional (2-D) measurements of fast (millisecond) events occurring simultaneously or at high frequency throughout the entire cell. However, if it is sufficient to measure Ca^{2+} cycling events serially in a much more restricted space, laser scanning confocal microscopy can achieve millisecond time resolution via so-called X-t line scanning in which the laser scans and fluorescence is acquired repeatedly (t dimension) from a "line" (x dimension) positioned in a myocyte. However, with repetitive scanning comes increased susceptibility to phototoxicity and photobleaching of the fluorophore, although in live cells more fluorophore can diffusively replace that which was photobleached

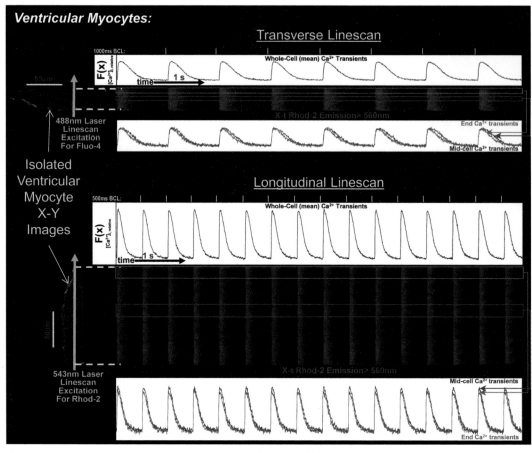

Figure 2.3 Laser scanning confocal microscope transverse versus longitudinal X-t line scanning in ventricular myocytes (yellow tics above mean whole-cell F(x)-t profile represent the electrical stimulus at the basic cycle length, BCL).

under the scan line. Spinning-disk confocal microscopy uses multiple pinholes arranged in an Archimedes' spiral array to provide 2-D measurements of Ca^{2+} cycling events with millisecond time resolution, but with less confocality and less ability to detect weaker fluorescence. Also, the disk pinholes of many commercially available spinning-disk confocal microscopes are not adjustable, and thus can only be used in conjunction with specifically matched objectives. Programmable array confocal microscopes are similar to spinning disks, but the disk pinholes can programmed to be open or closed so as to optimize images during high-speed acquisition, which requires more expensive instrumentation. Spinning-disk confocal microscopy is increasing in use particularly for live-cell imaging, but laser scanning confocal microscopy is still the more commonly used to study Ca^{2+} cycling in E-C

coupling. Advantages and disadvantages of each type of system need be thoroughly considered when devising experimental goals.

One other method that has recently come to some use in measuring Ca^{2+} cycling in cells is optical mapping. This methodology has typically been utilized to study voltage and Ca^{2+} signals (also using fluorescent dyes) over much larger, multicellular fields via employing light-emitting diodes (LEDs) for dye excitation and CCD cameras for dye-emission acquisition (see Chapter 7). Indeed, advances in CCD camera and LED technology have endowed optical mapping acquisition with much higher spatiotemporal resolution – portending the cellular level. However, because both in- and out-of-focal plan signal is acquired, truly single-cell/subcellular information is not obtained by this technique. On the other hand, the inherent signal averaging afforded by this technique provides for much higher signal-to-noise ratios to be obtained, which is quite essential for action potential measurement with the presently available voltage dyes – something confocal microscopy has struggled to achieve. Thus, this methodology allows for simultaneous Ca^{2+} and action potential measurements, which may be greatly advantageous and outweigh the high cellular/subcellular resolution but essentially Ca^{2+}-restricted acquisition provided by confocal microscopy. Of course this again is dependent on the overall goals of the investigator.

Conclusions

LSCM has become the gold-standard for obtaining subcellular-resolution measurement of Ca^{2+} cycling in isolated cardiac myocytes. It has and continues to provide detailed insight into the mechanisms governing E-C coupling (e.g., Ca^{2+} transients, sparks, blinks, puffs, etc.) and other cellular Ca^{2+} signaling (e.g., hypertrophy, arrhythmias, hypertension) requiring high spatiotemporal to delineate the multifaceted roles Ca^{2+} has in cardiovascular physiology and pathophysiology. The continued advances in confocal imaging will no doubt lend themselves to be indispensable in this regard for years to come.

References

1 Bers DM. Cardiac excitation-contraction coupling. *Nature* 2002; **415**: 198–205.

2 Bootman MD, Higazi DR, Coombes S, Roderick HL. Calcium signalling during excitation-contraction coupling in mammalian atrial myocytes. *J Cell Sci* 2006; **119**: 3915–3925.

3 Artman M, Henry G, Coetzee WA. Cellular basis for age-related differences in cardiac excitation-contraction coupling. *Prog Pediatr Cardiol* 2000; **11**: 185–194.

4 Louch WE, Ferrier GR, Howlett SE. Changes in excitation-contraction coupling in an isolated ventricular myocyte model of cardiac stunning. *Am J Physiol Heart Circ Physiol* 2002; **283**: H800–810.

5 Hintz KK, Norby FL, Duan J, et al. Comparison of cardiac excitation-contraction coupling in isolated ventricular myocytes between rat and mouse. *Comp Biochem Physiol A Mol Integr Physiol* 2002; **133**: 191–198.

6 Hobai IA, O'Rourke B. Decreased sarcoplasmic reticulum calcium content is responsible for defective excitation-contraction coupling in canine heart failure. *Circulation* 2001; **103**: 1577–1584.

7 Sjaastad I, Birkeland JA, Ferrier G, et al. Defective excitation-contraction coupling in hearts of rats with congestive heart failure. *Acta Physiol Scand* 2005; **184**: 45–58.

8 Lamb GD. Excitation-contraction coupling in skeletal muscle: Comparisons with cardiac muscle. *Clin Exp Pharmacol Physiol* 2000; **27**: 216–224.

9 Lipp P, Laine M, Tovey SC, et al. Functional insp3 receptors that may modulate excitation-contraction coupling in the heart. *Curr Biol* 2000; **10**: 939–942.

10 Sjaastad I, Wasserstrom JA, Sejersted OM. Heart failure – a challenge to our current concepts of excitation-contraction coupling. *J Physiol* 2003; **546**: 33–47.

11 Gomez AM, Guatimosim S, Dilly KW, et al. Heart failure after myocardial infarction: Altered excitation-contraction coupling. *Circulation* 2001; **104**: 688–693.

12 Zima AV, Blatter LA. Inositol-1,4,5-trisphosphate-dependent Ca(2+) signalling in cat atrial excitation-contraction coupling and arrhythmias. *J Physiol* 2004; **555**: 607–615.

13 Tanaka H, Masumiya H, Sekine T, et al. Involvement of ca2+ waves in excitation-contraction coupling of rat atrial cardiomyocytes. *Life Sci* 2001; **70**: 715–726.

14 Goldhaber JI, Qayyum MS. Oxygen free radicals and excitation-contraction coupling. *Antioxid Redox Signal* 2000; **2**: 55–64.

15 Scoote M, Poole-Wilson PA, Williams AJ. The therapeutic potential of new insights into myocardial excitation-contraction coupling. *Heart* 2003; **89**: 371–376.

16 Doggrell SA. Amiodarone – waxed and waned and waxed again. *Expert Opin Pharmacother* 2001; **2**: 1877–1890.

17 Kaestner L, Scholz A, Hammer K, et al. Isolation and genetic manipulation of adult cardiac myocytes for confocal imaging. *J Vis Exp* 2009; **31**: 1433.

18 Adams SR. How calcium indicators work. *Cold Spring Harbor Protocols*. 2010; **2010**: pdb.top70.

19 Paredes RM, Etzler JC, Watts LT, et al. Chemical calcium indicators. *Methods* 2008; **46**: 143–151.

20 Wu J, Biermann M, Rubart M, Zipes DP. Cytochalasin d as excitation-contraction uncoupler for optically mapping action potentials in wedges of ventricular myocardium. *J Cardiovasc Electrophysiol* 1998; **9**: 1336–1347.

21 Fedorov VV, Lozinsky IT, Sosunov EA, et al. Application of blebbistatin as an excitation-contraction uncoupler for electrophysiologic study of rat and rabbit hearts. *Heart Rhythm* 2007; **4**: 619–626.

22 Undrovinas AI, Maltsev VA. Cytochalasin d alters kinetics of Ca^{2+} transient in rat ventricular cardiomyocytes: An effect of altered actin cytoskeleton? *J Mol Cell Cardiol* 1998; **30**: 1665–1670.

23 Farman GP, Tachampa K, Mateja R, et al. Blebbistatin: Use as inhibitor of muscle contraction. *Pflugers Arch* 2008; **455**: 995–1005.

24 Pawley JB (ed.). *Handbook of Biological Confocal Microscopy*. New York: Plenum Press, 2006.

Generating a large animal model of persistent atrial fibrillation

Raphaël P. Martins[1,2] and José Jalife[1]

[1] University of Michigan, Ann Arbor, MI, USA

[2] University Hospital of Rennes, Rennes, France

Introduction

Atrial fibrillation (AF) is the most common, sustained cardiac arrhythmia seen in clinical practice [1]. Yet despite more than 100 years of basic and clinical research in AF, we still do not fully understand its fundamental mechanisms and we have not learned how to treat it effectively. Many drugs have been tried in persistent, long-lasting persistent, and permanent AF with very limited success [2]. On the other hand, the demonstration of AF triggers in the atrial sleeves of the pulmonary veins (PVs) has led to a significant improvement in therapy and today PV isolation using radiofrequency ablation (RF) is curative in about ~80% of paroxysmal AF patients. However, the success rate of RF ablation in the more prevalent and highly heterogeneous persistent and long-term persistent AF populations has, thus far, been a disappointing 30–50% [3–5]. Arguably, only a profound and complete understanding of the mechanisms involved in the maintenance and perpetuation of AF would allow us to generate more specific prevention and/or treatment of this dangerous and debilitating disease. Therefore, animal models have played, and will likely continue to play, an important role in the study of the pathophysiology of AF, including its molecular basis, its ion-current determinants, its anatomical features, and its macroscopic mechanisms, as well as in the development of new therapeutic approaches,

whether drug-based, molecular therapeutics, or device-related [6]. In this chapter we focus our attention on the description step-by-step of how to develop an ovine model of long-term persistent AF in which atrial tachypacing for ~9 weeks leads to stable, self-sustaining AF persisting for over 6 months. This novel, clinically relevant model is likely to open new paths toward the understanding of the mechanisms of persistent AF, as well as the development of more effective preventative approaches. We then switch gears to briefly review some of the animal models that have been used over the last 18 years to study the consequences of atrial tachycardia-induced electrical and structural remodeling that characterizes sustained AF.

Insights from tachypacing-induced AF models

When AF lasts continuously for more than 7 days it is designated as persistent AF. Spontaneous, pharmacological, or ablative resumption of sinus rhythm is infrequent in persistent AF, with prompt recurrences or commonly failed cardioversions in episodes lasting for more than 1 year, termed long-term persistent AF [2]. It is reasonable to speculate that continuous, high frequency, and heterogeneous bombardment of the atrial cells and tissues with fibrillatory waves during long-lasting AF leads to a modification of the molecular substrate on which waves propagate, with consequent electrical and structural remodeling, substantial enough to

Manual of Research Techniques in Cardiovascular Medicine, First Edition. Edited by Hossein Ardehali, Roberto Bolli, and Douglas W. Losordo.
© 2014 John Wiley & Sons, Ltd. Published 2014 by John Wiley & Sons, Ltd.

increase the likelihood of perpetuation of the electrical sources that maintain the arrhythmia. Therefore, since the mid-1990s investigators have endeavored to examine the mechanisms of remodeling and AF perpetuation using highly sophisticated and labor-intensive large animal models. The use of such models has greatly advanced our understanding of this highly prevalent arrhythmia.

In 1995, Morillo *et al.* [7] developed a novel canine chronic AF model, of right atrial tachypacing. For the first time, they demonstrated that the mean AF cycle length (1/dominant frequency) was significantly shorter in the left atrium compared with the right atrium. Such a consistent left-to-right dominant frequency gradient was similar to what was shown subsequently in optical mapping experiments in the isolated heart [8–10], and later contributed to the "mother rotor hypothesis" of AF [11]. In the experiments of Morillo *et al.* [7], cryoablation of the high-frequency area near the pulmonary veins (PVs) significantly prolonged AF cycle length and successfully restored sinus rhythm in most dogs, confirming the crucial role of localized sites with high activation frequency in the mechanism of AF. Such observations were later confirmed in humans by the seminal work of Haissaguerre *et al.* who demonstrated that ectopic beats originating within the PVs were capable of initiating and even maintaining AF, and that they could be eliminated by treatment with radiofrequency ablation [12].

In a similar model of atrial tachypacing-induced AF, Wijffels *et al.* [13], used goats that were chronically instrumented with electrodes sutured to both atria and connected to a modified external pacemaker that delivered rapid stimuli to the right atrium. These authors demonstrated electrical remodeling manifested as an abbreviation of the atrial effective refractory period (AERP), reversal of AERP rate adaptation, increase in AF rate and inducibility, and progressive increase in episodes duration. This led to the concept of "AF begets AF", which was shown to reverse to sinus rhythm upon switching the pacemaker off. Various groups later have used this model in dogs [14,15], sheep [16], or pigs [17,18].

In addition to electrical remodeling, contractile remodeling also occurs in atrial tachypacing as a consequence of the reduced contractility, and the decreased sarcoplasmic reticulum calcium load [19]

and release [20]. The contractile abnormality, also demonstrated in the fibrillating human atria [21], probably exacerbates the thromboembolic risk in AF patients. Moreover, structural remodeling of the atria is also a consequence of AF. The most common abnormalities observed are interstitial fibrosis [22] (although not in all species subjected to chronic atrial pacing), myocyte hypertrophy, accumulation of glycogen, mitochondrial abnormalities [23], and atrial dilation. Therefore, AF results in electrical, contractile, and structural remodeling, all of which leads to more AF and creates a vicious circle able to self-sustain the arrhythmia. This helps to provide a reasonable although unproven explanation for the progression from paroxysmal to persistent and eventually permanent AF that has been observed on occasion in clinical practice.

Protocol

Generating a tachypacing-induced AF model

In this section we provide details of the standard protocol used routinely in our laboratory to generate an ovine model of tachypacing-induced AF. The model derives from those used previously in other species [7,13]. The procedure requires the chronic implantation of a pacemaker and of a transvenous catheter. Yet it is safe, considered minor surgery, and is accompanied by very few complications. In humans, a similar surgical procedure is often performed under conscious sedation and local anesthesia.

Pre-op procedures. We use 6 to 12-month-old male Dorset sheep weighing 30–40 kg. Preprocedural injection of antibiotics is not given routinely. In case of preprocedural signs of infection (fever, cough, diarrhea, shortness of breath, etc.), the procedure is postponed to allow the treatment of the infection; the animal is implanted after full recovery. The length of the surgical fasting period is 12 hours (water restriction is not required).

Sheep are placed in sternal recumbency and safely handled. A 16 to 18-gauge venous catheter is placed for vascular access in a forelimb and secured to allow for the administration of i.v. fluids, induction agents, supplemental parenteral anesthetics, and analgesics. If the animal needs to be calmed before the insertion of the venous catheter, an intramuscular injection of xylazine (0.2 mg/kg) can be administered. The jugular vein is not catheterized; it is subsequently used for pacemaker lead implantation. Catheter patency is checked using saline solution. Once the catheter is successfully placed, heparin is flushed to avoid coagulation (this procedure is repeated after each drug injection via the catheter). Then, propofol i.v. (4–6 mg/kg) is injected for induction of anesthesia. A slow injection is required to avoid severe bradycardia, which could cause myocardial ischemia, and to minimize the risk of seizures. Buprenorphine (0.01 mg/kg, i.m. or s.c.) is injected at the beginning of the procedure to ensure analgesia.

Next, endotracheal intubation is performed placing the animal in the sternal recumbency or supine position. A laryngoscope is inserted to visualize the larynx and the vocal cords. A 33–37 cm endotracheal tube is then inserted and the cuff inflated; the cuff is checked for leaks before intubation. Ties are used to secure the tube to the lower jaw. The proper position of the tube is checked by auscultation of the chest with a stethoscope to ensure the presence of equal bilateral thoracic sounds and no sounds over the stomach area. In addition, equal bilateral rise and fall of the chest should occur when inflating/ deflating the breathing bag, and there should be vapor in the endotracheal tube. Isoflurane gas is initiated and the animal ventilated at 5–10 mL/kg (respiratory rate 20/min). A rumen tube is placed and ophthalmic ointment is applied to the eyes. Next, the surgical area (right part of the neck and of the upper chest) is clipped and scrubbed with three alternating chlorhexidine/ alcohol scrubs. The animal should be connected to the following monitors: pulse oximetry connected to one of the ears, respiration, body temperature, pulse rate, ECG, and blood pressure. The surgically prepped area is then isolated with sterile towels and sterile drapes.

Pacemaker implantation. The procedure is performed as follows. First, locate the right jugular vein by occluding manually the flow downstream from the future incision site. Then proceed to make an approximately 5-cm long incision on the skin along the jugular vein with a standard scalpel; the incision should be superficial to avoid direct vein incision. An electric scalpel is used to gently cut the skin layers to the subcutaneous tissue through the

previous incision. Carefully dissect the subcutaneous tissue using a small artery forceps; small bleeders should be cauterized using an electric cautery. Continue with progressive dissection until the external jugular vein is visualized, carefully avoiding vein damage. Proceed with the dissection to isolate the external jugular vein in its entire circumference all along the skin incision. If the jugular vein receives venous branches, they should be occluded downstream and upstream using non-absorbable silk and then cauterized. Once the jugular vein is perfectly isolated circumferentially from the subcutaneous tissue, it should be occluded upstream at the edge of the incision using non-absorbable silk (for safety reasons, we usually ligate the vein twice); the jugular vein is then totally flat. Thereafter, the canister pocket is molded in the subcutaneous tissue plane by careful blunt dissection using the fingers; the pocket should be filled with gauze pads to perform hemostasis and avoid blood penetration during lead insertion.

The fluoroscopy C-arm is prepared and centered in the chest area. The operator should replace surgical gloves before touching the pacemaker canister and lead.

Lead implantation. The endocardial lead should be a 6 to 8 Fr, 46 to 52 cm bipolar, active fixation and steroid-eluting lead (Figure 3.1). Before implantation, the mechanical function of the helix may be tested by screwing and unscrewing it; the helix should be

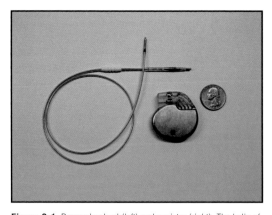

Figure 3.1 Pacemaker lead (left) and canister (right). The helix of the lead tip is extended. Shown is a dual-chamber pacemaker (atrial and ventricular ports).

completely retracted before inserting the lead into the vein. To insert the lead start by lifting the vein using a small tissue forceps, and making a small vein incision (2–3 mm) using Potts–Smith scissors to insert the lead (a vein-lifter can be used to facilitate the insertion). Under fluoroscopic guidance (anteroposterior view), push the lead gently and progressively through the jugular vein to the superior vena cava and then the right atrium. Due to the vertical position of the sheep heart, the lead is likely to slide directly from the superior to the inferior vena cava. At this point, insert a J-shaped stylet into the lead; as the stylet approaches the lead tip, retract progressively the lead into the right atrium; the lead tip will spontaneously glide into the right atrial appendage (RAA). Check the correct position of the lead using fluoroscopy. The electrode tip should slightly move from right to left in a windshield wiper-like movement. Then move the fluoroscopy to the lateral view: the J-curve of the lead should appear in profile. Slightly pull the lead/ stylet to give an L-shape to the lead; this movement stabilizes the tip of the lead in the appendage. Using the screw-driver tool, extend the helix to fix the lead to the RAA (clockwise rotation), making sure the helix is extended on the fluoroscopic image. Retract the stylet from the lead with a smooth and steady movement, while keeping the lead tip in position. Then slightly push the lead to give it a correct J-shape assessed in the anteroposterior view.

Intraoperative measurements. Three parameters should be verified during the implantation of the lead: the impedance, the sensitivity, and the stimulation threshold. Such measurements require connecting the pacemaker canister to the lead (or a pacing system analyzer through the programmer).
• Impedance: ideally between 200 and 2000 Ω (<200 Ω: insulation break, >2000 Ω: lead fracture).
• Sensitivity: this reflects the detection ability of the pacemaker in a given position of the lead. Ideally, a high voltage atrial signal (>2 mV) should be detected with a low amplitude ventricular far-field.
• Threshold: this reflects the pacing ability of the pacemaker in a given position of the lead. Ideally, a low stimulation threshold value (<1 V) should be obtained to avoid excessive battery drain during the follow-up and to prevent any loss of capture if the pacing threshold increases after the acute phase.

A good position of the lead is reflected by a high amplitude signal and a low pacing threshold. If the values are not correct, a different position of the lead should be targeted. To secure the lead, the suture sleeve should be firmly tied to the lead and the underlying tissue under fluoroscopic guidance to detect any displacement of the lead tip.

Insertion of the pacemaker canister. First, remove the gauze pads filling the pacemaker pouch. Then check if hemostasis is necessary. Please note that, at this point, the electric cautery should be used very carefully to avoid any damage to the lead. Next, connect the lead to the atrial port of the single chamber pacemaker (if a dual-chamber pacemaker is used and the ventricular port is not used, it should be occluded using specific plugs), and insert the pacemaker canister inside the pouch. Redundant leads should be looped underneath the device. Fluoroscopically examine the lead and the canister to check proper positioning before closure. Proceed with a standard two-layer closure to secure the device and close the pocket; synthetic absorbable suture is used to close the subcutaneous fascia and surgical staples are used to close the skin.

Short-term follow-up. Program the pacemaker for "atrial sensing-only" mode (OAO) and discontinue the anesthesia. The animal should remain intubated until there is evidence of sufficient spontaneous respiration. Daily physical examination should include checking the wound, the animal's weight, breathing and heart rates, and the temperature. Staples should be removed 7 days after pacemaker implantation. The pacemaker is programmed in order to induce AF after a 10-day recovery period.

Pacing protocols

Many different pacing protocols provided by the device industry may be used to induce AF in animals. The pacing protocol most commonly used in published studies is one that includes alternation between burst pacing and waiting periods. The protocol described here is available for St. Jude Medical (St. Paul, Minnesota, USA) pacemaker devices. In this specific pacing algorithm, four parameters can be programmed: (1) **Burst pacing rate**: from 4 to 50 Hz. (2) **Burst pacing period**: 6, 10, 30 s or continuous pacing. (3) **Waiting period**: the

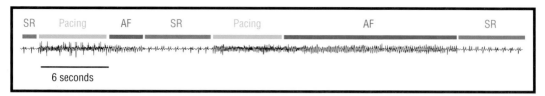

Figure 3.2 Auto mode switch algorithm activated in association with pacing. The pacing period in this example is 6 seconds. After the pacing period, the pacemaker "senses" the atrial activity and only resumes pacing if sinus rhythm (SR) is detected. AF, atrial fibrillation.

time between two burst pacing periods, may last between 2 and 10 s (or absent when in the continuous pacing mode). (4) **Suspension of pacing after the wait period if AF is detected, and resumption of pacing if reversion to sinus rhythm is detected**. This parameter can be activated by switching on the «Auto Mode Switch» (AMS) algorithm of the device, an example of which is presented in Figure 3.2.

The AMS algorithm reliably generates tachypacing-induced self-sustained AF because the pacemaker resumes pacing only if AF stops and sinus rhythm is detected. As such, the algorithm readily reproduces the phenomenon of "AF begets AF" described originally by Wijffels *et al.* [13] Importantly, the approach may be used to predict the evolution of AF that might occur in some human patients, from the initiation of premature atrial beats, to the establishment of paroxysmal and eventually persistent AF [24]. To this aim, the device stores valuable information that may be used to characterize the AF history of the animal, including the number and duration of AF episodes (Figure 3.3A,B), and the precise moment of each episode's occurrence. The device also has Holter capabilities that can be used to record the intracardiac electrogram during initiation and/or termination of a given AF episode. All such features can be used to create histograms and follow the evolution of the arrhythmia (Figure 3.3C).

In our experience, the time to AF stabilization is quite variable. The first AF episode occurs after a median of 5 days from the onset of pacing, sometimes immediately and sometimes up to 2 months after the first pacing burst. The time in paroxysmal AF (episodes <7 days' duration) is around 2 months. Thus, a period of 2.5 months of burst pacing is usually needed before persistent AF is established. A recording of the first AF episode in a sheep is given in Figure 3.4.

Electrical recordings (ECG or intracardiac electrograms) can be used to analyze the characteristics of the arrhythmia. At any time in the AF evolution, animals can be sacrificed to study electrical or structural remodeling from the molecule to the whole organ.

Ventricular rate during AF: to ablate or not to ablate

Conduction of atrial fibrillatory impulses through the atrioventricular (AV) node in animals with AF can be complicated by tachycardiomyopathy and heart failure [25,26]. Heart failure can itself lead to atrial remodeling (electrophysiological and structural), sometimes similar to AF-induced remodeling but sometimes different (see section "congestive heart failure model" later in the chapter) [27], and thus rate control may be necessary in some species. Therefore, some groups have proposed the need to perform His bundle ablation (HBA), together with the implantation of a ventricular lead to control the ventricular rate in the atrial tachypacing model. Radiofrequency energy may be used to perform this ablation [28]. Sequential atrial and ventricular pacing uses a single, or two separate pacemaker canisters. In a sheep model of tachypacing-induced AF, Anné *et al.* did not find any significant difference in terms of AF inducibility although sheep undergoing HBA developed persistent AF later than non-HBA sheep [16]. Furthermore, sheep with normal AV conduction displayed increased LA fibrosis compared to HBA-sheep. Markers of substrate remodeling (e.g. metalloproteinases) were also different in the two groups [28]. However, even though HBA allows investigators to elucidate the substrate and electrical remodeling that depend specifically on atrial tachypacing, it renders the model less clinically relevant.

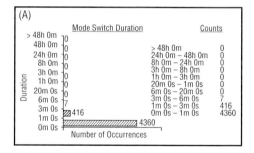

Date/Time	Duration
Apr 10 2011 4:42 pm	0d 12h 31m 10s
Apr 10 2011 1:57 am	0d 14h 44m 52s
Apr 9 2011 3:25 pm	0d 10h 31m 46s
Apr 9 2011 4:18 am	0d 11h 6m 48s
Apr 7 2011 9:37 pm	1d 6h 41m 24s
Apr 7 2011 9:13 am	0d 0h 23m 28s
Apr 7 2011 3:15 pm	0d 5h 57m 34s
Apr 7 2011 2:22 pm	0d 0h 53m 22s
Apr 7 2011 1:55 am	0d 0h 26m 20s
Apr 7 2011 8:33 am	0d 5h 21m 50s
Apr 7 2011 8:04 am	0d 0h 29m 26s
Apr 7 2011 8:04 am	0d 0h 0m 14s
Apr 7 2011 8:02 am	0d 0h 1m 22s
Apr 7 2011 2:59 am	0d 5h 3m 22s
Apr 6 2011 11:26 pm	0d 3h 32m 40s
Apr 6 2011 6:27 pm	0d 4h 58m 16s

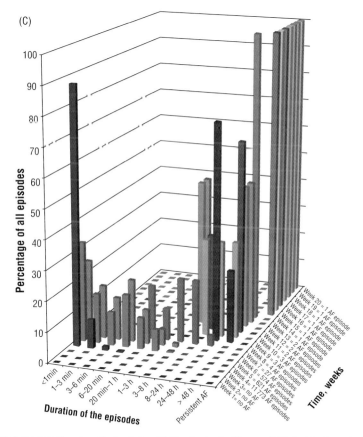

Figure 3.3 Information stored by the device. (A) AF episodes (in this case, 4783 short-lasting episodes in 1 week) are classified according to their duration. (B) The times episodes occur are also stored on the device's memory (two different sheep in A and B). (C) Weekly interrogation can be performed to create a histogram of the evolution of the arrhythmia. In this animal, the first AF episode occurred 4 weeks after the initiation of pacing. Episodes tended to last longer with time until self-sustained persistent AF developed. As this time, the pacemaker is does not resume pacing because sinus rhythm will not be detected.

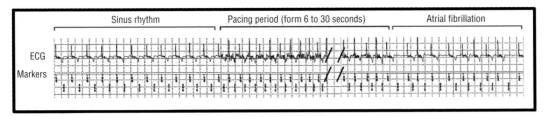

| Sinus rhythm | Pacing period (form 6 to 30 seconds) | Atrial fibrillation |

Figure 3.4 First episode of AF detected by an implantable loop recorder. After the wait period in sinus rhythm, pacing resumes for the programmed period (6 to 30 s, in this case 20 Hz during 30 s). At the end of the pacing period, AF is recorded.

Strengths and weaknesses of the model

The greatest strength of the tachypacing-induced AF model is its high reliability in undergoing atrial remodeling and reproducing the changes associated with sustained AF that are often observed in patients. The procedure is well tolerated by the animals and in experienced hands presents very few complications (see section Potential complications) [29]. Moreover, this type of model can provide a vast amount of information on AF, including its evolution, its relation to fibrosis, and when combined with other multidisciplinary approaches, its molecular and cellular mechanisms. Hence, for the last 16 years, atrial burst pacing models have provided important insights into the mechanisms of electrophysiological [13,14] and structural remodeling [23,30] in AF. They have also been used to evaluate the effects of drugs acting on the electrophysiological properties (e.g. antiarrhythmic drugs) or the structural remodeling of the atria (inhibitors of renin–angiotensin system [16], anti-inflammatory drugs [31], statins [32], etc.). However, a major disadvantage of the atrial burst pacing model is its relatively high cost, both in terms of resources and personnel and the need for a long-term commitment to the experiment, particularly when the experimental design calls for a model of long-term persistent AF (>6 months), which can bring the cost of each animal to more than $5000, including the purchase of the animal, surgical procedures, long-term follow up, and ancillary technologies (e.g. biochemistry, patch clamping, optical mapping, etc.).

Another potential disadvantage is that while the atrial burst pacing model nicely reproduces the "lone AF" seen in clinical practice, it does not necessarily apply to other forms of AF. Lone AF is not the same as AF in the context of hypertension or heart failure, or in the patient with ischemic heart disease. Therefore, extreme care must be exerted when attempting to extrapolate its results to the human. In fact, it may be argued that an important requirement for an appropriate animal model of AF is that it closely reproduces the substrate associated with the specific diseased that caused it. On the other hand, one should always keep in mind that this is only a model, which by no means accurately represented the clinical situation and this premise applies to any model. Hence we are convinced that the tachypacing-induced persistent AF model may be used to make predictions about AF mechanisms in general, as long as it is done cautiously and the investigation in question is accompanied by parallel research into the pathophysiological mechanisms associated with the aging process and/or the underlying disease as well as the pathologic processes that generated AF, including, fibrosis, adiposis, and inflammation.

Complications and alternative approaches to study AF

Potential complications

During the last 5 years, we have used this model in 80 sheep. Pacemaker implantation is extremely well tolerated in this species. We have not observed any significant hypotension, syncope, or evidence of device canister intolerance in our experiments, and the overall behavior of the animals is completely normal after the procedure. While persistent AF is induced in most animals, we have not seen any pacemaker infections, strokes, heart failure symptoms, or sudden cardiac deaths. The only complications we have observed are as follows: (1) wound healing: while rare, the major complication at this stage is extrusion of the canister through the unhealed wound; and (2) acute displacement of the lead: this can be in the form of microdisplacement within the right atrium, revealed by an increase in pacing threshold, a decrease in the amplitude of the detected signal, or a change in impedance. However, should this happen the pacing can still be activated using a higher-energy pacing output. Lead displacement to the right ventricle, revealed by a ventricular morphology when pacing, is tested at the postoperative measurement; fast pacing must not be switched ON since it would immediately induce ventricular fibrillation. A redo procedure is required to reposition the lead. Finally, miscellaneous extracardiac complications may also occur, including cold, pneumonia, parasite infection, etc.

Alternative AF models

Obviously, the choice of any given model should depend on the specific questions being asked. As discussed earlier, the atrial burst pacing model closely reproduces "lone AF" as seen in clinical practice. However, ideally, animal models should attempt to reproduce the conditions that prevail in the pathologies that produce the arrhythmia, including hypertension, heart failure, mitral valve disease, etc. Throughout the years, a number of experimental models have been developed in which AF pathophysiology may be studied in relation to a specific underlying disease. Data derived from all these models have contributed to improve our understanding of AF mechanisms in the clinical setting and have allowed for the development of novel therapeutic approaches. Here we touch on various models, developed over the last 15 years, to mimic the other conditions generating AF.

Congestive heart failure model. In 1999, Li *et al.* developed a canine model of heart failure by pacing the right ventricle at a fast heart rate (>200 bpm) [27]. They demonstrated structural and electrophysiological changes in atrial cardiomyocytes. A substantial increase in fibrosis was also noted, but no changes were found in the action potential duration (APD) or AERP [27]. The structural change led to conduction heterogeneity and increased duration of AF episodes, from seconds in the control group to minutes in the congestive heart failure group. Electrophysiological changes supporting the stability of APD were analyzed by the same group

[33]: they observed decreases in I_{CaL}, I_{to}, and I_{Ks} current densities and an increase in the transient inward Na^+/Ca^{2+} exchanger. However, they saw no changes in I_{CaT}, I_{Kur}, I_{Kr}, or I_{K1}. Interestingly, complete recovery of ionic remodeling was observed after 4 weeks without pacing, but structural remodeling (fibrosis) did not disappear, which explained in part the persistent vulnerability to AF after stopping the fast ventricular pacing [34]. Substrate remodeling seems to play an important role in maintaining AF in the congestive heart failure model. Remarkably, ionic modifications are different from what is observed in the atrial pacing model: this led Nattel and co-workers to study a model combining atrial and ventricular pacing (atrial tachycardia and congestive heart failure models, respectively), a common association often observed in clinical practice [35]. In this combined model, they demonstrated that the ionic remodeling pattern was different from that of heart failure or atrial pacing alone. They concluded that electrophysiological and substrate remodeling are not unique scenarios in AF but differ depending on the clinical situation.

Structural heart diseases: tricuspid [36] or mitral regurgitation [37–39]. Mitral regurgitation leads to atrial dilation, interstitial fibrosis, and homogeneously increased AERP [39]. In the mitral valve regurgitation model, conduction velocity during normal pacing was comparable between controls and dogs with regurgitation. However, conduction abnormalities were found during pacing at short cycle lengths and during premature extrastimuli, which may have been responsible for the increased AF inducibility in this model [38].

Sterile pericarditis. This model was developed and thoroughly characterized by the Waldo lab [40,41]. It reproduces predominantly atrial flutter, but AF can also occur. The surgical procedure consists of opening the pericardium by way of a right thoracotomy, and to dust the atrial surfaces with talcum powder. This model mimics the postoperative form of AF (occurring in up to 50% of patients after cardiac surgery). It has provided important insight and better understanding of flutter mechanisms and of the flutter–AF inter-relationship [42,43].

Complete AV block. This has been studied mainly in goats [44]. This model leads to progressive left atrial dilatation. However, there are no changes in AERP or AF cycle length, but the duration of AF episodes increased. Interestingly, histological analysis revealed myocyte hypertrophy but no fibrosis, and no changes in connexin expression were found.

Hypertension. Hypertension carries an important risk in AF patients. Hypertension is a predictor of AF induction and maintenance, and increases the risk of thromboembolic events. The relationship between AF and hypertension has been studied in spontaneously hypertensive rats [45] and in sheep exposed to corticosteroids during the prenatal period [46]. The presence of atrial fibrosis seems to participate in AF inducibility and stability in these models.

Arteriovenous shunts. These are responsible for chronic volume overload and have been studied in rabbits [47], goats [48], and sheep [49]. Although electrophysiological differences were noted in these different species, atrial dilation is a common feature and leads to an increase in AF vulnerability and stability.

Acute atrial injuries. Injuries such as acute stretch [50,51] or atrial ischemia [52] can increase atrial vulnerability to AF, and models of ischemia have been used to investigate experimental AF [53].

Aging. The prevalence of AF is known to increase with age. The atria of older animals display heterogeneous interstitial fibrosis [54,55], which may help to explain a decrease in conduction velocity and increased AF vulnerability. Electrophysiological investigation of right atrial cardiomyocytes from old dogs found no significant differences in resting membrane potential, AP amplitude or upstroke velocity, but the AP plateau was more negative and APD was longer in older animals [54]. Conduction velocity was normal for regular beats but reduced for premature beats.

Vagal nerve stimulation. In clinical practice, many patients present with vagally induced AF episodes; for instance, after vagal syncope, vomiting, or during the postprandial period. Vagal stimulation releases acetylcholine (ACh), which activates muscarinic receptors on the atrial cell and increases $I_{K,ACh}$,

leading to APD and AERP shortening. Consequently, the wavelength of re-entry (WL = conduction velocity × refractory period) decreases which prevents wavefront–wavetail interactions and increases the stability of the sources that maintain AF [11]. We previously demonstrated the existence of rotors, predominantly located in the left atrium, which is the region having the highest dominant frequency, in acetylcholine-induced AF [10,56]. These observations found in sheep hearts were supported by computer simulations [57], and later confirmed in patients in whom adenosine was used to test for the effects of increasing $I_{K,ACh}$ [58].

Pharmacologically induced AF. Aconitine crystals impregnated in the atrial muscle have been known to induce focal discharges maintaining AF in open-chest canine models [59,60]. Cesium infusion can also induce AF [61]. Acute asphyxia reproducibly induced AF in rats [62]. In clinical practice, many other drugs are known to induce AF [63].

Transgenic mouse models of AF. Many transgenic mice models have been developed over the last several years. A recent review details the characteristics and use of these different models [64].

Conclusion

Animal models of AF are here to stay. Since the independent publication of atrial tachypacing-induced AF models by two different laboratories more than 15 years ago [7,13], our knowledge of this arrhythmia has increased substantially. Animal models of AF have been an invaluable tool for studying atrial electrical and structural remodeling in AF. These models also offer great opportunities to study mechanisms and to develop novel therapeutic strategies. Knowledge derived from the various AF models will hopefully enable researchers to address important mechanistic questions, such as what processes underlie the transition from paroxysmal to persistent AF, whether there is any relationship between the development of atrial fibrosis and electrophysiological remodeling, and how one can take advantage of that knowledge to prevent AF progression. Animal models of AF are also likely to play crucial roles in the development and testing of new generations of antifibrillatory drugs. Such progress will be essential in our hope to avert the predicted huge increase in the incidence of this often devastating disease and its consequences [65].

Acknowledgement

Sources of funding: P01-HL087226 (J.J.) and the Leducq Foundation (J.J.). RPM received a grant from the Fédération Francaise de Cardiologie.

References

1 Kannel WB, Wolf PA, Benjamin EJ, Levy D. Prevalence, incidence, prognosis, and predisposing conditions for atrial fibrillation: Population-based estimates. *Am J Cardiol* 1998; **82**: 2N–9N.

2 Camm AJ, Kirchhof P, Lip GY, Schotten U, Savelieva I, Ernst S, *et al.* Guidelines for the management of atrial fibrillation: The task force for the management of atrial fibrillation of the European Society of Cardiology (ESC). *Europace* 2010; **12**: 1360–1420.

3 Matsuo S, Lim KT, Haissaguerre M. Ablation of chronic atrial fibrillation. *Heart Rhythm* 2007; **4**: 1461–1463.

4 Calkins H, Brugada J, Packer DL, Cappato R, Chen SA, Crijns HJ, *et al.* Hrs/ehra/ecas expert consensus statement on catheter and surgical ablation of atrial fibrillation: Recommendations for personnel, policy, procedures and follow-up. A report of the heart rhythm society (hrs) task force on catheter and surgical ablation of atrial fibrillation. *Heart Rhythm* 2007; **4**: 816–861.

5 Cappato R, Calkins H, Chen SA, Davies W, Iesaka Y, Kalman J, *et al.* Worldwide survey on the methods, efficacy, and safety of catheter ablation for human atrial fibrillation. *Circulation* 2005; **111**: 1100–1105.

6 Nishida K, Michael G, Dobrev D, Nattel S. Animal models for atrial fibrillation: Clinical insights and scientific opportunities. *Europace* 2010; **12**: 160–172.

7 Morillo CA, Klein GJ, Jones DL, Guiraudon CM. Chronic rapid atrial pacing. Structural, functional, and electrophysiological characteristics of a new model of sustained atrial fibrillation. *Circulation* 1995; **91**: 1588–1595.

8 Jalife J, Berenfeld O, Skanes A, Mandapati R. Mechanisms of atrial fibrillation: Mother rotors or multiple daughter wavelets, or both? *J Cardiovasc Electrophysiol* 1998; **9**: S2–12.

9 Berenfeld O, Mandapati R, Dixit S, Skanes AC, Chen J, Mansour M, *et al.* Spatially distributed dominant excitation frequencies reveal hidden organization in atrial fibrillation in the langendorff-perfused sheep heart. *J Cardiovasc Electrophysiol* 2000; **11**: 869–879.

10 Mandapati R, Skanes A, Chen J, Berenfeld O, Jalife J. Stable microreentrant sources as a mechanism of atrial

11 Jalife J, Berenfeld O, Mansour M. Mother rotors and fibrillatory conduction: A mechanism of atrial fibrillation. *Cardiovasc Res* 2002; **54**: 204–216.

12 Haissaguerre M, Jais P, Shah DC, Takahashi A, Hocini M, Quiniou G, *et al.* Spontaneous initiation of atrial fibrillation by ectopic beats originating in the pulmonary veins. *N Engl J Med* 1998; **339**: 659–666.

13 Wijffels MC, Kirchhof CJ, Dorland R, Allessie MA. Atrial fibrillation begets atrial fibrillation. A study in awake chronically instrumented goats. *Circulation* 1995; **92**: 1954–1968.

14 Gaspo R, Bosch RF, Talajic M, Nattel S. Functional mechanisms underlying tachycardia-induced sustained atrial fibrillation in a chronic dog model. *Circulation* 1997; **96**: 4027–4035.

15 Fareh S, Villemaire C, Nattel S. Importance of refractoriness heterogeneity in the enhanced vulnerability to atrial fibrillation induction caused by tachycardia-induced atrial electrical remodeling. *Circulation* 1998; **98**: 2202–2209.

16 Anné W, Willems R, Holemans P, Beckers F, Roskams T, Lenaerts I, *et al.* Self-terminating af depends on electrical remodeling while persistent af depends on additional structural changes in a rapid atrially paced sheep model. *J Mol Cell Cardiol* 2007; **43**: 148–158.

17 Dudley SC, Jr., Hoch NE, McCann LA, Honeycutt C, Diamandopoulos L, Fukai T, *et al.* Atrial fibrillation increases production of superoxide by the left atrium and left atrial appendage: Role of the nadph and xanthine oxidases. *Circulation* 2005; **112**: 1266–1273.

18 Chen CL, Huang SK, Lin JL, Lai LP, Lai SC, Liu CW, *et al.* Upregulation of matrix metalloproteinase-9 and tissue inhibitors of metalloproteinases in rapid atrial pacing-induced atrial fibrillation. *J Mol Cell Cardiol* 2008; **45**: 742–753.

19 Greiser M, Neuberger HR, Harks E, El-Armouche A, Boknik P, de Haan S, *et al.* Distinct contractile and molecular differences between two goat models of atrial dysfunction: Av block-induced atrial dilatation and atrial fibrillation. *J Mol Cell Cardiol* 2009; **46**: 385–394.

20 Sun H, Gaspo R, Leblanc N, Nattel S. Cellular mechanisms of atrial contractile dysfunction caused by sustained atrial tachycardia. *Circulation* 1998; **98**: 719–727.

21 Schotten U, Greiser M, Benke D, Buerkel K, Ehrenteidt B, Stellbrink C, *et al.* Atrial fibrillation-induced atrial contractile dysfunction: A tachycardiomyopathy of a different sort. *Cardiovasc Res* 2002; **53**: 192–201.

22 Everett THT, Olgin JE. Atrial fibrosis and the mechanisms of atrial fibrillation. *Heart Rhythm* 2007; **4**: S24–27.

23 Ausma J, Wijffels M, Thone F, Wouters L, Allessie M, Borgers M, *et al.* Structural changes of atrial myocardium

due to sustained atrial fibrillation in the goat. *Circulation* 1997; **96**: 3157–3163.

24 Cohen M, Naccarelli GV. Pathophysiology and disease progression of atrial fibrillation: Importance of achieving and maintaining sinus rhythm. *J Cardiovasc Electrophysiol* 2008; **19**: 885–890.

25 Armstrong PW, Stopps TP, Ford SE, de Bold AJ. Rapid ventricular pacing in the dog: Pathophysiologic studies of heart failure. *Circulation* 1986; **74**: 1075–1084.

26 Williams RE, Kass DA, Kawagoe Y, Pak P, Tunin RS, Shah R, *et al*. Endomyocardial gene expression during development of pacing tachycardia-induced heart failure in the dog. *Circ Res* 1994; **75**: 615–623.

27 Li D, Fareh S, Leung TK, Nattel S. Promotion of atrial fibrillation by heart failure in dogs: Atrial remodeling of a different sort. *Circulation* 1999; **100**: 87–95.

28 Anne W, Willems R, Holemans P, Beckers F, Roskams T, Lenaerts I, *et al*. Self-terminating af depends on electrical remodeling while persistent af depends on additional structural changes in a rapid atrially paced sheep model. *J Mol Cell Cardiol* 2007; **43**: 148–158.

29 Nishida K, Michael G, Dobrev D, Nattel S. Animal models for atrial fibrillation: Clinical insights and scientific opportunities. *Europace* 2010; **12**: 160–172.

30 He X, Gao X, Peng L, Wang S, Zhu Y, Ma H, *et al*. Atrial fibrillation induces myocardial fibrosis through angiotensin ii type 1 receptor-specific arkadia-mediated downregulation of smad7. *Circ Res* 2011; **108**: 164–175.

31 Shiroshita-Takeshita A, Brundel BJ, Lavoie J, Nattel S. Prednisone prevents atrial fibrillation promotion by atrial tachycardia remodeling in dogs. *Cardiovasc Res* 2006; **69**: 865–875.

32 Shiroshita-Takeshita A, Schram G, Lavoie J, Nattel S. Effect of simvastatin and antioxidant vitamins on atrial fibrillation promotion by atrial-tachycardia remodeling in dogs. *Circulation* 2004; **110**: 2313–2319.

33 Li D, Melnyk P, Feng J, Wang Z, Petrecca K, Shrier A, *et al*. Effects of experimental heart failure on atrial cellular and ionic electrophysiology. *Circulation* 2000; **101**: 2631–2638.

34 Cha TJ, Ehrlich JR, Zhang L, Shi YF, Tardif JC, Leung TK, *et al*. Dissociation between ionic remodeling and ability to sustain atrial fibrillation during recovery from experimental congestive heart failure. *Circulation* 2004; **109**: 412–418.

35 Cha TJ, Ehrlich JR, Zhang L, Nattel S. Atrial ionic remodeling induced by atrial tachycardia in the presence of congestive heart failure. *Circulation* 2004; **110**: 1520–1526.

36 Boyden PA, Hoffman BF. The effects on atrial electrophysiology and structure of surgically induced right atrial enlargement in dogs. *Circ Res* 1981; **49**: 1319–1331.

37 Guerra JM, Everett THT, Lee KW, Wilson E, Olgin JE. Effects of the gap junction modifier rotigaptide (zp123) on atrial conduction and vulnerability to atrial fibrillation. *Circulation* 2006; **114**: 110–118.

38 Verheule S, Wilson E, Banthia S, Everett THT, Shanbhag S, Sih HJ, *et al*. Direction-dependent conduction abnormalities in a canine model of atrial fibrillation due to chronic atrial dilatation. *Am J Physiol Heart Circ Physiol* 2004; **287**: H634–644.

39 Verheule S, Wilson E, Everett TT, Shanbhag S, Golden C, Olgin J, *et al*. Alterations in atrial electrophysiology and tissue structure in a canine model of chronic atrial dilatation due to mitral regurgitation. *Circulation* 2003; **107**: 2615–2622.

40 Page PL, Plumb VJ, Okumura K, Waldo AL. A new animal model of atrial flutter. *J Am Coll Cardiol* 1986; **8**: 872–879.

41 Kumagai K, Khrestian C, Waldo AL. Simultaneous multisite mapping studies during induced atrial fibrillation in the sterile pericarditis model. Insights into the mechanism of its maintenance. *Circulation* 1997; **95**: 511–521.

42 Roithinger FX, Karch MR, Steiner PR, SippensGroenewegen A, Lesh MD. Relationship between atrial fibrillation and typical atrial flutter in humans: Activation sequence changes during spontaneous conversion. *Circulation* 1997; **96**: 3484–3491.

43 Waldo AL, Feld GK. Inter-relationships of atrial fibrillation and atrial flutter mechanisms and clinical implications. *J Am Coll Cardiol* 2008; **51**: 779–786.

44 Neuberger HR, Schotten U, Verheule S, Eijsbouts S, Blaauw Y, van Hunnik A, *et al*. Development of a substrate of atrial fibrillation during chronic atrioventricular block in the goat. *Circulation* 2005; **111**: 30–37.

45 Choisy SC, Arberry LA, Hancox JC, James AF. Increased susceptibility to atrial tachyarrhythmia in spontaneously hypertensive rat hearts. *Hypertension* 2007; **49**: 498–505.

46 Kistler PM, Sanders P, Dodic M, Spence SJ, Samuel CS, Zhao C, *et al*. Atrial electrical and structural abnormalities in an ovine model of chronic blood pressure elevation after prenatal corticosteroid exposure: Implications for development of atrial fibrillation. *Eur Heart J* 2006; **27**: 3045–3056.

47 Hirose M, Takeishi Y, Miyamoto T, Kubota I, Laurita KR, Chiba S, *et al*. Mechanism for atrial tachyarrhythmia in chronic volume overload-induced dilated atria. *J Cardiovasc Electrophysiol* 2005; **16**: 760–769.

48 Remes J, van Brakel TJ, Bolotin G, Garber C, de Jong MM, van der Veen FH, *et al* Persistent atrial fibrillation in a goat model of chronic left atrial overload. *J Thorac Cardiovasc Surg* 2008; **136**: 1005–1011.

49 Deroubaix E, Folliguet T, Rucker-Martin C, Dinanian S, Boixel C, Validire P, *et al*. Moderate and chronic

hemodynamic overload of sheep atria induces reversible cellular electrophysiologic abnormalities and atrial vulnerability. *J Am Coll Cardiol* 2004; **44**: 1918–1926.

50 Kalifa J, Jalife J, Zaitsev AV, Bagwe S, Warren M, Moreno J, *et al.* Intra-atrial pressure increases rate and organization of waves emanating from the superior pulmonary veins during atrial fibrillation. *Circulation* 2003; **108**: 668–671.

51 Ravelli F, Allessie M. Effects of atrial dilatation on refractory period and vulnerability to atrial fibrillation in the isolated langendorff-perfused rabbit heart. *Circulation* 1997; **96**: 1686–1695.

52 Sinno H, Derakhchan K, Libersan D, Merhi Y, Leung TK, Nattel S, *et al.* Atrial ischemia promotes atrial fibrillation in dogs. *Circulation* 2003; **107**: 1930–1936.

53 Yamazaki M, Morgenstern S, Klos M, Campbell K, Buerkel D, Kalifa J, *et al.* Left atrial coronary perfusion territories in isolated sheep hearts: Implications for atrial fibrillation maintenance. *Heart Rhythm* 2010; **7**: 1501–1508.

54 Anyukhovsky EP, Sosunov EA, Plotnikov A, Gainullin RZ, Jhang JS, *et al.* Cellular electrophysiologic properties of old canine atria provide a substrate for arrhythmogenesis. *Cardiovasc Res* 2002; **54**: 462–469.

55 Hayashi H, Wang C, Miyauchi Y, Omichi C, Pak HN, Zhou S, Ohara T, *et al.* Aging-related increase to inducible atrial fibrillation in the rat model. *J Cardiovasc Electrophysiol* 2002; **13**: 801–808.

56 Mansour M, Mandapati R, Berenfeld O, Chen J, Samie FH, Jalife J, *et al.* Left-to-right gradient of atrial frequencies during acute atrial fibrillation in the isolated sheep heart. *Circulation* 2001; **103**: 2631–2636.

57 Kneller J, Zou R, Vigmond EJ, Wang Z, Leon LJ, Nattel S, *et al.* Cholinergic atrial fibrillation in a computer model of a two-dimensional sheet of canine atrial cells with realistic ionic properties. *Circ Res* 2002; **90**: E73–87.

58 Atienza F, Almendral J, Moreno J, Vaidyanathan R, Talkachou A, Kalifa J, *et al.* Activation of inward rectifier potassium channels accelerates atrial fibrillation in humans: Evidence for a reentrant mechanism. *Circulation* 2006; **114**: 2434–2442.

59 Scherf D. Studies on auricular tachycardia caused by aconitine administration. *Proc Soc Exp Biol Med* 1947; **64**: 233–239.

60 Hashimoto N, Yamashita T, Tsuruzoe N. Tertiapin, a selective ikach blocker, terminates atrial fibrillation with selective atrial effective refractory period prolongation. *Pharmacol Res* 2006; **54**: 136–141.

61 Satoh T, Zipes DP. Cesium-induced atrial tachycardia degenerating into atrial fibrillation in dogs: Atrial torsades de pointes? *J Cardiovasc Electrophysiol* 1998; **9**: 970–975.

62 Haugan K, Lam HR, Knudsen CB, Petersen JS. Atrial fibrillation in rats induced by rapid transesophageal atrial pacing during brief episodes of asphyxia: A new in vivo model. *J Cardiovasc Pharmacol* 2004; **44**: 125–135.

63 van der Hooft C3, Heeringa J, van Herpen G, Kors JA, Kingma JH, Stricker BH, *et al.* Drug-induced atrial fibrillation. *J Am Coll Cardiol* 2004; **44**: 2117–2124.

64 Nishida K, Michael G, Dobrev D, Nattel S. Animal models for atrial fibrillation: Clinical insights and scientific opportunities. *Europace* 2010; **12**: 160–172.

65 Schmid M, Khattab AA, Gloekler S, Meier B. Future epidemic impact of atrial fibrillation and a new interventional strategy for stroke prophylaxis. *Future Cardiol* 2011; **7**: 219–226.

Confocal imaging of intracellular calcium cycling in the intact heart

Neha Singh, Manvinder Kumar, James E. Kelly, Gary L. Aistrup, and J. Andrew Wasserstrom

Northwestern University Feinberg School of Medicine, Chicago, IL, USA

Introduction

Laser scanning confocal imaging has allowed for the investigation of cellular cardiac function with both high temporal and spatial resolution for nearly 20 years. Nearly all of the studies of cellular cardiac function to date have been performed in isolated cardiac myocytes, giving enormous insights into cardiac cellular electrical properties and intracellular Ca^{2+} cycling. Recently, however, a number of studies have used this technique to measure Ca^{2+} cycling in myocytes of intact heart *in situ* [1–3], often giving dramatically different results from those obtained from isolated myocytes, even from the same species. The focus of this chapter is to describe how confocal microscopy can be applied to measure intracellular Ca^{2+} cycling in intact hearts, particularly from rodents, although we have also used this approach successfully in atrial and ventricular preparations from larger animals as well. The advantages of this approach are the same as those in isolated myocytes: very high scan rates allow high-resolution temporal measurements of rapid Ca^{2+} cycling and selective line placement allows for high-resolution spatial measurements within cardiac myocytes but now in the intact heart. Furthermore, recordings made in intact hearts allow for measurements of Ca^{2+} cycling in many cells simultaneously so that the native heterogeneities in cellular function can be explored, which is especially important during rapid pacing and cardiac arrhythmias. Even higher spatial resolution is now becoming available with the use of rapid two-dimensional (2-D) imaging (e.g., the Zeiss 5/7Live confocal microscope), which permits imaging of microscopic Ca^{2+} events at micron resolution on a millisecond timescale. The applications of this form of Ca^{2+} imaging are only now being explored. So far they range from high-resolution Ca^{2+} imaging during physiological and pharmacological manipulations (altered heart rates, arrhythmia induction, ischemia and acidosis, drug effects on Ca^{2+} cycling, among others) to the determination of the extent of integration of exogenous cells transplanted in normal and injured hearts *in vivo*. No other currently available approach can provide definitive answers to the question of whether or not transplanted cells actually integrate into surrounding myocardium.

In addition, there is some evidence suggesting that imaging of transmembrane voltage, perhaps even simultaneously with Ca^{2+} imaging, may be accomplished in intact hearts using confocal microscopy. However, this approach is difficult and falls outside the scope of the current discussion, which is focused on the use of confocal microscopy for high-resolution Ca^{2+} imaging in the whole heart. The future development of combined voltage–Ca^{2+} imaging could provide an enormous advance in the imaging of cellular function in the intact heart.

Manual of Research Techniques in Cardiovascular Medicine, First Edition. Edited by Hossein Ardehali, Roberto Bolli, and Douglas W. Losordo.

Measurement of intracellular Ca²⁺ transients

The cardiac action potential (AP) is responsible for cardiac excitation and the resulting contraction and has unique properties necessary for mechanical function of the heart. The cardiac AP consists of several phases and varies in characteristics from region to region. In adult cardiomyocytes, a small Ca^{2+} influx through L-type Ca^{2+} channels during systole triggers a large Ca^{2+} release from storage in the sarcoplasmic reticulum (SR) through ryanodine receptors (RyR). Ca^{2+}-induced Ca^{2+} release (CICR) is the primary mechanism linking electrical excitation and mechanical contraction in cardiomyocytes. During diastole, Ca^{2+} is actively removed from the cytosol, mainly through SR Ca^{2+}-ATPase (SERCA) pumping Ca^{2+} back into SR and via the sodium/calcium exchanger (NCX), which restores the balance of Na^+ and Ca^{2+} across the sarcolemma. Therefore during the excitation–contraction (E-C) coupling cycle, intracellular Ca^{2+} concentration is maintained at a strict equilibrium. The ability to image Ca^{2+} signals at subcellular levels within the intact heart is important because it is the principal way of measuring the events underlying both normal and abnormal Ca^{2+} cycling, the latter of which can trigger cardiac arrhythmias. We now have nearly 20 years of experience using high-resolution confocal imaging to measure microscopic events during E-C coupling in isolated myocytes. More recently however, several investigators have begun to use this approach to measure Ca^{2+} cycling in the intact heart in order to study population behavior in addition to single-cell function. It is also possible to measure the timing of Ca^{2+} release among many myocytes, providing a means of evaluating the degree of synchronous activation among many cells in situ. This imaging technique in Langendorff-perfused hearts reveals intracellular Ca^{2+} transients, which can be used to distinguish between grafted fluorescent-tagged transplanted cells and host myocytes on the basis of their discrete emission profiles.

Principles and features of confocal microscopy

Confocal microscopy is an optical imaging technique with higher optical resolution and contrast than conventional epifluorescence microscopy. It also allows for careful control of the depth of imaging through planar sectioning of the object. The most distinguishing property of a confocal microscope is its use of a pinhole, which acts as a spatial filter in front of the detector thus reducing the effect of scattered light. This hinders extraneous light from entering the detector and allows for imaging with extremely high spatial resolution and signal-to-noise ratio. Extraneous light is also minimized by use of a laser light source. The system consists of a laser unit, a fixed stage microscope (inverted or upright), a laser-scanning head with a pinhole, a photomultiplier detector, and a host computer (Figure 4.1). The laser beam is focused on the preparation with an objective lens and excites an

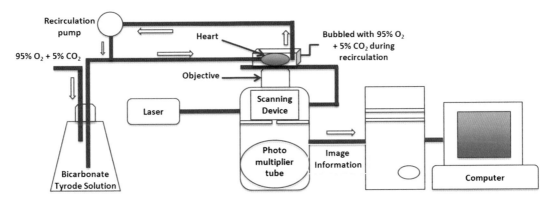

Figure 4.1 Confocal microscope setup: flow diagram of laser scanning microscope with Langendroff isolated heart preparation. Perfusion is maintained at constant flow and pressure by recirculation of Tyrode's solution through the heart.

exogenously delivered fluorophore within the specimen. The specialized detector then collects all image information point by point. Finally, this fluorescence image is digitized and stored in the main memory of the computer for further processing.

Procedure

This section will focus on general methods for measurements of single and multiple cells in the whole heart and then briefly describe how this approach can also be applied to measure host/graft integration following stem cell transplantation.

Materials and equipment

The following are required in order to measure Ca^{2+} transients in whole heart:

1. HEPES-buffered Tyrode's solution (HTS) contains (250 mL): 140 mM NaCl, 5.4 mM KCl, 1 mM $MgCl_2$, 0.4 mM NaH_2PO_4, 10 mM glucose, 10 mM N-2-hydroxyethylpiperazine N'-2-ethanesulphonic acid (HEPES). Adjust pH to 7.4. Add 450 μL of 1 M $CaCl_2$ for a final Ca^{2+} concentration of 1.8 mM and 250 μL of 1000 units/mL of Heparin to the 250 mL HTS and refrigerate. This solution will be used when the heart is first removed from the animal.
2. Sodium bicarbonate-buffered TS (BTS) contains (1 L): 140 mM NaCl, 5.4 mM KCl, 1 mM $MgCl_2$, 0.4 mM NaH_2PO_4, 10 mM glucose, and 24 mM $NaHCO_3$. Osmolarity should be 300 milliosmoles (adjust with NaCl). Add 20 g of BSA (2% w : w), stir for 20 minutes then filter through a pore size of 200 μ. Bubble with a mixture of 95% : 5% O_2 : CO_2 for 1 hour, then adjust pH to 7.35 with NaOH or HCl as needed, then add 1.8 mM $CaCl_2$.
3. Fluorescent Ca^{2+} indicator, Fluo-4AM (1 mg, F14201, Invitrogen) or rhod-2AM (1 mg, 21062, AAT Bioquest). Make 1 mM stock solution in ethanol solution for each experiment.
4. Fresh 20% Pluronic F-127 in ethanol (200 mg in 10 mL EtOH).
5. Perfusion chamber with heating capabilities (Figure 4.2) (we use an aluminum coil bath-insert through which warm water is circulated; alternatively, the chamber could be made so that water is circulated through the chamber block itself), mounted on the stage of a laser-scanning confocal microscope. The bottom of the chamber should have a #1 thickness

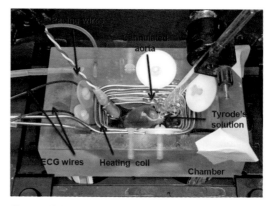

Figure 4.2 Langendorff heart setup showing cannulated heart immersed in bicarbonate Tyrode's solution. The heart is affixed with wire electrodes for electrical stimulation with ECG monitoring electrodes placed on either side of heart.

glass coverslip so that the heart can be imaged from below using an inverted microscope. The volume of the chamber should be as small as possible to accommodate the heart but minimize dead volume. If pseudo-ECG recordings are desired, a pair of Ag–$AgCl_2$ electrodes can be placed in the chamber situated on either side of the heart to obtain this recording. Psuedo-ECG recording electrodes are computer-interfaced via appropriate amplifier/ A-D converter and acquisition software (we use a World Precision Instruments Iso-DAM8A amplifier and Axon 1322A Digidata A-D converter with PClamp™ 8 signal acquisition software).
6. Confocal microscope (e.g. Zeiss LSM510 or 710) equipped with an Argon laser with 488 nm line for fluo-4 (or for EGFP excitation) or HeNe laser 543 nm line for rhod-2 (and if desired, simultaneous EGFP excitation with 488 nm line), and appropriate dichroic and band/long-pass filters for collecting emission signals at required wavelengths. For fluo-4AM, fluorescence is collected at wavelengths encompassing its emission maximum of ~525 nm (e.g. wavelengths >510 nm), whereas for rhod-2AM fluorescence is collected at wavelengths encompassing its emission maximum of ~580 nm (e.g. wavelengths >560 nm).

Experimental setup

Here we describe our approach for the Langendorff heart preparation and the experimental setup for rat and mouse hearts. The fluorescent dye we used in the following protocol is rhod-2AM, although the general methodology for fluo-4AM is same. It is important to design the experiment carefully before final choice of temperature and dye type. In our experience, fluo-4AM is poorly suited for use at temperatures above 30°C because signal intensity quickly diminishes after 30 minutes, presumably as anion transporters remove the dye at warm temperatures. Probenicid can be used to improve dye retention, although our experience has not been good with this transport inhibitor and Ca^{2+} transients are unstable and decline in magnitude. At lower temperatures (typically ~26°C), we are able to make stable recordings for several hours using fluo-4AM. However, if physiological temperatures are critical to the experiment, we have found that rhod-2AM is well-suited for stable recordings with bright signals for up to several hours.

1. Ten to fifteen minutes after intraperitoneal injection of heparin 2500 U/kg, anesthetize the rat with a combination of ketamine (80 mg/kg) and xylazine (5–8 mg/kg).

2. After deep anesthesia is achieved, rapidly excise the heart through a midsternal incision, making sure to leave enough of the aorta to allow a strong connection of the heart when tied to the cannula, usually up to but not including the bend of the aortic arch. Quickly plunge the heart into HTS and cannulate the ascending aorta with a glass cannula (WP Instruments) or customized number 18 hypodermic needle, with a raised lip so that a black braided silk surgical suture (#4) can be double-tied around the aorta. Time from cardiac excision to cannulation should be less than 5 minutes.

3. Once cannulation is completed, cardiac perfusion is initiated immediately in order to insure cardiac viability. The heart should start beating within about 1 minute after perfusion at 37°C with bicarbonate TS (bubbled with 95% O_2 and 5% CO_2). Perfusion pressure is maintained at 60–100 mmHg. The heart is equilibrated for about 15 minutes to insure that no infarcts develop (white or light patches) on the left ventricle (LV). The atria are either crushed, cut off, or tied off (with suture), which considerably slows the basal heart rate (due to AV or His-Purkinje system subordinate pacemaking) to expedite ventricular extrinsic pacing. The pseudo-ECG is monitored continuously to insure normal heart function. When placed in the chamber, the perfused heart is oriented such that the left ventricular epicardial surface faces down toward the objectives of the inverted microscope and this should be arranged at the time the heart is placed in the chamber. To optimize the focal plane, the heart is gently pressed against the bottom of the chamber by means of a manipulator-controlled metal spatula placed on the right ventricle.

4. Following successful perfusion, load the heart with rhod-2AM. The following procedure assumes ~25 mL of recirculating TS.
  • Add 15 µM rhod-2AM (374 µL of 1 mM rhod-2AM stock) + 0.3% pluronic acid (375 mL of 20% pluronic acid stock), mix thoroughly in the chamber and perfuse by recirculation for 20 minutes.
  • Add 12 µM rhod-2AM (300 µL of 1 mM rhod-2 stock) + 0.12% pluronic acid (150 µL of 20% pluronic stock), mix in chamber and recirculate for 20 minutes.
  • Add 10 µM rhod-2AM (250 µL of 1 mM rhod-2 stock) with no additional pluronic acid, mix in the chamber and perfuse the heart for 10–15 minutes.

After loading is complete, gently press the LV to the bottom of the chamber using a bent metal spatula or other positioning device. Scan for transients during the intrinsic rhythm using the HeNe (543 nm) laser. If bright signals are present, stop recirculation and perfuse with dye-free BTS for about 15 minutes. During this period, fine stainless steel or platinum needle electrodes (bent at the tips to produce a short hook) are inserted into the LV apex to provide for ventricular extrinsic pacing (see later). During this washout period, endogenous esterases hydrolyze AM-conjugated dyes and the de-esterified dye is retained inside the cells.

5. Heart rate is controlled by stimulation delivered through the pair of wire/needle electrodes inserted into the ventricular apex. Any isolated stimulator will suffice. Temperature inside the chamber is set to 37°C (unless fluo-4 is used in which case temperature is set to 26°C). The initial perfusion period of 15 minutes allows the heart to stabilize during pacing. This is the appropriate time to make fine adjustments to ensure constant temperature and pressure in the chamber.

6. Since spatial resolution is important in confocal imaging, it is necessary to block virtually all contraction in order to eliminate motion artifacts. Once the heart is stable and ready for recordings, a combination of cytochalasin D (50–60 μM) and blebbistatin (24–30 μM) is added to the chamber solution and recirculated to eliminate contraction-induced movement of the heart. The combination of these paralytic agents reduces the concentration that would be required for each alone to stop contraction, thus minimizing effects on Ca^{2+} transients.

7. Imaging is performed using high numerical aperture water (preferred or oil if necessary) immersion fluorescence optimized objectives with 10×, 25×, 40×, or 63× magnification, depending on requirements for image size and quality. With the 40× objective confocal imaging provides a sharp image at a depth of ±1.5 μm around the focal plane.

Video clip 4.1 shows a typical recording of intracellular Ca^{2+} transients during pacing at a basic cycle length of 700 ms. Note that all myocytes demonstrate nearly simultaneous increase in fluorescence intensity during systole in response to each electrical stimulus with a return to baseline low intensity during diastole. The position of the scan line during line scan imaging then determines which individual myocytes will be studied for high-resolution temporal and spatial Ca^{2+} imaging. Imaging can be performed in two modes: transverse and longitudinal. In a transverse recording, the scan line is drawn across the short axis of many cells. Recordings made with this method can be used to measure Ca^{2+} transients across many myocytes simultaneously. Figure 4.3A shows an example of a 2-D image of the epicardial surface of a rat heart stained with both di-4-ANEPPS (to show cell outlines) and loaded with fluo-4AM. The vertical

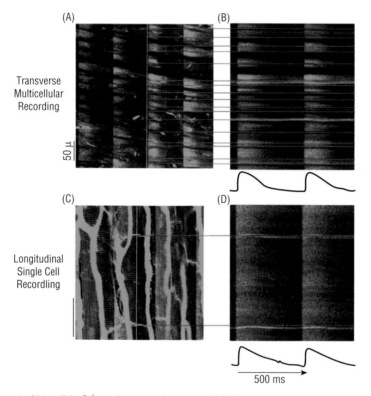

Figure 4.3 Measurements of intracellular Ca^{2+} transients in whole rat heart. (A) 2-D image of epicardial surface of rat heart loaded with fluo-4AM. Bright regions are periodic because of Ca^{2+} transients activated by pacing during image acquisition. (B) transverse line scan image of Ca^{2+} transients recorded across multiple cells at the site indicated by the vertical white line in (A). Red lines indicate cell borders. Profile of average fluorescence along the entire line is shown below. (C) 2-D image of individual myocytes outlined by di-4-ANEPPS. (D) longitudinal line scan image of the single cell indicated by the vertical white line shown in (C).

white line in the 2-D image shows the location where the scan line was positioned and the line scan image (Figure 4.3B) was recorded. Note that Ca^{2+} transients were activated simultaneously in all myocytes in the image (separated by horizontal red lines), indicating good electrical coupling in the heart. The average fluorescence intensity profile to the right of several myocytes indicates the variability in rise time, magnitude, and duration of Ca^{2+} cycling between cells. In general, this is the best approach for investigating population behavior among many myocytes, allowing measurements of Ca^{2+} transient characteristics (rise time, delay and initiation time after stimulation, magnitude, decay time, time to 50, 80, or 90% of total transient duration, and so forth) among many myocytes at different pacing rates. Once transients have been measured in one optical field, the spatula can be raised and the heart moved to another region and another field can be identified and studied, and so forth.

In a longitudinal recording, the scan line is drawn along the cell length, allowing high-resolution imaging of a single myocyte. This approach allows recordings over an extended period of time in a single cell, similar to recordings made in isolated cells. Figure 4.3C shows a 2-D image of a single myocyte and the location of the scan line for the line scan image of Ca^{2+} transients shown in Figure 4.3D. Note that the line scan image now reflects Ca^{2+} cycling throughout the length of a single cell (or as many as two to three myocytes, depending on choice of objective and zoom) much like conventional recordings in an isolated myocyte. In this case, intracellular spatial resolution is much greater than that in transverse recordings (Figure 4.3B) and it is even possible to measure Ca^{2+} cycling in specific subcellular regions (image profiles to the right of Figure 4.3D). Note that bleaching could become a problem, which is why it is better to keep the argon laser power at 10% (fluo-4AM recordings) or less if long recordings are essential.

It is also possible to use a membrane-staining dye (usually di-4- or di-8-ANEPPS) to show the precise location of cell borders. Depending on choice of indicators, however, there may be spectral overlap between the membrane and cytosolic (Ca^{2+}) dyes. In this case, the magnitude of Ca^{2+} transients cannot be accurately measured although it is still possible to measure the kinetic properties of Ca^{2+} release into

and removal from the cytoplasm. Rhod-2AM is superior to fluo-4AM in combination with di-4-ANEPPS because of less spectral interference for this purpose. Note that intracellular and membrane ultrastructure can be imaged using either 2-D or 3-D (z-stack) imaging in whole heart with extremely high resolution.

Limitations, potential pitfalls and alternative approaches

Single photon microscopy measures spontaneous and triggered Ca^{2+} transients in both isolated myocytes and intact tissue at a higher resolution than conventional epifluorescence microscopy. This method, however, does have two major limitations: fluorophore bleaching and depth of light penetration in intact tissue. Two-photon laser scanning microscopy (TPLSM)–based fluorescence imaging can potentially improve on these limitations [4,5]. Along with reduced photobleaching, TPLSM can measure Ca^{2+} transients in individual cardiomyocytes at a greater depth than traditional single-photon confocal imaging [6–8]. Because of this ability to image at greater tissue depths, TPLSM has been used as an alternative approach to monitor physiological coupling between transplanted cardiomyocytes and the host myocardium (see section Additional application) [9,10].

Another potential pitfall is excessive dye loading. This is evident when Ca^{2+} transient decay is slowed so that it takes several seconds to reach a minimum level of fluorescence after termination of pacing. Signals are extremely bright, and transients exhibit a saw tooth-like shape rather than a smooth, exponential decay. In a situation of excessive dye loading, look for other regions of the heart with less loading, and use less dye in future experiments (shorter loading periods, especially the last). Also, if cells demonstrate a large number of spontaneous Ca^{2+} waves immediately following pacing, it is likely that the heart is in distress, producing SR Ca^{2+} overload. The result is frequent spontaneous waves that usually occur as the result of developing infarction. This often occurs when intracoronary perfusion is compromised and is usually indicated by a rapid rise in perfusion pressure to 150 mmHg and above that is sustained. The heart should be examined to insure that no infarcts are present and that perfusion is normal. In this case waves may be interesting to observe but probably indicate abnormal function and poor myocyte and overall cardiac viability. If a high frequency of waves is observed under conditions in which Ca^{2+} overload should not occur (low heart rates, normal external $[Ca^{2+}]$, no pharmacological interventions), either look for other regions of the LV that do not demonstrate waves or terminate the experiment, as the heart should no longer be considered normal.

Because of the expense of materials, it is not practical to perform drug applications followed by drug washout. If this is required for the experimental design, the entire recirculation system must be flushed with fresh solution before recirculation can be re-initiated, at which point the cocktail of paralytic agents must also be added again.

Additional application: use of confocal imaging to determine efficacy of stem cell integration into host myocardium

The introduction of stem cells with cardiomyogenic properties has been investigated in recent years as a potential therapy to repair damaged myocardium. A number of studies now support the idea that stem cell transplantation improves overall cardiac function [11–13]. In most successful instances demonstrating therapeutic benefit, it is thought that transplanted cells release factors into host myocardium that stimulate neo-vascularization or cell differentiation. However, there has also been a great deal of interest in transplanting progenitor or even myocytes from adult or neonatal sources into damaged myocardium. The goal in this instance is to increase cardiac performance by re-populating damaged tissue with functional, contracting myocytes. When these cells are introduced into the damaged heart, they have the potential to replace injured cells with healthy ones, thus reducing or even reversing cardiac loss. After transplantation, it is important to track these cells to ensure that they survive and form new cardiomyocytes with the same functional properties as the host myocytes. There are a number of methodologies to differentiate these grafted cells from host cells for monitoring purposes. These include: (1) measuring tritiated thymidine or bromo-deoxyuridine (BrdU) of donor cells to determine the amount of cell proliferation; (2) use

of fluorescent lipophilic dye such as PHK26 to label grafted cells [14,15]; (3) transplanting male cardiomyocytes into female recipients then using fluorescent *in situ* hybridization (FISH) with a fluorescent probe for a specific region of the Y chromosome [13]; and (4) gene transfer either by transfecting foreign genes inside the cell or by using a transgenic animal as the donor [16–20] so that fluorescent markers, such as enhanced green fluorescent protein (EGFP), can be used in tracking the fate of transplanted stem cells [21–23].

After selecting one of these methodologies, the next step is to monitor the functional behavior of grafted cells in order to determine if these cells are integrated into the host myocardium. Highly regulated Ca^{2+} transients are one of the key signs of a normally functioning cardiomyocyte. Confocal microscopy can be used to demonstrate that cardiomyocytes arising from transplanted stem cells generate normal Ca^{2+} transients and thus can contribute to normal contractile function. Rubart *et al.* successfully used TPLSM to perform Ca^{2+} imaging [9] to study EGFP-expressing cardiomyocytes from transgenic mice that were transplanted into hearts of non-transgenic mice and used rhod-2 fluorescence imaging to distinguish donor cells (EGFP +rhod-2 emission) from host ones (rhod-2 emission only). When host tissue was subjected to confocal imaging, Ca^{2+} transients from each cell type were distinguished by taking advantage of the spectral differences between rhod-2 and EGFP. The wavelength of excitation was 810 nm, and EGFP fluorescence was captured at 500–550 nm while rhod-2 fluorescence was collected at 560–650 nm. This approach provides a dramatic improvement in our ability to determine viability and integration of individual myocytes transplanted into whole, damaged and working hearts.

Furthermore, recent studies using tissue engineering show promise in applying a patch over damaged myocardium that might lead to tissue repair. These engineered tissues consist of a basal cellular matrix (collagen, fibronectin, or gelatin), extracellular matrix protein (e.g. Matrigel, BD Biosciences) and cardiac progenitor or adult cells [24,25]. The goal is to use these grafts in many forms of treatment, including re-vascularization of ischemic or infracted myocardium and repair of congenital heart defects and end-stage heart failure.

Since scaffold-based myocardial patches may produce inflammation, scaffold-free cell sheet-based tissue engineering has also been developed recently [26]. The result is the production of cell sheets that are transplantable directly onto damaged heart as a myocardial patch. Several studies have demonstrated improvement in cardiac function by cell sheet transplantation [27,28]. It is likely that the confocal imaging can be used to determine the degree of both cell and tissue viability in these patches as well as their ability to integrate functionally into host myocardium by imaging along the periphery of the patch where it connects to native tissue. Voltage imaging would be especially useful in those instances where the goal is to produce an electrical bridge across damaged, electrically inert myocardium in order to prevent arrhythmogenesis, where functional Ca^{2+} cycling may be unnecessary. This application has not yet been attempted but could prove highly useful in the future as tissue engineering strategies are developed further.

References

1 Minamikawa T, Cody SH, Williams DA. In situ visualization of spontaneous calcium waves with perfused whole rat heart by confocal imaging. *Am J Physiol* 1997; **272**: 236–243.

2 Baader AP, Buchler L, Bircher-Lehmann L, Kleber AG. Real time, confocal imaging of Ca^{2+} waves in arterially perfused rat hearts. *Cardiovasc Res* 2001; **53**: 105–115.

3 Aistrup GL, Kelly JE, Kapur S, Kowalczyk M, Sysman-Wolpin I, Kadish AH, et al. Pacing-induced heterogeneities in intracellular Ca^{2+} signaling, cardiac alternans, and ventricular arrhythmias in intact rat heart. *Circ Res* 2006; **99**: e65–e73.

4 Denk W, Strickler JH, Webb WW. 2-Photon laser scanning fluorescence microscopy. *Science* 1990; **248**: 73–76.

5 Squirrell JM, Wokosin DL, White JG, Bavister BD. Long-term two-photon fluorescence imaging of mammalian embryos without compromising viability. *Nat Biotechnol* 1999; **17**: 763–767.

6 Rubart M, Wang E, Dunn KW, Field LJ. Two-photon molecular excitation imaging of Ca^{2+} transients in Langendorff-perfused mouse hearts. *Am J Physiol* 2003; **284**: C1654–C1668.

7 Centonze VE, White JG. Multiphoton excitation provides optical sections from deeper within scattering specimens than confocal imaging. *Biophys J* 1998; **75**: 2015–2024.

8 Rubart M, Pasumarthi KB, Nakajima H, Soonpaa MH, Nakajima HO, Field LJ, et al. Physiological coupling of donor and host cardiomyocytes after cellular transplantation. *Circ Res* 2003; **92**: 1217–1224.

9 Rubart M, Field LJ. Cardiac regeneration: repopulating the heart. *Annu Rev Physiol* 2006; **68**: 29–49.

10 Piao H, Youn TJ, Kwon JS, Kim YH, Bae JW, Bora S, et al. Effects of bone marrow derived mesenchymal stem cells transplantation in acutely infarcting myocardium. *Eur J Heart Fail* 2005; **7**: 730–738.

11 Grauss RW, Winter EM, Van TJ, Pijnappels DA, Steijn RV, Hogers B, Van der Geest RJ, et al. Mesenchymal stem cells from ischemic heart disease patients improve left ventricular function after acute myocardial infarction. *Am J Physiol Heart Circ Physiol* 2007; **293**: H2438–H2447.

12 Wang YQ, Wang M, Zhang P, Song JJ, Li YP, Hou SH, Huang CX, et al. Effect of transplanted mesenchymal stem cells from rats of different ages on the improvement of heart function after acute myocardial infarction. *Chin Med J (Engl.)* 2008; **121**: 2290–2298.

13 Reinecke H, Zhang M, Bartosek T, Murry CE. Survival, integration, and differentiation of cardiomyocyte grafts: a study in normal and injured rat hearts. *Circulation* 1999; **100**: 193–202.

14 Zhang XM, Du F, Yang D, Yu CJ, Huang XN, Liu W, et al. Transplanted bone marrow stem cells relocate to infarct penumbra and co-express endogenous proliferative and immature neuronal markers in a mouse model of ischemic cerebral stroke. *BMC Neurosci* 2010; **11**: 138.

15 Al-Timmemi H, Ibrahim R, Al-Jashamy K, Zuki A, Azmi T, Ramassamy R, et al. Neurobiology observation of bone marrow mesenchymal stem cell in vitro and invivo of injuried sciatic nerve in rabbit. *J Anim Vet Adv* 2011; **10**: 686–691.

16 Hruban RH, Long PP, Perlman EJ, Hutchins GM, Baumgartner WA, Baughman KL, et al. Fluorescence in situ hybridization for the Y-chromosome can be used to detect cells of recipient origin in allografted hearts following cardiac transplantation. *Am J Pathol* 1993; **142**: 975–980.

17 Orlic D, Kajstura J, Chimenti S, Jakoniuk I, Anderson SM, Li B, et al. Bone marrow cells regenerate infarcted myocardium. *Nature* 2001; **410**: 701–705.

18 Balsam LB, Wagers AJ, Christensen JL, Kofidis T, Weissman IL, Robbins RC, et al. Haematopoietic stem cells adopt mature haematopoietic fates in ischaemic myocardium. *Nature* 2004; **428**: 668–673.

19 Murry CE, Soonpaa MH, Reinecke H, Nakajima H, Nakajima HO, Rubart M, et al. Haematopoietic stem cells do not transdifferentiate into cardiac myocytes in myocardial infarcts. *Nature* 2004; **428**: 664–668.

20 Nygren JM, Jovinge S, Breitbach M, Sawen P, Roll W, Hescheler J, et al. Bone marrow-derived hematopoietic cells generate cardiomyocytes at a low frequency through

cell fusion, but not transdifferentiation. *Nat Med* 2004; **10**: 494–501.

21 Oh H, Bradfute SB, Gallardo TD, Nakamura T, Gaussin V, Mishina Y, *et al.* Cardiac progenitor cells from adult myocardium: homing, differentiation, and fusion after infarction. *Proc Natl Acad Sci USA* 2003; **100**: 12313–12318.

22 Muller-Ehmsen J, Peterson KL, Kedes L, Whittaker P, Dow JS, Long TI, *et al.* Rebuilding a damaged heart: long-term survival of transplanted neonatal rat cardiomyocytes after myocardial infarction and effect on cardiac function. *Circulation* 2002; **105**: 1720–1726.

23 Kehat I, Khimovich L, Caspi O, Gepstein A, Shofti R, Arbel G, *et al.* Electromechanical integration of cardiomyocytes derived from human embryonic stem cells. *Nat Biotechnol* 2004; **22**: 1282–1289.

24 Leor J, Cohen S. Myocardial tissue engineering: creating a muscle patch for a wounded heart. *Ann N Y Acad Sci* 2004; **1015**: 312–319.

25 Zimmermann WH, Melnychenko I, Eschenhagen T. Engineered heart tissue for regeneration of diseased hearts. *Biomaterials* 2004; **25**: 1639–1647.

26 Shimizu T, Yamato M, Kikuchi A, Okano T. Cell sheet engineering for myocardial tissue reconstruction. *Biomaterials* 2003; **24**: 2309–2316.

27 Masuda S, Shimizu T, Yamato M, Okano T. Cell sheet engineering for heart tissue repair. *Adv Drug Deliv Rev* 2008; **60**: 277–285.

28 Shimizu T, Sekine H, Yamato M, Okano T. Cell sheet-based myocardial tissue engineering: new hope for damaged heart rescue. *Curr Pharm Des* 2009; **15**: 2807–2814.

Recording and measurement of action potentials

Kenneth S. Ginsburg and Donald M. Bers

University of California, Davis, CA, USA

Introduction

In cardiac cells, the action potential (AP) is the time-dependent transmembrane potential (E_m) associated with excitation and contraction. The AP (Figure 5.1A) is shaped by, and also drives, time-dependent changes in ion fluxes through numerous ion channels and transporters. This chapter describes recording of APs from individual separated myocytes, using a glass pipette which provides direct contact between an electrode and intracellular space, along with an extracellular reference electrode. APs can also be detected using purely extracellular recording from either single or multicellular preparations. An inert electrode, typically a Pt wire etched to a sub-μm point or a microfabricated array of Au islands, can detect E_m changes via largely capacitive coupling, but accuracy is limited [1]. Potential-sensitive fluorophores such as RH237 can provide accurate photometric AP records [2,3]. We will not discuss extracellular recording further.

Protocol

Theory of AP recording

The fundamental macroscopic principle of electricity is Ohm's law. Like all flux laws it states that, at any instant, flow of ion X (current; I_X) is the product of ease of passage (conductance; G_X) and driving force or electrochemical potential ($E_X - E_m$), or $I_X = G_X(E_X - E_m)$. E_X is the Nernst potential (e.g. $E_K = RT/zF \ln ([K^+]_o / [K^+]_i)$) at which there is no net electrochemical driving force on ion X. E_m in almost all cells is negative (intracellular negative to extracellular). Negative E_m derives from an asymmetric distribution of [Na] and [K] (driven by the Na/K-ATPase) and a basal K^+ conductance higher than for Na^+ or Ca^{2+}. Overall cell membrane conductance (G_{memb}) reflects an ensemble of conductances of various channels and transporters whose individual G values depend on E_m, local ion concentrations and fluxes, and regulatory signaling. Furthermore, ionic flux through each pathway tends to dissipate the gradient which drives it, altering E_m, and affecting thereby the other pathways.

Understanding ion channel gating and conductance has been advanced greatly via voltage clamp (VC), wherein E_m is forced to chosen values and the resulting current is measured. VC allows otherwise interdependent ion channels to be analyzed separately with respect to E_m-dependent gating (e.g. opening, closing, inactivation), conductance (ion permeation), and effects of drugs, ligands, or secondary regulation (e.g. phosphorylation). VC has revealed the E_m-dependence of gating and permeation (i.e. rectification) for channels which underlie excitability and repolarization. These channels (e.g. I_{Na}, I_{Ca}, and I_{K1}) exhibit nonmonotonic current–voltage (I-V) functions which include regions of negative slope conductance where the current gets larger despite a reduction in driving force. E_m-dependent activation of I_{Na} and I_{Ca} defines excitability: once

Manual of Research Techniques in Cardiovascular Medicine, First Edition. Edited by Hossein Ardehali, Roberto Bolli, and Douglas W. Losordo.

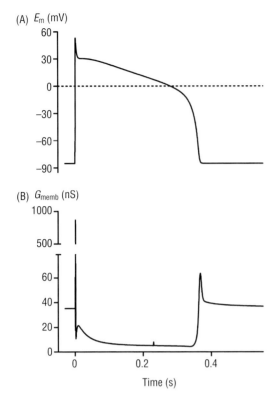

(A) E_m (mV)

(B) G_{memb} (nS)

Time (s)

Figure 5.1 AP waveform (A) and total membrane conductance G_{memb} (B) generated by model rabbit ventricular myocyte [5]. C_m was 150 pF; pacing rate was 1 Hz.

injects a small pulse of inward current to mimic the activating current, which in the intact heart would spread passively via gap junctions from neighboring cells which are actively producing APs. At any moment during the AP, G_{memb} represents the then-active channels. Model-simulated [5] G_{memb} for a cardiomyocyte (Figure 5.1B) was near 35 nS at rest or diastole, increased dramatically at peak I_{Na} opening to 850 nS, decreased as low as 4.3 nS during the plateau phases of the AP and then returned to the diastolic value during repolarization. The low G_{memb} during the AP plateau implies a delicate balance of multiple ionic currents. Even modest changes in ionic conductance can sensitively affect AP shape and duration (APD), accelerating or delaying repolarization.

The membrane capacitance C_m increases with surface area and complexity (typically 1 μF/cm²). C_m is the ability of the membrane to maintain a stable separation of charges. The distribution of charge at any instant represents E_m ($Q_m = C_m E_m$). The redistribution of charges that occurs when E_m changes represents physical work, and the finite rate at which this occurs is the rate of rise or fall of E_m during the AP, such that $dE_m/dt = I_m/C_m$. During the AP rise when I_{Na} activity dominates, the maximum dE_m/dt (420 V/s in Figure 5.1A) has been used to infer Na conductance [6].

activated, inward current shifts E_m positive, leading to yet further activation by positive feedback of enough current to drive the AP upstroke and peak.

By clamping the current through the recording pipette (current clamp, CC) to zero, instead of clamping the voltage (as in VC) one can follow E_m with minimal perturbation, both at rest and during the time-dependent changes that constitute the AP. Since distinct ion channels and transporters carry currents via by their own E_m-dependent conductance, driven by their own ion's gradient (and influenced by signaling), I = 0 means only that net (algebraically summed) transmembrane current is zero. Since any or all individual channels or transporters may be open (conductive) and may mediate current flow, G_{memb} is finite (>0). Membrane input resistance R_{memb} is the inverse of G_{memb}.

A cell can freely produce APs while under CC. Pacemaker cells can spontaneously fire APs [4]. Normally, for atrial and ventricular myocytes one

Procedure

Recording amplifier

For design and construction of an AP recording setup, investigators should consult topical reviews, manufacturers' literature, and web pages (for instance [7]) to guide choices for their intended studies. The choice of a CC amplifier is discussed here.

Traditionally, CC was done using a voltage follower, an amplifier design which behaves nearly like the ideal open circuit (Figure 5.2B) while measuring E_m. A high-quality voltage follower has input resistance near 10^{15} Ω and transfers only sub-pA currents, thus perturbing a preparation very minimally.

These days, it is common to record APs with a VC amplifier that has been switched to CC mode. A VC amplifier in VC mode (current to voltage converter; transconductance amplifier) has essentially zero

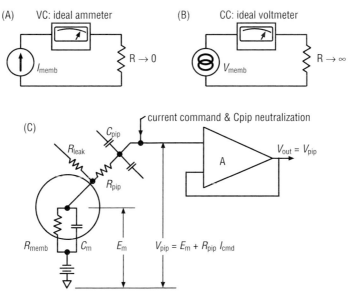

Figure 5.2 Concepts of ideal voltage clamp (A) and current clamp (B). (C) shows realistic current clamp situation. Consequences of parasitic elements R_{leak} and C_{pip} are described in the text.

input impedance. It presents a short circuit to a cell so as not to impede ion currents being measured; Figure 5.2A. When a VC amplifier is switched to CC, the normal user-chosen VC commands are replaced by an internal command derived from the pipette current. By feedback this command continually drives E_m toward the value which results in pipette current of zero or another specified value, accomplishing CC. A VC amplifier in CC configuration has a slower response time than a true voltage follower, and unlike the voltage follower is not unconditionally stable, especially with very low resistance pipettes [8].

Pipette capacitance C_{pip} strongly affects AP recording. Figure 5.2C shows C_{pip} and other factors that can affect CC quality. Pipette access resistance R_{pip} in series and C_{pip} in parallel form a low pass filter which causes recorded E_m (V_{pip}) to change more slowly than actual E_m. This can compromise measuring the AP, especially during the rapid upstroke. To overcome this, CC amplifiers include C_{pip} neutralization, in which current proportional to $C_{pip} \times dE_m/dt$ is fed back to fast-charge the C_{pip}. Neutralization speeds up the CC amplifier's response and is a form of feedback compensation, analogous with series R compensation used during VC to improve E_m control.

A high-fidelity CC amplifier should have a 10–90% response rise time that is 10% of the AP rise time under study. Cardiac ventricular myocyte APs typically have upstroke velocity of 200–500 V/s (depending on temperature [6,9]). Thus for a 100 mV AP rising within 200–500 μs, the amplifier rise time should be 20–50 μs ($\tau \approx 10$–25 μs). Lower resistance pipettes can improve rise time, as can coating pipettes with low dielectric constant varnish or silicone to reduce C_{pip}.

APs can be induced in a resting or nonpacemaker cell, and G_{memb} or excitability can be measured, by applying a perturbing transmembrane current. Current can be applied via the recording pipette (see section AP recording procedure). The pipette is in series with the membrane; thus whenever applied current is not zero, the voltage V_p at the pipette tip (Figure 5.3A,i) becomes the sum of actual E_m (Figure 5.3A,ii) and the drop across R_{pip} (Figure 5.3A,iii), resulting in a potentially large E_m error. The bridge balance function in CC amplifiers can correct for pipette voltage drop. Bridge balance cannot improve E_m fidelity, just as capacitance cancellation (sometimes wrongly called compensation) cannot improve VC quality, but both improve the appearance of records by removing artifacts.

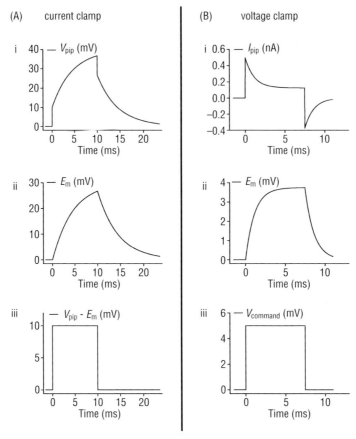

Figure 5.3 Modeled passive membrane responses to step pipette current injection in current clamp (A) and to step voltage command in voltage clamp (B). Ion channel activity or excitability are not depicted. In (A) the difference between the recordable response during 1 nA current injection (i) and true E_m (ii) is the pipette voltage drop (iii). In (B), i shows that the pipette and net membrane current has both C_m-dependent transient and G_{memb}-dependent steady components. R_{pip} was 10 megΩ, G_{memb} was 33 nS and C_m was 150 pF. To limit artifacts, CC stimuli are typically shorter and more intense than in (A).

Choices to make before an experiment

Pioneering researchers recorded APs with sharp (sub-μm) pipettes filled with 1–3M KCl (resistance 25 MΩ or larger). Now it is common to use patch pipettes filled with solutions mimicking intracellular composition (typical resistances 1–10 MΩ). Patch pipettes are used in either ruptured or perforated patch mode (Table 5.1).

In Table 5.1, compliance is the ability of the CC amplifier to pass suprathreshold current through high resistance pipettes to cells that are large and/or poorly excitable. Liquid junction potentials (LJP [10]) arise at interfaces among ions of different mobility and cause correctable errors in initial setting of zero current or voltage for pipettes in bath

solution. In perforated patch mode, the dialyzing properties of the patch can complicate correction. Micropipettes filled with concentrated KCl do not generate junctional potentials because K and Cl are almost equally mobile. Especially in ruptured patch mode, the statistical properties of APs often change over time due to diffusion of ions, metabolites and signal molecules between cytoplasm and pipette, and/or osmotic gradients.

Filling solutions for APs are K⁺ based, but other components depend on the pipette type. Almost always, Ag/AgCl electrodes provide the interfaces between pipette or bath solution and the recording electronics. These require Cl⁻ containing solutions to maintain reversibility. The user must also choose

Table 5.1 Comparison of approaches to single cell recording

Property	Micropipette	Patch pipette (ruptured)	Patch pipette (perforated)
Resistance	very high	low to medium	medium
Amplifier compliance required	very high	low to medium	medium
Liquid junction potential correction needed?	none	likely	likely
Stationarity	fair to good	poor	usually best
User's control of cell contents via pipette	none, except by iontophoresis	required and extensive; can be rapid (minutes)	limited by charge and / or size selectivity

Ca^{2+} and/or pH buffering, metabolic supports and modulators to match experimental aims. Agar bridge reference electrodes, similar in concept to double junction pH references, can be used in experiments requiring Cl^- free solutions.

When needed to induce APs, depolarizing current is passed through the pipette via the CC amplifier, or by external field stimulation. Pipette-delivered commands need to be large enough to trigger APs reliably, even if excitability changes, but not so large as to introduce noise and/or unintended E_m shifts in sensitive cells. The latter is a risk with computer-generated commands, so we typically use an analog stimulator. External field stimulation (via Pt or Pt–Ir wires in the bath) can be used if the stimulator output is isolated (not earth-referenced). Field stimuli in the range of ~50V/cm may be required, due to the volume and low resistivity of bath solution. Some stimulus energy will be capacitatively coupled into the recording system, causing artifacts in the AP record. Using the shortest duration effective stimuli will make these easier to remove (≤ 1 ms is ideal).

It is convenient to synchronize computer recording with AP stimuli where relevant. Popular data acquisition program/ interface packages can generate stimuli synchronous with recording via the same computer. However we prefer to use a separate stimulator, so that we can choose single versus periodic pacing, steady versus nonsteady state, or other features in real time. Modern stimulators and data acquisition subsystems use TTL logic standards and offer varied trigger, marker, and status inputs and outputs.

AP recording procedure

AP recording with sharp KCl-filled glass micropipettes and a voltage follower has a long history. In this method, a pipette was manipulated to contact the cell's surface and caused to penetrate by a light mechanical disturbance and/or brief application of high-frequency, high-amplitude current pulses. When a healthy cell was successfully penetrated, recorded E_m jumped from 0 to the expected rest or diastolic value (around −80mV). An experiment could begin once C_{pip} was neutralized and bridge balance was set as stated previously.

We here describe our approach using patch pipettes. If the recording amplifier allows it, we recommend starting in VC, to establish whole cell recording quality, then switching to CC.

1. Prepared cells should be bathed in a normal Tyrode or similar solution containing typically 4–5mM K and 1–2mM Ca in which reference electrode is placed.

2. Fill pipette, ensuring there are no air pockets in it, typically with 140mM K, 20mM Cl and 120mM Asp, Glu or similar impermeant ion. Dip pipette tip in solution, and then backfill with a fine needle. Place it in holder, and bring it under visual control near a candidate cell in the bath or chamber. Light positive pressure on the pipette suction port helps keep debris away from the tip.

3. Adjust pipette offset for zero current. Apply small rectangular test pulses (2–5mV; Figure 5.3B,iii) to verify pipette resistance (e.g. 5mV applied to a 2.5 megΩ pipette produces 2nA current). We link our test pulse application with data acquisition so that pulses are applied continuously, but only while not recording data. We observe test responses on an analog oscilloscope.

4. Manipulate pipette to contact cell surface, detected visually as a slight indentation and electrically as a reduced pipette current response to the test pulses when the pipette lumen becomes partly obscured. A pipette containing K may locally depolarize nearby cells, causing them to move or twitch. This is usually inconsequential.

5. Seal pipette to cell by suction. Required strength of suction will depend on pipette tip size, cell stiffness, and pressure losses. Once seal begins to form (substantial loss of pipette current response), clamping the pipette to negative voltage (near cell rest E_m, say 80 mV) can promote sealing. The best seals reduce pipette current response to just a few pA. Sealing may require a few seconds to several minutes.

6. Adjust pipette offset voltage to correct the LJP error previously determined for the solutions in use (details in [10]). If LJP is not corrected, a pipette filled with a typical low [Cl⁻] solution and zeroed in a bath with normal [Cl⁻] will report E_m about 10 mV positive of its actual value.

7. Next, the pipette needs to gain access to the interior of the cell. Unlike in most VC experiments, a very low pipette access resistance, evidenced by large C_m transients, is not essential or usually even desired in CC.

If using ruptured patch, apply additional suction to rupture the membrane patch under the pipette. On successful rupture, the transient response to the test pulses will increase dramatically as C_m becomes part of the pipette circuit (Figure 5.3B,i). Some cell membranes rupture more readily if hyperpolarized, for instance with a series of brief pulses to −140 mV. Some cells respond best to steady gentle suction while others respond to strong impulsive suction. Light positive pressure can often open a marginal ruptured patch further.

For perforated patch, we usually recommend amphotericin or β-escin added only to backfilled portion of pipette solution. Additional suction is not needed. Within 10–15 min, test pulse transients from a sealed cell will usually begin to grow, as perforation progresses.

8. The test pulse response will likely have a sustained component (Figure 5.3B,i) due to inward rectifier

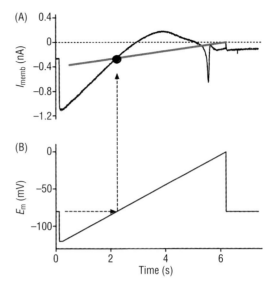

Figure 5.4 Composite current recorded from a rabbit myocyte in VC during setup of a CC experiment was dominated by inward rectifier current I_{K1}. Large then small inward spikes near 5.6 s represent I_{Na} and I_{Ca}(L) transiently activated during ascending voltage ramp. Grey line describes hypothetical pure leak current. At $E_m = -80$ mV, leak and I_{K1}-dominated current would be the same. Note that I_{K1} shifted outward in the −50 mV range.

current I_{K1}. To verify that the current is I_{K1} and not seal leakage, apply a voltage ramp, say −120 to 0 mV, for 1–2 seconds. The I_{K1} current–voltage relation is N-shaped and will reverse (cross 0) a few mV positive of E_K, while leakage is linear with voltage and will reverse at 0 (Figure 5.4).

9. Upon switching from voltage to current clamp, it is essential first to set clamp current to 0, to protect cells from damage by unintended current or voltage forcing. Typical CC amplifiers have an I=0 mode. At this time, the resting, diastolic, or spontaneous E_m should appear. If the previous VC period was prolonged, tens of sec or more may be required for ion re-equilibration and E_m stabilization.

10. Next, enable current commands and apply stimuli for AP triggering (if needed). Start small and increase toward a reliable suprathreshold response.

11. Finally, adjust C_{pip} neutralization and bridge balance and begin the experiment.

Frequent problems

1. Pipette seal leakage consistently increases and seal fails within several minutes. This may indicate overly fragile cell membranes. Check for poor cell isolation conditions or hypoxia during cardiac excision (caused, for example, by anesthetic overdosing). Seals may also fail because the pipette solution has an incorrect ion composition or osmolarity) or has degenerated.

2. Seal leakage (R_{leak} in Figure 5.2) is relatively stable but excessive. Review point (8) mentioned earlier. Actual leakage conductance, if appreciable compared with G_{memb} divides or dissipates E_m. If E_m is substantially positive of expected rest value, injecting steady hyperpolarizing current via pipette may renormalize E_m and allow the researcher to salvage some information from an otherwise lost preparation. However, this is not recommended as routine practice.

3. AP duration or other properties run up or down during an experiment. This is frequent in ruptured patch due to diffusion of signaling molecules from cell to pipette. Perforated patch may be needed.

4. Electrical noise appears. Whole cell CC or VC data are recorded unbalanced, relative to a reference, not differentially (like EKG), and so are susceptible to noise pickup. The near open circuit CC input easily picks up power line frequency noise by magnetic coupling, while the near short circuit VC input readily senses high frequency radiated noise. Where possible, identify and remove noise sources. Faraday cages are needed in most environments. Additional shielding (ferrous metal for magnetic fields) will help, but to avoid exacerbation of noise, all shields and other nearby metal objects must be securely bonded to a central earth ground.

5. Mechanical sensitivity. Seals can be lost when mechanically stressed or loose setup components transmit environmental vibration. Contaminated, dirty, leaky, or cracked pipette holders or recording chambers can transfer solutions by capillary, forming adventitious conductive pathways which introduce noise or offset errors. Dirt or loss of integrity in Ag/AgCl electrodes will cause noise, drifts, or jumps in the E_m record.

AP analysis

APs must be recorded with sufficient time and amplitude resolution for analysis. For a CC amplifier with 20–50 μs rise time, the Nyquist information criterion requires a sampling interval shorter than half of this, that is <10–25 μs or 40–100 KHz. With this the AP rise would be represented by ~20 samples. Amplitude resolution should be <0.1 mV; with

modern 16-bit computer data acquisition, ×10 postamplification is typical and sufficient.

For many studies, descriptive analysis of the AP waveform under steady state or stationary conditions is sufficient. Descriptors include rest or maximum diastolic potential, peak E_m, and the difference between them (AP amplitude, APA), as well as durations at fractional repolarizations such as APD_{50} and APD_{90}, and maximum rates of depolarization and final repolarization (dE_m/dt_{max}). Hypotheses on these features are amenable to difference-of-mean tests (t, z, ANOVA).

Waveforms of recorded APs can be reconstructed or simulated with computational models such as [5]. Numerous species and/or tissue-specific models have been proposed, including extensions to ligand/messenger phenomena and multiscaling [11]. While direct fitting of comprehensive multiequation models to data would be daunting, modern modeling has power to predictively assess the often high sensitivity of the AP to ion channel modulation [12].

Intervals between APs as well as AP waveform properties are statistical phenomena, which may relate to clinical features such as heart rate and QT interval variability. Time series and spectral analysis, prominent in neurophysiology, econometrics and engineering, are applicable. These approaches can treat not only spontaneous but also paced activity, where analyses typically concern the fidelity or coherency of response.

Alternative approaches and extensions

VC is usually used under ion-selective conditions with step stimuli to characterize channel properties that may be expected to occur during the AP. This approach can characterize ionic currents over a broad range of voltages and conditions but cannot discern dynamic interactions among ionic currents or other features such as Ca dependence, which are intrinsic to APs. We now mention four methods which support more physiological inferences about the underlying structure of the AP.

True AP-clamp, introduced in 1989 [13], and refined steadily [14], begins with recording in CC a particular cell's own AP in normal physiological solution. This same cell is then placed under VC, with the recorded AP used as the command E_m. Initially the zero net current balance of CC is reproduced. Adding a channel-selective blocker(e.g. for I_{Kr}) eliminates that channel's current from the balance. To maintain voltage control, the VC provides compensating current equal to the blocked current, with opposite sign. AP-clamp reveals each current as selectively as its blocker allows, minimizing disturbances to the others, but even so it cannot achieve absolute separation. It cannot control for feed-forward interactions. For instance, when L-type channel Ca influx is blocked, the Ca gradient driving Na/Ca exchange is unavoidably disturbed. AP-clamp is exacting and requires high-quality stable cells.

Dynamic clamp is similar to AP-clamp, but instead of treating the cell under study, manipulations like pharmacological block are simulated by adjusting a model-based VC command. The command can be analog [15] but is usually computer generated [16]. As with AP-clamp, a baseline model-derived AP command yields no current, insofar as that AP truly matches the natural AP of that cell. The command can then be reprogrammed to simulate experiments such as pharmacological block, altered waveforms, overexpressed channels, or current coupling between cells, but this process is necessarily inferential. Computational dynamic clamp requires fast feedback, a true real time operating system, and advanced programming.

A less ambitious approach, sometimes also called AP-clamp, uses an AP waveform (not necessarily from the cell under study) as the VC command, along with ion-selective solutions. Although it does no better at addressing channel interdependence than does VC with steps, it does reveal currents similar to those during APs, and allows testing for effects of Ca buffering, or of modified or foreign APs [17].

Interruption of an AP at any chosen time allows study of channel currents flowing under what become the initial conditions at that time. Either an AP-clamp waveform is imposed in VC [18] or the AP is recorded directly in CC, followed by a fast switch to VC [19]. In either case the VC command is set to activate selectively a particular type of channel such as Na/Ca exchange or I_{K1}. A simultaneous fast switch to ion-selective solution may be required. If reasonably selective activation can be attained, physiologically relevant state transitions can be studied.

Weaknesses and strengths

We have emphasized the interdependence of the ion channels, pumps and transporters whose behavior underlies the AP. Models in current literature contain 50 or more simultaneous equations (mostly differential and nonlinear equations). Models of this complexity are unlikely to be fit effectively to observed data, not the least due to the challenge of representing each ion flux pathway accurately. Realistic models of reduced complexity can be matched to data and complement experiments by elucidating the dynamic interplay among ionic channels and transporters during the AP.

Conclusion

We have shown the essential reasoning behind the study of APs and provided practical suggestions for recording and analysis. Whether analyzed using descriptive statistics or via modeling for detailed mechanistic inferences, AP studies complement traditional biophysically oriented VC studies using steps and ion-selective solutions. They represent a highly sensitive, physiologically relevant assay in cardiac physiology, just as in neuroscience and sensory physiology.

References

1 Connolly P, Clark P, Curtis ASG, Dow JAT, Wilkinson CDW. An extracellular microelectrode array for monitoring electrogenic cells in culture. *Biosens Bioelectron* 1990; **5**: 223–234.

2 Fast V, Ideker R. Simultaneous optical mapping of transmembrane potential and intracellular calcium in myocyte cultures. *J Cardiovasc Electrophys* 2000; **11**: 547–556.

3 Burton F. *Optical mapping*, 2010. Available at: http://www.heartrhythmcongress.com/files/file/HRC2010_Presentations_Sunday/BasicSciences1400_F_Burton.pdf

4 Lakatta EG, Maltsev VA, Vinogradova TM. A coupled SYSTEM of intracellular Ca^{2+} clocks and surface membrane voltage clocks controls the timekeeping mechanism of the heart's pacemaker. *Circ Res* 2010; **106**: 659–673.

5 Shannon TR, Wang F, Puglisi J, Weber C, Bers DM. A mathematical treatment of integrated Ca dynamics within the ventricular myocyte. *Biophys* 2004; **J87**: 3351–3371.

6 Roberge FA, Drouhard J-P. Using Vmax to estimate changes in the sodium membrane conductance in cardiac cells. *Comp Biomed Res* 1987; **20**: 351–365.

7 Molecular Devices (MDS Analytical Technologies). *The Axon Guide: A Guide to Electrophysiology and Biophysics Laboratory Techniques*. #2500-0102 Rev. C, 2008. Available at: www.moldev.com.

8 Magistretti J, Mantegazza M, Guatteo E, Wanke E. Action potentials recorded with patch-clamp amplifiers: are they genuine? *Trends Neurosci* 1996; **9**: 530–544.

9 Callewaert G, Carmeliet E, Vereecke J. Single cardiac Purkinje cells: general electrophysiology and voltage-clamp analysis of the pace-maker current. *J Physiol* 1984; **349**: 643–661.

10 Kenyon J. *Revised primer on junction potentials*, 2008. Available at: http://www.medicine.nevada.edu/physio/docs/revised_primer_on_junction_potentials_3e.pdf

11 Yang JH, Saucerman JJ. Computational models reduce complexity and accelerate insight into cardiac signaling networks. *Circ Res* 2011; **108**: 85–97.

12 Grandi E, Puglisi JL, Wagner S, Maier LS, Severi S, Bers DM, et al. Simulation of Ca-calmodulin-dependent protein kinase II on rabbit ventricular myocyte ion currents and action potentials. *Biophys J* 2007; **93**: 3835–3847.

13 Doerr T, Denger R, Trautwein W. Calcium currents in single SA nodal cells of the rabbit heart studied with action potential clamp. *Pflugers Arch* 1989; **413**: 599–603.

14 Banyasz T, Horvath B, Jian Z, Izu LT, Chen-Izu Y. Sequential dissection of multiple ionic currents in single cardiac myocytes under action potential-clamp. *J Mol Cell Cardiol* 2011; **50**: 578–581.

15 Tan RC, Joyner RW. Electrotonic influences on action potentials from isolated ventricular cells. *Circ Res* 1990; **67**: 1071–1081.

16 Goaillard JM, Marder E. Dynamic clamp analyses of cardiac, endocrine, and neural function. *Physiology (Bethesda)* 2006; **21**: 197–207.

17 Yuan W, Ginsburg KS, Bers DM. Comparison of sarcolemmal calcium channel current in rabbit and rat ventricular myocytes. *J Physiol* 1996; **493**: 733–746.

18 Linz KW, Meyer R. Control of L-type calcium current during the action potential of guinea-pig ventricular myocytes. *J Physiol* 1998; **513**: 425–442.

19 Egan TM, Noble D, Noble SJ, Powell T, Spindler AJ. Sodium calcium exchange during the action potential in guinea-pig ventricular cells. *J Physiol* 1989; **411**: 639–661.

6

Patch-clamp recordings from isolated cardiac myocytes

Kai-Chien Yang, Wei Wang, and Jeanne M. Nerbonne

Washington University School of Medicine, Saint Louis, MO, USA

Introduction

Contraction of the mammalian heart depends on proper electrical functioning: the generation of action potentials in individual cardiomyocytes, the sequential activation of cells in the specialized conducting system, and the propagation of electrical activity throughout the ventricles [1,2]. The normal cardiac cycle begins with action potentials originating in the sinoatrial node, propagating through the atria to the atrioventricular node; the electrical activity then spreads through the His bundle and conducting Purkinje fibers to excite the working ventricular myocardium [1].

Myocardial action potentials are generated by the sequential activation and inactivation of ion channels conducting depolarizing (inward) Na^+ and Ca^{2+} and repolarizing (outward) K^+ currents [1–3]. Voltage-gated inward Na^+ currents contribute to the upstroke of action potentials in atrial and ventricular myocytes, which is followed by a rapid phase of repolarization, mediated by transient outward K^+ currents, to the action potential plateau, resulting from the delicate balance between inward currents through voltage-gated Na^+ and Ca^{2+} channels and outward currents through voltage-gated K^+ channels. The latter phase of repolarization reflects a shift in this balance, due to increased outward K^+ currents through voltage-gated K^+ channels, as well as through inwardly rectifying K^+ channels, which also contribute

to the maintenance of resting membrane potential [2,3]. During the cardiac action potential, Ca^{2+} influx through voltage-gated Ca^{2+} channels triggers the release of Ca^{2+} from the sarcoplasmic reticulum into the cytosol, activating the intracellular contractile machinery and leading to myocyte shortening [4]. The synchronized shortening of ventricular myocytes results in the contraction of the heart (systole) and the ejection of blood through the aorta.

A variety of inherited [5,6] and acquired [7,8] cardiac diseases are associated with changes in the expression and/or the biophysical properties of myocardial ion channels, changes that can lead to alterations in the waveforms and/or the propagation of action potentials in different regions of the heart, predisposing individuals to potentially life-threatening arrhythmias and sudden cardiac death [2]. Detailed understanding of disease-linked alterations in cardiac ion channel expression and/or properties is clearly needed to facilitate accurate diagnosis of risk and the development of optimal treatment strategies. Unlike the detailed analyses of action potential waveforms, which requires current-clamp recordings (see Chapter 5), characterizing the functional expression and properties of myocardial ion channels requires voltage-clamp, an experimental approach designed to provide precise temporal and spatial control of the cellular membrane potential (voltage) to allow current flow through membrane ion channels to be measured directly.

Manual of Research Techniques in Cardiovascular Medicine, First Edition. Edited by Hossein Ardehali, Roberto Bolli, and Douglas W. Losordo.

Theory of patch-clamp recording

Over past six decades, voltage-clamp recording techniques have been developed, refined, and exploited extensively to allow the measurement and detailed characterization of the currents through ion channels in myocardial cells, as well as in a host of other excitable and nonexcitable cells. The first voltage-clamp experiment was conducted on the squid giant axon by Kenneth Cole [9] using a space clamp and electronic feedback circuit developed by George Marmont [10]. Working in parallel, Alan Hodgkin and Andrew Huxley refined the design of the voltage-clamp circuit and exploited this technique elegantly to detail the time- and voltage-dependent properties of the ionic conductances underlying action potential generation in the squid giant axon [11].

In the ground-breaking work of Hodgkin and Huxley [11], two axial electrodes were inserted in the axon, one to control voltage, one to measure current. Although revolutionary, the approach was not widely applicable to other smaller biological preparations. Vaseline-gap and sucrose-gap voltage-clamp methods [12,13], without the use of axial wires, were later developed for voltage-clamp studies of smaller elongated and/or multicellular preparations, such as myelinated axons [12], vertebrate skeletal, and cardiac muscle fibers [13]. Although these methods use large electrodes of very low resistance, allowing rapid clamping of the membrane voltage and reliable current recordings, the types of preparations that can be studied are also limited. The desire to apply voltage-clamp techniques to single cells led to the development of two-microelectrode voltage clamp [11,14,15]. The application of this technique, however, is limited as the insertion of two microelectrodes without producing substantial damage can only be done routinely in relatively large (>70 μm) cells. A further advance was the development of the single-microelectrode voltage clamp, which involves using a (fast) feedback circuit to switch the microelectrode (rapidly) between voltage sensing and current passing modes [16]. Although the single-microelectrode technique made it possible to record from relatively small cells, as well as from cells in intact tissues, the high pipette resistance and capacitance were quickly recognized as substantive limitations. The voltage-clamp technique was revolutionized by the

development of patch-clamp recording technique [17,18], which combines a low-noise, high-resistance feedback amplifier with a low-resistance patch pipette and requires a high-resistance "gigaseal" between the recording pipette and the cell membrane [19] that combine to minimize noise and permit the measurements of currents, including currents through single ion channels [17–21], across the membranes of small, as well as large, cells.

The voltage-clamp technique allows the measurement of macroscopic membrane currents, and the detailed characterization of the properties of these currents including: (1) time- and voltage-dependent properties; (2) ion permeability and selectivity; and (3) reversal potentials. Patch-clamp recording techniques, however, also provide the opportunity to control the compositions of both the intracellular and extracellular solutions, as well as to measure microscopic membrane currents, enabling quantification of single-channel conductances, selectivities, voltage-dependent properties, and open and closed probabilities [19–21]. The ability to manipulate the intracellular medium and to remove the channel from its normal cellular environment also enables studies focused on exploring channel modulation by intracellular and extracellular signaling pathways [19–21].

There are multiple configurations of the patch-clamp recording method designed to enable analyses of macroscopic and microscopic membrane currents. These are described in the following text in the experimental order in which the different configurations are achieved.

Cell-attached configuration

For all patch-clamp recordings, the first step involves establishing a high-resistance seal between the cell membrane and the recording pipette (Figure 6.1). With the patch pipette placed in close proximity to the cell membrane, the application of suction allows the establishment of a tight "gigaseal". If the quality of the seal in this cell-attached configuration (Figure 6.1A) is high (≥ 1–$10\,G\Omega$), the current flowing through single or multiple channels within the small patch of membrane can be measured directly. Because the cell membrane remains intact and contents of the cytosol are not disturbed, recordings in the cell-attached configuration allow the measurement of ion channel activity under "physiological" conditions. However, the downside of this configuration is that the membrane potential cannot be measured directly and the intracellular constituents cannot be manipulated.

Whole-cell recording configuration

The whole-cell recording configuration (Figure 6.1B) is achieved by rupturing the cell membrane by applying negative suction or high-frequency voltage pulse across the membrane patch while in the cell-attached configuration (Figure 6.1A), establishing a low-resistance pathway between the cell cytoplasm and the solution inside the pipette. The whole-cell configuration allows control of the composition of both the intracellular and extracellular compartments, permitting the measurement of whole-cell membrane

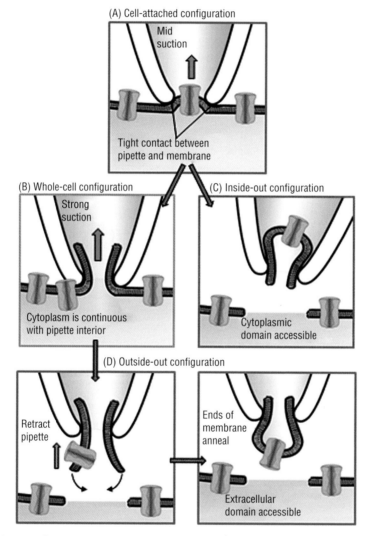

(A) Cell-attached configuration

Mid suction

Tight contact between pipette and membrane

(B) Whole-cell configuration

Strong suction

Cytoplasm is continuous with pipette interior

(C) Inside-out configuration

Cytoplasmic domain accessible

(D) Outside-out configuration

Retract pipette

Ends of membrane anneal

Extracellular domain accessible

Figure 6.1 Patch-clamp recording configurations. For both whole-cell and single-channel current recordings, the first step is the formation of a tight, gigaohm (GΩ) seal between the recording pipette and the cell membrane (A). This is accomplished by applying suction to the back of the pipette after making contact with the cell membrane. If the seal resistance is high (several GΩ), single channel recordings can be obtained in the "cell-attached" configuration (A). With the application of additional suction, the membrane patch under the recording pipette ruptures, establishing the whole-cell configuration (B). Alternatively, pulling back the pipette (while in the cell-attached configuration) excises the membrane patch to enable single channel recordings in the "inside-out" configuration (C). Alternatively, if the pipette is retracted while in the whole-cell configuration, the membrane that is removed (still attached to the pipette) anneals (D) and the "outside-out" configuration is achieved.

potential changes (in the current-clamp mode) as well as whole-cell macroscopic currents (in the voltage-clamp mode) under a variety of conditions. A variation of the whole-cell configuration is the perforated patch recording method [22,23], in which pore-forming hydrophobic agents, such as nystatin [22] or amphotericin B [23], are included in the pipette (tip) solution. Rather than rupturing the membrane under the patch pipette, electrical access is achieved in the perforated patch method when the nystatin and amphotericin B translocate from the pipette tip to the cell membrane. The pore properties of nystatin and amphotericin B allow only the movement of monovalent cations and anions and the problems with the "wash-out" of cytoplasmic factors that occur in the whole-cell configuration are avoided.

Inside-out excised patch configuration

The inside-out excised patch configuration is obtained from the cell-attached configuration by pulling back the pipette after forming gigaseal (Figure 6.1C). Excision of the membrane patch exposes the cytosolic surface of transmembrane ion channels to the bath solution, the composition of which can be controlled and manipulated. The inside-out configuration permits detailed studies of the effects of intracellular small molecules and proteins on the properties of membrane ion channels.

Outside-out excised patch configuration

The outside-out excised patch configuration is obtained from the whole-cell configuration by pulling back the patch pipette (Figure 6.1D). If the seal is stable, the membrane will reseal and the extracellular surface will now be facing the bath solution (Figure 6.1D). The outside-out configuration permits detailed studies of the impact of the application of extracellular molecules on channel properties at the resolution of single-channel events.

Instrumentation for patch-clamp recordings

The equipment requirements for constructing a patch-clamp recording set up are relatively simple and few: all of the typical components of any electrophysiological recording set-up, including an air table, upright or inverted microscope, micromanipulator(s), recording amplifier, and microelectrode puller. Depending on the specific experiments to be conducted, it might also be useful to have the microscope equipped for epifluorescence, as well as a camera and other imaging hardware. The most critical components needed for successful patch-clamp recordings are the recording pipettes and the recording amplifier. Pipettes are typically fabricated from borosilicate glass, selected because it has a low softening temperature and low electrical noise, and, in addition, seals readily to biological membranes. The geometry of the shank and the size of the tip of the pipette are readily controlled by the specific glass selected and temperature and timing of the heating and pulling the glass in much the same manner as in the construction of microelectrodes, although two-stage, not one-stage, pullers are typically used. In general, pipettes are pulled immediately prior to use and are stored in a sealed container to avoid dust and other particulate contamination of the tips. The shanks, up to the tips, can be coated prior to use with an insulating material, such as Sylgard™ (Dow Corning), to reduce pipette capacitance [19]; the improvement provided is a function of the glass and the shape of the shank and, is, therefore, evaluated empirically. It has also be argued that fire-polishing the pipette tip improves formation of a membrane seal [19]; this can be accomplished using a microforge, although many of the two-stage pipette pullers available provide some degree of fire-polishing, reducing the need for this additional step.

High-quality patch-clamp recording amplifiers are available commercially from a number of sources. The key components of the circuit are illustrated in Figure 6.2. The recording pipette, illustrated in contact with an isolated myocyte, is connected to the negative input of a high-gain, high-input resistance operational amplifier. The applied voltage to the pipette (V_p) follows the command voltage (V_{com}) of the amplifier and the pipette current (I_p), which is proportional to the voltage output (V_{Rf}) of the amplifier, flows through the feedback resistor (R_f). Typically, the circuit will contain a frequency correction current circuit (FR) that allows reduction (or elimination) of the stray capacitance (C_f) and R_f. The analog signals from the headstage are passed through an analog-to-digital

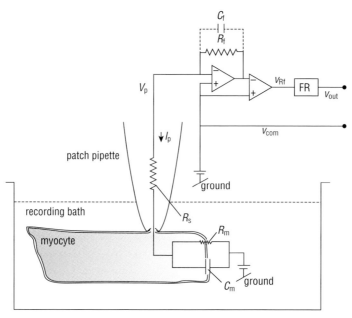

Figure 6.2 Schematic of the patch-clamp amplifier (with a resistive head stage) in the whole-cell voltage-clamp configuration in contact with an isolated mammalian cardiac myocyte. The patch recording pipette is connected to the negative input of a high-gain, high-input resistance operational amplifier and the pipette voltage (V_p), therefore, follows the command voltage (V_{com}). The pipette current (I_p) flows through the feedback resistor (R_f) and is proportional to the voltage output (V_{Rf}) of the amplifier. The frequency correction current circuit (FR) allows correction for the stray capacitance (C_f) and R_f. V_{com}, command voltage; R_s, series resistance; R_m, membrane resistance; and C_m, membrane capacitance.

converter, the signal is digitized and sent to a computer for storage and offline analysis. Conversely, digital outputs from the computer are converted to analog signals to vary the voltages applied to the cell (see Section Experimental aspects of patch clamp recordings, Whole cell recordings). Most commercially available amplifiers can also be used in the current-clamp mode to control the membrane current and allow the measurement of membrane voltage. A number of patch-clamp amplifiers with a capacitative feedback circuit that improves the speed of the clamp, particularly in the current-clamp mode, are now available. The performance of patch-clamp recording amplifiers can be further improved using "supercharging", which renders the speed of the clamp independent of the electrode and feedback resistance over a rather large range [24].

Experimental aspects of patch-clamp recordings

A critical factor in all electrophysiological studies is the optimization of the recording conditions to permit the reliable and accurate measurement of the voltage and current signals of interest. Optimization of the contents of the bath solution to allow action potentials (in current-clamp mode) or macroscopic/ microscopic ionic currents (in voltage-clamp mode) to be recorded reliably is readily accomplished [11,14,15]. Using the patch-clamp recording method, however, it is also possible to control the composition of the intracellular pipette solution [19]. In combination with well-designed voltage-clamp protocols, the ability to control the compositions of the extracellular bath and the intracellular pipette solution facilitates the isolation of individual current components [19] for detailed analyses of kinetic and voltage-dependent properties of macroscopic/ microscopic currents (see Experimental aspects of patch clamp recordings, Whole-cell voltage-clamp protocols, Data acquisition and analysis).

Gigaseal formation

Once the bath and pipette solutions have been selected and pipettes have been fabricated and filled, the next step is the formation of a high resistance seal between the pipette tip and the cell membrane, which is essential for the successful recording of macroscopic and microscopic (single channel) currents using the patch-clamp technique. The amplitudes of random fluctuations in background membrane currents and instrument/ system electrical noise dramatically influence the ability to resolve and record biologically relevant ionic currents. Increasing the signal to noise ratio (S/N) to acceptable level was a long sought goal that was realized with the development of methods to establish high-resistance, "giga" ($>10^9 \Omega$ or GΩ) seal between the recording electrode and the cell (myocyte) membrane [17–19]. To begin, the pipette is lowered into the bath solution with positive pressure applied, to help to keep the tip clean. To facilitate formation of gigaseals, the cell surface membrane should be devoid of debris or damage and both the bath and the recording pipette solutions should be filtered (at 0.2 μm) to avoid clogging of the tip. With the application of a potential across the tip, the pipette resistance can be measured (Figure 6.3A) and monitored continuously. Contact between the pipette tip and the cell membrane is signaled by an abrupt increase (two to tenfold) in pipette resistance. At this point, application of gentle suction

facilitates the formation of a seal between the pipette and the cell membrane, signaled by a marked increase, from MΩ to GΩ, in pipette resistance (Figure 6.3B) and the cell-attached configuration is achieved (Figure 6.1A).

Whole-cell recordings

After forming a gigaseal, the pipette capacitance should be compensated electronically, while still in the cell attached configuration. The whole-cell configuration is achieved by the application of a brief pulse of suction and is signaled by the appearance of large current transients in response to the (10 mV) test pulse (Figure 6.3C), reflecting the whole-cell capacitative current. If the abrupt suction does not rupture the membrane patch, a brief, large amplitude voltage pulse can be used as an alternative. Once the whole-cell configuration is achieved, the cell membrane potential is clamped to the desired, negative voltage, typically at or near the cell resting membrane potential, that is in the range of −70 to −80 mV.

In the whole-cell configuration, using the conventional or the perforated patch method, the access resistance and the cell input resistance and capacitance can be calculated from records like those in Figure 6.3C, and then compensated electronically.

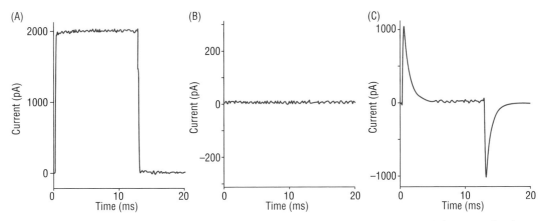

Figure 6.3 Illustration of gigaseal formation and establishment of the whole-cell configuration using a model cell. Current recordings from a model cell with an input resistance of 500 MΩ and a capacitance of 33 pF, using a 5 MΩ patch pipette with an applied (test) voltage at +10 mV. (A) Current recorded with the pipette in the bath solution prior to seal formation. (B) High-resistance ("gigaseal") seal formation is indicated by an abrupt decrease in the current response to the same +10 mV test pulse. Acquisition of the whole-cell configuration (C) is evidenced by the appearance of the large capacitive transients. In whole-cell recordings from myocytes, records such as those in (C) can be used to calculate whole-cell membrane capacitances and series resistances. Using the compensation circuit, the currents due to the series resistance and the whole-cell capacitance can be compensated, typically to 60–90%, depending on the size of the pipette and the cell.

Integration of the capacitative transient, evoked in response to a low-amplitude voltage step, provides the capacitative current (I_C), from which the whole cell membrane capacitance (C_m), can be calculated according to the formula $I_C = C_m(dV/dT)$. For mammalian cardiac myocytes, the capacitance compensation is only partial as these cells are large and the compensation circuits in most commercially available amplifiers are limited to 100 pF; cell input resistances are typically >200 MΩ. The access or series resistance (R_s) (Figure 6.2), which reflects the resistances of all components in series with the cell membrane, should be measured and compensated electronically. It is important to measure the extent of the compensation achieved as voltage drops across the uncompensated R_s will result in (voltage) errors that could be substantial, particularly for large amplitude currents. It is also important to report the uncompensated R_s and the resulting voltage errors. Most patch-clamp amplifiers provide a positive feedback R_s(%) compensation circuit (at least in the voltage-clamp mode), in which a signal proportional to the measured current is added to the command potential. It is essential to adjust R_s compensation properly to achieve maximum % compensation.

Whole-cell voltage-clamp protocols, data acquisition, and analysis

The whole-cell voltage-clamp technique has proven to be very useful in experiments aimed at detailing the properties of myocyte membrane currents. Specific strategies have been developed and are now widely used to isolate and characterize individual current components. To begin, experimental (recording) conditions are established to eliminate all of the currents other than the current of interest. As noted earlier, for example, the intracellular pipette and extracellular bath solutions are optimized to facilitate the isolation of the current of interest, sometimes involving the inclusion of selective pharmacological blockers of the different types of ion channels. In some cases, currents are measured before and after exposure to the blocker and are subtracted from one another, yielding the sub-tracted, "blocker-sensitive" currents. In addition, specific voltage-clamp protocols, involving step depolarizations or hyperpolarizations of fixed durations are designed and used, alone and in combination with blockers, to facilitate the isolation of the specific current component of interest.

Representative voltage-clamp recordings, obtained from isolated adult mouse ventricular myocytes, are presented to illustrate these points (Figure 6.4). With K^+ in the recording pipette and voltage-gated inward Na^+ and Ca^{2+} currents blocked with the inclusion of tetrodotoxin (TTX) and Cd^{2+}($CdCl_2$), respectively, in the bath, voltage-gated outward K^+ (Kv) currents are routinely recorded from these cells in response to 4.5 s depolarizing voltage steps to potentials between −60 and +40 mV from a holding potential of −70 mV, presented at an interval of 15 s (Figure 6.4A); the voltage-clamp paradigm is illustrated below the current records. The maximal (peak) and the steady-state (plateau) outward currents evoked at each test potential were measured and normalized to the whole-cell membrane capacitance (measured in the same cell), and peak and plateau current densities as a function of the test potential are plotted (Figure 6.4A, right panel). In addition to current-voltage plots as shown here, the Kv current records displayed can be analyzed to determine the kinetics of current activation and inactivation. The voltage-clamp protocol can be modified in experiments designed to determine reversal potentials, as well as the voltage-dependences of current activation and steady-state inactivation.

For recording inward Na^+(I_{Na}) (Figure 6.4B) and Ca^{2+}(I_{Ca}) (Figure 6.4C) currents, the K^+ in the recording pipette solution is replaced by equimolar Cs^+ to eliminate outward K^+ currents. In experiments focused on measuring/characterizing I_{Na}, Cd^{2+} ($CdCl_2$) was also added in bath solution and I_{Na}, evoked in response to brief (20 ms) depolarizing voltage steps to potentials between −70 mV and +50 mV (in 5 mV increments at 2 s intervals) were recorded (Figure 6.4B); the voltage-clamp paradigm is illustrated below the current records. Peak I_{Na} amplitudes at each test potential were measured, normalized to the cell membrane capacitance (measured in the same cell and peak I_{Na} density plotted as a function of the test potential (Figure 6.4B, right panel). It should be noted that the recordings displayed were obtained with low (20 mM) Na^+ in the extracellular bath solutions to reduce the amplitudes of the currents to allow for adequate voltage clamp control and recording of Na^+ currents, which is otherwise difficult/ impossible

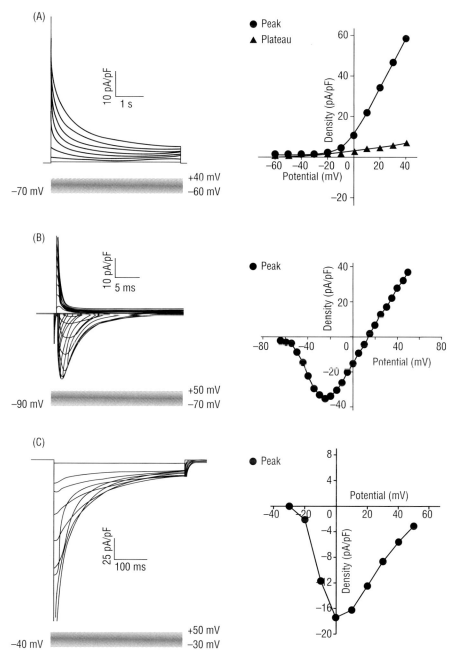

Figure 6.4 Representative voltage-clamp recording from isolated (mouse) ventricular myocytes. (A) With inward Na^+ and Ca^{2+} currents blocked and K^+ in the recording pipette, whole-cell voltage-gated outward K^+ currents, evoked in response to depolarizing voltage steps to −60 to +40 mV (in 10 mV increments) from a holding potential (HP) of −70 mV, are recorded. The peak and plateau (at 4.5 s) current densities measured at each test potential are shown in the current-voltage (IV) plot to the right of the records. With Cs^+ in the recording pipette (in place of K^+), voltage-gated Na^+ (B) and Ca^{2+} (C) currents can be recorded. (B) For this representative myocyte, whole-cell Na^+ currents were recorded in response to brief (20 ms) test depolarizations to −70 to +50 mV (in 5 mV increments) from a HP of −90 mV. The peak current densities are shown in the IV plot on the right. (C) With tetrodotoxin in the bath to block voltage-gated Na^+ currents, inward currents through voltage-gated Ca^{2+} channels are recorded in response to voltage steps to test potentials between −30 and +50 mV (in 10 mV increments) from a HP of −40 mV. Peak inward Ca^{2+} currents are plotted as a function of the test potential in the IV plot in the panel on the right.

to achieve for adult cardiomyocytes. For recording currents through L type Ca^{2+} ($I_{Ca,L}$), the Cd^{2+} ($CdCl_2$) was eliminated from the bath and TTX was added. In addition to the Cs^+ in the pipette solution, tetraethylammonium (TEA) is also added to the bath to provide more complete block of outward K^+ currents, facilitating the reliable measurement of $I_{Ca,L}$, evoked in response to (400 ms) depolarizing voltage steps to test potentials ranging from -30 mV to $+50$ mV in 10 mV increments at 5 s intervals (Figure 6.4C). Currents were evoked from a holding potential of -40 or -50 mV (Figure 6.4C), which was done to inactivate residual Na^+ currents not completely blocked by the presence of the TTX in the bath. The current–voltage relation for peak $I_{Ca,L}$ density is illustrated in the right panel of Figure 6.4C.

An interesting alternative to the fixed voltage steps that are typically used (Figure 6.4) has been the development and application of action potential voltage-clamp paradigms, in which the currents evoked in response to voltage deflections that correspond to action potential waveforms are measured [25–27]. This approach, therefore, allows direct assessment of the currents under voltage-clamp during the normal trajectory of the cardiac action potential [27].

As noted previously, current-clamp recordings of myocyte membrane potentials and action potential waveforms can also be accomplished using the whole-cell configuration of the patch-clamp recording technique. Voltage recordings can be obtained from the resting membrane potential, that is without any added depolarizing or hyperpolarizing currents injected, or with current added to manipulate the membrane potential and determine the effects of these manipulations on action potential thresholds, amplitudes, and durations.

Conclusions and future directions

Patch-clamp recording techniques, used extensively in cardiovascular research for more than three decades now, have provided many details of the properties of cardiomyocyte membrane currents and the mechanisms involved in the regulation and modulation of these currents. In addition, a number of techniques, particularly imaging methods, have been combined with patch-clamp recordings to enable simultaneous analyses of myocyte membrane currents and intracellular, particularly intracellular Ca^{2+}-mediated pathways. Although not yet applied to large cells, such as mammalian cardiomyocytes, new patch-clamp methods, such as the "PatchChip", hold the promise of enabling two or more simultaneous whole-cell recordings to be obtained at high bandwidth and with low noise [28]. Advances in nanotechnology are also being exploited increasingly to improve patch camp recording efficiency and resolution [29]. Another important step forward has been demonstrated with the application of the dynamic-clamp technique, which combines mathematical simulations of ion channel currents with patch-clamp recordings and allows the introduction of simulated conductances into cells during electrophysiological recordings [30,31]. Although originally developed and exploited in studies of synaptic currents [32], several investigators have begun to use the dynamic-clamp approach, in combination with conventional whole-cell recordings and with perforated patch recordings, to probe directly the physiological roles of specific conductance pathways in regulating the resting and active membrane properties of cardiac myocytes [30–33]. These approaches seem certain to be used increasingly to probe directly the physiological roles of cardiac membrane currents and the pathophysiological consequences of alterations in these currents associated with inherited and acquired cardiac and noncardiac diseases.

References

1 Fozzard HA. Excitation-contraction coupling in the heart. *Adv Exp Med Biol* 1991; **308**: 135–142.

2 Nerbonne JM, Kass RS. Molecular physiology of cardiac repolarization. *Physiol Rev* 2005; **85**: 1205–1253.

3 Roden DM, Balser JR, George AL, Jr., Anderson ME. Cardiac ion channels. *Annu Rev Physiol* 2002; **64**: 431–475.

4 ter Keurs HE. Electromechanical coupling in the cardiac myocyte; stretch-arrhythmia feedback. *Pflugers Arch* 2011; **462**: 165–175.

5 Nademanee K, Veerakul G, Nimmannit S, Chaowakul V, Bhuripanyo K, Likittanasombat K, *et al*. Arrhythmogenic marker for the sudden unexplained death syndrome in Thai men. *Circulation* 1997; **96**: 2595–2600.

6 Morita H, Wu J, Zipes DP. The QT syndromes: long and short. *Lancet* 2008; **372**: 750–763.

7 Beuckelmann DJ, Nabauer M, Erdmann E. Alterations of K$^+$ currents in isolated human ventricular myocytes from patients with terminal heart failure. *Circ Res* 1993; **73**: 379–385.

8 Volk T, Nguyen THD, Schultz JH, Faulhaber J Ehmke H. Regional alterations of repolarizing K$^+$ currents among the left ventricular free wall of rats with ascending aortic stenosis. *J Physiol* 2001; **530**: 443–455.

9 Cole KS. Dynamic electrical characteristics of the squid axon membrane. *Archives des Sciences Physiologiques* 1949; **3**: 253–258.

10 Marmont G. Studies on the axon membrane; a new method. *J Cell Physiol* 1949; **34**: 351–382.

11 Hodgkin AL, Huxley AF. A quantitative description of membrane current and its application to conduction and excitation in nerve. *J Physiol* 1952; **117**: 500–544.

12 Nonner W. A new voltage clamp method for Ranvier nodes. *Pflugers Arch* 1969; **309**: 176–192.

13 Hille B, Campbell DT. An improved vaseline gap voltage clamp for skeletal muscle fibers. *J Gen Physiol* 1976; **67**: 265–293.

14 Meech RW, Standen NB. Potassium activation in Helix aspersa neurones under voltage clamp: a component mediated by calcium influx. *J Physiol* 1975; **249**: 211–239.

15 Adams DJ, Gage PW. Ionic currents in response to membrane depolarization in an Aplysia neurone. *J Physiol* 1979; **289**: 115–141.

16 Finkel AS, Redman S. Theory and operation of a single microelectrode voltage clamp. *J Neurosci Meth* 1984; **11**: 101–127.

17 Neher E, Sakmann B. Single channel currents recorded from membrane of denervated frog muscle fibres. *Nature* 1976; **260**: 799–802.

18 Neher E, Sakmann B, Steinbach JH. The extracellular patch clamp: a method for resolving currenrts through individual open channels in biological membranes. *Pflügers Archiv* 1978; **375**: 229–238.

19 Hamill OP, Marty A, Neher E, Sakmann B, Sigworth FJ. Improved patch-clamp techniques for high-resolution current recording from cells and cell-free membrane patches. *Pflugers Arch* 1981; **391**: 85–100.

20 Sakmann B, Neher E. Patch clamp techniques for studying ionic channels in excitable membranes. *Annu Rev Physiol* 1984; **46**: 455–472.

21 Kornreich BG The patch clamp technique: Principles and technical considerations. *J Vet Cardiol* 2007; **9**: 25–37.

22 Horn R, Marty A. Muscarinic activation of ionic currents measured by a new whole-cell recording method. *J Gen Physiol* 1988; **92**: 145–159.

23 Rae J, Cooper K, Gates P, Watsky M. Low access resistance perforated patch recordings using amphotericin B. *J Neurosci Meth* 1991; **37**: 15–26.

24 Armstrong CM, Chow RH. Supercharging: a method for improving patch-clamp performance. *Biophys J* 1987; **52**: 133–136.

25 Bouchard RA, Clark RB, Giles WR. Effects of action potential duration on excitation-contraction coupling in rat ventricular myocytes. Action potential voltage-clamp measurements. *Circ Res* 1995; **76**: 790–801.

26 Bányász T, Fülöp L, Magyar J, Szentandrássy N, Varró A, Nánási PP, *et al.* Endocardial versus epicardial differences in L-type calcium current in canine ventricular myocytes studied by action potential voltage clamp. *Cardiovasc Res* 2003; **58**: 66–75.

27 Szentandrássy N, Nagy D, Ruzsnavszky F, Harmati G, Bányász T, Magyar J, *et al.* Powerful technique to test selectivity of agents acting on cardiac ion channels: the action potential voltage-clamp. *Curr Med Chem* 2011; **18**: 3737–3756.

28 Weerakoon P, CulurcIello E, Yang Y, Santos-Sacchi J, Kindlmann PJ, Sigworth FJ, *et al.* Patch-clamp amplifiers on a chip. *J Neurosci Method.* 2010; **192**: 187–192.

29 Zhao Y, Inayat S, Dikin DA, Singer JH, Ruoff RS, Troy JB, *et al.* Patch clamp technique: review of the current state of the art and potential contributions from nanoengineering. *Proc Inst Mech Eng Part N: J Nanoeng Nanosys* 2009; **223**: 121–131.

30 Sun X, Wang, HS. Role of the transient outward current (Ito) in shaping canine ventricular action potential–a dynamic clamp study. *J Physio* 2005; **564**: 411–419.

31 Dong M, Niklewski PJ, Wang HS. Ionic mechanisms of cellular electrical and mechanical abnormalities in Brugada syndrome. *Am J Physiol Heart Circ Physiol* 2011; **300**: H279–H287.

32 Goaillard JM, Marder E. Dynamic clamp analyses of cardiac, endocrine, and neural function. *Physiol* 2006; **21**: 197–207.

33 Berecki G, Zegers JG, Bhuiyan ZA, Verkerk AO, Wilders R, van Ginneken AC, *et al.* Long-QT syndrome-related sodium channel mutations probed by the dynamic action potential clamp technique. *J Physiol* 2006; **570**: 237–250.

Optical mapping of the heart

Di Lang, Sarah Gutbrod, Jacob Laughner, and Igor R. Efimov

Washington University, St. Louis, MO, USA

Introduction

Optical mapping has evolved in the last several decades to become the gold standard of electrophysiology mapping at the tissue and organ level *in vitro* [1]. This chapter presents an overview of the optical mapping procedure with voltage-sensitive dyes applied to mouse, rabbit, and human heart preparations as well as some specific applications. This methodology has engendered advancements in our understanding of excitation–contraction coupling and arrhythmia in the mammalian heart. Optical mapping methodology is endowed with unique spatial and temporal resolution, which allows optical recordings from up to tens of thousands of sites from fields of view as small as a single cell and as large as the entire epicardium of intact heart. Another important feature of the methodology is the ability to conduct multiparametric imaging of multiple parameters such as sarcolemma transmembrane potential, intracellular calcium, mitochondria inner membrane potential, etc. [2]. Optical mapping of metabolism–excitation–contraction is likely to undergo a transformational change in the near future due to dramatic advancements in genetic methods for encoding fluorescent reporters, novel light sources and detectors, and image processing techniques.

The principle behind this methodology is based on capturing the spectral shift of the fluorescence emitted from a membrane-embedded voltage-sensitive dye. The fractional fluorescence intensity corresponds to the spatially averaged voltage changes (or other parameter of interest) in the tissue (Figure 7.1A). In order to generate this signal the tissue must be excited with the appropriate wavelength of light, typically from a laser, tungsten–halogen lamp, or LED light source. The emitted light is then recorded with a photodetector through an emission filter. Photodetector options include PDA, CCD, or CMOS cameras. For multiparametric or panoramic imaging, multiple detectors are necessary (Figure 7.1B,C).

Protocols

Experimental set-up

1. Prepare Tyrode's solution (Table 7.1) fresh for each experiment to perfuse the tissue. Fill the holding reservoir with 2 L and warm the solution to 37°C.

2. Bubble 95% O_2/5% CO_2 gas into the solution. Monitor the pH and adjust the gas flow rate to maintain a pH of 7.35 ± 0.05.

3. Use peristaltic pumps to maintain a constant fluid level in the chamber and perfuse the tissue with constant flow or constant pressure (60 ± 5 mmHg) monitored with a pressure transducer.

4. Set up the CMOS camera systems with the appropriate filters (Table 7.2) and field of view.

Manual of Research Techniques in Cardiovascular Medicine, First Edition. Edited by Hossein Ardehali, Roberto Bolli, and Douglas W. Losordo.

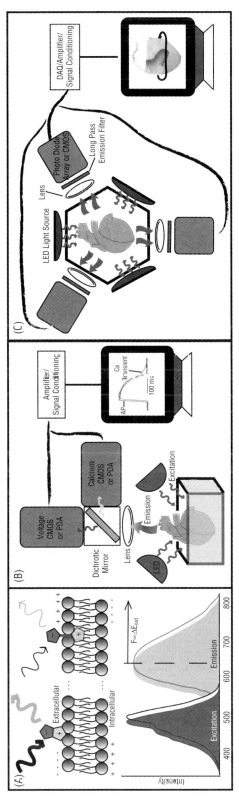

Figure 7.1 Mechanism of optical mapping. (A) Theory behind how the fractional change in fluorescence of dye represents the local average of a transmembrane action potential. (B) Experimental set-up for simultaneous calcium and voltage recording. (C) Experimental set-up for panoramic 3D imaging of the epicardium.

5. Adjust the excitation lights (halogen or LED) to illuminate the desired field of view.

6. Place two Ag/AgCl paddle electrodes into the bath and connect to a bioamplifier to record the ECG.

Tissue preparations (Figure 7.2)

Intact mouse heart (Figure 7.2A)

1. Anesthetize the mouse with ketamine/ xylazine (ketamin, 80 mg/kg; xylazine, 10 mg/kg) and heparin

Table 7.1 Solutions for optical mapping set-up

Name	Components (mM in DI water)
Tyrode's	NaCl: 128.2, CaCl$_2$: 1.3, KCl: 4.7, MgCl$_2$: 1.05, NaH$_2$PO$_4$: 1.19, NaHCO$_3$: 20, Glucose: 11.1
Cardioplegia	NaCl: 110, CaCl$_2$: 1.2, KCl: 16, MgCl$_2$: 16, NaHCO$_3$: 10

Table 7.2 Dyes

Name	Concentration	Emission filter
di-4 ANEPPS	10–25 µM	> 650 nm
RH237	10–25 µM	>700 nm
Di-4 ANBDQBS	20–40 µM	>715 nm
RHO2-AM (1 : 1 with Pluronic F127)	5–15 µM	585 ± 20 nm

(100 units) by intraperitoneal injection. Assure appropriate level of anesthesia by the lack of pain reflex.

2. After a midsternal incision, quickly remove the heart and wash it in Tyrode's solution.

3. Using a dissecting microscope, rapidly identify the aorta and make a clean cut across the ascending aorta below the right subclavian artery. A short section of aorta is then attached to a 21-gauge cannula with a rounded beveled tip for silk attachment. 4-0 black-braided silk is used to fix the heart onto the cannula. After cannulation, the heart is retrogradely perfused and superfused with Tyrode's solution.

4. After the heart is cannulated, carefully remove the lung, thymus, and fat tissue.

5. Pin the isolated heart at the apex to the bottom of the silicone coated perfusion chamber to prevent stream-induced movement. Stretch and pin the right and left atrial appendages to the bottom of the chamber to provide maximal surface area for optical measurements.

6. Insert a small silicone tube into the left ventricle through the pulmonary veins and suture it to nearby connective tissue. This prevents solution congestion and acidification of the perfusate trapped in the left ventricle.

Intact rabbit hearts

1. Restrain rabbit with towel or rabbit restrainer. Deliver a combination of 1–5% inhaled isoflurane

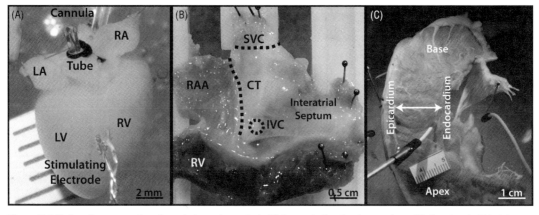

Figure 7.2 Various tissue preparations for optical mapping analysis. (A) Langendorff-perfused mouse heart. (B) Superfused rabbit right atrial preparation. (C) Left ventricular human wedge preparation. CT, christa terminalis; IVC, inferior vena cava; LA, left atrium; LV, left ventricle; RA, right atrium; RAA, right atrial appendage; RV, right ventricle; SVC, superior vena cava. (Source: (A) Lang 2011 [6]. (B) Laughner 2012 [7]. Reproduced with permission from Wolters Kluwer Health).

to effect through a mask and 400 units/kg of heparin intravenously to the ear vein. Assess unresponsiveness by evaluating the rabbit's pain reflex.

2. Keeping the isoflurane on, open the thoracic cavity of the rabbit. Begin by creating a lateral incision below the xiphoid process and diaphragm. Cut into the diaphragm to expose the heart. Open the thoracic cavity to allow room to excise the heart by cutting into the rib cage on both sides.

3. Cut the ascending and descending portions of the circulatory system. Lift the apex of the heart and separate the heart from surrounding tissues. Remove the heart from the thoracic cavity.

4. Transfer heart to a noncirculating Langendorff perfusion system. Cut the ascending portion of the aortic arch and cannulate the remaining aorta with a 16-gauge cannula attached to a bubble trap. Care must be taken to avoid introducing air bubbles into the heart. Once cannulated, remove the pericardium. Remove all remaining fat, lung, trachea, and connective tissue from the heart and flush heart of all blood. Warning: this step is time sensitive. Prolonged dissection can cause ischemic damage to the heart.

5. Transfer heart to circulating chamber for imaging.

Isolated right atria (Figure 7.2B)

1. Follow steps 1–4 mentioned earlier and stain with appropriate dye.

2. Transfer cannulated heart to a dissection tray with a silicone bottom and fill with Tyrode's solution.

3. Restrain heart, anterior side up, by pinning the aorta and apex of the heart. Separate the ventricles from the atria by cutting laterally, inferior to the atrioventricular groove.

4. Insert a grooved director into the tricuspid valve and out the superior vena cava (SVC). Cut along the grooved director starting at the tricuspid valve near the right atrial appendage (RAA). Cut along the ridge of the RAA from the tricuspid valve to the SVC to open the endocardial cavity of the right atrium.

5. Remove the left atrium and excess ventricular tissue.

6. Transfer isolated atrial preparation to superfusion system for imaging.

Human left ventricle wedge (Figure 7.2C)

1. Perfuse explanted hearts through left and right coronary arteries with cold cardioplegia solution in the operating room immediately after the removal of the heart from chest to wash out the blood and protect the hearts during the subsequent period of wedge isolation.

2. Hearts are bathed in cold cardioplegia solution during transportation to the laboratory.

3. Isolate a transmural wedge from the posterior-lateral left ventricular (LV) free wall supplied by left marginal artery.

4. Dissect the preparation several centimeters below the base of the ventricles and extend about 3 cm towards the apex.

5. Make sure wedge preparation contains a section of coronary artery (diameter ≥1 mm) along its length, which is cannulated with the custom-made flexible plastic cannula.

6. Ligate major arterial leaks in the wedges with 0-0 black-braided silk.

7. Inject methylene blue dye to verify the quality of perfusion. Poorly perfused tissue is trimmed from the wedges.

8. Mount the isolated tissues in a warm chamber with the exposed transmural surface up, facing the optical apparatus, and begin perfusion with Tyrode's solution.

Staining and image acquisition

There are many excellent voltage- and calcium-sensitive dyes on the market with distinct advantages and disadvantages for each. It is important to select the dye that is most appropriate for a study on an individual basis. Here we have included a short list of popular dyes and uncouplers and how to use them (Tables 7.2 and 7.3). Concentrations will vary depending on the size of tissue preparation and should be calibrated for an optimal signal to noise ratio throughout the experiment. Note: the isolated

Table 7.3 Excitation–contraction uncouplers

Name	Abbreviation	Concentration
Blebbistatin	BB	10 μM
2,3-butanedione monoxime	BDM	15 mM
Diacetylmonoxime	DAM	15 mM
Cytochalasin D	Cyto-D	5 μM

atrial preparation is stained prior to dissecting away the ventricles due to the fact that it is only superfused in the dish. Here we will use blebbistatin (BB) and di-4-ANEPPS as examples [3].

1. Bring the stock solutions of BB (~2 mg/mL in DMSO) and dye (1.25 mg/mL in DMSO) to room temperature. Warning: continue the remainder of the protocol with the lights off to minimize photobleaching.
2. Add 80–90% of the final concentration of uncoupler directly to the holding reservoir. Dilute the final amount (1:10) in Tyrode's solution and slowly inject it through a drug port directly into the aortic cannula over a 20-minute period.
3. Dilute the appropriate amount of dye in 1 mL of Tyrode's and inject through a drug port into the aortic cannula over 5–7 minutes. If two dyes are being used, start with the voltage dye and allow 5 minutes of equilibration before injecting the secondary dye.
4. Wait 25–30 minutes for the chemicals to take effect. Add more BB if necessary to suppress motion. Continuously monitor pressure and ECG recordings to assess electrical function of heart.
5. Adjust the excitation lights to establish uniform illumination and adequate dye.
6. Place a clear cover glass over the field of view to minimize the motion of the fluid surface
7. Acquire each optical recording with the excitation lights on and the superfusion pump turned off. The length of the file and sampling rate can be adjusted for experimental needs.
8. Apply custom protocol and continue to monitor ECG and pH to determine if the tissue begins to deteriorate. Depending on cannulation quality and tissue preparation, the tissue should last 3–6 hours.

Special case: panoramic imaging
There are several additional steps for panoramic imaging (note: step 6 is skipped).

1. Take 36 pictures of the heart, one every 10 degrees.
2. Reconstruct the 3D geometry using Niem's method.
3. Match the area of the unwrapped surface with the field of view from each of the three cameras (spaced 120 degrees apart) to project optical recordings onto the entire epicardial surface.

Data processing and analysis
Valuable physiological information in the temporal and spatial domain can be extracted from the optical recordings. Although there is a long list of processing techniques, here we will provide a short sample of analysis techniques for activation, action potential duration (APD), conduction velocity, calcium transient delay, and phase analysis.

1. Filter the matrix of optical data with an appropriate digital band-pass filter (e.g. 0.5 Hz–200 Hz) and spatially bin (e.g. 3×3) if necessary to improve signal quality. Normalize the amplitude values from 0 to 1.
2. *Creation of activation map:* Window the data to include the earliest and latest upstroke. Calculate the maximum derivative in the time domain for each point. Plot these time points in a two-dimensional (2D) map relative to the time of earliest activation.
3. *Creation of APD80 map:* Window the data to include a complete action potential. Calculate the delay between the maximum derivative in the time domain and the time at which the amplitude returns 80% of the way back to baseline for each point. Plot these time delays in a 2D map.
4. *Conduction velocity map:* Calculate the 2D spatial gradient of the activation map in the X and Y directions. Calculate local conduction velocity in X and Y coordinates by dividing X and Y spatial derivatives by the sum of the X and Y components squared. To ensure unique activation times and noninfinite conduction velocities, a 2D surface can be fit to the activation map before the calculation of the spatial gradient as described by Bayly *et al.* [4].
5. *Calcium transient delay:* Window calcium and voltage signals to include the earliest and latest upstroke. Calculate the maximum positive derivative for both the calcium and voltage signals. Subtract the calcium activation time from the voltage activation time and plot in a 2D map.
6. *Phase map and phase singularity:* For each point in space use the Hilbert transform to generate a phase shifted signal. Find the ratio between the original and shifted signal to calculate the instantaneous phase using the following equation:

$$\theta(x, y, t) = \arctan\left(\frac{V'(x, y, t)}{H[V'(x, y, t)]}\right),$$

plot in 2D map [5]. The spatial gradient of the phase will help identify wave breaks and phase singularities in arrhythmia studies.

Representative results

Quantitative electrophysiological functional data can be investigated from optical mapping. In Figure 7.3, we show different studies done in heart preparations of different species. The left column (Figure 7.3A) shows action potential (AP) and calcium transient (CaT) signals from a single pixel recorded from mouse atrium and ventricle, respectively. APD of each pixel from the whole preparation can be calculated and displayed as a map. Such APD maps are shown as lower two panels

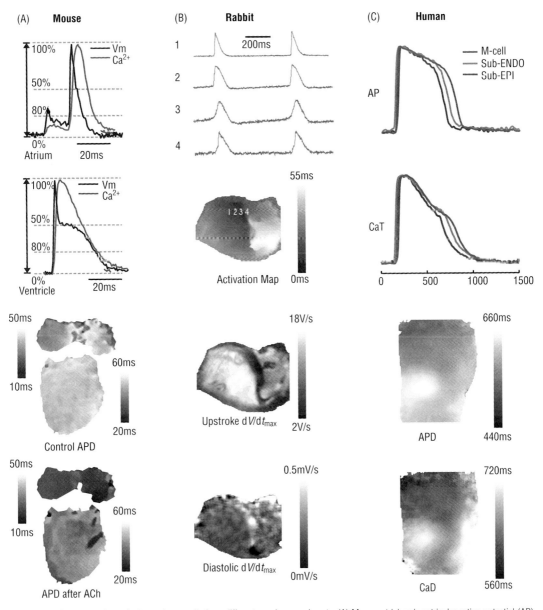

Figure 7.3 Representative optical mapping results from different species experiments. (A) Mouse: atrial and ventricular action potential (AP) and Ca transient (CaT) signals; APD shortening after ACh in *Pyk2-/-* mouse. (B) Rabbit: atrial AP signals from locations marked by 1–4 in the activation map; upstroke, diastolic slope characterization of whole atrium. (C) Human: AP and CaT signals from human left ventricle wedge preparation; M-cell detected from action potential duration (APD) and Ca duration (CaD) map. (Source: (A) Lang 2011 [6]. (B) Lang D 2011 [8]. Reproduced with permission of Springer. (C) Lou Q 2011 [9]. Reproduced with permission of Wolters Kluwer Health).

of the left column. One can appreciate significant APD shortening in both atria and ventricles of a *Pyk2*$^{-/-}$ mouse during ACh perfusion, which does not occur in wild type mouse ventricles. Electrophysiology study of pacemakers from rabbit right atrium preparation are shown in the middle column (Figure 7.3B). The raw optical APs recorded from four representative locations labeled in the lower figure are plotted. Different electrophysiology indicated by different morphology of the signals from atrium, subsinus node area, sinus node, and the block zone are shown. For each pixel, the time point of maximum derivative for the AP upstroke can be calculated. By plotting this time point, activation map that indicates the propagation pattern of AP is presented below. The upstroke dV/dt_{max} map indicates that sinus node cells have much slower rate of rise of their AP upstrokes as compared to the rest of the right atrium due to its calcium but not sodium dependence of activation. Higher diastolic dV/dt_{max} value in sinus node seen in the diastolic dV/dt_{max} map indicated the contribution of I_f current in phase 4. Simultaneous AP-CaT dual optical mapping on human left ventricle wedge preparation is shown in the right column (Figure 7.3C). The transmural heterogeneity can be investigated. In the APD and CaD map, a small region of cells with long APD is observed in subendocardium.

Figure 7.4 shows the representative results of a Langendorff-perfused rabbit experiment using the panoramic optical mapping system. In Figure 7.4 A we showed the anterior view of the rabbit heart. The rabbit heart geometry was reconstructed in the form of a 3D mesh-grid surface. The epicardial surface color-coded by the phase was unwrapped indicating the wavefront during an episode of tachyarrhythmia (Figure 7.4B). The optical action potential recordings from five locations around the phase singularity marked by 1–5 in panel B were plotted out showing different phases in Figure 7.4C. We plotted eight snapshots of activation wavefront propagation during a cycle of a stable re-entrant arrhythmia in Figure 7.4D. The wavefront circles clockwise around a phase singularity, which is visible at the anterior surface of the heart. The gray bar for repolarization (gray) is set to be partially transparent so that the posterior wavefront is visible.

Alternative approaches

Common alternative technologies for electrical mapping in the heart include: (1) microelectrodes, monophasic action potentials (MAPs), and (2) bipolar/ unipolar electrode arrays. Microelectrode recordings involve plunging a machine-pulled, glass capillary electrode into the myocardium to measure transmembrane potential. While microelectrode recordings represent a "gold-standard" technique for measuring action potentials, comparison of action potentials recorded with microelectrodes and optical techniques show excellent correlation [2]. MAPs are extracellularly recorded electrical signals that are also used to record transmembrane electrical activity using suction or contact electrodes. While both microelectrodes and MAPs provide local electrical activity, they are limited to a single location or sparse locations and cannot be used for high-resolution mapping. Multielectrode bipolar/ unipolar arrays have been successfully employed to improve spatial resolution and study spatial activation and repolarization patterns in healthy and arrhythmogenic substrates. However, extracellular electrograms do not directly represent transmembrane potential and are sometimes challenging to interpret, especially with respect to repolarization.

Weaknesses and strengths of method

Optical mapping techniques allow the measurement of electrophysiological parameters from multiple sites with high spatiotemporal resolution. Such visualization of action potential propagation revolutionizes the investigation of physiological (e.g. pacemaker activities) and pathological (e.g. arrhythmias) electrical activities in cardiac tissues. Although electrode arrays as mentioned earlier in the alternative methods section can also detect activation sequences, it is difficult to achieve the same degree of spatial resolution due to electrode size constraints. This may present difficulties in assessing the information of repolarization as well as interpreting complicated or imperceptible remodeling of electrical activities. The ability of optical mapping to report variation of membrane potentials by fluorescence also facilitates the studies of defibrillation, since electrical artifacts induced by shock

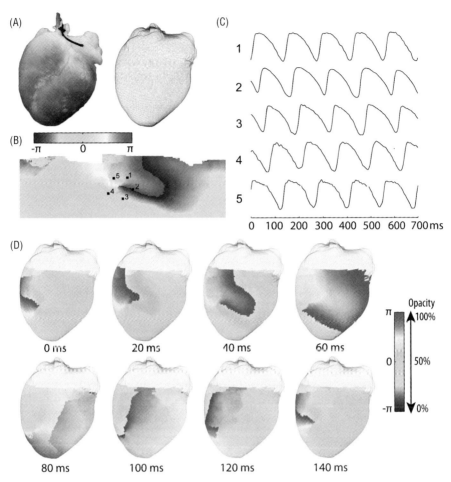

Figure 7.4 Representative results of rabbit experiment using the panoramic optical mapping system. (A) Anterior view and reconstructed geometry in the form of a three-dimensional mesh-grid surface. (B) Unwrapped epicardial surface gray scale-coded by the phase during an episode of tachyarrhythmia. (C) Recordings around the rotor marked by 1–5 in B. (D) Activation wavefront propagation during a cycle of a stable re-entrant arrhythmia. (Source: Lou Q 2011 [10]).

always invalidate recordings by conventional electrical measurement techniques. Simultaneous applications of other fluorescence indicators with voltage-sensitive dyes in optical mapping can uncover real-time dynamics and relevance of electrical activity to other factors, such as calcium and NADH.

However, there are several limitations of optical mapping with the current state of the technology. The need for fluorescent dye is the major limitation as it restricts *in vivo* application and could preclude the use of the technology in the clinic. Motion of either the preparation or detector relative can cause

large changes in optical signals. As described earlier, excitation–contraction uncouplers, such as blebbistatin, are wildly used in optical mapping experiments to mitigate motion artifact in optical recordings. This intervention makes it difficult to simultaneously study mechanics and electrical propagation and may have unwanted effects on the metabolic state of the heart. Although the spatial resolution can be very high, for large preparations like intact heart, a single pixel still detects the averaged fluorescence signal from thousands of cells. Additionally, the nature of fluorescent imaging may cause scattering, which should be considered during data interpretation. Perhaps the most significant limitation is that the excitation light does not penetrate deep inside the tissue preparations. This makes it difficult to interpret propagation in 3D space. Several groups are working on the creation of new dyes and creative lighting tricks to address this concern.

Conclusions

Optical mapping of fluorescent dyes in basic and translational cardiac research has increased exponentially in recent years – a trend likely to continue with emerging novel molecular probes and camera systems. The ability to describe electrical activity with high spatial and temporal resolution has made optical mapping techniques invaluable tools for investigations of normal and pathologic cardiac physiology. Here, we present a broad description of current state-of-the-art optical mapping techniques: experimental systems and protocols, processing techniques, and analysis methods. The methodology described herein is essential to any researcher involved in cardiac optical mapping studies and will hopefully aid in the development of novel therapeutic strategies for cardiac arrhythmias.

References

1 Salama G, Morad M. Merocyanine 540 as an optical probe of transmembrane electrical activity in the heart. *Science* 1976; **191**: 485–487.

2 Efimov IR, Nikolski VP, Salama G. Optical imaging of the heart. *Circ Res* 2004; **95**: 21–33.

3 Lou Q, Li W, Efimov IR. The role of dynamic instability and wavelength in arrhythmia maintenance as revealed by panoramic imaging with blebbistatin vs. 2,3-butanedione monoxime. *Am J Physiol Heart Circ Physiol* 2012; **302**: H262–269.

4 Bayly PV, KenKnight BH, Rogers JM, Hillsley RE, Ideker RE, Smith WM. Estimation of conduction velocity vector fields from epicardial mapping data. *IEEE Trans Biomed Eng* 1998; **45**: 563–571.

5 Bray MA, Lin SF, Aliev RR, Roth BJ, Wikswo JP, Jr. Experimental and theoretical analysis of phase singularity dynamics in cardiac tissue. *J Cardiovasc Electrophysiol* 2001; **12**: 716–722.

6 Lang D, Sulkin M, Lou Q, Efimov IR. Optical Mapping of Action Potentials and Calcium Transients in the Mouse Heart. *J. Vis Exp* 2011; (**55**): e3275.

7 Laughner JI, Sulkin MS, Wu Z, Deng CX, Efimov IR. Three potential Mechanisms for Failure of HIFU Ablation in Cardiac tissue. *Circ Arrhythm Electophysio.* 2012; **5**(2): 409–416.

8 Lang D, Petrov V, Lou Q, Osipov G, Efimov IR. Spatiotemporal control of heart rate in a rabbit heart. *J Electrocardio.* 2011; **44**(6): 626–634.

9 Lou Q, Federov VV, Glukov AV, Moazami N, Fast VG, Efimov IR. Transmural heterogeneity and remodelling of ventricular excitation-contraction coupling in human heart failure. *Circulation.* 2011; **123**(17): 1881–1890.

10 Lou Q, Li W, Efimov IR. Multiparametic Optical Mapping of the Langendorff-perfused Rabbit Heart. *J. Vis. Exp.* 2011 (**55**), e3160.

Part 2

Isolation and Maintenance of Primary Stem Cells

Isolation of colony-forming endothelial progenitor cells

Haruchika Masuda[1] and Takayuki Asahara[1,2]

[1] Tokai University School of Medicine, Isehara, Kanagawa, Japan
[2] Institute of Biomedical Research and Innovation, Kobe, Hyogo, Japan

Introduction

Circulating endothelial progenitor cell (EPC) are now regarded as subdivided into two categories, hematopoietic and nonhematopoietic lineage EPCs (after controversy during the decade following their initial isolation [1]), as there is no definitive delineation of EPCs, no clear differentiation hierarchy, or unambiguous defined isolation protocol. Hematopoietic EPCs (hEPCs) have been reported to originate from a provasculogenic subpopulation of hematopoietic stem cells (HSCs) in bone marrow (BM). hEPCs have been quantified and qualified as either circulating cell populations identified by cell surface markers such as CD34, CD133, and vascular endothelial growth factor receptor-2 (VEGFR-2) [2–11] or "colonies" [12], using conventional EPC culture methods to produce spindle adherent cells from peripheral blood (PB), BM, or umbilical cord blood (UCB) mononuclear cells (MNCs) with endothelial growth factors and cytokines. These assays using conventional EPC culture protocols were simple and satisfactory to speculate on the vasculogenic properties of EPC-enriched fractions, but have recently been criticized with respect to the quality and quantity of EPCs derived from primary cells. These assays further group heterogeneous EPCs into one qualitative category, "adhesive cultured EPCs," without any hierarchical discrimination and proper characterization of contaminating cell populations, which consist mainly of hematopoietic cells [13].

Ingram and Yoder *et al.* have demonstrated circulating endothelial differential stages, high and low proliferative potential endothelial colony-forming cells (HPP-ECFCs and LPP-ECFCs), using their original culture parameters, demonstrating clonal colony-forming units (CFUs) in outgrowth EPCs, cultured adhesive EPCs, or differentiated endothelial cells (ECs)[14,15]. This carefully conceived culture assay system, demonstrating thorough insight into stem cell biology, is contributing significantly to the development of EPC biology via the introduction of a differential hierarchy system for ECs. It is relevant to the isolation of CFUs from cultured adhesive cells of tissue-derived ECs or EPCs (i.e. nonhematopoietic EPCs) but it does not appear to address the identification of primary circulating EPCs from PB, BM, or UCB (i.e. hEPCs). In response to the need for a defined assay to detect hEPCs qualitatively and quantitatively from primary blood samples, we have developed a new colony assay system.

Our methodology utilizes the conventional methylcellulose assay used for stem/ progenitor cell identification, and is modified to resemble the previously developed semisolid colony assay system for the determination of EPC-CFUs [16–18]. As we

Manual of Research Techniques in Cardiovascular Medicine, First Edition. Edited by Hossein Ardehali, Roberto Bolli, and Douglas W. Losordo.
© 2014 John Wiley & Sons, Ltd. Published 2014 by John Wiley & Sons, Ltd.

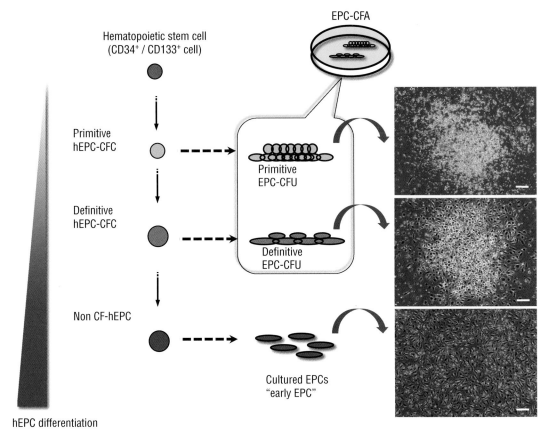

hEPC differentiation

Figure 8.1 The concept of EPC-CFA to assess the hEPC differentiation cascade.
hEPCs originate from HSCs. During hEPC differentiation, hEPCs lose their colony-forming potential and become vasculogenic. Based on this, hEPCs exhibit individual colony-forming features: primitive EPC-CFUs or definitive EPC-CFUs, which are morphologically defined as small round colony cells or spindle-like colony cells. These are provasculogenic or vasculogenic, respectively, thereby providing the characteristic to estimate the proportion of colonies with vasculogenic potential of the investigated cell populations. HSC, hematopoietic stem cell; hEPC-CFC, hematopoietic EPC colony-forming cell; non CF-EPC, noncolony-forming EPC. The upper, middle, and lower pictures indicate primitive EPC-CFUs, definitive EPC-CFUs, or cultured EPCs, respectively. Scale bar = 200 μm. (Source: Masuda H. 2013 [2]. Reproduced with permission from Elsevier).

have recently reported, the present assay system differentiates the two types of EPC-CFUs, morphologically identified by the respective colony cells with the features of small (10–20 μm) round cells and large (50–200 μm) spindle-like cells [19,20]. The smaller colony cells with proliferative capability, in secondary semisolid colony assay system, convert into the latter larger spindle-shaped cells with vasculogenic property. Thus this assay defines EPC colonies as *primitive EPC-CFU (PEPC-CFU)* and *definitive EPC-CFU (DEPC-CFU)*. The essential findings provide a novel and fundamental concept of the EPC colony-forming assay (EPC-CFA) to

quantitatively assess each colony in terms of the hEPC differentiation cascade (Figure 8.1, Table 8.1).

The advantage of this semisolid colony assay lies in its ability to estimate the number of immature progenitors that will go on to form colony units from a single cell and the possibility to assess the differential quality of colonies without any contamination by differentiated cells. Furthermore, we devised a semisolid media condition capable of evaluating the adhesive potential of endothelial lineage colonies.

The methodological concepts of hEPC biology were examined using: (1) EPC-CFU analysis of

Table 8.1 Functional characteristics of hEPC colonies in hEPC differentiation

	Primitive EPC CFU (PEPC-CFU)	Definitive EPC-CFU (DEPC-CFU)
Colony-forming cell features	Weakly adhesive round cells (10–20 μm)	Strongly adhesive spindle-like cells with monolayer structure (50–200 μm)
Cell density per colony	High	Low
2nd colony-forming potential	High	Low~ Absence
Gene expression:		
CD31	Low	High
VEGFR-2,VE-Cad, eNOS, Tie2, vWF	Low	High
CD45, CD14 immunocytochemistry:		
VEGFR-2, VE-Cad, eNOS	Yes	Yes
acLDL-Dil uptake and	Yes	Yes
UEA1 lectin-FITC binding		
Angiogenic/ vasculogenic activity:		
Proliferation	Dominant	
Adhesion		Dominant
Tube formation promotion		Dominant
Sprouting activity		Dominant
In vivo vascular regeneration		Dominant

Low, High, and Dominant indicates the comparison between PEPC-CFU and DEPC-CFU. Yes indicates the positive feature in each item of immunocytochemistry.

single cells or bulk cells from hEPC-enriched, arbitrary fractions, their cultured cells or nonselected populations; and (2) cell fate analysis of single cells or bulk cells following suspension conditions. Our newly introduced analytical system clarifies the cell fate of each sample cell, reviews the differentiation hierarchy of hEPCs, and identifies the determinants of hEPC proliferation, commitment, and differentiation *in vitro* and *in vivo* (Figure 8.2). In this chapter, we present a step by step protocol for the hEPC-CFA of isolated cell populations from UCB, PB, or BM.

Materials

Laboratory reagents

1. Cells: The experimental protocol of fresh PB, UCB, or BM should be performed under the approval of the institutional ethical committees of the Cord Blood and/or Clinical Investigation Committee.

Alternatively, isolated MNCs, CD34⁺, or CD133⁺cells in UCB, PB, or BM can be purchased (e.g. ALLCELLS™: http://www.allcells.com).

All blood samples should be handled under the biological guideline for human samples. Investigators should work with a class 2 safety cabinet, and wear gloves and other personal protective clothing, which should be disinfected with bleach before being discarded.

2. MethoMethoCult™ GF⁺H4435 (Stem Cell Tec, cat. no. 04435)

3. Iscove's Modified Dulbecco's Medium (IMDM) (Invitrogen, cat. no. 31980-030)

4. BSA (Sigma-Aldrich, cat. no. A4503)

5. PBS without calcium and magnesium (Sigma-Aldrich, cat. no.P4417-100TB)

6. 0.5 M EDTA solution (Nacalai Tesque, cat. no.14362-24)

7. 0.05% (wt/vol) Trypsin/ 0.2% (wt/vol) EDTA ·4Na solution (Sigma-Aldrich, cat. no. T3924)

8. Ammonium chloride, NH₄Cl (Wako Pure Chemical Industries Ltd., cat. no. 017-02995)

9. Potassium bicarbonate, KHCO₃ (Wako Pure Chemical Industries Ltd., cat. no.166-03275)

10. EDTA-2Na (Wako Pure Chemical Industries, Ltd., cat. no. 345-01865)

11. Histopaque-1077 (Sigma-Adrich, cat. no. 10771)

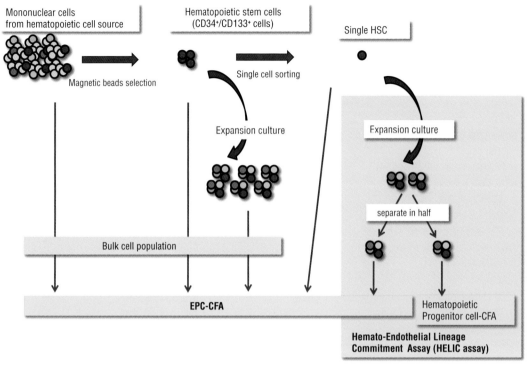

Figure 8.2 Application of EPC-CFA for primary or expansion cultured cell populations.
EPC-CFA is applicable to primary or expansion cultured cells, not only for bulk non-selected MNCs or selected CD34+/CD133+ cells, but also for single selected CD34+/CD133+ cells. In particular, the hematoendothelial lineage commitment assay (HELIC assay), which is applicable to EPC-CFA, uses single hematopoietic stem cells to analyze their commitment into hematopoietic and/or endothelial lineages. In brief, EPC-CFA and a conventional hematopoietic progenitor cell-CFA can be performed by using half of the expanded cells from a single hematopoietic stem cell. Subsequently, the cell fate of the single stem cells into endothelial and/or hematopoietic cell lineages can be quantitatively evaluated by analyzing the frequency of the stem cells generating EPC-CFUs in EPC-CFA and/or hematopoietic lineage-CFUs (e.g. erythrocyte-CFU, granulocyte/ macrophage-CFU, monocyte/ macrophage-CFU) in hematopoietic progenitor cell-CFA. (Source: Masuda H. 2013 [2]. Reproduced with permission from Elsevier).

12. CD34 MicroBead Kit (Miltenyi Biotec., cat. no. 130-046-702)

13. CD133 MicroBead Kit (Miltenyi Biotec., cat. no. 130-050-801)

14. Cellbanker (Nippon Zenyaku Kogyo Co., Ltd., cat. no. BLC-1)

15. Reagents of semisolid culture medium for EPC-CFA (Table 8.2)

16. Reagents for expansion culture (EX-culture), and hematoendothelial lineage commitment (HELIC) assay (Table 8.3)

17. $CaCl_2 \cdot 2H_2O$ (Wako Pure Chemical Industries, Ltd, cat. no. 031-00435)

Laboratory equipment

1. Culture dishes or plates (Table 8.4)

2. Polypropylene conical tubes, 15 mL (TPP, cat. no. 91015)

3. Polypropylene conical tubes, 50 mL (TPP, cat. no. 91050)

4. Screw-cap sampling tubes, 1.5 mL (Assist, cat. no. A.1500)

5. 14-mL polypropylene round-bottom tubes (BD falcon, 352059)

6. CryoTube™ vials (Nunc, cat. no. 366656)

7. Bio freezing vessels, Bicell (Nihon Freezer Co., Ltd.)

Table 8.2 Reagents for semisolid master mixture for EPC-CFA

Reagents	Company, Cat. no.	Final concentration
MethoCult™ SF^BIT H4236	Stem Cell Tec, 04236	
rhSCF	Peprotec, 300-07	100 ng/mL
rhVEGF	Peprotec, 100-20	50 ng/mL
rhbFGF	Peprotec, 100-18B	50 ng/mL
rhEGF	Peprotec, 100-15	50 ng/mL
rhIGF-1	Peprotec, 100-11	50 ng/mL
rhIL-3	Peprotec, 200-03	20 ng/mL
Heparin	Ajinomoto Pharma, 699053417	2 U/mL
FBS	SAFC Biosciences, 12303	30% (vol/vol)
Penicillin/ streptomycin	Invitrogen, 5140-122	1/100 (vol/vol)

rhbFGF, recombinant human basic fibroblast growth factor; rhEGF, recombinant human epidermal growth factor; rhIGF-1, recombinant human insulin like growth factor-1; rhIL-3, recombinant human interleukin-3; rhSCF, recombinant human stem cell factor; rhVEGF, recombinant human vascular endothelial growth factor.

Table 8.3 Reagents of EX-culture medium

Reagents	Company, Cat no.	Final concentration
Stem Span™ SFEM	Stem Cell Tec, 09650	
rhSCF	Peprotec, 300-07	100 ng/mL
rhFlt-3 ligand	Peprotec, 300-19	100 ng/mL
rhTPO	Peprotec, 300-18	20 ng/mL
rhVEGF	Peprotec, 100-20	50 ng/mL
rhIL-6	Peprotec, 200-06	20 ng/mL
Penicillin/ streptomycin	Invitrogen, 5140-122	1/100 (vol/vol)

rhFlt-3 ligand, recombinant human FMS-like tyrosine kinase 3 ligand; rhIL-6, recombinant human interleukin-6; rhSCF, recombinant human stem cell factor; rhTPO, recombinant human thrombopoietin; rhVEGF, recombinant human vascular endothelial growth factor; SFEM, serum-free expansion medium.

Table 8.4 Materials for EX-culture, EPC-CFA, and HELIC assay

Culture vessels	Company, Cat. no.	Application
35-mm Primaria™ tissue culture dish	BD Falcon, 353801	EPC-CFA of bulk cells
96-well Primaria™ tissue culture plate	BD Falcon, 353872	EPC-CFA of single cells, EX-culture of HELIC assay
24-well Primaria™ tissue culture plate	BD Falcon, 353847	EX-culture of bulk cells, EPC-CFA of HELIC assay
24-well suspension culture plate	Greiner, 662102	HPC-CFA of HELIC assay
18-gauge blunt end needle	NIPRO, 02-161	Seeding cells for EPC-CFA or HPC-CFA
Gridded scoring dish	Stem Cell Tec., 27500	Counting EPC-CFUs or SAU
14-mL Polypropylene round-bottom tube	BD Falcon, 352059	Storage of semisolid medium for EPC-CFA or HPC-CFA

8. Polystyrene microcentrifuge tube with plug cap, 1 mL for fluorescence-activated cell sorting (FACS) (Fisher Scientific, cat. no. 04-978-145)

9. 20-μL pipette tip (MbP, cat. no. 2069)

10. 200-μL pipette tip (MbP, cat. no. 2069)

11. 1000-μL pipette tip (MbP, cat. no. 2079E)

12. 20-μL pipette (Gilson, cat. no. F123600)

13. 200-μL pipette (Gilson, cat. no. F123601)

14. 1000-μL pipette (Gilson, cat. no. F123602)

15. Tuberculin syringe, 1 mL (Terumo, cat. no. SS-01T)

16. Syringe, 5 mL (Terumo, cat. no. SS-05LZ)

17. Syringe, 20 mL (Terumo, cat. no. SS–20ESZ)

18. Syringe, 50 mL (Terumo, cat. no. SS–50ESZ)

19. 2-gauge winged infusion set (Terumo, cat. no. SV-21DLK)

20. 23-gauge winged infusion set (Terumo, cat. no. SV-23DLK)

21. 18-gauge needle (Terumo, cat. no. NN-1838R)

22. Bottle top vacuum filtration system (Iwaki, cat. no. 11-067-008)

23. Disposable Pasteur pipette, 9 inch (Iwaki, cat. no. IK-PAS-9P)

24. Centrifuge (Hitachi, cat. no. Himac CF 8DL) for 15-mL or 50-mL conical tube

25. Centrifuge (Tomy, cat. no. MX-160) for 1.5-mL screw-cap tube

26. Vacuum pump for negative-pressure filtration or aspiration (ULVAC, cat. no. DAP-15)

27. Parafilm (Hitech Inc., cat. no. F-20001)

28. Cell filtration column of 30-μm nylon mesh (Consul, cat. no. 130-33S)

29. Polystyrene tubes (BD Falcon, cat. no. 352008)

30. Cell strainer capped polystyrene tube (BD Falcon, cat. no. 352235)

31. Vortex-Genie 2 (M&S Instruments Inc.)

32. Phase-contrast light microscope (Eclipse TE300, Nikon)

33. Fluorescent microscopy (IX70, Olympus)

34. autoMACS™ Separator (Miltenyi Biotec.)

35. FACSAria™ cell sorter(BD)

36. LSRFortessa™ cell analyzer (BD)

Methods

MNC isolation from fresh PB or UCB
Preparation of working solution

1. Ammonium chloride solution (0.15 M NH_4Cl) for hemolysis:

a. Measure 8.26 g NH_4Cl, 1.0 g $KHCO_3$, and 0.037 g EDTA-2Na.

b. Dissolve together in 1000 mL of sterilized MilliQ water.

c. Adjust the solution to pH 7.3 and store at 4°C after autoclave and cooling down.

2. PBS:

a. Dissolve one PBS tablet in 1000 mL MilliQ water.

b. Adjust to pH 7.4, and store at 4°C after autoclaving and cooling down.

3. PBS/ 2 mM EDTA: Add 0.5 M EDTA solution to autoclaved PBS (pH 7.4) at the ratio of 1:250 (vol/vol).

4. 10% (w/vol) BSA/PBS:

a. Measure 50 g of BSA and dissolve in 500 mL PBS.

b. Sterilize by filtration through bottle top vacuum filtration system with a vacuum pump.

c. Aliquot and store at −20°C until use.

For preparation of 0.1% BSA/PBS, dilute 10% BSA/PBS solution with PBS at the ratio of 1:100 (w/vol) prior to use.

5. MACS™ buffer: Adjust 2 mM EDTA/ 0.5% BSA/ PBS solution, sterilize by filtration through bottle top vacuum filtration system with a vacuum pump and store at 4°C until use.

Procedure
Guideline. Depending on an experimental design, the required PB volume will vary, e.g. 10 mL for EPC-CFA alone or more than 50 mL for isolation of CD34+/CD133+ cells. The protocol described here is for the isolation of CD34+ or CD133+ cells as a large-scale experiment, requiring 15 mL of Histopaque-1077 per 50-mL conical tube. The small-scale protocol for EPC-CFA alone requires 5 mL of Histopaque-1077 per 15-mL conical tube. In the case of UCB, use the large-scale protocol.

1. Prepare at room temperature (RT) 15 mL of Histopaque-1077 per 50-mL conical tube.

2. Gently layer 30 mL of PB or UCB on 15 mL Histopaque-1077 in a 50-mL conical tube.

3. Centrifuge at 400 g at RT for 30 minutes without acceleration and with low deceleration.

4. Confirm a clear white monolayer.

Tips. Blood samples and Histopaque-1077 should be preincubated at RT (15°C to 25°C) to form a clear monolayer of MNCs and acquire sufficient MNC numbers. Note that a blurred white monolayer will yield insufficient MNCs.

5. Aspirate upper a plasma layer with a 9-inch sterilized Pasteur pipette attached to a vacuum pump.

Tip. Leave an upper plasma layer to 1 cm above the visible white monolayer containing MNCs to avoid the aspiration of MNCs.

6. Carefully transfer the entire layer of MNCs to 50-mL conical tube with a 1000-μL pipette.

Tip. Thoroughly harvest the part of the monolayer attached to the inside wall of the conical tube to isolate as many MNCs as possible.

7. Completely resuspend the harvested MNC suspension to 15 mL with 2 mM EDTA/PBS solution.
8. Centrifuge at 850 g at 4°C for 20 minutes.
9. Aspirate the supernatant with a sterilized Pasteur pipette attached to a vacuum pump.
10. Warm NH$_4$Cl solution at 37°C in advance.
11. Add 5 mL of 0.15 M NH$_4$Cl solution to lyse erythrocytes, resuspend the cell pellet completely and incubate at 37°C for 7 minutes.

Tip. If a large number of erythrocytes seem to be contaminated in advance, add NH$_4$Cl solution up to half of the maximal volume in tube and incubate at 37°C for 7 minutes.

12. Fill up to maximal volume with 2 mM EDTA/PBS solution.
13. Centrifuge at 320 g, 4°C for 10 minutes.
14. Carefully aspirate the supernatant until the cell pellet alone remains; then completely resuspend the cell pellets with 1 mL of 2 mM EDTA/PBS solution.
15. Fill up to maximal volume with 2 mM EDTA/PBS solution.
16. Centrifuge at 200 g, 4°C for 10 minutes.
17. Carefully aspirate the supernatant until the cell pellet alone remains, and resuspend MNCs completely with 2 mL of either working medium for EPC-CFA or MACS™ buffer for isolation of CD34$^+$ or CD133$^+$ cells by AutoMACS™.
18. Count the suspended MNCs for downstream application.
19. When performing EPC-CFA of PBMNCs, suspend the cell pellet with 30% FBS/ IMDM at 2×10^5 cells /100 μL per dish for three dishes.
20. Isolate CD34$^+$ or CD133$^+$ cells by using commercially available antibody-coated beads (CD34 MicroBead Kit, CD133 MicroBead Kit from Miltenyi Biotec).
21. Evaluate the purities of the positive cells by flow cytometry (e.g. LSRFortessa™ cell analyzer (BD)). The antibodies for evaluation should be different clones from the ones for cell isolation. The example antibody clones are listed in Table 8.5.

Tips. Freshly isolated CD34$^+$ or CD133$^+$ cells may be cryopreserved until use. We usually cryopreserve

Table 8.5 Antibodies for confirmation of selected CD34$^+$/CD133$^+$ cells

Antibodies etc.	Clone	Isotype	Company, Cat. no.
CD34-FITC	581	Mouse IgG1	BD Biosciences, 555821
CD34-FITC	AC136	Mouse IgG2a	Miltenyi Biotec, 130-081-001
CD133/1-PE	AC133	Mouse IgG1	Miltenyi Biotec, 130-080-801
CD133/1-APC	AC133	Mouse IgG1	Miltenyi Biotec, 130-090-826
CD133/2-PE	293C3	Mouse IgG2b	Miltenyi Biotec, 130-090-853
CD133/2-APC	293C3	Mouse IgG2b	Miltenyi Biotec, 130-090-854
Mouse IgG1-FITC	A851	Mouse IgG1	BD Biosciences, 555748
Mouse IgG2a-FITC	S43.10	Mouse IgG2a	Miltenyi Biotec, 130-091-837
Mouse IgG1-PE	IS5-21F5	Mouse IgG1	Miltenyi Biotec, 130-092-212
Mouse IgG1-APC	IS5-21F5	Mouse IgG1	Miltenyi Biotec, 130-092-214
Mouse IgG2b-PE	ISE6-11E5.11	Mouse IgG2b	Miltenyi Biotec, 130-092-215
Mouse IgG2b-APC	ISE6-11E5.11	Mouse IgG2b	Miltenyi Biotec, 130-092-217

fractionated cells to detach the antibody coated MicroBeads before use. When using cryopreserved CD34⁺ or CD133⁺ cells after isolation, the same isotype antibody as coated on MicroBeads (QBEND/10 or AC133) are also available for the subsequent applications (e.g. cell sorting or EX-culture).

EPC-CFA of bulk cell populations in PB, GmPB, BM, or UCB

Preparation of working medium

1. EPC-CFA working semisolid medium

   a. Reconstitute and aliquot each growth factor/ cytokine solution (Table 8.2) according to the manufacturer's data sheets, then store at −20°C until use. Aliquot and store FBS at −20°C until use.

   b. One day prior to adjustment of EPC-CFA working medium, defrost one bottle of MethoCult™ SF^{BIT} H4236 (80 mL).

   c. Add each aliquot of growth factor/ cytokine, FBS, and penicillin/ streptomycin to the bottle; thoroughly mix the whole solution by vigorously shaking the master mix (Table 8.2).

   d. Place the bottle for 20 minutes at RT to eliminate small air bubbles appearing in the mixed solution.

   e. Aliquot 2 mL semisolid solution into each 14-mL Polypropylene round-bottom tubes with a 5-mL syringe attached to a blunt-end needle.

   f. Add 1 mL of 30% (vol /vol) FBS/IMDM with a 1000-μL pipette, and seal the lid with Parafilm to avoid volume loss by evaporation, then store at −20°C until use. The final volume of 3 mL EPC-CFA working medium should be prepared for three dishes of 35-mm Primaria™ Tissue culture dishes (BD Falcon, Cat. no. 353801) per group.

2. EX-culture medium

   a. Dissolve 500 mL of Stem Span™ serum-free expansion medium (SFEM) in one bottle at 4°C over night.

   b. Aliquot 20 mL each of Stem Span SFEM per 50-mL conical tube, and store at −20°C until further use.

   c. After melting in a water bath at 37°C, adjust EX-culture medium by mixing each aliquot of growth factor /cytokine (Table 8.3).

3. Hematopoietic progenitor cell CFA (HPC-CFA) working semisolid medium for HPC-CFA or HELIC assay (optional)

   a. Dissolve one bottle of MethoMethoCult™ GF⁺H4435.

   b. Aliquot 3 mL into each 14-mL polypropylene round-bottom tube and store at −20°C until use.

Preparation of cell suspension of bulk cell populations

1. Primary cell populations in PB, GmPB, BM, or UCB: Suspend the freshly isolated or cryopreserved bulk cells (MNCs, CD34⁺, or CD133⁺ cells) with 30% FBS/IMDM at the relevant cell number/100 μL per dish, for three dishes, in a 1.5-mL screw-cap sampling tube.

Tip. Note that EPC-CFA is irrelevant for the vasculogenic evaluation of BMMNCs, due to the interference of EPC-colony formation by the growth of contaminated BM stromal cells (Figure 8.3E).

2. EX-cultured CD34⁺ or CD133⁺ cells

   a. Adjust the suspension of CD34⁺ or CD133⁺ cells with EX-culture medium (1 × 10⁴ cells/500 μL) for EX-culture (Table 8.3).

   b. Seed 500 μL per well of a 24-well Primaria™ tissue culture plate (BD Falcon, Cat. no. 353847), and EX-culture for 7 days.

   c. Harvest EX-cultured cells and adjust the cell suspension with 30% FBS/IMDM at the relevant cell number /100 μL per dish, for three dishes, in a 1.5-mL screw-cap sampling tube.

Tips. The last medium or buffer suspending the cells should be completely replaced with 30% FBS/ IMDM for EPC-CFA, and not with the other solution, e.g. PBS or the different % FBS/IMDM. Replacement with a different medium or buffer interferes with the optimal growth of EPC-CFUs. Prepare more than the 300 μL of the whole cell suspension volume required for the three dishes per sample or group; we usually prepare 350 μL or more for safety.

Semisolid culture for EPC colony formation in EPC-CFA

1. Add 300 μL of the adjusted cell suspension (as in section Preparation of cell suspension of bulk cell

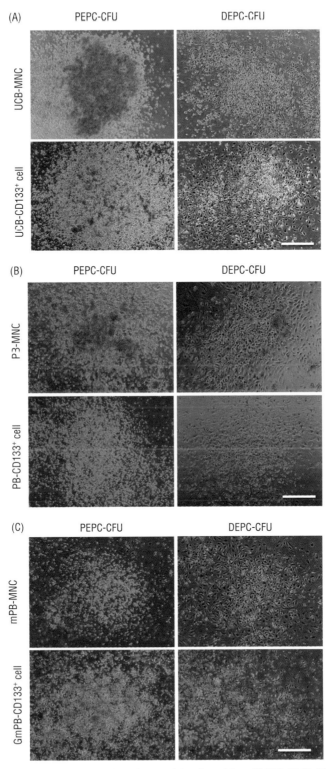

Figure 8.3 The features of EPC-CFUs generated from primary hematopoietic cell populations: (A) UCB, (B) PB, (C) GmPB, (D) BM, (E) stromal cells in EPC-CFA of BM-MNC. Scale bar = 500 μm. (Source: Masuda H 2011 [19]. Reproduced with permission from Wolters Kluwer Health).

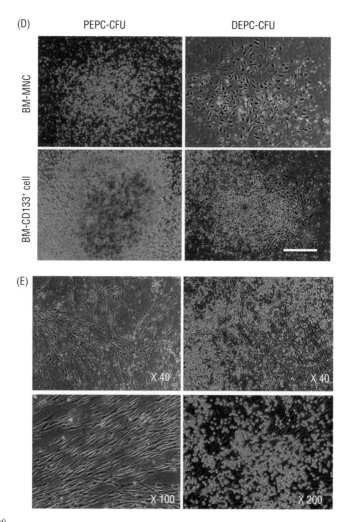

Figure 8.3 (*Continued*)

populations) into 3 mL of EPC-CFA working medium in a polypropylene round-bottom tube.

2. Vortex the tubes for 10 seconds and leave at RT for 10 minutes to eliminate small air bubbles in the medium.

3. Seed 1 mL of the semisolid cell suspension per dish into three 35-mm Primaria™ tissue culture dishes.

Tip. When seeding, pipette up and down the semisolid cell suspension three times in the tube with a 1-mL tuberculin syringe attached to a 18-gauge blunt-end needle, carefully avoiding the generation of small air bubbles.

4. Set a maximum of six semisolid culture dishes into a 15-cm nontreated culture dish as a container

and put in the center a 6-cm tissue culture dish with 5 mL of sterilized MilliQ water for humidification, and close the lid of the 15-mL tissue culture dish.

5. Culture at 37°C in CO_2 incubator until the EPC-CFU measurement. Assay plates should be kept in the CO_2 incubator until immediately before observation under microscope.

Tips. (1) When observing the growth of EPC-CFU through the culture period, handle the dishes gently to avoid scattering the colony cells. They are still nonadhesive or lightly adhesive at early time points. Otherwise, it may produce irregular-shaped EPC-CFUs with nondistinct foci, e.g. EPC-CFUs fused with nearby ones or elongated, which makes it difficult to count the exact number of EPC-CFU. (2)

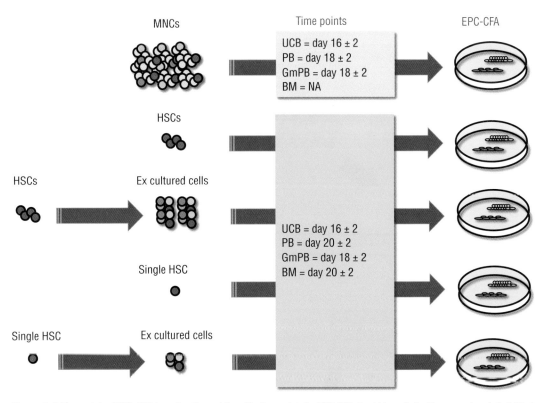

Figure 8.4 Time points of EPC-CFA in each cell population. The time points for EPC-CFA should be optimized by researchers in individual laboratories. The optimized time points necessary for EPC-CFA in our laboratory are shown in this figure. NA, not available.

Culture periods until counting EPC-CFUs are different among the cell populations (Figure 8.4).

Step by step counting procedure of EPC-CFU under phase-contrast microscopy

1. Check the color of the semisolid medium megascopically to assess the growth of EPC-CFU. In case of reddish medium, the growth of EPC-CFUs may be poor. On the other hand, when the medium is yellowish, the growth of EPC-CFUs, especially PEPC-CFUs, may be excellent.

Tips. (1) Note that when seeding MNCs, the growth of noncolony-forming EPCs with spindle-like shape or other hematopoietic colonies may also make the medium yellowish. (2) PEPC-CFUs with highly proliferative cells may be frequently observed as white spot colonies even by the naked eye.

2. Under phase-contrast light microscopy, identify adhesive cell colonies spreading two-dimensionally on the bottom of dish. This discriminates the EPC-CFUs units from the other hematological colonies, which do not adhere to the bottom of the dish.

3. Detect individual EPC-CFUs with a cell density of more than 100 cells per colony.

4. Identify the focus of each EPC-CFU, which is the origin of EPC-CFU. When counting the colonies whose growth is partly limited by the edge of dish, detect the border between colonies to their neighbors to distinguish them from each other and count each as an individual colony.

5. Define the identified colonies as either PEPC-CFU or DEPC-CFU, based on the morphological characteristics depicted in Figure 8.3 and Table 8.1.

6. Count the number of PEPC-CFU and DEPC-CFU per dish.

7. Evaluate the quantification and differentiation of EPC-CFC, as described in Figure 8.5.

Tips. (1) See Figure 8.4 to set the time points for counting the number of EPC-CFUs. (2) In the

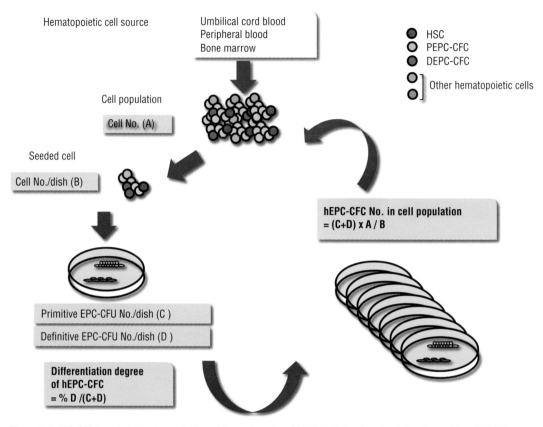

Figure 8.5 EPC-CFA to evaluate the degree of differentiation and number of hEPC-CFCs in a hematopoietic cell population. EPC-CFA allows us to evaluate the differentiation degree and number of hEPC-CFCs in a cell population from hematopoietic cell sources. When performing EPC-CFA, the cell number (A) and seeded cell number per dish (B) of the cell population are first determined. Using the counted numbers of primitive and definitive EPC-CFUs/dish (C and D), the differentiation degree is calculated as the percentage ratio of D to total EPC-CFUs (C + D). Further, total hEPC-CFCs in the whole cell population are simply estimated by the equation (C + D) × A/B. (Source: Masuda H 2013 [20]. Reproduced with permission from Elsevier).

preliminary trials, researchers should optimize the EPC-CFU number generated from each target population by dose-escalation studies in their own laboratories. The results of dose-escalation studies in our laboratory are shown in Figure 8.6.

Optional-1: EPC-CFA of single CD34⁺ or CD133⁺ cells in PB, GmPB, BM, or UCB

1. Prepare CD34⁺ or CD133⁺ cell suspension in 30% FBS/IMDM (e.g. 1×10^5 cells/mL) and leave on ice until sorting.
2. Apply 100 µL of EPC-CFA working semisolid medium per well of a 96-well Primaria™ tissue culture plate (BD Falcon, Cat. no. 353872).

3. Sort a single CD34⁺ or CD133⁺ cell into each well by cell sorter (e.g. FACSAria™ cell sorter(BD)), after staining the cell population with their surface antibodies listed in Table 8.5.
4. Perform EPC-CFA according to the procedure in section Semisolid culture for EPC colony formation in EPC-CFA and section Step by step counting procedure of EPC-CFU under phase-contrast microscopy.

Optional-2: HELIC assay of single CD34⁺ or CD133⁺ cells as cell fate assay of HSC

1. Prepare CD34⁺ or CD133⁺ cell suspension in EX-culture medium (e.g. 1×10^5 cells/mL) and leave on ice until sorting.

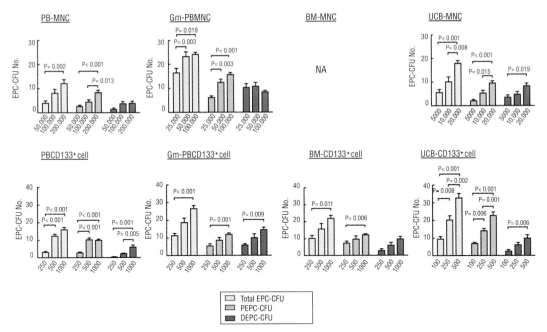

Figure 8.6 Methodological evaluation of EPC-CFA in primary cell populations of hematopoietic samples (PB, mPB, BM, UCB). The bar graphs represent values for each EPC-CFU number in MNC and CD133+ cell with the corresponding seeded primary cell number indicated on the x-axis. Data are means ± SEM. n = 9 per cell population. NA, not available. (Source: Masuda H 2011 [19]. Reproduced with permission from Wolters Kluwer Health).

2. Apply 100 μL of EX-culture medium per well of a 96-well Primaria™ tissue culture plate.

3. Sort a single CD34+ or CD133+ cell into each well by cell sorter (e.g. FACSAria™ cell sorter (BD)), after staining the cell population with their surface antibodies listed in Table 8.5.

4. EX-culture to expand sorted single cells at 37°C for 7 days in a CO_2 incubator.

5. Confirm that only one cell is sorted into each well under phase-contrast light microscopy 12–16 hours after sorting.

6. Count EX-cultured cell number per well at day 7 (optional).

Tip. To save time when counting at day 7, confirm the wells with EX-cultured cells in advance at day 6.

7. Prepare tissue culture plates for HELIC assay. Apply 300 μL of EPC-CFA working medium per well of Primaria™ 24-well plates for EPC-CFA. Simultaneously, apply 300 μL of MethoCult™ H4435 into wells of 24-well suspension culture plates (Greiner, Cat. no. 662102) for HPC-CFA.

8. Gently mix EX-cultured cell suspensions in each well of 96-well Primaria™ tissue culture plates with a 200 μl pipette three times.

9. Reseed half of the suspension (50 μL) into 300 μL of EPC-CFA working medium per well and the another half (50 μL) into 300 μL of MethoCult™ H4435 per well.

Tip. When mixing EX-cultured cell suspension, avoid making air bubbles to disturb the exact pipetting.

10. Culture the separated EX-cultured cells for EPC-CFA and HPC-CFA at 37°C in a CO_2 incubator.

Tips. To maintain appropriate humidity level, apply 1 mL of sterilized MilliQ water into each of the four wells located at the corner of both plates. Also, the spaces among wells should be filled with sterilized MilliQ water in both kinds of plates for EPC-CFA and HPC-CFA. Thus, 20 wells per plate are available for HELIC assay.

11. Count the colony numbers of colony-forming unit–erythroid (CFU-E), burst forming unit–erythroid (BFU-E), CFU–granulocyte/ macrophage

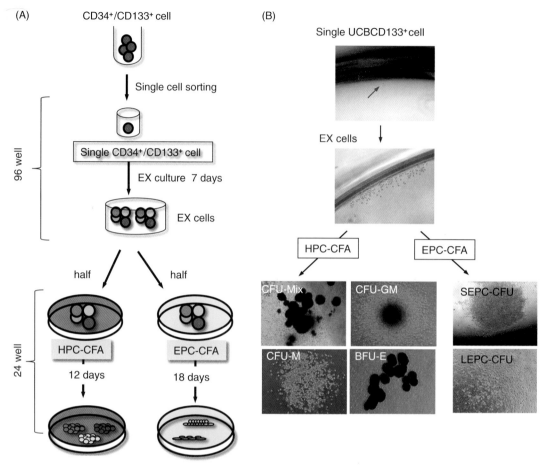

Figure 8.7 HELIC assay for single cell fate determination of the hematoendothelial lineage. (A) The schematic protocol of the HELIC assay, combining EPC-CFA with HPC-CFA for each half of the EX-cultured cells from single HSC (CD34+/CD133+ cell). (B) Representative cells and colonies at each step of the HELIC assay (×10 high power field (HPF)). BFU-E, burst forming unit erythroid; CFU-GM, CFU-granulocyte/ macrophage; CFU-M, CFU-macrophage; CFU-Mix, CFU-granulocyte/ erythrocyte/ monocyte/ macrophage. (Source: Masuda H 2011 [19]. Reproduced with permission from Wolters Kluwer Health).

(CFU-GM), CFU– macrophage (CFU-M), and/or CFU–granulocyte/ erythrocyte/ monocyte/ macrophage (mixed) per well at 12–14 days for HPC-CFA.

12. Count the colony numbers of PEPC-CFUs and/ or DEPC-CFUs per well at 14–18 days for EPC-CFA. The whole procedure and example data of a HELIC assay are shown in Figures 8.7 and 8.8.

Application

EPC-CFA provides the methodology for accurate research into basic scientific or clinical EPC biology. The applications include the following.

1. Basic research:
   a. evaluation of the effect of target factors on EPC expansion and/or differentiation
   growth factors, cytokines, hormones, cell signaling regulators, etc.;
   b. clarification of the EPC differentiation cascade;
   c. cell fate analysis of HSC in hematopoiesis and vasculogenesis.

2. Clinical research:
   a. evaluation of pathophysiology in cardio-vascular diseases etc. in terms of EPC biology;
   b. evaluation of vascular regenerative potential of cell sources for cell-based therapy.

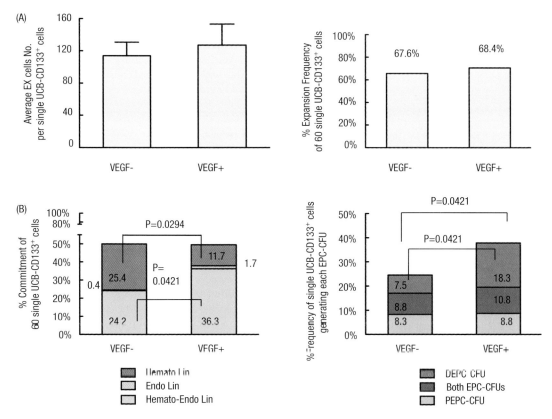

Figure 8.8 Example of an HELIC assay using UCB-CD133⁺ cells. (A) Left graph: Representative cell numbers per EX-cultured single UCB-CD133⁺ cell. Right graph: Percentage frequencies of EX-cultured cells from single UCB-CD133⁺ cells. (B) Left graph: Percentage commitment ratios of single UCB-CD133⁺ cells into hematopoietic (Hemato Lin), endothelial (Endo Lin), and both lineages (Hemato-Endo Lin). Percentage commitment frequency into Hemato Lin was estimated by counting single UCB-133 cells producing any colonies of BFU-E, CFU-GM, CFU-M and/or CFU-Mix. Right graph: Percentage frequencies of PEPC-CFUs and/or DEPC-CFUs in single UCB-CD133⁺ cells. Data are mean ± SEM (A left) or mean alone (A right, B); n = 4–6. (Source: Masuda H 2011 [19]. Reproduced with permission from Walters Kluwer Health).

Acknowledgements

EPC-CFA and HELIC assay were established under the dedicated preparation of equipments and reagents by Tomoko Shizuno, BS, Atsuko Sato, BS, Rie Ito, BS, and Michiru Kobori, BS in our laboratory. We also thank the outstanding technical support at the Teaching and Research Support Center of Tokai University School of Medicine.

UCB or PB samples from healthy volunteers were obtained according to institutional guidelines under the approval of the ethical committees of the Cord Blood Bank and Clinical Investigation Committee at the Tokai University School of Medicine. This work was supported by grants from the Riken Center for Developmental Biology Collaborative Research Fund, Kobe, Japan (08001475); National Institutes of Health, Bethesda, MD (HL53354 and HL57516); the Ministry of Health, Labor and Welfare (H14-Trans-001, H14-Trans-002, H17-Trans-002, H17-Trans-014, H20-Regenerative Medicine-General-001); and the Ministry of Education, Culture, Sports, Science and Technology, Japan (Academic Frontier Promotion Program and Basic Research Grant 22590796 and 25461091).

Competing interests statement

The authors declare that they have no competing financial interests.

References

1 Asahara T, Kawamoto A, Masuda H. Concise review: Circulating endothelial progenitor cells for vascular medicine. *Stem Cells* 2011; **29**: 1650–1655.

2 Asahara T, Murohara T, Sullivan A, Silver M, van der Zee R, Li T, *et al.* Isolation of putative progenitor endothelial cells for angiogenesis. *Science* 1997; **275**: 964–967.

3 Asahara T, Kalka C, Isner JM. Stem cell therapy and gene transfer for regeneration. *Gene Ther* 2000; **7**: 451–457.

4 Murohara T, Ikeda H, Duan J, Shintani S, Sasaki K, Eguchi H, *et al.* Transplanted cord blood-derived endothelial precursor cells augment postnatal neovascularization. *J Clin Invest* 2000; **105**: 1527–1536.

5 Gehling UM, Ergun S, Schumacher U, Wagener C, Pantel K, Otte M, *et al.* In vitro differentiation of endothelial cells from ac133-positive progenitor cells. *Blood* 2000; **95**: 3106–3112.

6 Peichev M, Naiyer AJ, Pereira D, Zhu Z, Lane WJ, Williams M, *et al.* Expression of vegfr-2 and ac133 by circulating human cd34(+) cells identifies a population of functional endothelial precursors. *Blood* 2000; **95**: 952–958.

7 Quirici N, Soligo D, Caneva L, Servida F, Bossolasco P, Deliliers GL, *et al.* Differentiation and expansion of endothelial cells from human bone marrow cd133(+) cells. *Br J Haematol* 2001; **115**: 186–194.

8 Eggermann J, Kliche S, Jarmy G, Hoffmann K, Mayr-Beyrle U, Debatin KM, *et al.* Endothelial progenitor cell culture and differentiation in vitro: A methodological comparison using human umbilical cord blood. *Cardiovas Res* 2003; **58**: 478–486.

9 Handgretinger R, Gordon PR, Leimig T, Chen X, Buhring HJ, Niethammer D, *et al.* Biology and plasticity of cd133+ hematopoietic stem cells. *Ann N Y Acad Sci* 2003; **996**: 141–151.

10 Alessandri G, Emanueli C, Madeddu P. Genetically engineered stem cell therapy for tissue regeneration. *Ann N Y Acad Sci* 2004; **1015**: 271–284.

11 Friedrich EB, Walenta K, Scharlau J, Nickenig G, Werner N. Cd34-/cd133+/vegfr-2+ endothelial progenitor cell subpopulation with potent vasoregenerative capacities. *Circ Res* 2006; **98**: e20–25.

12 Hill JM, Zalos G, Halcox JP, Schenke WH, Waclawiw MA, Quyyumi AA, *et al.* Circulating endothelial progenitor cells, vascular function, and cardiovascular risk. *N Engl J Med* 2003; **348**: 593–600.

13 Rohde E, Bartmann C, Schallmoser K, Reinisch A, Lanzer G, Linkesch W, *et al.* Immune cells mimic the morphology of endothelial progenitor colonies in vitro. *Stem Cells* 2007; **25**: 1746–1752.

14 Ingram DA, Mead LE, Tanaka H, Meade V, Fenoglio A, Mortell K, *et al.* Identification of a novel hierarchy of endothelial progenitor cells using human peripheral and umbilical cord blood. *Blood* 2004; **104**: 2752–2760.

15 Ingram DA, Caplice NM, Yoder MC. Unresolved questions, changing definitions, and novel paradigms for defining endothelial progenitor cells. *Blood* 2005; **106**: 1525–1531.

16 Eichmann A, Corbel C, Nataf V, Vaigot P, Breant C, Le Douarin NM, *et al.* Ligand-dependent development of the endothelial and hemopoietic lineages from embryonic mesodermal cells expressing vascular endothelial growth factor receptor 2. *Proc Natl Acad Sci U S A* 1997; **94**: 5141–5146.

17 Benndorf RA, Gehling UM, Appel D, Maas R, Schwedhelm E, Schlagner K, Silberhorn E, *et al.* Mobilization of putative high-proliferative-potential endothelial colony-forming cells during antihypertensive treatment in patients with essential hypertension. *Stem Cells Dev* 2007; **16**: 329–338.

18 Rustemeyer P, Wittkowski W, Greve B, Stehling M. Flow-cytometric identification, enumeration, purification, and expansion of cd133+ and vegf-r2+ endothelial progenitor cells from peripheral blood. *J Immunoassay Immunochem* 2007; **28**: 13–23.

19 Masuda H, Alev C, Akimaru H, Ito R, Shizuno T, Kobori M, *et al.* Methodological development of a clonogenic assay to determine endothelial progenitor cell potential. *Circ Res* 2011; **109**: 20–37.

20 Masuda H, Asahara T. Clonogenic assay of endothelial progenitor cells. *Trends Cardiovasc Med* 2013; **23**: 99–103.

Cardiac resident stem cells

João Ferreira-Martins, Fumihiro Sanada, and Marcello Rota

Brigham and Women's Hospital, Harvard Medical School, Boston, MA, USA

Introduction

In the last decade, large emphasis has been placed on the possibility that the adult heart harbors primitive cells with some of the characteristics of stem/progenitor cells. Several laboratories have identified cardiac cells with variable ability to self-renew, form multicellular clones, and/or generate cardiomyocytes, smooth muscle cells, and endothelial cells [1–11]. These findings raise important questions regarding the role played by resident progenitor cells in the normal and diseased heart and the possibility to implement therapeutic strategies promoting myocardial regeneration via activation of this primitive cell pool.

Cardiac stem cells (CSCs) expressing the stem cell antigen c-kit have been found in several species, including humans [1,12–16]. These cells possess the fundamental properties of stem cells and generate functionally competent myocardium in animal models of cardiac disease [1,14–23]. Importantly, initial clinical results indicate that intracoronary infusion of CSCs is effective in improving LV function and reducing infarct size in patients with ischemic cardiomyopathy [24], suggesting the validity of CSC-based regenerative therapies for the failing heart.

Increasing evidence supports the notion that cell turnover is an essential variable in cardiac biology and that CSCs underlie this homeostatic process [23,25,26]; acquired defects in the primitive cell pool may lead to an imbalance between newly formed parenchymal cells and myocardial cell loss [27–29], resulting in deposition of fibrotic tissue and deterioration of LV function. A principal aspect that CSCs share with stem cells found in other organs is their limited spontaneous regenerative capacity and their inadequate response to tissue damage. The identification of signaling cascades promoting CSC survival, growth, and activation may be critical in enhancing the intrinsic reparative potential of this primitive cell category [17,28,30]. Thus, several aspects of CSC biology remain to be clarified; in this regard, critical information may be obtained from small animal models in which genetic engineering and/or pharmacological interventions allow perturbation of molecular pathways impacting on progenitor cell biology. Thus, isolation of CSCs from the rodent heart represents an indispensable methodology to define the properties of this progenitor cell pool.

This chapter focuses on the isolation of c-kit-positive CSCs from the mouse heart. This protocol involves a preliminary phase in which single-cell preparations are obtained by enzymatic digestion of the myocardium; subsequently, small cells are separated from myocytes by filtration and centrifugation, and, finally, CSCs are selected by fluorescence-activated cell sorting (FACS) using the surface epitope c-kit (CD117) as a marker. Freshly isolated or multipassage cultured cells are suitable for experiments ranging from immunocytochemistry to transplantation assays.

Manual of Research Techniques in Cardiovascular Medicine, First Edition. Edited by Hossein Ardehali, Roberto Bolli, and Douglas W. Losordo.
© 2014 John Wiley & Sons, Ltd. Published 2014 by John Wiley & Sons, Ltd.

Protocol

Preparation of basic solutions and culture medium

One liter of Perfusion Buffer is necessary for digestion of ~10 mouse hearts. Each experiment will require 100 mL of Perfusion Buffer aliquoted into two 50-mL tubes. Additionally, a 0.5 M CaCl$_2$ stock solution is prepared to rise [Ca^{2+}] of the perfusate.

On the day of the enzymatic digestion, Perfusion Buffer is warmed at 37°C and supplemented with 2,3-butanedione monoxime (BDM) and/or 0.1 mM CaCl$_2$ and/or a cocktail of enzymes to be employed in the different phases of the perfusion:

1. Rinse Buffer (50 mL): Perfusion Buffer + BDM;
2. Digestion Buffer (15 mL): Perfusion Buffer + BDM + CaCl$_2$ + cocktail of enzymes;
3. Wash Buffer (35 mL): Perfusion Buffer + BDM + CaCl$_2$.

Following enzymatic digestion and mechanical dissociation of the heart, 50 mL of Blocking Buffer will be required to separate small cells. Subsequently, collected FACS sorted cells will be cultured in F-12K based medium.

What you will need

Equipment: analytical balance, magnetic stir plate, pH meter, class II biosafety cabinet with vacuum line, heated water bath.

Tools: a 1-L volumetric flask, a 1-L beaker, a 100-mL beaker, magnetic stir bar, spatula, adjustable-volume pipetters (0.1–10 µL).

Supplies: weighing papers, transfer pipettes, a sterile vacuum filter unit (1-L funnel with filter and 1-L receiver, Millipore Stericup), parafilm, 50-mL and 15-mL sterile tubes, permanent marker, 0.1–10 µL pipette tips, two 50-mL filter unit (pore size 0.22 µm, Steriflip, Millipore).

Chemicals and solutions: Double distilled water (dd-H$_2$O), NaCl, D-(+)-glucose, HEPES, MgCl$_2$, KCl, taurine, creatine, Na pyruvate, NaH$_2$PO$_4$, BDM, collagenase type 2 (300 U/mg), protease type XIV (4.4 U/mg), bovine serum albumin suitable for cell culture (BSA), 0.5 M EDTA solution, phosphate buffered saline w/o calcium and magnesium (PBS), 10 N NaOH solution, 1 N HCl solution.

Culture medium compounds: F-12K Nutrient Mixture Kaighn's Modification (Gibco), fetal bovine serum (FBS), human erythropoietin (cell culture tested, 10 U/vial), recombinant human fibroblast growth factor-basic (bFGF), penicillin-streptomycin (penicillin 10,000 U/mL, streptomycin 10 mg/mL), recombinant mouse leukemia inhibitory factor (LIF), cell culture grade water.

Procedures

1. Pour ~900 mL of dd-H$_2$O in a 1-L volumetric flask and add the following compounds: NaCl, 7.36 g, D-(+)-glucose, 3.96 g, HEPES, 5.72 g, MgCl$_2$, 0.476 g, KCl, 0.328 g, taurine, 2.5 g, creatine, 0.656 g, Na pyruvate, 0.55 g, NaH$_2$PO$_4$, 0.12 g. Adjust volume to 1 L, seal the flask with parafilm and mix the preparation 15–20 times.

2. Transfer a magnetic stir bar and the buffer into a 1-L beaker. Use a magnetic stirrer plate and a pH meter to mix and monitor pH of the solution. With a NaOH solution, slowly bring pH to 7.4.

3. Sterilize the buffer by filtration with sterile vacuum filter unit (Millipore) under a biosafety cabinet. Label and date the container, and store Perfusion Buffer at 4°C. On an as-needed basis, two 50 mL aliquots of Perfusion Buffer in two sterile 50-mL tubes are prepared under the biosafety cabinet for digestion of one mouse heart.

4. Enzymatic digestion of the heart will require Perfusion Buffer supplemented with 0.1 mM CaCl$_2$. For this purpose, a 0.5 M CaCl$_2$ stock solution is prepared by placing 3.675 g of CaCl$_2$ in a 50-mL tube filled with dd-H$_2$O. The stock is stored at 4°C.

5. Prepare aliquots and stock solutions for culture medium:

   a. Transfer 5-mL aliquots of penicillin–streptomycin in 15-mL tubes and store at −20°C.

   b. Transfer 1 mL of cell culture grade water in the vial containing 10 U of human erythropoietin; after mixing, prepare four aliquots of 250 µL using 0.5 mL Eppendorf tubes; label and store them at −20°C.

   c. Pour 80 mL of dd-H$_2$O in a 100-mL beaker and add 1.21 g of Tris base. While stirring with a magnet and monitoring the pH, add drops of HCl using a transfer pipette to adjust pH to 7.6. Adjust volume to 100 mL (final concentration is 100 mM). Transfer 2 mL of 100 mM Tris base solution in a 50-mL tube, add 38 mL of dd-H$_2$O and 40 mg of BSA. Mix this 5 mM Tris buffer and filter with a 50-mL filter unit. Finally, transfer 500 μL of 5 mM Tris buffer in a vial containing 50 μg of bFGF; prepare 50 μL aliquots using 0.5-mL Eppendorf tubes and store at −20°C.

6. Add 50 mL of FBS, 250 μL human erythropoietin stock solution, 50 μL recombinant human fibroblast growth factor-basic (bFGF), 5 mL penicillin–streptomycin stock solution, and 500 μL recombinant mouse leukemia inhibitory factor (LIF) to 450 mL of F-12K medium.

One hour before the experiment:

7. With a thermostat-controlled bath, warm two 50-mL tubes containing Perfusion Buffer at 37°C.

8. Add 62.6 mg of BDM in each of the two vials. Shake the mixture until completely dissolved. Label one of the two tubes as Rinse Buffer and return it to the water bath.

9. Add 10 μL of 0.5 M CaCl$_2$ stock solution to the second 50 mL tube. Label the tube as Wash Buffer and place it in the water bath.

10. Place 15 mg of collagenase and 1.5 mg of protease into a 15 mL tube, label as Digestion and place it at 4°C. Before starting perfusion of the heart, add 15 mL of Wash Buffer to the tube containing enzymes and mix it until completely dissolved. This is the Digestion Buffer. Place the vial at 37°C.

11. Prepare Blocking Buffer: using a biosafety cabinet, transfer 50 mL of PBS in a 50-mL sterile tube using a 25-mL serological pipette and add 200 μL of 0.5 M EDTA solution. Subsequently, weight and add 250 mg of BSA and mix until BSA is completely dissolved. Sterilize the preparation using 50-mL filter unit.

12. Prepare a 4′,6-diamidino-2-phenylindole (DAPI) stock solution by adding 1 mL of dd-H$_2$O to 1 mg of DAPI powder. After mixing, store the stock at 4°C.

Enzymatic digestion of the mouse heart

For myocardial digestion, the mouse is sacrificed, the aorta cannulated, and the heart explanted and perfused retrogradely. This is accomplished using a constant flow, recirculating Langendorff apparatus consisting of a water-jacked organ bath equipped with bubbler in which solution is warmed and oxygenated. Using the drain port, warmed fluids are withdrawn by a tube connected to a peristaltic pump, and used to perfuse the heart, which is positioned inside the bath. This closed circuit allows recirculation of the perfusate at constant flow. Following enzymatic digestion, the heart is cut in four to six small pieces and pipetted to obtain single a cell preparation.

What you will need

Equipment: Langendorff apparatus composed of a water-jacked organ bath with oxygen bubbler (Radnoti), heated water bath circulator (Thermo Scientific Haake), peristaltic pump (Cole-Parmer), tubing (Masterflex), compressed gas mixture (nitrogen 15% balanced oxygen), inverted microscope.

Surgical tools: operating table, two forceps, fine scissors, spring scissors, 4-0 silk suture, 2 × 2 inch gauze, cotton tipped applicators, PE-50 tubing, 23-gauge needles, miniature file, a timer.

Supplies: 1 mL syringes, heparin sodium injection 1000 U/mL, Institutional Animal Care and Use Committee (IACUC) approved anesthetic, ethyl alcohol 70%, 60-mm and 35-mm Petri dishes, transfer pipettes.

Procedures

13. An aortic cannula is prepared and used for several experiments by polishing a 23-gauge needle with a miniature file and inserting it in a PE-50 tubing. The tube is cut with an oblique angle to facilitate insertion in the aorta. Luer locking system is used to connect to the cannula to the perfusion apparatus.

14. One hour before the experiment, the Langendorff apparatus is washed by adding ethyl alcohol 70%, and then dd-H$_2$O to the organ bath, and by activating the system in nonrecirculating mode (open circuit, fluids not returning to the organ bath). The heated water bath circulator, set at 37°C, is turned on.

15. Rinse, Digestion, and Wash Buffers are prepared and warmed (see 7–10).

16. Preparation of the Langendorff system: bubble the oxygen/ nitrogen mixture in the organ bath, remove completely dd-H$_2$O, pour Rinse Buffer (50 mL), and activate the system in recirculating mode (Rinse Buffer returns to the organ bath). Connect the cannula to the system and remove bubbles trapped in the tubing.

17. Inject the mouse with 0.2 mL heparin (ip) using a 1-mL syringe.

18. Five minutes after heparin injection, anesthetize the animal following an approved IACUC protocol. Wipe chest and abdomen with 70% ethyl alcohol and secure the animal on the surgical table.

19. Transfer ~15 mL of warm Rinse Buffer from the organ bath to a 60-mm Petri dish with a pipette. Disconnect the cannula from the apparatus and immerse it in the dish.

20. *In situ* cannulation of the aorta: with forceps and fine scissors, produce a transversal incision of the mouse abdomen to expose the diaphragm. Cut the anterolateral border the diaphragm and proceed with a double lateral thoracotomy to completely remove the thoracic cage and expose the heart. Open the pericardium and pull apart the two lobes of the thymus with forceps. Using gauze and cotton tipped applicators, clear the aortic arch from blood and remaining tissue. When cleared, pass a 4-0 silk suture under the aorta between its origin and the first innominate (the first branch of the aortic arch) and create a loose knot. While holding the aorta with a forceps where the first innominate originates, cut perpendicularly one-third of the vessel in the region close to the origin of the left common carotid arteries (second branch of the aortic arch) with spring scissors. Remove excess of blood with a cotton tipped applicator, insert the cannula in the aorta, tighten the knot around the tubing and secure it with a second knot. Excise the heart and place it in warm Rinse Buffer inside the Petri dish. Repeatedly, apply a gentle pressure on the ventricles to remove blood from the chambers.

21. Connect the cannula to the Langendorff system and keep the heart outside of the organ bath. Start the timer and set flow of perfusion to 1 drop every 1.5–2 s. After 1 minute, when blood has been removed from the coronary system, immerse the heart in the organ bath and continue recirculating mode of Rinse Buffer for additional 4 minutes.

22. At 5 minutes from the beginning of perfusion, remove Rinse Buffer from the organ bath with a transfer pipette, and pour the 15 mL of Digestion Buffer. After initial 10 minutes, inspect the heart frequently for signs of completed digestion, i.e. softness and mushiness of the tissue. When digestion is completed, remove the heart from the organ bath (nonrecirculating mode), take out Digestion Buffer

with a transfer pipette, and pour ~25 mL of Wash Buffer in the bath.

23. After 1 minutes of perfusion with Wash Buffer, place the heart in the organ bath and continue perfusion for additional 4 minutes. Then, remove the heart from the perfusion apparatus and place it in a 35-mm Petri dish and add ~4 mL of Wash Buffer.

24. With forceps and spring scissors, excise large vessels and cut the heart. Using a transfer pipette, mechanically dissociate the myocardium by gentle pipetting. Put a drop of the preparation in a Petri dish and rapidly examine at the microscope for the presence of rod-shaped myocytes and absence of cell aggregates.

Separation of small cells

Following enzymatic digestion of the heart, small cells are separated from other myocardial cells by filtration and centrifugation.

What you will need

Equipment: class II biosafety cabinet with vacuum line, refrigerated centrifuges with rotor for 15 and 50-mL tubes and 1.5-mL Eppendorf tubes, inverted microscope.

Tools: hemocytometer, pipetter, adjustable-volume pipetters (10–100 μL), tally counter, a timer.

Supplies: 50-mL and 15-mL sterile tubes, sterile transfer pipettes, 2 and 25-mL sterile serological pipettes, 1.5-mL sterile Eppendorf tubes, 10–100-μL sterile pipette tips, 40-μm nylon cell strainer (BD Falcon), 0.4% trypan blue solution.

Procedures

25. Working under a biosafety cabinet, transfer the cell suspension through a 40-μm nylon cell strainer in a sterile 50-mL tube (tube #1), using a sterile transfer pipette. With a 25-mL serological pipette, dilute the preparation with Blocking Buffer to adjust volume to 15 mL.

26. Centrifuge at $100\,g$ for 1 minute at 4°C.

27. Transfer supernatant into a second sterile 50-mL tube (tube #2) and resuspend pellet of tube #1 in 15 mL of Blocking Buffer.

28. Centrifuge tube #1 at $100\,g$ for 1 minute at 4°C.

29. Transfer supernatant of tube #1 in tube #2. The pellet of tube #1 contains mainly myocytes and may be discarded or used for other purposes.

30. Centrifuge tube #2 at $300\,g$ for 5 minutes at 4°C to obtain a pellet of small cells.

31. Discard supernatant and resuspend pellet in 2 mL of Blocking Buffer, with a 2-mL serological pipette.

32. Cell counting: mix 20 µL of the cell suspension and 20 µL of trypan blue in a 0.5-mL Eppendorf tube using a pipetter. Pipet 10-µL of the cell suspension/ trypan blue mixture into the counting chamber of a hemocytometer. Using a microscope (10× objective) and a tally counter, determine the number of viable cells (not stained by trypan blue) in the four large 1 mm^2 corner squares. The total number of cells in tube #2 is equal to the number of cells counted multiplied by ×10^4 (this takes into account the number of squares analyzed, the dilution factor and the volume of cell suspension in tube #2).

33. To adjust the total number of cells in tube #2 to a density suitable for immunolabeling, the cell preparation is centrifuged at $300\,g$ for 5 minutes at 4°C; supernatant is discarded and volume is adjusted to a density of 1×10^6 cells/100 µL with Blocking Buffer. Then transfer the cell suspension into a 1.5-mL Eppendorf tube.

Sorting c-kit-positive cells using FACS

To select c-kit-positive CSCs by FACS, the small cell population is stained using an anti-CD117 primary-conjugated antibody. Additionally, to adjust parameters for sorting (gating), a negative control sample will be employed to exclude the fluorescence signal originating from small cells stained with a nonspecific IgG antibody (isotype control).

What you will need
Flow cytometer sorter.

Equipment: class II biosafety cabinet with vacuum line, refrigerated centrifuges with rotor for 1.5-mL Eppendorf tubes, tube rotator with rotisserie for 1.5-mL Eppendorf tubes.

Tools: pipetter, adjustable-volume pipetters (10–100 µL), a permanent marker, a timer.

Supplies: 10–100-µL sterile pipette tips, sterile 1.5-mL Eppendorf tubes, sterile 5-mL polystyrene round-bottom test tubes (dual-position snap cap) with and without mesh-strainer (35-µm pore size, BD Biosciences), CD117 antibody (BD Biosciences), isotype antibody, two 50-mL filter unit (pore size 0.22 µm, Steriflip, Millipore), 3-mL syringe with luer lock tip, cell culture dishes, ice.

Procedures
34. After mixing the small cell suspension, transfer an aliquot corresponding to 2×10^4 cells into a 1.5-mL tube. Add the isotype antibody and label the tube as Isotype. Then, add anti-CD117 antibody to the remaining small cell suspension and label the tube as CD117. For the two antibodies, an equal dilution varying from 1:30 to 1:100 is applied.

35. Mount the two vials on a tube rotator, and incubate cells at 4°C for 1 hour at a rotation speed of 8 rpm.

36. During the incubation time, a DAPI solution is prepared by adding 1 µL of DAPI stock solution (see point 12) to 10 mL of PBS using a 50-mL tube. Sterilize the preparation with a 50-mL filter unit. Additionally, Collecting Solution to be employed during sorting is prepared: mix 2.5 mL of FBS and 7.5 mL of PBS in a 50-mL tube; after filtration with a 50-mL filter unit, 2-mL aliquots of Collecting Solution are transferred into two 5-mL polystyrene round-bottom test tube that will serve as collecting tubes.

37. After 1 h of incubation, add 1 mL of Blocking Buffer to each of the two cell suspensions and centrifuge at 300 g for 5 minutes at 4°C.

38. Discard supernatant from the two vials and resuspend pellets in 1 mL of Blocking Buffer.

39. Centrifuge at $300\,g$ for 5 minutes at 4°C.

40. Discard supernatant from the two vials and resuspend pellets in 200 µL of DAPI solution.

41. Prior to sorting, each of the two cell suspensions has to be filtered. Under the biosafety cabinet, two filtering units are prepared by mounting a 3-mL syringe with luer lock tip on a 5-mL polystyrene round bottom test tube with cell-strainer cap. Remove the plunge from the syringe, transfer the Isotype cell suspension into the barrel with a pipetter, insert the plunge, and flush cells through the mesh. Replace the cell-strainer cap with a regular cap and label the vial. Using a second filtering unit, filter the CD117 cell suspension. Tubes are then kept on ice.

42. At the FACS facility, examine the Isotype cell suspension first. Cell debris, clumps of two or more cells, and dead cells are excluded based on forward/

side scatter and DAPI staining. Subsequently, the fluorescence signal of the Isotype preparation is determined. The CD117 cell suspension is then processed based on the gating parameters obtained from the Isotype sample. The sorted positive and negative fractions are collected in tubes prepared previously (see Step 36).

43. For primary cell culture purposes, centrifuge cell suspensions at $300\,g$ for 5 minutes at 4°C. Resuspend pellets in culture medium and plate cells in culture dishes at a density meeting your experimental plans.

Alternative approaches

A fundamental property of c-kit-positive CSCs is their ability to self-renew and to originate multicellular clones. Thus, serially passaged clonal or nonclonal cell pools can be expanded *in vitro* and used in substitution for freshly isolated cells. However, the spontaneous tendency of murine CSCs to undergo commitment may result in the progressive loss of c-kit expression and accumulation of differentiated cardiovascular cells. Thus, the purity of the cell population should be routinely determined by immunostaining and/or FACS sorting when serially passaged cells are employed.

An alternative protocol for the selection of CSCs from small cell preparations is represented by magnetic activated cell sorting (MACS) [12,23,27,31]. This is a fast and accessible methodology, which employs microbeads conjugated to a CD117 antibody. Following incubation with the antibody, the small cell suspension is transferred into columns placed in a magnetic field. While unlabeled cells run through the column, c-kit-positive CSCs are retained by the attraction of the microbeads to the magnetic field, and therefore can be collected. While FACS is superior in providing high purity selection of the sample, MACS offers other advantages, including fast processing and reduced stress imposed on the cells. Additionally, it may represent the methodology of choice when flow cytometer sorter facilities are not available.

Weaknesses and strength of the method

The described procedures present minor challenges for the researcher, since they involve preparation of solutions, nonsurvival surgery in mice, and basic

immunolabeling. While cannulation of the aorta and proper digestion of the myocardium may necessitate some practice, selection of the CD117-positive population by flow cytometry require a skilled operator. One intrinsic limitation of the experiment is represented by the small number of CSCs present in the rodent myocardium, precluding studies requiring large number of cells. However, this aspect can be easily overcome by combining cell preparations obtained from several animals. Alternatively, the procedure can be adapted to other species by slight modifications of the volume of perfusate and selection of a suitable CD117 antibody.

The provided protocol does not describe the lineage negative selection of c-kit-positive CSCs using surface markers specific for hematopoietic and mesenchymal cells. Although these epitopes have been found to be minimally expressed in the CD117-sorted cells obtained from normal mouse hearts [23,31], a thorough characterization of the cell population is recommended, particularly when conditions promoting mobilization of other cell types to the heart have been employed.

Conclusion

The described protocol allows the researcher to obtain c-kit-positive cells from the mouse heart, which can be employed for molecular, physiological, and biological *in vitro* characterization together with *in vivo* transplantation assays.

Acknowledgements

This work was supported by National Institutes of Health grants.

References

1 Beltrami AP, Barlucchi L, Torella D, Baker M, Limana F, Chimenti S, *et al*. Adult cardiac stem cells are multipotent and support myocardial regeneration. *Cell* 2003; **114**: 763–776.

2 Oh H, Bradfute SB, Gallardo TD, Nakamura T, Gaussin V, Mishina Y, *et al*. Cardiac progenitor cells from adult myocardium: homing, differentiation, and fusion after infarction. *Proc Natl Acad Sci USA* 2003; **100**: 12313–12318.

3 Martin CM, Meeson AP, Robertson SM, Hawke TJ, Richardson JA, Bates S, *et al*. Persistent expression of the ATP-binding cassette transporter, Abcg2, identifies

cardiac SP cells in the developing and adult heart. *Dev Biol* 2004; **265**: 262–275.

4 Matsuura K, Nagai T, Nishigaki N, Oyama T, Nishi J, Wada H, *et al*. Adult cardiac Sca-1-positive cells differentiate into beating cardiomyocytes. *J Biol Chem* 2004; **279**: 11384–11391.

5 Laugwitz KL, Moretti A, Lam J, Gruber P, Chen Y, Woodard S, *et al*. Postnatal isl1+ cardioblasts enter fully differentiated cardiomyocyte lineages. *Nature* 2005; **433**: 647–653.

6 Messina E, De Angelis L, Frati G, Morrone S, Chimenti S, Fiordaliso F, *et al*. Isolation and expansion of adult cardiac stem cells from human and murine heart. *Circ Res* 2004; **95**: 911–921.

7 Pfister O, Mouquet F, Jain M, Summer R, Helmes M, Fine A, *et al*. CD31- but not CD31+ cardiac side population cells exhibit functional cardiomyogenic differentiation. *Circ Res* 2005; **97**: 52–61.

8 Rosenblatt-Velin N, Lepore MG, Cartoni C, Beermann F, Pedrazzini T. FGF-2 controls the differentiation of resident cardiac precursors into functional cardiomyocytes. *J Clin Invest* 2005; **115**: 1724–1733.

9 Tomita Y, Matsumura K, Wakamatsu Y, Matsuzaki Y, Shibuya I, Kawaguchi H, *et al*. Cardiac neural crest cells contribute to the dormant multipotent stem cell in the mammalian heart. *J Cell Biol* 2005; **170**: 1135–1146.

10 Oyama T, Nagai T, Wada H, Naito AT, Matsuura K, Iwanaga K, *et al*. Cardiac side population cells have a potential to migrate and differentiate into cardiomyocytes in vitro and in vivo. *J Cell Biol* 2007; **176**: 329–341.

11 Smith RR, Barile L, Cho HC, Leppo MK, Hare JM, Messina E, *et al*. Regenerative potential of cardiosphere-derived cells expanded from percutaneous endomyocardial biopsy specimens. *Circulation* 2007; **115**: 896–908.

12 Urbanek K, Cesselli D, Rota M, Nascimbene A, De Angelis A, Hosoda T, *et al*. Stem cell niches in the adult mouse heart. *Proc Natl Acad Sci USA* 2006; **103**: 9226–9231.

13 Hosoda T, D'Amario D, Cabral-Da-Silva MC, Zheng H, Padin-Iruegas ME, Ogorek B, *et al*. Clonality of mouse and human cardiomyogenesis in vivo. *Proc Natl Acad Sci USA* 2009; **106**: 17169–17174.

14 Linke A, Müller P, Nurzynska D, Casarsa C, Torella D, Nascimbene A, *et al*. Stem cells in the dog heart are self-renewing, clonogenic, and multipotent and regenerate infarcted myocardium, improving cardiac function. *Proc Natl Acad Sci USA* 2005; **102**: 8966–8971.

15 Bearzi C, Rota M, Hosoda T, Tillmanns J, Nascimbene A, De Angelis A, *et al*. Human cardiac stem cells. *Proc Natl Acad Sci USA* 2007; **104**: 14068–14073.

16 Bearzi C, Leri A, Lo Monaco F, Rota M, Gonzalez A, Hosoda T, *et al*. Identification of a coronary vascular progenitor cell in the human heart. *Proc Natl Acad Sci USA* 2009; **106**: 15885–15890.

17 Rota M, Padin-Iruegas ME, Misao Y, De Angelis A, Maestroni S, Ferreira-Martins J, *et al*. Local activation or implantation of cardiac progenitor cells rescues scarred infarcted myocardium improving cardiac function. *Circ Res* 2008; **103**: 107–116.

18 Ferreira-Martins J, Rondon-Clavo C, Tugal D, Korn JA, Rizzi R, Padin-Iruegas ME, *et al*. Spontaneous calcium oscillations regulate human cardiac progenitor cell growth. *Circ Res* 2009; **105**: 764–774.

19 D'Alessandro DA, Kajstura J, Hosoda T, Gatti A, Bello R, Mosna F, *et al*. Progenitor cells from the explanted heart generate immunocompatible myocardium within the transplanted donor heart. *Circ Res* 2009; **105**: 1128–1140.

20 Hosoda T, Zheng H, Cabral-da-Silva M, Sanada F, Ide-Iwata N, Ogórek B, *et al*. Human cardiac stem cell differentiation is regulated by a mircrine mechanism. *Circulation* 2011; **123**: 1287–1296.

21 Goichberg P, Bai Y, D'Amario D, Ferreira-Martins J, Fiorini C, Zheng H, *et al*. The ephrin A1 EphA2 system promotes cardiac stem cell migration after infarction. *Circ Res* 2011; **108**: 1071–1083.

22 D'Amario D, Cabral-Da-Silva MC, Zheng H, Fiorini C, Goichberg P, Steadman E, *et al*. Insulin-like growth factor-1 receptor identifies a pool of human cardiac stem cells with superior therapeutic potential for myocardial regeneration. *Circ Res* 2011; **108**: 1467–1481.

23 Ferreira-Martins J, Ogórek B, Cappetta D, Matsuda A, Signore S, D'Amario D, *et al*. Cardiomyogenesis in the developing heart is regulated by c-kit-positive cardiac stem cells. *Circ Res* 2012; **110**: 701–715.

24 Bolli R, Chugh AR, D'Amario D, Loughran JH, Stoddard MF, Ikram S, *et al*. Cardiac stem cells in patients with ischaemic cardiomyopathy (SCIPIO): initial results of a randomised phase 1 trial. *Lancet* 2011; **378**: 1847–1857.

25 Kajstura J, Urbanek K, Perl S, Hosoda T, Zheng H, Ogórek B, *et al*. Cardiomyogenesis in the adult human heart. *Circ Res* 2010; **107**: 305–315.

26 Kajstura J, Gurusamy N, Ogórek B, Goichberg P, Clavo-Rondon C, Hosoda T, *et al*. Myocyte turnover in the aging human heart. *Circ Res* 2010; **107**: 1374–1386.

27 Rota M, LeCapitaine N, Hosoda T, Boni A, De Angelis A, Padin-Iruegas ME, *et al*. Diabetes promotes cardiac stem cell aging and heart failure, which are prevented by deletion of the p66shc gene. *Circ Res* 2006; **99**: 42–52.

28 Gonzalez A, Rota M, Nurzynska D, Misao Y, Tillmanns J, Ojaimi C, *et al*. Activation of cardiac progenitor cells reverses the failing heart senescent phenotype and prolongs lifespan. *Circ Res* 2008; **102**: 597–606.

29 Cesselli D, Beltrami AP, D'Aurizio F, Marcon P, Bergamin N, Toffoletto B, *et al*. Effects of age and heart failure on

human cardiac stem cell function. *Am J Pathol* 2011; **179**: 349–366.

30 Urbanek K, Rota M, Cascapera S, Bearzi C, Nascimbene A, De Angelis A, *et al*. Cardiac stem cells possess growth factor-receptor systems that after activation regenerate the infarcted myocardium, improving ventricular function and long-term survival. *Circ Res* 2005; **97**: 663–673.

31 Urbanek K, Cabral-da-Silva MC, Ide-Iwata N, Maestroni S, Delucchi F, Zheng H, *et al*. Inhibition of notch1-dependent cardiomyogenesis leads to a dilated myopathy in the neonatal heart. *Circ Res* 2010; **107**: 429–441.

Cardiospheres

Rachel Ruckdeschel Smith

Cedars-Sinai Medical Center, Heart Institute and Capricor, Inc., Los Angeles, CA, USA

Introduction

Right around the turn of the current century, proof that the adult mammalian heart contained an endogenous population of stem cells emerged from several independent laboratories [1–3]. The cardiosphere method was developed by Messina and Giacomello, thereafter adopted by the Marbán laboratory, and was among the first means by which cardiac stem cells were isolated and cultured from the human heart. The method is modeled after the neurosphere method [4] and generates structures *in vitro* that resemble the *in vivo* cardiac stem cell niche. Cardiospheres consist of cardiac stem cells, partially differentiated progenitor cells, and supporting cell types coupled together and surrounded by extracellular matrix proteins.

Since the original study, cardiospheres have been cultured repeatedly from humans [5–13], as well as from rats [14–17] and pigs [18,19] by the Marbán and Giacomello laboratories, and by others from species ranging from mouse to monkey [20–37]. The method lends itself to generating either multicellular cardiospheres or single cells that are either precursors to or derivatives of the cardiospheres. Cardiospheres themselves are a useful *in vitro* system in which to study the process of cardiac stem cell differentiation. Without exogenous manipulation, the cardiosphere system will achieve a steady-state fraction of cardiac stem cells, partially differentiated progenitor cells, and supporting cell types. Under stimulating conditions, for example coculture with neonatal rat ventricular myocytes, differentiation will progress such that a fraction of cells adopt a more terminally differentiated phenotype (e.g. sarcomeric organization, synchronous contractions, calcium cycling) and the adaptation of the *in vitro* cardiac stem cell niche can be observed.

Cardiospheres and their single cell counterparts have also proven to be a safe and effective therapy when used in animal models of heart disease. These animal studies have led to the initiation of several human clinical trials registered on http://www.clinicaltrials.gov. The first has been recently completed (NCT00893360) [38], the second is still recruiting (NCT01273857), and two others have been registered but not yet initiated (NCT01458405, NCT01496209).

Protocols

Preparation for explant creation

1. Prepare a cardioplegic solution or obtain a commercial solution (i.e. Viaspan, DuPont Pharma). A volume sufficient to submerge the tissue of choice times three is sufficient.

2. Keep the cardioplegic solution cold prior to (4°C) and during (wet ice) tissue transport. For situations where the intact vascularized heart is explanted to obtain tissue, but is not first perfused *in situ* with cardioplegic solution, the addition of 10 units/mL heparin will help prevent the formation of blood clots in the explanted tissue.

3. Prepare the number of dishes required for the amount of tissue being used by coating them with fibronectin. A fibronectin stock solution (1 mg/mL) can be prepared, aliquoted, and stored at −20°C.

Manual of Research Techniques in Cardiovascular Medicine, First Edition. Edited by Hossein Ardehali, Roberto Bolli, and Douglas W. Losordo.

Care should be taken when preparing the stock solution to mix by tilting gently rather than pipetting or shaking vigorously. A working solution (25 μg/mL) should be prepared as needed and used immediately. Table 10.1 is provided as a guide. To keep from wasting any source tissue, prepare extra dishes, freezing any that go unused.

4. Cover the surface of the dishes with the fibronectin solution and allow to coat for 1 hour at room temperature. Make sure the surfaces never dry out by tilting occasionally. Dishes can be prepared ahead of time and stored frozen. Wrap the coated dishes in Parafilm and place level at −20°C to freeze. When needed, dishes can be removed, left at room temperature to thaw, and used.

5. Remove and discard the fibronectin solution after 1 hour of coating or thawing. Add an equal volume of PBS (phosphate-buffered saline) to the dish surface. Take care not to disrupt the fibronectin coating by adding the PBS slowly with the pipette tip against the side of the dish. Take care to also not allow the fibronectin coating to dry out. If necessary, keep the dishes in PBS until needed, but not longer than 1 hour.

6. Prepare a volume of collagenase sufficient for the amount of tissue being used. A working solution (1 mg/mL) can be prepared, aliquoted, and stored at −20°C. Collagenase will be added to the tissue in appropriately sized dishes. Table 10.2 is provided as a guide.

Table 10.1 Fibronectin volumes required per dish

Tissue mass	Dishes	Volume of fibronectin
25 mg	1 100-mm dish	5 mL
250 mg	10 100-mm dishes	50 mL (5 mL per dish)
1 g	2 150-mm dishes	40 mL (20 mL per dish)

Table 10.2 Collagenase volumes required per dish

Tissue mass	Dishes	Volume of collagenase
25 mg	1 60-mm dish	1 mL
250 mg	1 100-mm dish	5 mL
1 g	1 150-mm dish	15 mL

7. Prepare media for explants. Batches are typically 0.5 L and consist of: 400 mL Iscove's Modified Dulbecco's Medium (IMDM), 100 mL fetal bovine serum (FBS), 100 units/mL penicillin and 100 μg/mL streptomycin, 2 mM L-glutamine, and 0.1 mM 2-mercaptoethanol combined. Batches should be stored cold (4°C), in the dark, and any excess discarded ~1 month after the date of preparation.

Explant creation

1. Obtain source tissue (e.g. whole heart, cardiac biopsy, surgical discard) from species of interest (e.g. human, pig, rat) and immediately submerge in cold cardioplegic solution.

2. Ideally, tissue should be stored for as brief a period as possible; however, 24 hours of storage has no known consequences and up to 96 hours of storage results in an insignificant decrease in total yield.

3. Maintain sterile conditions or aseptic technique as best as possible during tissue collection. For situations where tissue is stored for prolonged periods of time, the addition of antibiotics (e.g. 100 units/mL penicillin and 100 μg/mL streptomycin) will help prevent growth of micro-organisms.

4. Transfer the tissue to a sterile biological safety cabinet for explant creation.

5. Place the tissue in an appropriately sized Petri dish. Keep tissue moist with cardioplegic solution during handling.

6. Begin by dissecting and discarding any connective tissue, adipose tissue, major blood vessels, or valves, leaving only myocardium. Handle myocardium with forceps as gently as possible. Dissection can be performed with scissors and/or a scalpel.

7. Weigh out the amount of tissue desired from any region (e.g. septum, atrium, ventricle). Tissue obtained from the atria will show a slight growth advantage. For small amounts of tissue (i.e. <100 mg), a wet weight obtained with the tissue submerged in cardioplegic solution from which the weight of the container and cardioplegic solution can be subtracted, may be more accurate.

8. Keep tissue cold in cardioplegic solution if time is taken for coating dishes. Tissue should be transferred at this point to uncoated dishes selected for use with collagenase (refer to Table 10.2). Cut tissue into cubes ~0.5 cm along each side using scissors and/or a scalpel. Keeping cardioplegic solution shallow during the cutting process will help keep tissue from floating around.

9. Remove and discard cardioplegic solution and wash tissue cubes briefly in warm (37°C) PBS by swirling. Remove and discard PBS and add warm collagenase solution, swirling tissue cubes again briefly.

10. Cover dishes and transfer to an incubator (37°C) for 5–15 minutes. Monitor the digestion, observing the tissue under a microscope every 5 minutes, and returning to the incubator as needed. The tissue will begin to look loose and will become fuzzy around the edges as the digestion progresses. At the point when single cells are beginning to be released from the tissue, the digestion is complete.

11. Remove and discard collagenase solution (along with released single cells) and add an equal volume of warm media (with FBS) to stop the digestion, swirling tissue cubes again briefly.

12. Cut tissue cubes into pieces ~0.5 mm along each side using scissors and/or a scalpel. Keeping media shallow during the cutting process will help keep tissue from floating around.

13. Tissue will be transferred at this point to fibronectin coated dishes (refer to Table 10.1). Remove and discard the PBS from the surface of the coated dishes. Add a shallow volume of media to the surface of the coated dishes (e.g. 2 mL to each 100-mm dish, 8 mL to each 150-mm dish). Take care not to disrupt the fibronectin coating by adding the media slowly with the pipette tip against the side of the dish. Take care to also not allow the fibronectin coating to dry out.

14. Using forceps, transfer the tissue pieces one at a time to the coated dishes with shallow media. Place each piece of tissue gently onto the surface of the dish taking care not to scratch the fibronectin coating. Pieces should be spaced at least 1 cm from one another and from the edge of the dish and should be evenly distributed on the dish. If tissue is floating, reduce the volume of media in each dish until the tissue settles to the surface.

15. Transfer the dishes slowly to an incubator, taking care not to disturb the placement of the tissue pieces (explants).

16. Do not disturb the dishes until the next day, allowing 12–24 hours time for the explants to attach.

17. Check to see that the majority of the explants have attached. If necessary, a scalpel can be used to

force attachment of any floating explants. Keeping the media shallow, run the scalpel through the explant at a 45° angle with the surface of the dish, pressing hard so as to scrape the surface of the dish and force a portion of the explant into the groove made.

18. Once the majority of the explants have been attached, media should be added to cover the explants (e.g. +3 mL to each 100-mm dish, +10 mL to each 150-mm dish). Take care not to disrupt the explants by adding the media slowly with the pipette tip against the side of the dish.

19. Do not disturb the dishes until the next day. At this point, all explants that will attach will now be attached. Discard any floating explants. If more than 70% of the explants originally plated are now attached, the culture will likely succeed. Add media to achieve the full volume in each dish (e.g. +7 mL to each 100-mm dish, +12 mL to each 150-mm dish).

20. Every 2–3 days, perform a 50% change of the media. Remove and discard half of the total volume from each dish and replace with warm media. This process leaves behind 50% conditioned media with each media change. Table 10.3 is provided as a guide.

21. Explants should be observed under the microscope every day or at a minimum at every media change. An outgrowth of cells will begin to surround each explant. When the cells surrounding each explant are at least 80% confluent and cover the area within 0.5 cm radius of each explant (Figure 10.1), it is time to collect the cardiosphere-forming cells. The duration of the explant outgrowth stage will vary depending primarily on the species. Table 10.4 is provided as a guide.

Table 10.3 Media volumes required per dish for explant creation

Tissue mass	Dishes	Volume of media
25 mg	1 100 mm dish	12 mL total
250 mg	10 100 mm dishes	120 mL total (12 mL total per dish)
1 g	2 150 mm dishes	60 mL total (30 mL total per dish)

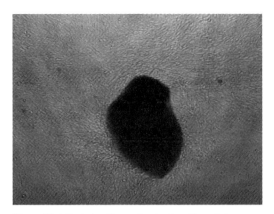

Figure 10.1 Explants with a confluent outgrowth, ready for collection of cardiosphere-forming cells, shown at 4× magnification.

Table 10.4 Expected durations of explant outgrowth stage by species

Species	Duration of explant outgrowth stage
Human	14–28 days
Pig	10–14 days
Rat	7–10 days

Preparation for cardiosphere formation

1. Prepare the number of plates required for the amount of tissue being used by coating them with poly-D-lysine *at least 2 days in advance*. A poly-D-lysine stock solution (0.5 mg/mL) can be prepared, aliquoted, and stored at −20°C. A working solution (20 μg/mL) should be prepared as needed and filtered prior to use. Table 10.5 is provided as a guide. To keep from wasting any cardiosphere-forming cells, prepare extra plates, discarding any that go unused.

2. Cover the surface of the plates with the poly-D-lysine solution and allow to coat for 2–4 days in an incubator. Make sure the surfaces never dry out by tilting occasionally.

3. Remove and discard the poly-D-lysine solution after 2–4 days of coating. Add an equal volume of PBS to the plate surface. Take care not to disrupt the poly-D-lysine coating by adding the PBS slowly with the pipette tip against the side of the plate. If necessary, keep the plates in PBS until needed, but not longer than 1 hour.

Table 10.5 Poly-D-dlysine volumes required per dish

Tissue mass	Dishes	Volume of poly-D-lysine
25 mg	2 6-well plates	18 mL (9 mL per plate)
250 mg	1 150-mm dish	20 mL
1 g	4 150-mm dishes	80 mL (20 mL per dish)

4. Note: Trypsin is used to collect the cardiosphere-forming cells. The trypsin used should be 0.05%. Animal-free trypsin replacements can also be used, typically without modifying the protocol.

5. Prepare media for cardiospheres. Batches are typically 100 mL and consist of: 35 mL IMDM, 65 mL DMEM/F-12 (Dulbecco's Modified Eagle Medium: Nutrient Mixture F-12), 3.5 mL FBS, 100 units/mL penicillin and 100 μg/mL streptomycin, 2 mM L-glutamine, 0.1 mM 2-mercaptoethanol, 2% B27 supplement, 4 nM cardiotrophin-1, 10 ng/mL bFGF (basic fibroblast growth factor), 5 ng/mL EGF (epidermal growth factor), and 20 nM thrombin combined. In lieu of B27, cardiotrophin, bFGF, EGF, and thrombin, FBS can be increased to a volume of 10 mL. Batches should be stored cold (4°C), in the dark, and any excess discarded ~2 weeks after the date of preparation.

Cardiosphere formation

1. Remove and discard the majority of the media from each dish of explants, leaving behind the volume needed to cover the surface (refer to Table 10.1). Remove and save the remaining volume of media, setting aside in a tube for centrifugation. Add warm PBS in a volume needed to cover the surface. Tilt the dishes to gently wash the explants and outgrowth of cells. Remove and save the PBS wash, adding to the media. Add warm trypsin in a volume equivalent to PBS.

2. Cover dishes and transfer to an incubator for 5 minutes. After 5 minutes, observe the explants under a microscope. The majority of the cells surrounding each explant should have detached and should be floating as single cells. If this is not the case, gently tilt the dish while continuing to observe under the microscope. Large, flat cells should remain attached

Table 10.6 Recommended concentrations of cardiosphere-forming cells by species

Species	Cardiosphere-forming cell concentration
Human	6×10^4 cells/mL (for 3×10^4 cells/mL final)
Pig	8×10^4 cells/mL (for 4×10^4 cells/mL final)
Rat	1×10^5 cells/mL (for 5×10^4 cells/mL final)

Table 10.7 Media volumes required per dish for cardiosphere formation

Tissue mass	Dishes	Volume of media
25 mg	2 6-well plates	24 mL (12 mL per plate)
250 mg	1 150-mm dish	30 mL
1 g	4 150-mm dishes	120 mL (30 mL per dish)

to the surface of the dishes along with the explants. Should the cell outgrowth detach as an intact sheet, the explants were likely over-confluent and should have been collected sooner. Brief pipetting can help dissociate the sheets into single cells.

3. Add the trypsin and cells to the collected media and PBS. Remove any explants that may have inadvertently detached during the trypsinization process, filtering cells if necessary through a tube-top mesh (with pore size $\geq 100\,\mu m$). Centrifuge the collected washes at room temperature for 5 minutes at 1000 rpm.

4. A full volume of media can be added back to each dish (refer to Table 10.3) and the dishes returned to the incubator. An outgrowth of cells will again emerge from each explant in about half the time originally required (refer to Table 10.4). The process of collecting cardiosphere-forming cells can be repeated up to three times if desired.

5. Resuspend the pelleted cardiosphere-forming cells in a small volume of media and perform a cell count. The targeted cell concentration will vary depending on species. Table 10.6 is provided as a guide. Adjust the volume of media accordingly such that the concentration of the cell suspension is twice that desired as a final concentration.

6. Cells will be transferred at this point to poly-D-lysine coated plates (refer to Table 10.5). Remove and discard the PBS from the surface of the coated plates. Add a half full volume of media to the surface of the coated plates (e.g. 6 mL to each 6-well plate, 15 mL to each 150-mm dish). Take care not to disrupt the poly-D-lysine coating by adding the media slowly with the pipette tip against the side of the plate.

7. Add an equal volume of cell suspension to each plate to achieve the full volume and the desired final cell concentration. Table 10.7 is provided as a guide.

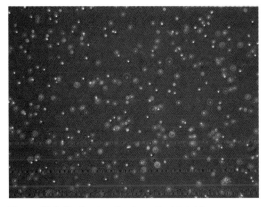

Figure 10.2 Cardiosphere-forming cells plated at 5×10^4 cells/mL, shown at 4× magnification.

8. The cell density should be visually verified (comparing one well to another in a plate and one dish to another; using prior experience and Figure 10.2 as a guide) and adjusted if necessary. Plating density is critical to the success of cardiosphere formation: too dense and a monolayer will form in lieu of cardiospheres, too sparse and cardiospheres may never form.

9. Transfer the plates to an incubator.

10. Cardiospheres should be observed under the microscope every day and the plates shaken gently (or contents pipetted) every day.

11. Every other day, add a small volume of media (e.g. 1.5 mL to each 6-well plate, 4 mL to each 150-mm dish) to each plate.

12. Cardiosphere formation will require only 3–6 days. Cardiospheres will begin to form preferentially along the edges of the plate, but will cluster together, floating in the center when formation is complete. Cells may be loosely adherent to plates in the first few days, shaking and/or pipetting will aid in

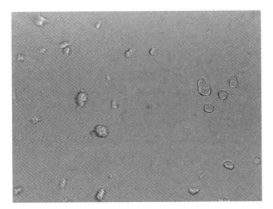

Figure 10.3 Cardiospheres ready for collection, shown at 10× magnification.

detaching them, but cardiospheres will eventually grow in suspension.

13. When the majority of cardiospheres are ~50 μm in diameter (Figure 10.3), it is time to collect the cardiospheres. Cardiospheres should not be allowed to grow larger than ~200 μm in diameter as the centers will begin to become necrotic.

14. Cardiospheres are collected by pipetting the media in each plate several times to aid in final detachment. Media can be removed by centrifuging the collected cardiospheres at room temperature for 8 minutes at 800 rpm.

Alternative approaches

Cardiac stem cells have been identified by a variety of cell surface markers (e.g. c-Kit, Sca-1) [1,2], which can be used to select for a population pure on the basis of that marker. Antibodies against the surface marker of interest, directly conjugated or indirectly bound to either a magnetic particle or fluorescent molecule, can be used for antigenic selection by magnetic-activated or fluorescence-activated cell sorting, respectively. This selection process can be performed on single cells obtained from dissociated primary tissue, an outgrowth of cells grown from explant culture, or cells derived from cardiospheres. Single cells can be derived from cardiospheres either by dissociation [3] or more readily by returning the cardiospheres to adherent culture conditions (i.e. fibronectin-coated dishes) for subsequent passaging [5]. Following antigenic selection, the maximum

purity of the resulting population will be defined by the exclusivity of the marker used. That is, should the marker identify both cardiac stem cells and partially differentiated progenitor cells, the resulting population will consequently contain both. Selection methods would be more appropriate than the cardiosphere method for studies aimed at characterizing a cell population uniformly defined by the expression of a single marker (or multiple markers, in which case selection would be a multistep process).

Cardiospheres can also be clonally derived [3,6]. Cardiosphere-forming cells can be plated at limiting dilutions, wells containing one cell can be visually verified, and cloning efficiency can be expected to be >10%. Using the traditional method, cardiospheres will form both by cell aggregation and clonal proliferation.

Weaknesses and strengths of the method

Cardiospheres are multicellular and are a heterogeneous collection of cells (cardiac stem cells, partially differentiated progenitor cells, supporting cell types). This can be viewed as both a strength and a weakness. The end product of the method is certainly inappropriate for studies focused on defining the properties of any one cell population. However, the cardiosphere method can be a useful means of culturing and expanding a population that may be limited in number when selected from an original source, as the method maintains a relatively constant proportion of each cell population even as cells expand in number. Furthermore, evidence suggests that for therapeutic use in animal models, the heterogeneous mixture of cell populations is more effective than one purified on the basis of a single marker [13].

Cardiospheres are a useful *in vitro* mimic of the *in vivo* cardiac stem cell niche, capturing the essential features, including differentiating progenitor cells. This makes them an attractive model in which to study the process of differentiation. Cardiospheres offer an *in vitro* environment that encourages partial differentiation of cardiac stem cells without the need for exogenous application of nonspecific differentiating agents (e.g. dexamethasone). However, as a model for the *in vivo* cardiac stem cell niche, cardiospheres should continue to be regarded as just that, an *in vitro* model. The degree to which cardiospheres recapitulate the cardiac stem cell niche under different disease conditions or for different donors warrants further investigation. When possible, correlations with the *in vivo* niche should be sought and discrepancies defined. Cardiospheres can however serve as a useful *in vitro* tool for characterizing donors or disease conditions on the basis of their response to a given agent under investigation, particularly when characterizing a human response to an agent not yet approved for use in humans or when access to animal models is limited.

Conclusions

The cardiosphere method is less than a decade old, but has been utilized in nearly three dozen studies, including one completed clinical trial. While cardiospheres are a valuable model system for studying the process of cardiac stem cell differentiation and the interplay of cardiac stem cells, differentiating progenitors, and supporting cell types, their greatest utility may be for therapeutic use. The majority of studies conducted to date have employed cardiospheres in animal models of disease and have proven successful. Interestingly, the mechanisms of action of cardiospheres *in vivo* are not primarily related to differentiation of the transplanted cells. Instead, following transplantation, cardiospheres initiate a cascade of events that lead overall to improvements in cardiac function, reduction of scar size, and regeneration of healthy myocardium. Likely mediated by secreted growth factors, these events include prevention of apoptosis, recruitment of endogenous cardiac stem cells, stimulation of cardiomyocyte cell cycle reentry, and angiogenesis. The methods detailed herein will hopefully enable widespread adoption of the cardiosphere technique, allowing for a more thorough understanding of their biology and the mechanisms surrounding their regenerative capacity.

References

1 Beltrami AP, Barlucchi L, Torella D, Baker M, Limana F, Chimenti S, *et al.* Adult cardiac stem cells are multipotent and support myocardial regeneration. *Cell* 2003; **114**: 763–776.

2 Oh H, Bradfute SB, Gallardo TD, Nakamura T, Gaussin V, Mishina Y, *et al.* Cardiac progenitor cells from adult myocardium: homing, differentiation, and fusion after infarction. *Proc Natl Acad Sci U S A* 2003; **100**: 12313–12318.

3 Messina E, De Angelis L, Frati G, Morrone S, Chimenti S, Fiordaliso F, *et al.* Isolation and expansion of adult cardiac stem cells from human and murine heart. *Circ Res* 2004; **95**: 911–921.

4 Reynolds BA, Weiss S. Generation of neurons and astrocytes from isolated cells of the adult mammalian central nervous system. *Science* 1992; **255**: 1707–1710.

5 Smith RR, Barile L, Cho HC, Leppo MK, Hare JM, Messina E, *et al.* Regenerative potential of cardiosphere-derived cells expanded from percutaneous endomyocardial biopsy specimens. *Circulation* 2007; **115**: 896–908.

6 Davis DR, Zhang Y, Smith RR, Cheng K, Terrovitis J, Malliaras K, *et al.* Validation of the cardiosphere method to culture cardiac progenitor cells from myocardial tissue. *PLoS One* 2009; **4**: e7195.

7 Chimenti I, Smith RR, Li TS, Gerstenblith G, Messina E, Giacomello A, *et al.* Relative roles of direct regeneration versus paracrine effects of human cardiosphere-derived cells transplanted into infarcted mice. *Circ Res* 2010; **106**: 971–980.

8 Davis DR, Ruckdeschel Smith R, Marban E. Human cardiospheres are a source of stem cells with cardiomyogenic potential. *Stem Cells* 2010; **28**: 903–904.

9 Chimenti I, Rizzitelli G, Gaetani R, Angelini F, Ionta V, Forte E, *et al.* Human cardiosphere-seeded gelatin and collagen scaffolds as cardiogenic engineered bioconstructs. *Biomaterials* 2011; **32**: 9271–9281.

10 White AJ, Smith RR, Matsushita S, Chakravarty T, Czer LS, Burton K, *et al.* Intrinsic cardiac origin of human cardiosphere-derived cells. *Eur Heart J* 2013; **34**: 68–75.

11 Cheng K, Shen D, Smith J, Galang G, Sun B, Zhang J, *et al.* Transplantation of platelet gel spiked with cardiosphere-derived cells boosts structural and functional benefits relative to gel transplantation alone in rats with myocardial infarction. *Biomaterials* 2012; **33**: 2872–2879.

12 Shen D, Cheng K, Marban E. Dose-dependent functional benefit of human cardiosphere transplantation in mice with acute myocardial infarction. *J Cell Mol Med* 2012; **16**: 2112–2116.

13 Li TS, Cheng K, Malliaras K, Smith RR, Zhang Y, Sun B, *et al.* Direct comparison of different stem cell types and

subpopulations reveals superior paracrine potency and myocardial repair efficacy with cardiosphere-derived cells. *J Am Coll Cardiol* 2012; **59**: 942–953.

14 Davis DR, Kizana E, Terrovitis J, Barth AS, Zhang Y, Smith RR, *et al*. Isolation and expansion of functionally-competent cardiac progenitor cells directly from heart biopsies. *J Mol Cell Cardiol* 2010; **49**: 312–321.

15 Cheng K, Li TS, Malliaras K, Davis DR, Zhang Y, Marban E, *et al*. Magnetic targeting enhances engraftment and functional benefit of iron-labeled cardiosphere-derived cells in myocardial infarction. *Circ Res* 2010; **106**: 1570–1581.

16 Bonios M, Terrovitis J, Chang CY, Engles JM, Higuchi T, Lautamäki R, *et al*. Myocardial substrate and route of administration determine acute cardiac retention and lung bio-distribution of cardiosphere-derived cells. *J Nucl Cardiol* 2011; **18**: 443–450.

17 Malliaras K, Li TS, Luthringer D, Terrovitis J, Cheng K, Chakravarty T, *et al*. Safety and efficacy of allogeneic cell therapy in infarcted rats transplanted with mismatched cardiosphere-derived cells. *Circulation* 2012; **125**: 100–112.

18 Johnston PV, Sasano T, Mills K, Evers R, Lee ST, Smith RR, *et al*. Engraftment, differentiation, and functional benefits of autologous cardiosphere-derived cells in porcine ischemic cardiomyopathy. *Circulation* 2009; **120**: 1075–1083.

19 Lee ST, White AJ, Matsushita S, Malliaras K, Steenbergen C, Zhang Y, *et al*. Intramyocardial injection of autologous cardiospheres or cardiosphere-derived cells preserves function and minimizes adverse ventricular remodeling in pigs with heart failure post-myocardial infarction. *J Am Coll Cardiol* 2011; **57**: 455–465.

20 Aghila Rani KG, Jayakumar K, Srinivas G, Nair RR, Kartha CC. Isolation of ckit-positive cardiosphere-forming cells from human atrial biopsy. *Asian Cardiovasc Thorac Ann* 2008; **16**: 50–56.

21 Takehara N, Tsutsumi Y, Tateishi K, Ogata T, Tanaka H, Ueyama T, *et al*. Controlled delivery of basic fibroblast growth factor promotes human cardiosphere-derived cell engraftment to enhance cardiac repair for chronic myocardial infarction. *J Am Coll Cardiol* 2008; **52**: 1858–1865.

22 Tang YL, Zhu W, Cheng M, Chen L, Zhang J, Sun T, *et al*. Hypoxic preconditioning enhances the benefit of cardiac progenitor cell therapy for treatment of myocardial infarction by inducing CXCR4 expression. *Circ Res* 2009; **104**: 1209–1216.

23 Zakharova L, Mastroeni D, Mutlu N, Molina M, Goldman S, Diethrich E, *et al*. Transplantation of cardiac progenitor cell sheet onto infarcted heart promotes cardiogenesis and improves function. *Cardiovasc Res* 2010; **87**: 40–49.

24 Aghila Rani KG, Kartha CC. Effects of epidermal growth factor on proliferation and migration of cardiosphere-derived cells expanded from adult human heart. *Growth Factors* 2010; **28**: 157–165.

25 Maxeiner H, Krehbiehl N, Muller A, Woitasky N, Akintürk H, Müller M, *et al*. New insights into paracrine mechanisms of human cardiac progenitor cells. *Eur J Heart Fail* 2010; **12**: 730–737.

26 Bonios M, Chang CY, Pinheiro A, Dimaano VL, Higuchi T, Melexopoulou C, *et al*. Cardiac resynchronization by cardiosphere-derived stem cell transplantation in an experimental model of myocardial infarction. *J Am Soc Echocardiogr* 2011; **24**: 808–814.

27 Bonios M, Chang CY, Terrovitis J, Pinheiro A, Barth A, Dong P, *et al*. Constitutive HIF-1alpha expression blunts the beneficial effects of cardiosphere-derived cell therapy in the heart by altering paracrine factor balance. *J Cardiovasc Transl Res* 2011; **4**: 363–372.

28 Carr CA, Stuckey DJ, Tan JJ, Tan SC, Gomes RS, Camelliti P, *et al*. Cardiosphere-derived cells improve function in the infarcted rat heart for at least 16 weeks – an MRI study. *PLoS One* 2011; **6**: e25669.

29 Lautamaki R, Terrovitis J, Bonios M, Yu J, Tsui BM, Abraham MR, *et al*. Perfusion defect size predicts engraftment but not early retention of intra-myocardially injected cardiosphere-derived cells after acute myocardial infarction. *Basic Res Cardiol* 2011; **106**: 1379–1386.

30 Li Z, Guo X, Matsushita S, Guan J. Differentiation of cardiosphere-derived cells into a mature cardiac lineage using biodegradable poly(N-isopropylacrylamide) hydrogels. *Biomaterials* 2011; **32**: 3220–3232.

31 Martens A, Gruh I, Dimitroulis D, Rojas SV, Schmidt-Richter I, Rathert C, *et al*. Rhesus monkey cardiosphere-derived cells for myocardial restoration. *Cytotherapy* 2011; **13**: 864–872.

32 Tan SC, Carr CA, Yeoh KK, Schofield CJ, Davies KE, Clarke K, *et al*.Identification of valid housekeeping genes for quantitative RT-PCR analysis of cardiosphere-derived cells preconditioned under hypoxia or with prolyl-4-hydroxylase inhibitors. *Mol Biol Rep* 2012; **39**: 4857–4867.

33 Mishra R, Vijayan K, Colletti EJ, Harrington DA, Matthiesen TS, Simpson D, *et al*. Characterization and functionality of cardiac progenitor cells in congenital heart patients. *Circulation* 2011; **123**: 364–373.

34 Koninckx R, Daniels A, Windmolders S, Carlotti F, Mees U, Steels P, *et al*. Mesenchymal stem cells or cardiac progenitors for cardiac repair? A comparative study. *Cell Mol Life Sci* 2011; **68**: 2141–2156.

35 Machida M, Takagaki Y, Matsuoka R, Kawaguchi N. Proteomic comparison of spherical aggregates and adherent cells of cardiac stem cells. *Int J Cardiol* 2011; **153**: 296–305.

36 Chen L, Ashraf M, Wang Y, Zhou M, Zhang J, Qin G, *et al*. The role of Notch1 activation in cardiosphere derived cell differentiation. *Stem Cells Dev* 2012; **21**: 2122–2129.

37 Ye J, Boyle A, Shih H, Sievers RE, Zhang Y, Prasad M, *et al*. Sca-1 cardiosphere-derived cells are enriched for isl1-expressing cardiac precursors and improve cardiac function after myocardial injury. *PLoS One* 2012; **7**: e30329.

38 Makkar R, Smith RR, Cheng K, Malliaras K, Thomson LE, Berman D, *et al*. Intracoronary cardiosphere-derived cells for heart regeneration after myocardial infarction (CADUCEUS): a prospective, randomized phase 1 trial. *Lancet* 2012; **379**: 895–904.

Mesenchymal stem cells

Jose S. Da Silva and Joshua M. Hare

University of Miami, Miami, FL, USA

Introduction

Cardiac remodeling and left ventricular (LV) dysfunction are the major consequences of a myocardial infarction (MI) because of the inability or inadequacy of the heart to self regenerate [1]. Today, the therapeutic method of choice to treat end-stage heart failure is heart transplantation or mechanical circulatory assistance [2,3]. Nevertheless, novel therapeutic options to generate cardiac tissue and restore cardiac function have been studied over the past decade. Cell-based therapies represent a novel therapeutic option in which cells (either autologous or allogeneic) are used for the repair or replacement of cells, tissues, or organs that have been damaged due to disease or injury [4]. Mesenchymal stem cells (MSCs) from bone marrow (BM) were discovered several decades ago [5] and have become a leading candidate for cardiac repair.

The abilities of MSCs to self renew, undergo multiple passages of *ex vivo* expansion, give rise to specialized cell types, and to be used as an allogeneic graft make this cell type a highly promising candidate as a therapy to treat the damaged heart [6–9]. Several studies have demonstrated the use of MSCs effectively *in vivo* [10]. Our group has reported the successful use of both allogeneic and autologous MSCs in swine [10–14]. In one of the studies, allogeneic BM MSCs were used in an adult miniature swine model of chronically infarcted myocardium in order to test the hypothesis that these cells engraft and differentiate in the chronically infarcted

myocardium [11]. Indeed, in this study, we demonstrated the ability of allogeneic MSCs to engraft and differentiate into three cell lineages (cardiomyocytes and vascular smooth muscle and endothelial cells). It also demonstrated that injection of MSCs led to infarct size reduction and reverse remodeling resulting in the restoration of cardiac function and tissue perfusion. Our group also conducted a randomized, blinded, placebo-controlled trial of BM MSCs in adult miniature swine to assess whether autologous MSCs safely reduce infarct size and improve cardiac function in post-MI heart failure [10]. This study demonstrated that autologous MSCs can be safely delivered epicardially by injections into and surrounding kinetic or hypokinetic areas of the heart, resulting, over time, in a decrease in scar size, an increase in wall thickness in the infarct region, increase improvement in contractile function, increased perfusion, improve global LV function, and increase in ejection fraction compared to the placebo group.

Based on our results of reverse remodeling obtained from our extensive translational findings in the swine model, phase I/II clinical trials are under way to test the safety and efficacy of autologous and allogeneic BM MSCs. These studies are:

1. A Phase I/II, Randomized, Double-Blinded, Placebo-Controlled Study of the Safety and Efficacy of Transendocardial Injection of Autologous Human Cells (Bone Marrow or Mesenchymal) in Patients with Chronic Ischemic Left Ventricular Dysfunction

Manual of Research Techniques in Cardiovascular Medicine, First Edition. Edited by Hossein Ardehali, Roberto Bolli, and Douglas W. Losordo.
© 2014 John Wiley & Sons, Ltd. Published 2014 by John Wiley & Sons, Ltd.

and Heart Failure Secondary to Myocardial Infarction (TAC-HFT) [15];

2.. A Phase I/II, Randomized Pilot Study of the Comparative Safety and Efficacy of Transendocardial Injection of Autologous Mesenchymal Stem Cells Versus Allogeneic Mesenchymal Stem Cells in Patients With Chronic Ischemic Left Ventricular Dysfunction Secondary to Myocardial Infarction (POSEIDON) [16];

3. A Phase I/II, Randomized, Double-Blinded, Placebo-Controlled Study of the Safety and Efficacy of Intramyocardial Injection of Autologous Human Mesenchymal Stem Cells (MSCs) in Patients With Chronic Ischemic Left Ventricular Dysfunction Secondary to Myocardial Infarction (MI) Undergoing Cardiac Surgery for Coronary Artery Bypass Grafting (PROMETHEUS) [17];

4. A Phase I/II, Randomized Pilot Study of the Comparative Safety and Efficacy of Transendocardial Injection of Autologous Mesenchymal Stem Cells Versus Allogeneic Mesenchymal Stem Cells in Patients With Nonischemic Dilated Cardiomyopathy (POSEIDON-DCM) [18].

Protocols

Isolation of human MSCs from BM aspirates

Here we describe the isolation of human MSCs from BM aspirates as well as their expansion, cryopreservation, and thawing. This protocol reflects the processes used for the production of BM MSCs for our clinical trials. All open processes are performed inside of an ISO5 biosafety cabinet (BSC). Bioburden checks (sterility testing), which are normally taken during processing, have been omitted from the protocol in the following text.

Isolation of BM mononuclear cells (MNC) by density gradient

Reagents

1. Lymphocyte separation medium (LSM)
2. Plasma-Lyte A (Baxter) 1×
3. Human serum albumin (HSA), 25%

Media preparation

Wash media:
1. Plasma-Lyte A, 1×
2. 25% HSA, 1% final concentration

Processing

1. Transfer the bone marrow aspirate into 250-mL conical tubes and dilute it 1 : 1 with Plasma-Lyte A and mix well. After dilution, determine the number of 50-mL conical tubes into which the diluted marrow should be aliquoted to have 30 mL per tube.

2. Aliquot 15 mL of LSM into each of the 50-mL tubes and overlay 30 mL of the diluted bone marrow aspirate on top of LSM.

3. Centrifuge at 800 *g* for 30 minutes, at room temperature, with the centrifuge brake "OFF".

4. After centrifugation, collect the interface from each 50-mL conical tube and transfer it into the same number of clean 50-mL conical tubes. Bring the volume in each tube up to 50 mL with Wash Media.

5. Centrifuge at 500 *g* for 10 minutes, at room temperature.

6. Remove all the supernatant leaving 1–2 mL in each tube. Resuspend the cell pellet in each conical tube and combine the cells from all the conical tubes into a single 50-mL conical tube. Bring the total volume up to 50 mL with wash media.

7. Centrifuge at 500 *g*, for 10 minutes, at room temperature.

8. Remove all the supernatant leaving 1–2 mL of the supernatant in the conical tube. Resuspend the cell pellet and bring the volume up to 50 mL using fresh Wash Media.

Culture and expansion of human BM MSCs

Reagents

1. Alpha minimal essential media (MEM), 1×
2. Penicillin–streptomycin–glutamine (100×), liquid
3. Fetal bovine serum (FBS), gamma irradiated
4. Trypsin EDTA, 1×; 0.12% gamma irradiated
5. Phosphate buffered saline (DPBS), Ca^{2+} and Mg^{2+} free
6. L-Glutamine 200 mM (100×)
7. Human serum albumin (HSA), 25%

Media preparation

Wash Media:
1. DPBS (Ca^{2+} and Mg^{2+} free)
2. 25% Human serum albumin, final concentration 1%

Complete Culture Media with Antibiotics:
1. Alpha MEM media
2. Penicillin–streptomycin–glutamine (100×), liquid

3. FBS, gamma irradiated and heat inactivated, final concentration 20%

Complete Culture Media without antibiotics:
1. Alpha MEM media
2. L-Glutamine 200 mM (200×), liquid
3. FBS, gamma irradiated and heat inactivated, final concentration 20%

Expansion (P0)
1. Once the mononuclear cells (MNCs) are prepared, seed ten T-185 flasks by dividing the MNCs equitably among the 10 flasks and bring to a final volume of 25 mL with Complete Culture Media with Antibiotics.
2. Incubate at 37°C and 5% CO_2 for at least 72 hours in order to allow the cells to adhere to the flask.
3. After 72 hours, remove the media from the flask.
4. Add 25 mL of Complete Culture Media with Antibiotics and incubate at 37°C and 5% CO_2.

Feeding the cells
1. Feed the cells every 3–4 days until harvest. Use Complete Culture Media with Antibiotics. The cells will be split when they are >80% confluent. In addition, examine each tissue culture flask for absence of contamination. If contamination is present, discard the flask or the whole preparation.
2. Remove the culture media from the T-180 flasks.
3. Add fresh 25 mL of Complete Culture Media with antibiotics.
4. Incubate at 37°C with 5% CO_2, for further culture.

Harvesting cells using trypsin EDTA
1. When the cells are approximately >80% confluent (≈day 14 of culture), remove the media from each flask and add 25 mL of Wash Media and swirl it around the flask.
2. Aspirate off the Wash Media and add 10 mL of trypsin EDTA to each flask. Return the flask to the incubator at 37°C and 5% CO_2 for no more than 8 minutes.
3. Neutralize trypsin activity by adding 15 mL of Complete Culture Media without Antibiotics to each flask. Swirl the media around the flask to make sure all the cells are in suspension.
4. Transfer the cell suspension from each flask to a sterile 50-mL conical tube.

5. Add 25 mL of Wash Media to the flask and swirl to remove any remaining cells. Collect the Wash Media from the flask and add it to the 50-mL conical tube with the detached cells.
6. Centrifuge the 50-mL conical tubes at 500 g for 10 minutes at room temperature.
7. Aspirate the supernatant and leave 1–2 mL of media. Resuspend the pellet in the 50-mL conical tube and bring the volume up to 50 mL with Complete Culture Media without Antibiotics.

Expansion (P1) and final harvest
1. Seed T-185 flasks by equitably dividing the cell suspension from each of the 50-mL conical tubes into four tissue culture flasks, i.e. 12.5 mL of cell suspension in each flask. Bring to a final volume of 25 mL with Complete Culture Media without Antibiotics.
2. Culture the cells for an additional 7 days, feeding the cells 3–4 days after seeding or until cells are >80% confluent.
3. When cells are >80% confluent, harvest the cells as described earlier.
4. Resuspend the cells in 50 mL of Wash Media and centrifuge at 500 g for 10 minutes.
5. Aspirate supernatant, pull all cell pellets together into a single 50-mL conical tube and resuspend in another 50 mL of Wash Media.
6. Take a 100 μL sample and perform a cell count and viability.
7. If the cell number is less than 250×10^6 total cells, culture and expansion must continue.
8. If cell number is sufficient, proceed to cryopreservation. If not, continue with culture and expansion.
9. Remove 2×10^6 cells for CFU-F analysis and 1×10^6 cells for flow cytometric analysis (CD105[POS]/CD45[Neg]).
10. Proceed to the cryopreservation of MSCs.

Cryopreservation of human MSCs
Reagents
1. Dimethyl sulfoxide (DMSO) (Cryoserve)
2. Phosphate buffered saline (DPBS), Ca^{2+} and Mg^{2+} free (Miltenyi)
3. 25% Human serum albumin (HSA), USP grade
4. Hespan (B Braun)
5. Water for irrigation

Media preparation
Wash Media
1. DPBS buffer, Ca^{2+} and Mg^{2+} free
2. 25% HSA, 1% final concentration

Cryopreservation Media without DMSO (Freeze Media 1)
1. Hespan (6% Hetastarch in 0.9% sodium chloride)
2. 25% HSA, 2% final concentration

Cryopreservation Media with 10% DMSO (Freeze Media 2)
1. Hespan (6% Hetastarch in 0.9% sodium chloride)
2. 25% HSA, 2% final concentration
3. DMSO, 10% final concentration

Note. Once prepared, cryopreservation media must be maintained at 4–8°C until and while being used.

Cryopreservation of BM MNC
1. Centrifuge MNCs obtained earlier in a 50-mL conical tube at $500\,g$, for 10 minutes, at room temperature.
2. Remove the supernatant with a sterile aspirating pipette. Gently resuspend the cells with 10 mL of Freeze Media 1. Then, add an equal volume (10 mL) of Freeze Media 2. This will result in a final concentration of 5% DMSO.
3. Cell suspension in a final volume of 20 mL will be cryopreserved in 50-mL Cryocyte bag (Baxter).
4. Cryopreserve the cells with a controlled rate freezer.

Cryopreservation of MSCs
1. Centrifuge the MSCs obtained before in a 50-mL conical tube at $500\,g$, for 10 minutes, at room temperature.
2. Remove the supernatant. Calculate the total resuspension volume to resuspend the cells to a final concentration (1.5×10^6–15×10^6 cells/mL) of your choice (stock cell suspension).
3. Resuspend the cells in up to 50% of the total resuspension volume with Freeze Media 1.
4. Add Freeze Media 2 up to the total resuspension volume, for a final concentration of your choice. The cells will be aliquoted into 50-mL Cryocyte bags, for cryopreservation. The final volume in the Cryocyte bag must not exceed 20 mL.

5. Cryopreserve the cells using a controlled rate freezer.
6. Following cryopreservation, transfer the product bags to liquid nitrogen storage.

Thawing of MSC products
Reagents
1. Plasma-Lyte A, 1×
2. Human serum albumin, 25%
3. Water for irrigation

Media preparation
Thawing Media:
1. Plasma-Lyte A
2. 25% HSA, 1% final concentration

Product thawing
1. Remove the product bag(s) from the liquid nitrogen storage tank.
2. Place a metal cassette with product in a Steri-Drape isolation bag (Medline), and place in the water bath for a few seconds and gently but quickly, remove the Cryocyte bag with the product from the metal cassette.
3. Place the product bag in the Steri-Drape isolation bag (use two bags) and place the Cryocyte bag with the product back in the water bath.
4. Thaw the product until crystals can no longer be observed in the bag. This process should not take longer than 5 minutes.
5. After the product is completely thawed, confirm the total product volume in the bag. This step is necessary to determine the volume of thawing media (which must be equal to the product volume) required for washing (e.g. when the final product volume is 20 mL, 20 mL of the thawing media is required).

Washing the product in a 50-mL Cryocyte bag
1. Aseptically, insert a COBE coupler into the injection port of the Cryocyte bag and connect a sterile 60 mL syringe containing 20 mL of Thawing Media.
2. Slowly introduce the Thawing Media into the product bag and by gently mixing the contents.
3. After all the Thawing Media is added to the bag, remove the contents of the bag using the syringe and transfer to a 50-mL conical tube.

4. Rinse the Cryocyte bag 3× using 10 mL of thawing media each time. Add the rinse to the same 50 mL conical tube.

5. Remove 100 μL of the cell suspension to perform a cell count and viability.

6. Centrifuge the conical tube at 500 g for 10 minutes, at 22°C.

7. Discard the supernatant and adjust the cell concentration as to deliver your total cell amount in a total volume of your choice.

8. Resuspend the pellet gently by using a sterile 10-mL regular tip pipette.

9. Continue to disperse the pellet until it is completely resuspended, and there are no clumps. Avoid formation and/or introduction of air bubbles.

Conclusions

MSCs represent a lead candidate for a novel cell-based therapeutic strategy for cardiac repair. They have the ability to halt and reverse cardiac remodeling due to MI as proven in swine preclinical studies. Further support for this strategy derives from a clinical phase I pilot study for the TAC-HFT trial conducted by our group, where the initial results demonstrated that infused BM MSCs caused reverse remodeling, decreased scar size, and increased contractility in patients [19]. The fact that MSCs are easy to isolate from BM and are simple to expand due to their ability to self renew, gives us the capacity to use adequate cell doses necessary to obtain significant therapeutic results. It also enables us to manufacture high cell numbers from a single donor to be used in allogeneic transplants for different patients, thus eliminating cell variability between infused patients. Together these properties, coupled with emerging encouraging results from preclinical and clinical studies, provide encouraging support for the ongoing development of MSCs as a novel cell-based therapeutic.

Acknowledgements

Work is funded by National Institutes Health grants U54-HL081028 (Specialized Center for Cell Based Therapy), P20-HL101443, and R01- grants HL084275, HL110737-01, HL107110, and HL094849 to Dr. Hare.

References

1 Pfeffer MA, Braunwald E. Ventricular remodeling after myocardial infarction: experimental observations and clinical implications. *Circulation* 1990; **81**: 1161–1172.

2 Husnain KH, Haider MA. Bone marrow cell transplantation in clinical perspective. *J Mol Cell Cardiol* 2004; **38**: 225–235.

3 Muller YD, Seebach JD, Bühler LH, Pascual M, Golshayan D. Transplantation tolerance: Clinical potential of regulatory T cells. *Self Nonself* 2011; **2**: 26–34.

4 Ratcliffe E, Thomas RJ, Williams DJ. Current understanding and challenges in bioprocessing of stem cell-based therapies for regenerative medicine. *Br Med Bull* 2011; **100**: 137–155.

5 Friedenstein AJ, Chailakhjan RK, Lalykina KS. The development of fibroblast colonies in monolayer cultures of guinea-pig bone marrow and spleen cells. *Cell Tissue Kinet* 1970; **3**: 393–403.

6 Kemp KC, Hows J, Donaldson C. Bone marrow-derived mesenchymal stem cells. *Leuk Lymphoma* 2005; **11**: 1531–1544.

7 Togel F, Westenfelder C. Adult bone marrow-derived stem cells for organ regeneration and repair. *Dev Dyn* 2007; **236**: 3321–3331.

8 Biehl JK, Russell B. Introduction to stem cell therapy. *J Cardiovasc Nurs* 2009; **24**: 98–103; quiz 104–105.

9 Boyle AJ, McNiece IK, Hare JM. Mesenchymal stem cell therapy for cardiac repair. *Methods Mol Biol* 2010; **660**: 65–84.

10 Schuleri KH, Feigenbaum GS, Centola M, Weiss ES, Zimmet JM, Turney J, et al. Autologous mesenchymal stem cells produce reverse remodelling in chronic ischaemic cardiomyopathy. *Eur Heart J* 2009; **30**: 2722–2732.

11 Quevedo HC, Hatzistergos KE, Oskouei BN, Feigenbaum GS, Rodriguez JE, Valdes D, et al. Allogeneic mesenchymal stem cells restore cardiac function in chronic ischemic cardiomyopathy via trilineage differentiating capacity. *Proc Natl Acad Sci U S A* 2009; **106**: 14022–14027.

12 Amado LC, Saliaris AP, Schuleri KH, St John M, Xie JS, Cattaneo S, et al. Cardiac repair with intramyocardial injection of allogeneic mesenchymal stem cells after myocardial infarction. *Proc Natl Acad Sci U S A* 2005; **102**: 11474–11479.

13 Amado LC, Schuleri KH, Saliaris AP, Boyle AJ, Helm R, Oskouei B, et al. Multimodality noninvasive imaging demonstrates in vivo cardiac regeneration after mesenchymal stem cell therapy. *J Am Coll Cardiol* 2006; **48**: 2116–2124.

14 Schuleri KH, Amado LC, Boyle AJ, Centola M, Saliaris AP, Gutman MR, et al. Early improvement in cardiac

tissue perfusion due to mesenchymal stem cells. *Am J Physiol Heart Circ Physiol* 2008; **294**: H2002–H2011.

15 http://clinicaltrials.gov/ct2/show/NCT00768066?term= tac-hft&rank=1

16 http://clinicaltrials.gov/ct2/show/NCT01087996?term= poseidon&rank=5

17 http://clinicaltrials.gov/ct2/show/NCT00587990?term= prometheus&rank=1

18 http://clinicaltrials.gov/ct2/show/NCT01392625?term= poseidon&rank=4

19 Williams AR, Trachtenberg B, Velazquez DL, McNiece I, Altman P, Rouy D, *et al.* Intramyocardial stem cell injection in patients with ischemic cardiomyopathy: functional recovery and reverse remodeling. *Circ Res* 2011; **108**: 792–796.

Generation and differentiation of human iPS cells

Sebastian Diecke,[1] Lei Ye,[2] Sophia Zhang,[2] and Jianyi Zhang[2]

[1] Stanford University School of Medicine, Palo Alto, CA, USA

[2] University of Minnesota Medical School, Minneapolis, MN, USA

Introduction

Perhaps one of the most significant achievements in science was the discovery of induced pluripotent stem (iPS) cells [1,2]. iPS cells are a type of pluripotent stem cell derived from adult somatic cells that have been genetically reprogrammed back to an embryonic stem-cell-like state through the forced expression of genes and factors important for maintaining the defining properties of embryonic stem (ES) cells [3]. Human iPS cells were first produced from human fibroblasts by two independent groups – the Yamanaka lab at Kyoto University and the Thomson lab at University of Wisconsin, Madison. iPS cells are similar to ES cells in many aspects, including the expression of ES cell markers, chromatin methylation patterns, embryoid body formation, teratoma formation, viable chimera formation, and pluripotency in differentiation. The basic concept of somatic cell reprogramming was discovered in the late nineties through the cell fusion and somatic cell nuclear transfer experiments [4–6]. Based on these findings, Shinya Yamanaka and his coworkers were able to show that mouse embryonic fibroblasts (MEFs) could be converted into germline-competent induced pluripotent stem cells by retroviral expression of four transcription factors: OCT4, SOX2, KLF4, and c-MYC [3,7]. The reprogramming process is based on the ectopic expression of these transcription factors, which initiate a rare reactivation of the endogenous pluripotency genes OCT4, SOX2, and NANOG [8]. This reactivation leads to a resetting of the epigenetic profile of a terminally differentiated somatic cell and activates the molecular circuitry of pluripotency [9,10]. Thereafter, the derived iPS cells are similar to embryonic stem cells with regard to their morphology, growth characteristics, differentiation capacities, and expression of various marker genes [11]. The transition from a somatic to a pluripotent state could be further enhanced through chromatin-modifying chemicals and microRNAs [12,13]. Subsequent studies revealed that the induction of pluripotency was also possible with different transcription factor combinations and could be improved by activation or inhibition of different signaling pathways [14–18].

The unique property of iPS cells to differentiate into all other cell types of the human body opened up new clinical perspectives for developing successful stem-cell-based therapies. However, the use of retroviral and lentiviral vectors for reprogramming carries a high risk of DNA incorporation into chromosomes and can lead to the disruption of gene transcription and tumor formation [19]. Therefore, it is important to develop further nonintegrating reprogramming techniques for future applications in the field of regenerative

Manual of Research Techniques in Cardiovascular Medicine, First Edition. Edited by Hossein Ardehali, Roberto Bolli, and Douglas W. Losordo.

medicine. These techniques are based on an almost complete removal of the integrated virus from the genome or on nonintegrating viruses [20,21]. More recently, different virus-independent reprogramming approaches, like transient vector expression, protein- or mRNA-based, have also been developed, which will further improve the quality of iPS cells [22–24]. The breakthrough discovery of iPS cells has allowed researchers to obtain pluripotent stem cells without the controversial use of embryos, providing a novel and powerful method to "de-differentiate" cells whose developmental fates had been traditionally assumed to be determined. Furthermore, tissues derived from iPS cells will be a nearly identical match to the cell donor, an important factor in the research of disease modeling, drug screening, and potentially repairing the injured organs in the human body. This chapter provides protocols to generate human iPS cells from fibroblasts and their subsequent differentiation into cardiac myocytes.

Protocol I: Generation of hiPSC from fibroblasts

So far, the efficiency of the alternative reprogramming approaches have been low. Here, we describe a protocol in detail that uses the most efficient Lentiviral reprogramming technique. This protocol is subdivided into a detailed description how to produce the lentivirus and the actual reprogramming protocol (Figure 12.1).

The target fibroblast cell line should be thawed and cultured for 1 week before the reprogramming experiment is started.

Production of the VSV-G Lentivirus (6 days)
Day 0 (in the morning)
• Coat a 10-cm dish with 5 mL of diluted poly-L-lysine solution (0.01 % Sigma P4832-50 mL) for 1 hour (fill up 1.2 mL poly-L-lysine solution to 5 mL using PBS).

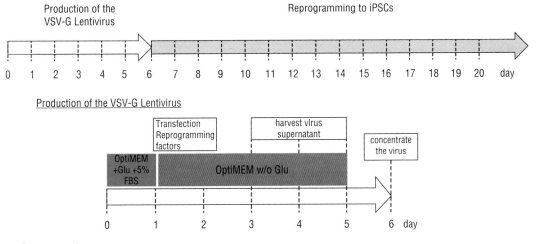

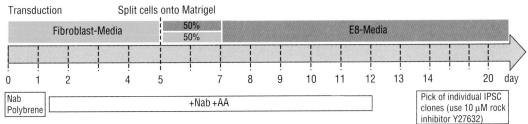

Figure 12.1 Timeline of a normal lentiviral reprogramming experiment. The overall protocol can be subdivided into the production of the lentivirus and reprogramming parts.

• Remove the solution completely and let the dishes dry for several hours.

Day 0 (in the afternoon)
• Wash the dishes with MQ directly before use.
• Seed 6×10^6 HEK293TN cells in 10 mL Opti-MEM with Glutamax (Life Technologies 51985034) + 5% FBS (all the media in this protocol are without antibiotics) per 10-cm dish.

Day 1 (in the morning):
• Change the medium to Opti-MEM without Glutamax (Life Technologies 31985070) supplemented with 25 µM chloroquine (Sigma C6628-25g) to reduce plasmid degradation, increasing the effective plasmid concentration in the cells.
• Prewarm 50 mL Opti-MEM to RT and the rest of the bottle to 37°C.
• Mix the Opti-MEM with the DNAs according to Table 12.1 (all maxipreps were performed with the Qiagen endotoxin-free plasmid kit) and incubate at RT for 5 minutes.
• Mix the Opti-MEM with the Lipofectamine 2000 (Life Technologies 11668027) and incubate at RT for 5 minutes.
• Mix the two solutions together.
• Incubate 20 minutes at RT.
• Add the transfection mixture to each dish dropwise, gently swirl the dish crosswise.
• Put the dishes back in the incubator and incubate for at least 6 hours or over night.

Table 12.1 Transfection mixture for lentivirus production

	1 × 10-cm dish	5 × 10-cm dish
1. DNA-Mix:		
Opti-MEM(µL)	1000	5000
pMD2G	3 µg	15 µg
pAX2	9 µg	45 µg
4 in 1 Tomato Reprogramming Vector	12 µg	60 µg
2. Lipo2000-Mix:		
Opti-MEM (µL)	1000	5000
Lipo2000	50	250
total (µL)	~ 2000	~ 10500

Day 2 (in the morning):
• After the 6 hours incubation or the next morning, change the medium to 5–10 mL Opti-MEM (without Glutamax) supplemented with 10 µM sodium butyrate (Sigma 5887-250G) (0.5 µL sodium butyrate stock solution (200 mM) in 10 mL medium)
• Incubate the cells for 24 hours.

Day 3–5 (in the morning):
• Virus harvest: collect the medium in 50-mL falcons (pool the supernatant) and add 5–10 mL Opti-MEM *without* serum.
• Incubate the cells for an additional 24 hours.
• Store virus supernatant in an ice bucket in the fridge.

Day 5 (Lenti-X-Concentrator):
• Centrifuge collected supernatant at $500g$ for 15 minutes to remove cells and cell debris (supernatant can also be filtered through a 0.45-µm PVDF, filtration may decrease the amount of virus).
• Transfer supernatant to a sterile 50-mL tube and add 1 volume of cold Lenti-X Concentrator (Clontech Laboratories 631231) to every 3 volumes of lentivirus-containing supernatant and mix by gentle inversion. (Example: 7 mL Lenti-X with 21 mL viral supernatant.)
• Refrigerate overnight (at least 4 hours). Lentivector-containing supernatants mixed with Lenti-X Precipitation Solution are stable for up to 3 days at 4°C.
• use PEG-*it* Virus Precipitation Solution (SBI).

Day 6:
• Centrifuge supernatant/ Lenti-X mixture at $1500g$ for 45 minutes at 4°C. After centrifugation, the lentiviral particles appear as a white pellet.
• Aspirate supernatant.
• Resuspend lentiviral pellet in 1:100 of original volume using cold, sterile phosphate buffered saline (PBS) (e.g.1:100 of the initial volume, i.e. 300 µL if you started with 30 mL supernatant).
• Aliquot in cryogenic vials and store at −70°C until ready for use.

Reprogramming of human fibroblasts (~14 days)
Day 0:
• Plate 3×10^4 human fibroblast 1 day before starting the reprogramming into each well of a 6-well dish.

Day 1 (afternoon):
• Use different multiplicity of infection (MOI) between 1 and 10 for the transduction of fibroblasts (alternatively, use increasing doses of untitered virus supernatant) in 2 mL per well (usually 30 μL of 1/100 concentrated virus).
• Spin inoculate (700 g) the cells for 1 hour at 37°C.
• Place plate in incubator overnight.

Medium for transduction: Fibroblast Media + Polybrene (10 μg/mL; Santa Cruz Biotechnology sc-134220) + 50 μg/mL ascorbic acid.

Day 2 (morning):
• Media change to Fibroblast Media + sodium butyrate (0.2 mM) + 50 μg/mL ascorbic acid.

Day 4:
• Media change to Fibroblast Media + sodium butyrate (0.2 mM) + 50 μg/mL ascorbic acid.

Day 5:
• Split the induced fibroblast 1:3, 1:6, 1:9 on Matrigel (BD Biosciences 356231) and cultivate the cells in half Fibroblast Media + half E8 + sodium butyrate 0.2 mM + 50 μg/mL ascorbic acid.

Day 7:
• Media change to E8 + sodium butyrate 0.2 mM + 50 μg/mL ascorbic acid (first colonies visible, Figure 12.2).

Day 8–13:
• Media change to E8 + sodium butyrate 0.2 mM + 50 μg/mL ascorbic acid.

Day 14:
• Media change to E8.

After reprogramming Day 14 change E8 Media every day until the iPS colonies are big enough for manual picking (Day 20, Figure 12.2) under the

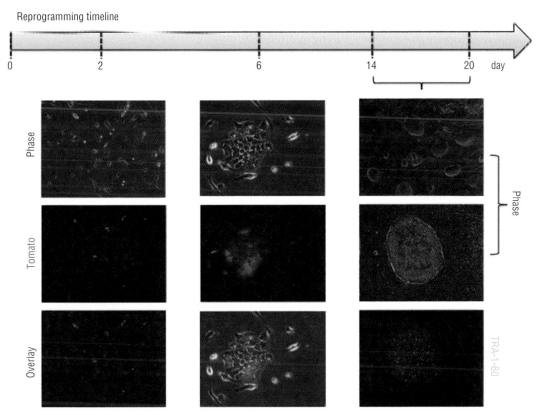

Figure 12.2 Representative images showing the transformation of transduced human fibroblast over time during the reprogramming. Two days after transduction, induced fibroblast turn red and 4 days later the first small colonies appear. At the earliest, 14 days after starting the induction of pluripotency fully reprogrammed iPSC (Tra-1-60 marker staining) are ready for picking.

microscope. Pick six individual iPS clones and transfer them into six different wells of a Matrigel-coated plate with E8 Media and in presence of 10 μM ROCK Inhibitor (Stemgent Y-27632, 04-0012).

Plasmids and media

The packaging plasmids pPAX2 (Plasmid 12260) and pMD2.G (Plasmid 12259) can be ordered from Addgene. The reprogramming plasmid was kindly provided by Dr. Axel Schambach [25].

Fibroblast media:

DMEM/GlutaMAX (Life Technologies 10569-010)

20% FCS (Hyclone; Thermo Scientific SH30071.03)

1× Non-essential amino acids (NEAA; Life Technologies 11140-050)

100 μM mercaptoethanol (Life Technologies 21985)

E8 media:

DMEM/F12 L-glutamine, HEPES (Life Technologies 11330-057)

543 μg/mL NaHCO$_3$ (Life Technologies 25080-094)

64 μg/mL L-Ascorbic acid-2-phosphate (Sigma A8960-5g)

140 ng/mL Sodium selenite (Sigma 5261-10g)

10.7 μg/mL Transferrin (Sigma T3705-5g)

20 μg/mL Insulin (Life Technologies 12585-014)

100 ng/mL bFGF (Peprotech 100-18B)

2 ng/mL TGFβ (Peprotech 100-21)

Titration of the virus

Preparation of a serial dilution of the lentiviral preparation

• Add 2 μL virus to 198 μL PBS to generate a 1 : 100 dilution.

• Prepare five tubes with 100 μL PBS each.

• Pipette 100 μL of the 1 : 100 virus dilution to the first Eppendorf tube, mix by vortexing.

• Repeat this for every tube (resulting dilutions are 1 : 100, 1 : 200, 1 : 400, 1 : 800, 1 : 1600, 1 : 3200, and so forth).

• Seed 1×10^5 HEK cells in each well of a 24-well plate.

• Add exactly 50 μL of each viral dilution to the cells, mix thoroughly.

• After 72 hours at 37°C remove medium, trypsinize the cells, pellet, and resuspend in PBS (0.5 mL) by

pipetting gently up and down and transfer to fluorescence-activated cell sorting (FACS) tubes.

• Determine the percentage of Tomato-positive cells by FACS analysis.

Biological titer calculation (TU, transducing units)

$$TU/\mu L = (P \times N/100 \times V) \times 1/DF$$

P = % Tomato$^+$ cells, N = number of cells at time of transduction, V = volume of dilution added to each well = 40 μL, and DF = dilution factor = 1 (undiluted), 10^{-1} (diluted 1/10), 10^{-2} (diluted 1/100), and so on.

Only dilutions yielding to 1–20% of Tomato-positive cells in a linear range should be used for titer calculations (below 1% FACS may not be accurate, above 20% the chance for multiple infections increases).

TU/mL (transduction units/mL) or viral titer – the relative concentration of transduction-competent pseudoviral particles;

MOI (multiplicity of infection) – the ratio of transduction pseudoviral particles (TU) to the number of cells being infected.

For example, if 1×10^6 cells are to be infected at an MOI of 1, then 1×10^6 TU should be added to the cells.

Protocol II: differentiation hiPSCs to myocytes

We describe here a protocol for the monolayer differentiation of cardiac myocytes from human iPS (hiPS) cells (Figure 12.3).

Day −4

• Wash hiPS cells with Dulbecco's Phosphate-Buffered Saline (DPBS; Life Technologies 14190-144) and incubate with Versene (Life Technologies 15040-066) for 5 minutes at 37°C in an incubator.

• After aspiration of Versene, wash hiPS cells with DPBS and hiPS cells culture medium (each once). Dissociate hiPS cells into single cells by gently pipetting in hiPS cell culture medium. Collect cells into 15-mL centrifuge tube that contains fresh hiPS cell culture medium.

• Harvest hiPS cells by centrifuge at 1200 rpm for 5 minutes. Resuspend cells in hiPS cell culture medium and centrifuge again.

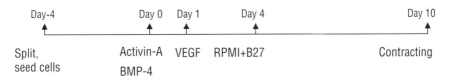

Figure 12.3 An outline of the protocol used for hiPS-CM differentiation.

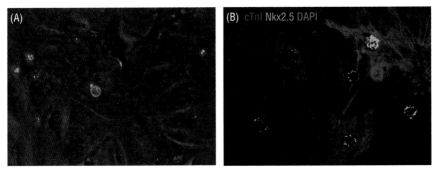

Figure 12.4 (A) Phase contrast image of hiPS cell differentiated cardiac myocytes. The contracting area of differentiated cells was mechanically selected and cultured for 10 days with RMPI1640 supplemented with B27 complete. (See Video clip 12.2.) (B) Sarcomeric (cardiac troponin I (cTnI)) organization and Nkx2.5 expression in cardiac myocytes derived from hiPS cells. (Magnification: A – 200×, B = 400×.)

• Resuspend hiPS cells in mTeSR1 medium (StemCell Technologies, Inc.) that is supplemented with 10 μM ROCK inhibitor and count cell density using a hemocytometer.
• Seed 1×10^6 iPS cells into each well of a 6-well plate that has been precoated with growth factor reduced Matrigel (BD Biosciences CB40234, CB40234).

Day −3 to −1
• Exchange mTeSR1 medium daily with 2.5 mL/well.
• When cells reach 100% confluence, it is ready for differentiation.

Day 0 of differentiation
• Wash cells with RPMI1640 medium (Life Technologies 11875-085) twice.
• Prepare RPMI1640 medium supplemented with B27 minus (without insulin; Life Technologies 0050129SA), 50 ng/mL Activin A (R&D Systems 338-AC-010) and 25 ng/mL BMP-4 (R&D Systems 314-BP-010).

Day 1 of differentiation
• Replace the culture medium with RPMI1640 medium supplemented with B27 minus and 5 ng/mL VEGF (R&D Systems 293VE).

Day 4 of differentiation
• Wash cells with RPMI1640 and feed the cells with RPMI1640 supplemented with B27 complete (Life Technologies 17504044).

Day 7 afterwards
• Exchange medium every 3 days (day 7, day 10, etc.) with RPMI supplemented with B27 complete.
  We have observed contracting cells starting at day 10, which can continue for 60 days (Figure 12.4 and Video clips 12.1 and 12.2).

Future perspectives

iPS cells are among the most significant scientific achievements in modern biological research. The technology restores pluripotency to fully differentiated cells through the ectopic co-expression of reprogramming factors and, consequently, promises to personalize regenerative therapy by enabling patients to be treated with stem-like cells that have been obtained from their own tissues. However, research on therapeutic applications for iPS cells is in its infancy, and there remains a lack of consensus about how closely iPS cells replicate the genomes and functions of ESCs. Recent reports have identified significant genetic and epigenetic differences, and concerns have also been expressed about alterations in karyotype and about point mutations in the protein-coding regions of iPS-cell DNA. Alternative methods for inducing pluripotency, including virus-independent reprogramming techniques, must continue to be investigated, and the genetic profiles of cells that are derived from iPS cells must be thoroughly characterized to determine whether this technology can be safely evaluated in clinical trials.

References

1 Takahashi K, Tanabe K, Ohnuki M, Narita M, Ichisaka T, Tomoda K, et al. Induction of pluripotent stem cells from adult human fibroblasts by defined factors. Cell 2007; **131**: 861–872.

2 Yu J, Vodyanik MA, Smuga-Otto K, Antosiewicz-Bourget J, Frane JL, Tian S, et al. Induced pluripotent stem cell lines derived from human somatic cells. Science 2007; **318**: 1917–1920.

3 Takahashi K, Yamanaka S. Induction of pluripotent stem cells from mouse embryonic and adult fibroblast cultures by defined factors. Cell 2006; **126**: 663–676.

4 Cowan CA, Atienza J, Melton DA, Eggan K. Nuclear reprogramming of somatic cells after fusion with human embryonic stem cells. Science 2005; **309**: 1369–1373.

5 Tada M, Takahama Y, Abe K, Nakatsuji N, Tada T. Nuclear reprogramming of somatic cells by in vitro hybridization with ES cells. Curr Biol 2001; **11**: 1553–1558.

6 Wilmut I, Schnieke AE, McWhir J, Kind AJ, Campbell KH. Viable offspring derived from fetal and adult mammalian cells. Nature 1997; **386**: 810–813.

7 Okita K, Ichisaka T, Yamanaka S. Generation of germline-competent induced pluripotent stem cells. Nature 2007; **448**: 313–317.

8 Mitalipov S, Wolf D. Totipotency, pluripotency and nuclear reprogramming. Adv Biochem Eng Biotechnol 2009; **114**: 185–199.

9 Feng B, Ng JH, Heng JC, Ng HH. Molecules that promote or enhance reprogramming of somatic cells to induced pluripotent stem cells. Cell Stem Cell 2009; **4**: 301–312.

10 Maherali N, Sridharan R, Xie W, Utikal J, Eminli S, Arnold K, et al. Directly reprogrammed fibroblasts show global epigenetic remodeling and widespread tissue contribution. Cell Stem Cell 2007; **1**: 55–70.

11 Wernig M, Meissner A, Foreman R, Brambrink T, Ku M, Hochedlinger K, et al. In vitro reprogramming of fibroblasts into a pluripotent ES-cell-like state. Nature 2007; **448**: 318–324.

12 Amabile G, Meissner A. Induced pluripotent stem cells: current progress and potential for regenerative medicine. Trends Mol Med 2009; **15**: 59–68.

13 Anokye-Danso F, Trivedi CM, Juhr D, Gupta M, Cui Z, Tian Y, et al. Highly efficient miRNA-mediated reprogramming of mouse and human somatic cells to pluripotency. Cell Stem Cell 2011; **8**: 376–388.

14 Heng J.-C.D, Feng B, Han J, Jiang J, Kraus P, Ng JH, et al. The nuclear receptor Nr5a2 can replace Oct4 in the reprogramming of murine somatic cells to pluripotent cells. Cell Stem Cell 2010; **6**: 167–174.

15 Marson A, Foreman R, Chevalier B, Bilodeau S, Kahn M, Young RA, et al. Wnt signaling promotes reprogramming of somatic cells to pluripotency. Cell Stem Cell 2008; **3**: 132–135.

16 Nakagawa M, Koyanagi M, Tanabe K, Takahashi K, Ichisaka T, Aoi T, et al. Generation of induced pluripotent stem cells without Myc from mouse and human fibroblasts. Nat Biotechnol 2008; **26**: 101–106.

17 Redmer T, Diecke S, Grigoryan T, Quiroga-Negreira A, Birchmeier W, Besser D, et al. E-cadherin is crucial for embryonic stem cell pluripotency and can replace OCT4 during somatic cell reprogramming. EMBO Reports 2011; **12**: 720–726.

18 Silva J, Barrandon O, Nichols J, Kawaguchi J, Theunissen TW, Smith A, et al. Promotion of reprogramming to ground state pluripotency by signal inhibition. PLoS Biol 2008; **6**: e253.

19 Sommer CA, Sommer AG, Longmire TA, Christodoulou C, Thomas DD, Gostissa M, et al. Excision of reprogramming transgenes improves the differentiation potential of iPS cells generated with a single excisable vector. Stem Cells 2010; **28**: 64–74.

20 Stadtfeld M, Hochedlinger K. Induced pluripotency: history, mechanisms, and applications. Genes Dev 2010; **24**: 2239–2263.

21 Stadtfeld M, Nagaya M, Utikal J, Weir G, Hochedlinger K. Induced pluripotent stem cells generated without viral integration. Science 2008; **322**: 945–949.

22 Jia F, Wilson KD, Sun N, Gupta DM, Huang M, Li Z, et al. A nonviral minicircle vector for deriving human iPS cells. Nat Methods 2010; **7**: 197–199.

23 Warren L, Manos PD, Ahfeldt T, Loh YH, Li H, Lau F, et al. Highly efficient reprogramming to pluripotency and directed differentiation of human cells with synthetic modified mRNA. Cell Stem Cell 2010; **7**: 618–630.

24 Zhou H, Wu S, Joo JY, Zhu S, Han DW, Lin T, et al. Generation of induced pluripotent stem cells using recombinant proteins. Cell Stem Cell 2009; **4**: 381–384.

25 Warlich E, Kuehle J, Cantz T, Brugman MH, Maetzig T, Galla M, et al. Lentiviral vector design and imaging approaches to visualize the early stages of cellular reprogramming. Mol Ther 2011; **19**: 782–789.

Isolation of neonatal and adult rat cardiomyocytes

Md. Abdur Razzaque and Jeffrey Robbins

Cincinnati Children's Hospital Medical Center, Cincinnati, OH, USA

Introduction

For the last three-quarters of a century, investigators have attempted to prepare and maintain stable cell lines that recapitulate the cardiac phenotype. With rare exceptions, and those exceptions are severely limited as well, they have been unsuccessful. Because of these failures, almost all laboratories studying basic cellular processes that are cardiomyocyte-based have found it necessary to routinely prepare primary cell cultures of either neonatal or adult rat cardiomyocytes. The neonatal and adult rat cardiomyocyte primary cultures enable the investigator to study and understand the morphological, biochemical, and electrophysiological characteristics of isolated cells. These cells exhibit most of the characteristics of cardiomyocytes *in vivo*, but may be studied in an isolated and reductionist fashion, free of the confounding effects of extracellular matrix, paracrine, endocrine, and, to a large extent, autocrine effects. Thus, cardiomyocyte-based signaling pathways, metabolism, cell death, ion flux, biochemistry, physiology, and pathology can be determined in a cell autonomous fashion [1].

Despite the intensive use of transgenically altered hearts to understand the cause and effect relationships underlying cardiac function, cardiomyocyte cell culture has been and will remain highly relevant to heart research. Its versatility, economy and convenience, as compared to whole animal experiments, ensure its continued utility. Like many primary cultured cells, investigators have found it more convenient and easier to derive the cells from embryonic or neonatal hearts, with the rat being the animal of choice as it offers higher yields (as compared to the mouse) on a per heart basis. Neonatal rat cardiomyocytes, derived from the ventricles (NRVMs), are postmitotic, terminally differentiated cells, which do not divide, beat spontaneously, and respond to different pharmacological stimuli. Reports documenting the preparation of cardiomyocyte cultures that showed contractile properties began appearing in the late 1960s and early 1970s but these early cultures were severely limited, both in terms of their ability to be maintained in a healthy state and their purity, as they were rapidly overgrown by contaminating fibroblasts. The modern era of cardiomyocyte cell culture was ushered in by the Simpson laboratory, which, in the early 1980s, initiated a series of reports documenting the practical and reproducible preparation of primary cultures that were highly purified and could be maintained in a contractile state for 7 days or longer. These cells were first used to study the pathways and mechanisms that underlie the development of ventricular hypertrophy [2–5]. The ability to culture NRVMs for an extended period has allowed the study of other complex pathways, such as the cardiomyocyte's response to hypoxia [6,7], cardiomyocyte apoptosis [8,9], or cardiac gene expression [10–12]. A few cell lines

Manual of Research Techniques in Cardiovascular Medicine, First Edition. Edited by Hossein Ardehali, Roberto Bolli, and Douglas W. Losordo.
© 2014 John Wiley & Sons, Ltd. Published 2014 by John Wiley & Sons, Ltd.

(AT1 andHL-1) derived from atrial tumor cells have also been established [13,14]. However, their intrinsic limitations, which are considered in more detail later in the text have restricted their application. Thus, primary cells have been and will remain the system of choice for most *in vitro* cardiomyocyte-based studies. Isolated cells can be cultured for up to 2 weeks and the cells efficiently transfected or pharmacologically manipulated to modulate metabolism or specific cell signaling pathways as desired. Because of the relatively high yields, NRVMs [15–17] allow a large number of experiments to be carried out using a relatively small number of animals, with the data being evaluated quickly at relatively low cost. Although cardiomyocytes do not represent the majority of cells in the rat heart, they represent the main cell mass and determine the function of the ventricle as a pump. Cardiomyocyte isolation techniques are therefore of critical importance, as are methods for cell culture that preserve as closely as possible the *in vivo* structural integrity and function of the myocytes.

Protocols

Isolation of neonatal rat ventricular cardiomyocytes

We describe here a standard protocol for the isolation and maintenance of cardiomyocytes obtained from neonatal rat hearts. This preparation is convenient and, in our hands, routinely and repeatedly yields high quality and high purity (>90–95%) cardiomyocyte cultures in our laboratory.

Day #1

Prepare:

1. Hanks Balanced Salt Solution (HBSS, calcium and magnesium free): at least 30 mL for each batch of 10–12 neonate rat hearts. One 50-mL conical tube for each batch of hearts. 500 mL HBSS, ice cold for rinsing hearts.
2. 0.05% trypsin–EDTA kept on ice.

Harvest:

1. To maintain rapidity in the initial stages of isolation, we usually process 10–12 hearts at one time. This is referred to as a "batch." Harvest 1 batch of rat pup hearts (1–3 days old) in necropsy.

Decapitate and surgically remove hearts and immediately put into ice cold HBSS.
2. Under a class IIA safety hood, pour the hearts and the 30 mL of HBSS into a 10-cm tissue culture plate that is sitting on an ice block.
3. While the hearts are in the ice cold HBSS, remove both atria and the major vessels with forceps. Separate each heart in half using the forceps to help rinse the blood out of the chambers.
4. Move the bisected hearts to a fresh 10-cm plate containing 10–12 mL of ice cold HBSS per 10–12 hearts, leaving the atria and vessels behind.
5. Put 0.05% trypsin into a 50-mL conical tube with filter cap; 1 mL for each heart collected.
6. Move rinsed hearts to the tube with trypsin. Incubate overnight at 4°C.

Day #2

Prepare:
1. Ice cold HBSS.
2. Ice cold calcium-containing media, such as M119 or Dulbecco's Modified Eagle Medium (DMEM)/F12.
3. Collagenase; reconstitute with media to 2000 U/mL media.
4. AlphaMEM with 10% fetal bovine serum (FBS), warmed in a 37°C water bath.

Tissue culture:
1. Aspirate trypsin from cells very carefully and gently rinse hearts with ice cold HBSS. Let the hearts settle.
2. Aspirate HBSS from cells and repeat rinse with ice cold calcium-containing medium.
3. Aspirate medium and replace with media and collagenase solution. Final volume should be about 20 mL (per batch). Add 10 μL of DNase (concentration 20 mg/mL) to collagenase solution and hearts. Use 1600–2000 units of collagenase per batch of 10–12 hearts.
4. Warm hearts to 37°C in waterbath for 15 minutes. Place tube on an Adams nutator (or equivalent) at 37°C and incubate for 30 minutes. Gently triturate 3–4 times using a wide-bore 10 mL serological pipette, filling and emptying the barrel at a rate of about 3.0 mL/second, and incubate longer if needed.
5. Triturate cells 7–10 times as mentioned previously and let cells settle for about 4–5 minutes.

6. Rinse a 40-μm nylon cell strainer (BD Falcon, 352340), with 1 mL of the calcium-containing medium (no serum).

7. Filter the cell supernatant through the cell strainer into a fresh 50-mL conical tube.

8. Add an additional 5 mL media to tissue residue and repeat Steps 5–7. Rinse strainer with 2 mL medium.

9. Centrifuge cells for 5 minutes at 50–100 g.

10. Resuspend the cell pellet in AlphaMEM with 10% FBS. Use 1.5 mL of media per heart and add 10 μL of 20 mg/mL DNase.

Preplating:

Transfer to a 75-cm² tissue culture flask (or 2–3 10-cm plates) and incubate for 30 minutes. Fibroblasts preferentially will adhere to the plate, increasing the proportion of cardiomyocytes in the final plated cultures. We use 10-cm plates (not coated) with about 10 mL of cells per plate. Transfer media from plate to 50-mL conical tube. Rinse flask with 5 mL of AlphaMEM with 10% FBS and transfer that to the 50-mL conical tube. Mix well but gently prior to counting cells. Check cell viability by dye exclusion technique. One drop of trypan blue is mixed with one drop of cell suspension and the mixture allowed to sit for 1–2 minutes for absorption. The total number of cells and the number of stained cells are then counted using a hemocytometer. Cell viability is calculated:

$$\text{Percent viability} = (\text{total cells counted} \\ - \text{stained cells})/\text{total cells counted} \times 100$$

Some cautionary notes:
• The optimal concentration of trypsin must be established for every new lot as trypsin activity changes from one lot to another.
• To avoid loss of activity, the trypsin solution has to be made fresh, just before the beginning of the preparation, as prolonged equilibration at 37°C results in trypsin autodigestion.
• Preparations from older animals often result in lower yield and cell viability.
• Remove the heart as quickly as possible, since unnecessary delays result in lower myocyte viability.
• The size of the pieces is a critical parameter for cardiomyocyte yield and viability. Cell damage can occur (a) during mincing and digestion if the pieces

are too small, or (b) during a slower trypsin digestion if the pieces are too large. Mincing should be performed as quickly as possible.
• The presence of cell clumps or cells with irregular membranes denotes that digestion was not complete, or that mechanical dissociation was too harsh.
• Most of the cardiomyocytes are usually isolated in the first 10 dissociations. The digestion is complete when the tissue becomes mostly white and clumpy and the supernatant contains only damaged cells. If the digestion is not complete after 3 hours, the concentration of trypsin needs to be increased for the next cardiomyocyte preparation, since longer exposure to trypsin will damage the cells.
• Cell filtration (Step 7, mentioned earlier) is an important step because the filter retains unwanted cell clumps containing cardiac fibroblasts. Because of their rapid growth, fibroblasts can become the predominant cell population in the cultures within 3–5 days if filtration is not effectively used.
• During the preplating step, healthy cardiomyocytes can adhere quite rapidly as well, so the optimal time for this step should be experimentally determined by frequently monitoring the process under the microscope.
• If one is interested in culturing fibroblasts, the settled, attached cells from the preplating contain the nonmyocyte cell population contaminated by a small number of NRVMs. A few passages will remove NRVMs and leave mostly cardiac fibroblasts.
• NRVM attachment can be enhanced by precoating the tissue culture plates with gelatin. A 0.1% sterile gelatin solution is added to the plates, and the bottom covered completely using a rubber policeman or equivalent spreading utensil, allowed to dry, and used within 5 days.

Isolation of adult rat cardiomyocytes

1. Prepare Perfusion Buffer (approximately 150 mL/adult heart): 113 mM NaCl, 4.7 mM KCl, 0.6 mM KH_2PO_4, 0.6 mM Na_2HPO_4, 1.2 mM $MgSO_4·7H_2O$, 0.032 mM phenol red, 12 mM $NaHCO_3$, 10 mM $KHCO_3$, 10 mM HEPES buffer, 30 mM taurine, 10 mM 2,3-butanedione monoxime (BDM), 5.5 mM glucose (final concentration in water, pH 7.46).

2. Laminin (2 mg/mL stock solution, BD Bioscience) is diluted to 12 μg/mL in PBS and used to coat any plates that are going to be used. It is best to leave them coated for about 2 hours before plating myocytes.

3. Set up the heart perfusion apparatus [18] by running some Perfusion Buffer through all parts of it, making sure that there are no air bubbles. Also heat up the circulating water bath so that the temperature of the buffer leaving the cannula is 37°C. The size of the cannula must be carefully chosen based on the size of the aorta. The typical size of cannula used for rats varies from 14 to 8 gauge (1.6–3.2 mm).

4. Fill one 6-cm dish with warmed Perfusion Buffer (to rinse the heart before cannulation). Then fill one dish partially with warmed Perfusion Buffer, and have the cannula immersed in it. Make three knots with 4-0 silk and hang them on the end of the cannula floating in the Perfusion Buffer.

5. Inject the rat with heparin and sodium pentobarbital as per your institutional guidelines. Allow about 5 minutes for the drugs to take effect. If the rat isn't completely sedated put its nose in a sedation cone with some isoflurane for complete sedation.

6. Pin the rat down, and make a cut in the skin and muscles in order to access the diaphragm. Cut the diaphragm and then cut up through both sides of the rib cage so that it can be removed. Remove the thymus and lungs as well. Remove any blood that is blocking your view of the aorta with either a small sponge or cotton swab. Cut the heart from the rat's chest by cutting the aorta right below where it starts to branch. Also cut the vena cava. Then place the heart in the first dish to wash off some of the excess blood. Transfer the heart to the second dish and pull the aorta over the cannula; use two knots to fasten the heart to the cannula. If you only use one knot, sometimes it won't hold and the heart will shoot off when you start the perfusion.

7. Start the perfusion at a rate of one drop per second with the Perfusion Buffer, and then immediately prepare the Digestion Buffer by adding to the Perfusion Buffer the following: 0.25 mg/mL Liberase blendzyme 1 (Roche), 0.14 mg/mL trypsin (Invitrogen) and $CaCl_2$ to a final concentration of 12.5 μM. Take 2.5 mL of Digestion Buffer and place it in a 6-cm dish for after the digestion. Then add the rest of the Digestion Buffer to the rig and start the digestion. The digestion should proceed for 20–30 minutes and about 40 mL should perfuse

through the heart. Sometimes, with very dilated hearts the perfusion goes very rapidly (<15 minutes), in which case you need to make a second batch of buffer up to run through the heart so that it is adequately digested.

8. After the digestion is complete, remove the heart from the cannula and place in the 6-cm dish with the Digestion Buffer. The rest of the procedure should be done in a sterile hood.

9. Manually tear apart the heart into very tiny pieces. The heart should come apart very easily. After it is completely dissociated you can triturate it a few times to break the heart up the rest of the way by pipetting at a rate of about 3.0 mL per second using a 10-mL serological pipette. Then filter the cells through a 200 μ nylon mesh (Spectrum Labs 146487) into a 15-mL conical tube to remove any remaining clumps. Wash the dish with 2.5 mL of Myocyte Stopping Buffer 1 (10% bovine calf serum, 12.5 μM calcium chloride final concentration added to the Perfusion Buffer) and pass the wash through the same mesh into the conical tube.

10. Allow the cells to settle by gravity for about 10 minutes. The dead cells should float, and the living cells should sink to the bottom of the tube.

11. Remove the supernatant and add 10 mL of Myocyte Stopping Buffer 2 (5% bovine calf serum, 12.5 μM $CaCl_2$ final concentration in Perfusion Buffer). Triturate and then begin the calcium add-backs as outlined here:

Calcium reintroduction:

1. Add 50 μL of 10 mM $CaCl_2$, triturate and wait 4 minutes.

2. Add 50 μL of 10 mM $CaCl_2$, triturate and wait 4 minutes.

3. Add 100 μL of 10 mM $CaCl_2$, triturate and wait 4 minutes.

4. Add 30 μL of 100 mM $CaCl_2$, triturate and wait 4 minutes.

5. Add 50 μL of 100 mM $CaCl_2$, triturate and wait 15 minutes.

6. Plate cells on precoated laminin dishes (Step 2).

Even in laboratories with long-term experience in the isolation of cardiomyocytes, from time to time the quality of cell preparations declines. Some general guidelines for troubleshooting are as follows:

• Avoid the use of detergents in cleaning the glassware used for cell isolation. Use cleaning agents specially designated for tissue culture that leave no residue.

• It is important to keep the perfusion system clean. Therefore, the system should be washed first with clean water, then with 70% ethanol for 30 minutes, and dried using a stream of clean gas.

• Sometimes, after the initial 30 minutes perfusion with collagenase, the heart is still not soft. This usually indicates that the blood was not totally removed during the initiation of perfusion and has coagulated. Try to reduce the time between opening the thorax to remove the heart and connecting the heart to the perfusion system, or inject heparin into the animal in accordance with institutional guidelines before starting to prepare the heart.

• Another problem that often occurs is that the heart is soft but the cells are rounded up. The usual reason for this is that the calcium gradient is too steep. View the morphology of the myocytes after each centrifugation step and increase the gradient more carefully.

• The number of damaged (round) cells can be reduced by trypsinization (10 mg trypsin per 50 mL buffer). Trypsin should be added to the suspension treated after perfusion. Rounded and damaged cells are more easily digested than intact cells. The amount of trypsin must be adjusted to the batch used and the combined effect to the collagenase that is used in parallel. The number of damaged cells in the final cultures can also be reduced by gently washing the cultures 2 hours after plating. Rounded cells are less well attached to the cell culture dish and are dislodged more easily during this initial wash.

Alternative approaches

Cardiomyocyte cell lines provide an alternative for at least some of the experimental studies. A small number of established cardiomyocyte cell lines, such as HL-1 and H9C2 [14,19], have been used. HL-1 cells are derived from mouse atrial tumors and have been used successfully to investigate atrial fibrillation [20]. In contrast, the H9C2 cell line (ATCC, CRL-1446) was originally derived from embryonic rat ventricular tissue, which may be potentially important as cardiac hypertrophy resulting from hypertension mainly occurs in the ventricular

muscle of the heart. Although H9C2 cells do not contract, they still show many similarities to primary cardiomyocytes, including aspects of their morphology, expression of the proteins involved in the G protein signaling cascade, and electrophysiological properties [21,22]. Importantly, they can display hypertrophy-associated traits when stimulated with hypertrophic agents *in vitro* [23–25]. However, the value of H9C2 cells as an *in vitro* model of cardiac hypertrophy is questionable as they, by definition, proliferate, in contrast to the nonproliferating nature of the hypertrophied cardiomyocyte.

Adult cardiomyocytes can be studied for longer times when cultured in the creatinine–carnitine–taurine (CCT) medium supplemented with 20% FBS. The cells initially undergo a period of atrophy, round up, and change their morphology completely [26]. However, after 6 days, they reach a stable morphology in which the cells spread around their centers and show expression of the contractile proteins. These cells do lose some of their *in vivo* characteristics, including their characteristic rod-shaped morphology. However, energy metabolism and coupling of specific receptors such as α-adrenoceptors functioning in the regulation of protein synthesis, are still intact [27]. They also form new cell–cell contacts [28] and secrete growth factors, such as transforming growth factor β, which is then activated by proteases in the FBS. Therefore, these cultures represent a suitable model for studying certain questions in the cardiovascular field.

Weaknesses and strengths of the method

Isolated ventricular myocytes provide a largely homogenous population free of neural and humoral influences in a controllable environment. However, at the present time, the intact cells cannot be effectively separated from damaged ones with any reproducible efficiency. Many studies can be affected by the presence of damaged cells, with the exception of electrophysiological studies performed on single cells or certain biophysical analyses. The investigator can, however, fully control the conditions to which the cells are exposed, and can analyze the functional behavior of ventricular cells irrespective of the influence of other cells. This is both a strength and weakness of the method. Isolated cells are well suited for visualizing cellular structure and the precise localization of intracellular molecules. Isolated cardiomyocytes are also routinely used for examining intracellular Ca^{2+} homeostasis, cellular mechanics, and protein biochemistry. Genetic output can be easily and quickly modified via gene transfer studies or knocking down a gene of interest with small inhibitory RNA (siRNA). However, as the heart exists as a functional syncytium, whose physiology is completely dependent upon cell–cell interactions, those critical aspects of cardiomyocyte function are necessarily lost in culture.

Ventricular cardiomyocytes are terminally differentiated and do not divide *in vitro*. Therefore, cells must be newly isolated for each individual experiment. This requires the establishment of highly reproducible techniques that guarantee a reproducible quality of the cardiomyocyte preparations. Despite rigorous attempts to standardize the process and procedures, a certain amount of variation both between cell preparations and in the cells from a single preparation is unavoidable. This leads to significant (and sometimes unacceptable) scatter in the data such that the noise overwhelms the signal and the data become uninterpretable. At that point the investigator has little choice and must often turn to a different cell type to study the process or pathway under investigation.

Conclusions

Isolated rat (or mouse) cardiomyocytes are an invaluable tool for studying cardiac function, regulation, and pathology at the autonomous cellular level. These cells are widely used to study the electrophysiology, intracellular calcium fluxes, immunohistochemistry, contractile mechanics, genetic networks of activation and silencing, and protein expression. More recently, techniques for cardiomyocyte culture have gained additional importance with the advent of our ability to carry out gain- and/or loss-of-function via transfection or gene silencing. The ability to culture myocytes, even for short times, is often informative and represents a first step in the development of novel therapeutics, serving as "proof-of-principle" in defining causality for a novel gene, gene product, or biological agent. Although myocytes have been isolated and cultured for a number of years by standard techniques, it remains somewhat of an art to consistently produce high-quality cells. However, with care, cells can be prepared that, over a period of a few days, will develop well-formed sarcomeres, apparent as regular striations when viewed under light microscopy (Figure 13.1). Knowledge of the described reagents and protocols, and the critical points raised in this chapter will hopefully enable researchers to more easily establish cell-based

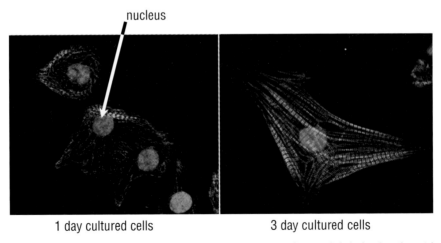

nucleus

1 day cultured cells   3 day cultured cells

Figure 13.1 Cultured cardiomyocytes. Myocytes were prepared as described in the text. Over a period of a few days, the proteins that make up the contractile apparatus are synthesized and form well defined sarcomeres.

research strategies, and advance the pursuit of mechanism of diseases.

References

1 Sutherland FJ, Hearse DJ. The isolated blood and perfusion fluid perfused heart. *Pharmacol Res* 2000; **41**: 613–627.

2 Simpson P, Savion S. Differentiation of rat myocytes in single cell cultures with and without proliferating nonmyocardial cells. Cross-striations, ultrastructure, and chronotropic response to isoproterenol. *Circ Res* 1982; **50**: 101–116.

3 Simpson P, McGrath A, Savion S. Myocyte hypertrophy in neonatal rat heart cultures and its regulation by serum and by catecholamines. *Circ Res* 1982; **51**: 787–801.

4 Simpson P. Norepinephrine-stimulated hypertrophy of cultured rat myocardial cells is an alpha 1-adrenergic response. *J Clin Invest* 1983; **72**: 732–738.

5 Simpson P. Stimulation of hypertrophy of cultured neonatal rat heart cells through an alpha 1-adrenergic receptor and induction of beating through an alpha1- and beta 1-adrenergic receptor interaction. Evidence for independent regulation of growth and beating. *Circ Res* 1985; **56**: 884–894.

6 Musters RJ, Post JA, Verkleij AJ. The isolated neonatal rat cardiomyocyte used in an in vitro model for 'ischemia'. A morphological study. *Biochem Biophys Acta* 1991; **1091**: 270–277.

7 Iwaki K, Chi SH, Dillmann WH, Mestril R. Induction of HSP70in cultured rat neonatal cardiomyocytes by hypoxia and metabolic stress. *Circulation* 1993; **87**: 2023–2032.

8 Tanaka M, Ito H, Adachi S, Akimoto H, Nishikawa T, Kasajima T, *et al*. Hypoxia induces apoptosis with enhanced expression of Fas antigen messenger RNA in cultured neonatal rat cardiomyocytes. *Circ Res* 1994; **75**: 426–433.

9 Shimojo T, Hiroe M, Ishiyama S, Ito H, Nishikawa T, Marumo F, *et al*. Nitric oxide induces apoptotic death of cardiomyocytes via a cyclic-GMP dependent pathway. *Exp Cell Res* 1999; **247**: 38–47.

10 Van der Lee KA, Vork MM, De Vries JE, Willemsen PH, Glatz JF, Reneman RS, *et al*. Long-chain fatty acid-induced changes in gene expression in neonatal cardiac myocytes. *J Lipid Res* 2000; **41**: 41–47.

11 Liu T, Lai H, Wu W, Chinn S, Wang PH. Developing a strategy to define the effects of insulin-like growth factor-1 on gene expression profile in cardiomyocytes. *Circ Res* 2001; **88**: 1231–1238.

12 Charron F, Tsimiklis G, Arcand M, Robitaille L, Liang Q, Molkentin JD, *et al*. Tissue-specific GATA factors are transcriptional effectors of the small GTPaseRhoA. *Genes Dev* 2001; **15**: 2702–2719.

13 Steinhelper ME, Lanson NA Jr, Dresdner KP, Delcarpio JB, Wit AL, Claycomb WC, *et al*. Proliferation in vivo and in culture of differentiated adult atrial cardiomyocytes from transgenic mice. *Am J Physiol* 1990; **259**: H1826–1834.

14 Claycomb WC, Lanson NA Jr, Stallworth BS, Egeland DB, Delcarpio JB, Bahinski A, *et al*. HL-1 cells: a cardiac muscle cell line that contracts and retains phenotypic characteristics of the adult cardiomyocyte. *Proc Natl Acad Sci USA* 1998; **95**: 2979–2984.

15 Estevez MD, Wolf A, Schramm U. Effect of PSC 833,Verapamil and Amiodarone on adriamycin toxicity in cultured rat cardiomyocytes. *Toxicol in Vitro* 2000; **14**: 17–23.

16 Harary I, Farley B. *In vitro* studies on single beating rat heart cells. *Exp Cell Res* 1963; **29**: 451–465.

17 Grynberg A, Athias P, Degois M. Effect of change in growth environment on cultured myocardial cells investigated in a standardized medium. *In Vitro Cell Dev Biol* 1986; **22**: 44–50.

18 Louch WE, Sheehan KA, Wolska BM. Methods in cardiomyocyte isolation, culture, and gene transfer. *J Mol Cell Cardiol* 2011; **51**: 288–298.

19 Kimes BW, Brandt BL. Properties of a clonal muscle cell line from rat heart. *Exp Cell Res* 1976; **98**: 367–381.

20 Rao F, Deng CY, Wu SL, Xiao DZ, Yu XY, Kuang SJ, *et al*. Involvement of Src in L-type Ca^{2+} channel depression induced by macrophage migration inhibitory factor in atrial myocytes. *J Mol Cell Cardiol* 2009; **47**: 586–594.

21 Hescheler J, Meyer R, Plant S, Krautwurst D, Rosenthal W, Schultz G, *et al*. Morphological, biochemical, and electrophysiological characterization of a clonal cell (H9c2) line from rat heart. *Circ Res* 1991; **69**: 1476–1486.

22 Sipido KR, Marban E. L-type calcium channels, potassium channels, and novel nonspecific cation channels in a clonal muscle cell line derived from embryonic rat ventricle. *Circ Res* 1991; **69**: 1487–1499.

23 Koekemoer AL, Chong NW, Goodall AH, Samani NJ. Myocyte stress 1 plays an important role in cellular hypertrophy and protection against apoptosis. *FEBS Lett* 2009; **583**: 2964–2967.

24 Huang CY, Chueh PJ, Tseng CT, Liu KY, Tsai HY, Kuo WW, *et al*. ZAK reprograms atrial natriuretic factor expression and induces hypertrophic growth in H9c2 cardiomyoblast cells. *Biochem Biophys Res Commun* 2004; **324**: 973–980.

25 Zhou Y, Jiang Y, Kang YJ. Copper inhibition of hydrogen peroxide induced hypertrophy in embryonic rat cardiac

H9c2 cells. *Exp Biol Med (Maywood)* 2007; **232**: 385–389.

26 Piper HM, Jacobsen SL, Schwartz P. Determinants of cardiomyocyte development in long-term primary culture. *Mol Cell Cardiol* 1988; **20**: 825–835.

27 Schluter KD, Goldberg Y, Taimor G, Schäfer M, Piper HM, *et al.* Role of phosphatidyl 3-kinase activation in the hypertrophic growth of adult ventricular cardiomyocytes. *Cardiovasc Res* 1998; **40**: 174–181.

28 Schwartz P, Piper HM, Spahr R, Hütter JF, Spieckermann PG. Development of new intracellular contacts between adult cardiac myocytes in culture. *Basic Res Cardiol* 1985; **80** (**Suppl. 1**): 75–78.

Isolation and culture of vascular smooth muscle cells

Milton Hamblin,[1] Lin Chang,[2] and Y. Eugene Chen[2]

[1] Tulane University School of Medicine, New Orleans, LA, USA

[2] University of Michigan Medical Center, Ann Arbor, MI, USA

Introduction

Smooth muscle cells (SMCs), critical components of the vessel wall, are highly-specialized cells that arise through cell–cell and cell–matrix signaling events during normal mouse embryonic development [1]. SMCs provide structural stability to newly developed blood vessels and, in mature arteries, provide further structural support, regulate blood pressure, and synthesize extracellular matrix proteins [2]. Vascular smooth muscle cells (VSMCs) can readily adapt to changes in environmental stimuli, which is critical for maintaining normal vascular function [3]. In response to vessel injury, VSMCs undergo phenotypic adaptation or modulation to a synthetic state, which is characterized by increased proliferation, migration, and matrix production along with decreased expression of SMC differentiation marker genes [4]. Vascular plasticity plays an important role in the pathogenesis and development of vascular lesion formation, atherosclerosis, and restenosis following angioplasty [1,2,4]. As a result, there is increasing interest in elucidating regulatory and signaling mechanisms mediating phenotypic modulation of smooth muscle cells to a contractile or synthetic state in response to altered environmental conditions.

The isolation and culture of smooth muscle cells from vascular tissue provides an important platform for studying cell biology, function and molecular circuitry of differentiated, and de-differentiated smooth muscle cell subpopulations. Furthermore, the particular methodology used for isolating VSMCs has critical importance in determining the initial fate or phenotype of a cell culture population. Here, we describe a method for establishing rat and mouse primary aortic and mesenteric artery VSMC culture systems.

Protocol

Reagents

• Animals: 180-g male rats and/or 8-week-old male mice. Before commencing experiments, rodents should be housed in a temperature-controlled animal facility with a 12 h : 12 h light : dark cycle. Rodents should be allowed *ad libitum* access to a standard diet and drinking water.
• Dulbecco's Modified Eagle Medium: Nutrient Mixture F-12 (D-MEM/F-12 Media) (Invitrogen, #11320-033)
• Hanks balanced salt solution without $CaCl_2$, $MgCl_2$, and $MgSO_4$ (HBSS) (Invitrogen, #14170-112)
• Fetal bovine serum (FBS) (Gibco, #10437-010)
• Penicillin/streptomycin, 100× solution (Gibco, #15140122)
• Collagenase, type II, (Worthington Biochemical Corporation, #LS004174)
• Elastase, type IV, 6 U/mg (Sigma-Aldrich, #E-0258)
• 70% (v/v) ethanol

Manual of Research Techniques in Cardiovascular Medicine, First Edition. Edited by Hossein Ardehali, Roberto Bolli, and Douglas W. Losordo.

- Antiseptic skin cleanser, Betadine surgical scrub (povidone-iodine, 7.5%) or swab sticks
- Sylgard silicone elastomer (World Precision Instruments, #SYLG184)
- Graphite fine powder (Sigma-Aldrich, #15553)

Equipment

- Dissecting microscope
- Phase-contrast microscope
- 37°C cell culture incubator with 95% air/5% CO_2
- Sterile dissection hood
- Table top centrifuge
- Large (100 mm × 20 mm) tissue culture dishes (Falcon, #353003)
- 35-mm cell culture dishes
- Six-well, flat bottom culture plates (Falcon, #353046)
- 15-mL conical tubes – polystyrene (Falcon, #352095)
- 50-mL conical tubes – polypropylene (Falcon, #352070)
- Pair of 14.5-cm straight blunt–blunt Metzenbaum baby scissors (F.S.T., #14018-14) or equivalent
- Pair of 10.5-cm straight sharp–sharp Moria fine scissors (F.S.T., #14370-22) or equivalent
- Pair of 8.5-cm straight sharp Spring scissors (F.S.T., #15009-08) or equivalent
- Pair of 15-cm straight 1 × 2 teeth Gillies forceps (F.S.T., #11028-15) or equivalent
- Pair of 10-cm straight serrated Graefe forceps (F.S.T., #11050-10) or equivalent
- Pair of 9-cm 45° angled smooth Delicate forceps (F.S.T., #11063-07) or equivalent
- Micro-serrefines (F.S.T, #18055-05)
- Plastic Pasteur pipettes
- Gauze sponges
- Cotton-tipped applicators, autoclaved
- Insect pins, autoclaved.

Reagent setup

- FBS 50-mL aliquots stored at −20°C
- Wash medium (DMEM/F12)
- Culture medium (DMEM/F12 + 10% (v/v) FBS + 1% (v/v) penicillin/ streptomycin solution) add 50 mL FBS and 5 mL penicillin/ streptomycin solution (100×) to 445 mL DMEM/F-12
- Dissecting instruments: all microdissecting instruments (scissors, forceps, micro-serrefines) should be autoclaved before use.

Preparation and equipment setup

To construct a Sylgard dissection pad, please follow the manufacturer's instructions. To allow for optimal visualization of vessels during dissection procedures, add fine graphite powder to make the silicone elastomer (Sylgard) black. A black background allows for optimal visualization of the vessel during dissection. Keep the dissection dish in a sterilized culture hood.

Procedure
Enzymatic dissociation method
Steps 1–8: Animal preparation (about 10 minutes) (same for SMC isolation from rat and mouse thoracic aortas and rat mesenteric arteries)
1. Autoclave all necessary instruments (scissors, forceps, etc.).
2. Add 2 mL of wash medium (DMEM/F12 without FBS and penicillin/ streptomycin) in each well of a 6-well plate under sterile conditions. (*Note: perform this step in a culture hood.*).
3. Fill a dissecting dish (100 mm × 20 mm tissue culture dish) with 2 mL of wash medium under sterile conditions.
4. Anesthetize the rat/mouse with an intraperitoneal injection of a ketamine (100 mg/kg)/xylazine (10 mg/kg) combination.
5. Remove hair on chest and abdominal regions using hair removal cream (Nair) or clippers.
6. Swab the skin with Betadine using a cotton-tipped applicator.
7. Wipe the skin with 70% (v/v) ethanol using a cotton-tipped applicator.
8. Make a midline incision in the skin starting at the middle abdomen and proceeding up to the neck region (Figure 14.1A) using sterile scissors (F.S.T., #14018-14). Retract and pin the skin flaps to expose the chest (for thoracic SMC isolation) and abdominal regions (for mesenteric SMC isolation).

Steps 9–14: dissection of thoracic aorta (about 3 minutes)
9. Open the chest cavity using a second set of sterile scissors (F.S.T., #14018-14).
10. Remove blood from the chest cavity with autoclaved gauze sponges.
11. Using sterile micro-serrefines (F.S.T., #18055-05), block blood flow from the heart by clamping the aortic arch.

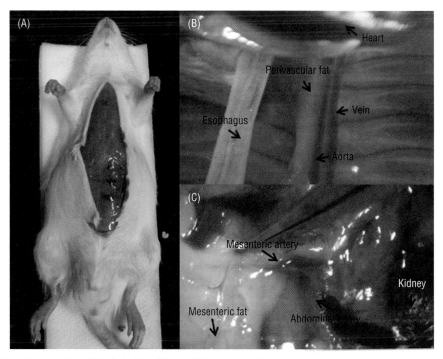

Figure 14.1 Anatomy of arteries: (A) skin incision; (B) aorta; (C) mesenteric artery.

12. Using small sterile scissors (F.S.T., #14370-22) and forceps (F.S.T., #11050-10), dissect the descending aorta (area between aortic arch and diaphragm) together with surrounding perivascular connective tissue (Figure 14.1B). (*Note: be able to differentiate between the aorta and esophagus – the aorta connects to the heart and the esophagus connects to the stomach.*).

13. Skip to Step 17 or proceed with Steps 14–16 if also dissecting mesenteric artery.

Steps 14–16: dissection of mesenteric artery (about 3 minutes)

14. Open the abdominal cavity using a second set of sterile scissors (F.S.T., #14018-14).

15. Carefully manipulate intestines with sterile forceps to expose the abdominal aorta.

16. Dissect the mesenteric artery (second arterial branch from the abdominal aorta below the diaphragm) and adjacent tissue starting at the abdominal aorta to its branches using small sterile scissors (F.S.T., #14370-22) and forceps (F.S.T., #11050-10) (Figure 14.1C).

Steps 17–21: cleaning of dissected vascular tissue (about 10 minutes)

17. Transfer excised vascular tissue to a 6-well plate containing 2 mL of wash medium in each well and remove blood from the tissue surface by successive transfer of tissue to each of the six wells.

18. Transfer excised vascular tissue to a dissecting dish containing 2 mL of wash medium.

19. Transfer the dissecting dish containing excised vascular tissue to the culture hood.

20. Using sterile insect pins, fix both ends of the vessel tissue to a Sylgard pad.

21. Under a dissecting microscope, carefully dissect and remove all surrounding adipose and connective tissue using fine scissors (F.S.T., #14370-22).

Steps 22–28: removal of the adventitial layer (about 80 minutes)

22. Prepare the first digesting enzyme solution-dissolve 2 mg collagenase (365 U/mg) in 2 mL of HBSS.

23. Using a Pasteur pipette, transfer dissected artery to a 35-mm culture dish containing 2 mL of the collagenase enzyme solution.

24. Cover culture dish with a lid before placing inside 37°C incubator.

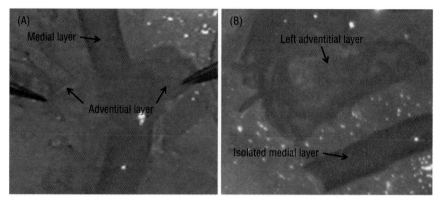

Figure 14.2 Removal of adventitial layer. (A) Strip off adventitia from aorta. (B) Check to ensure that adventitia is separated from medial layer.

25. Incubate dissected vessels in collagenase enzyme solution for 1 hour (or 30 minutes for a mouse artery).

26. Transfer the partially digested tissue to a new 35-mm culture dish containing 1 mL HBSS and then rinse three times for 1 minutes each time. Do not transfer an excessive amount of the collagenase enzyme solution with the vessel.

27. Transfer the vessel to a dissecting dish containing 2 mL of wash medium and with sterile pins, gently fix the ends of the artery.

28. Using a dissecting microscope, remove the adventitial layer of the vessel with fine curved forceps (F.S.T., #11063-07) to avoid contaminating the smooth muscle cell culture with fibroblasts (Figure 14.2A,B). (*Note: if the adventitial layer is difficult to remove, go back step to Step 25 and reincubate vessels in collagenase solution for an additional 10 minutes.*)

Steps 29–30: removal of the endothelial layer (about 2 minutes)

29. With spring scissors (F.S.T., #15009-08), longitudinally cut open the artery to expose the lumen.

30. Denude the endothelium through gentle rubbing of the intimal surface with a sterile cotton-tipped applicator.

Steps 31–34: enzymatic digestion (overnight)

31. Prepare second enzyme solution: dissolve 2 mg collagenase (365 U/mg) and 1 mg elastase (6 U/mg) in 2 mL HBSS.

32. Add 2 mL of the second enzyme solution to a 35-mm culture dish.

33. Transfer vessel to culture dish containing enzyme solution and cut the vessel into 1 mm × 1 mm pieces.

34. Cover the culture dish with a lid and place in the 37°C incubator overnight.

Steps 35–40: VSMC dissociation (about 20 minutes)
The next day:

35. The following morning, transfer the partially digested artery and enzyme solution to a 15-mL conical tube (Falcon, #352095).

36. Using a Pasteur pipette, dissociate the cells by mild trituration. (*Note: tissue should be less evident during cell dissociation. If dissociation proves to be difficult, the enzyme concentrations should be optimized by increasing collagenase and elastase 0.5–5 times.*).

37. Add 10 mL of culture medium (DMEM/F12 + 10% (v/v) FBS + 1% (v/v) penicillin/streptomycin solution) to the cell suspension to halt digestion.

38. Spin cells at 1800 rpm for 10 minutes using a table top centrifuge.

39. Remove and discard the supernatant.

40. Resuspended the visible cell pellet in 2 mL of 37°C prewarmed culture medium.

The dissociated smooth muscle cells can be plated on a cell culture plate for experiments or a 100-mm dish for splitting. Split the smooth muscle cells every 3–4 days (Figure 14.3A). Smooth muscle cell α-actin staining should be performed every two passages to identify the cell purity (Figure 14.3B).

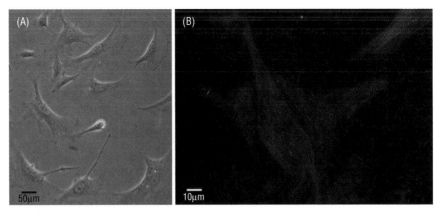

Figure 14.3 Enzymatic dissociation method. (A) Split the smooth muscle cells every 3–4 days. (B) Smooth muscle cell α-actin staining.

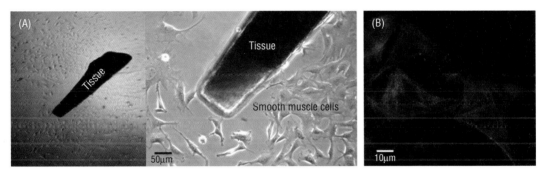

Figure 14.4 Explant method. (A) Migration of smooth muscle cells from explanted vessels; left: 40× magnification; right: 200× magnification. (B) Smooth muscle cell α-actin staining.

Alternative approaches

Explant method

The particular methodology of isolation is often critical for determining the initial phenotype of cultured VSMC cells. Besides enzymatic dissociation, another technique commonly employed for isolation of VSMC is explantation. This method utilizes outgrowth of medial layer tissue to yield VSMC in the synthetic state.

Preparation of aortic and mesenteric tissue for the Explant Method, including removal of the adventitia and endothelium, is the same as in Steps 1–30 described before in the Enzymatic Dissociation Method. Following Steps 1–30 as described previously, proceed with the following steps for explant culture:

1. Place the adventitia and endothelium removed-artery on a dissecting board and cover artery with wash medium (DMEM/F12 without FBS and penicillin/streptomycin) to keep the artery physiologically moist.

2. Wash vessel medial layer two times with 1 mL of wash medium, and then transfer the vessel medial layer to a new 100-mm Petri dish.

3. Using a scalpel blade or scissors, cut vessel strips into 1–2 mm pieces. (*Caution: excessive cutting will damage tissue, making it difficult for cells to migrate from tissue.*).

4. Add 500 μl of wash medium to vessel pieces.

5. With a 1-mL sterile Pasteur pipette, transfer all vessel pieces to a 100-mm Petri dish, and then homogeneously disperse the vessel pieces to the Petri dish bottom (Figure 14.4B). (*Note: after the vessel pieces are homogeneously dispersed, any extra medium can be aspirated.*)

6. Place 1 mL of culture medium (DMEM/F12 containing 10% FBS and 1% penicillin/streptomycin) in the lid of a 100-mm Petri dish.

7. Place the Petri dish in an upside-down (inverted) position.

8. Transfer the inverted Petri dish to a 37°C, 95% air/5% CO_2 chamber.

9. Once the inverted Petri dish is placed in the incubator, maintain the Petri dish in an upside-down position for 4 hours. This will allow the vessel pieces to firmly adhere to the Petri dish bottom.

10. After 4-hour incubation, take out the Petri dish from the chamber, then carefully turn over the inverted Petri dish from upside-down to right-side-up position in hood, and carefully add 8 mL of culture medium to the Petri dish. Next, transfer the Petri dish to chamber. (*Note: to avoid detachment of vessel pieces, carefully add culture medium at the edge of the dish.*)

11. Every 4 days, replace one-half of the culture medium in the Petri dish with fresh prewarmed culture medium. (*Note: vessels should be inspected each day for possible infection without disturbing outgrowth process.*).

12. Within 9–10 days, smooth muscle cell migration from explanted vessels should be evident. (*Note: if cell migration from explanted vessels is observed within 6–7 days, the adventitial layer, in all likelihood, was not completely removed and the cell culture is contaminated with fibroblasts.*).

13. After 13–14 days, the smooth muscle cell density surrounding explanted tissues should be ample (Figure 14.4A).

14. Remove culture medium and wash cells and vessel pieces with PBS to remove serum. Cover cells with prewarmed trypsin/EDTA and incubate at 37°C for 2–5 minutes.

15. Check all cells detached from dish, and add 5 mL culture medium and gently triturate cell suspension with a Pasteur pipette.

16. Transfer cells to a new culture dish, and wait for 3–4 days until evidence of monolayer cells.

17. Split cells in a 1:4 ratio every 3–4 days. Smooth muscle cell α-actin staining should be performed every two passages to identify the cell purity (Figure 14.4B).

Strengths and weaknesses of method

Enzymatic dissociation tends to yield a small quantity of smooth muscle cells with a quiescent, contractile phenotype. This particular method is ideal for conducting studies on dispersed single cells. However, enzyme-dispersed smooth muscle cells in subculture conditions do not readily proliferate and phenotypic switching of vascular smooth muscle cells following enzyme dissociation does not usually occur until after cell passaging has been completed. Conversely, tissue explantation does not readily yield smooth muscle cells in the contractile state; vascular smooth muscle cells grown from explants often exhibit a synthetic or de-differentiated phenotype. Furthermore, development of explant culture is slower versus smooth muscle cell isolation by enzymatic dispersion. Nevertheless, the utilization of explant cultures is ideal in cases of limited vascular tissue.

Conclusion

We describe a reliable and reproducible method for isolating and culturing vascular smooth muscle cells for *in vitro* studies of cellular properties and environmental responses in both large conduit vessels and small resistance arteries. Following isolation of smooth muscle cells from rat or mouse vascular tissue, we utilize enzymatic dissociation for obtaining confluent cell monolayers suitable for subculturing or passaging. The establishment of our cell culture system allows for the acquisition of homogenous primary vascular smooth muscle cell populations necessary for studying vascular remodeling and vascular-related pathophysiology.

References

1 Owens GK, Kumar MS, Wamhoff BR. Molecular regulation of vascular smooth muscle cell differentiation in development and disease. *Physiol Rev* 2004; **84**: 767–801.

2 Long X, Slivano OJ, Cowan SL, Georger MA, Lee TH, Miano JM, *et al.* Smooth muscle calponin: an unconventional CArG-dependent gene that antagonizes neointimal formation. *Arterioscler Thromb Vasc Biol* 2011; **31**: 2172–2180.

3 Xie C, Ritchie RP, Huang H, Zhang J, Chen YE. Smooth muscle cell differentiation in vitro: models and underlying molecular mechanisms. *Arterioscler Thromb Vasc Biol* 2011; **31**: 1485–1494.

4 Mack CP. Signaling mechanisms that regulate smooth muscle cell differentiation. *Arterioscler Thromb Vasc Biol* 2011; **31**: 1495–1505.

Isolation and culture of cardiac endothelial cells

Asish K. Ghosh, Joseph W. Covington, and Douglas E. Vaughan

Northwestern University Feinberg School of Medicine, Chicago, IL, USA

Introduction

Endothelial cells originate from splanchnopleuric mesoderm and form the endothelium, found in the endocardial surface and the inner surface of the blood vessels of the entire circulatory system. Endothelial cells derived from different vascular origins however, show different molecular, bio chemical, cellular, and functional characteristics [1]. Endothelial cells form complex intercellular connections through tight gap and adherens junctions in the endothelium and act as a selective barrier between the lumens of blood vessels and the surrounding tissue controlling the transport of materials including fluid filtration and neutrophil recruitment [2]. It is also known that during embryonic organogenesis, endothelial cells have the capacity to differentiate into fibroblast-like cells and contribute to the development of the embryonic heart cushion, the future heart valves [3].

Although it is well established that endothelial cells originate from mesodermal progenitor cells, existing evidence also shows that the vascular endothelial cells may originate from bone marrow-derived circulating endothelial progenitor cells (EPCs) in response to vascular endothelial growth factor (VEGF) signaling. Different views and theories on the ontogenetic and phylogenetic origin of endothelial cells have been elegantly reviewed by Muñoz-Chápuli and colleagues [4]. Endothelial cells secrete a wide variety of factors and play a significant role in controlling lipid homeostasis, immunity, blood vessel tone, signal transduction, angiogenesis, vasculogenesis, and blood flow by regulating vasoconstriction and vasodilatation [2]. McIntire and colleagues demonstrated that the gene expression profile in endothelial cells is altered in response to pulsatile arterial flow compared to steady flow [5–8]. Vascular endothelial cell injury leads to inflammation, a major contributor to diseases such as arthrosclerosis, thrombosis, and organ fibrosis. Endothelial cells are characterized by the presence of signature genes such as adhesion molecules, VE Cadherin; CD31/PECAM-1, von Willebrand factor, endoglin, an endothelial-specific transforming growth factor-beta type III receptor, ASPP1, a p53-binding protein, and 31 microRNAs (Table 15.1) [9–11]. Endothelial cells can also be identified from cardiac fibroblast/myofibroblast cell populations by the absence of α-SMA staining and from cardiomyocytes by the absence of α-MHC and other myocyte-specific markers. Recently, McCall et al. [11] demonstrated that while a wide variety of microRNAs are common in endothelial, epithelial, and hematologic cells, a subset of microRNAs are unique to the endothelial cells. Therefore, in order to gain knowledge about endothelial cell biology, pure populations of endothelial cells in cultures are essential. Although, several attempts have been taken for isolation of endothelial cells for *in vitro* culture [12, discussed in 16], the first successful isolation and characterization of endothelial cells from human umbilical veins was reported in early seventies by Jafe et al. [13,14] and Gimborne et al. [15]. The chronological history of

Manual of Research Techniques in Cardiovascular Medicine, First Edition. Edited by Hossein Ardehali, Roberto Bolli, and Douglas W. Losordo.

Table 15.1 Endothelial signature genes

CD31/PCAM-1: cell surface protein, involved in cell adhesion, migration, and angiogenesis

CD102/ICAM-2: constitutively expressed in endothelial cells and mediates cell adhesion

vWF: a glycoprotein, involved in blood clotting

VE-Cadherin: an endothelial specific transmembrane protein, involved in cell–cell adhesion

Endothelial-specific transforming growth factor-beta type III receptor: highly expressed in microvascular but not in macrovascular endothelial cells; involved in TGF-β2-induced endothelial cell–cell separation during EndMT

ASPP1: apoptosis-stimulating protein of p53 is an activator of p53 and expressed largely in endothelial cells

Endothelial cells specific microRNAs (approximately 31 miRNAs): short ~22 nt RNA molecule; involved in the regulation of eukaryotic gene expression at the translational level

---

endothelial cell isolation was elegantly described by Nachman and Jafe [16] in their *Journal of Clinical Investigation* article entitled "Endothelial cell culture: beginning of modern vascular biology."

It is well documented in the literature that endothelial cell functions are regulated by a wide variety of cytokines and growth factors like VEGF-B and TGF-β [17–19]. Recent studies also demonstrate that the ERK5 MAPK/KLF4 axis plays a pivotal role in the maintenance of endothelial integrity and normal vascular function and deregulation in ERK5 leads to endothelial dysfunction [20–23]. Endothelial dysfunction, or the loss of normal endothelial function, is a salient feature of inflammation-associated vascular diseases, and is regarded as a key early event in the development of reduced vasodilation-related vascular disease like atherosclerosis. Impaired endothelial function, causing hypertension and thrombosis, is often seen in patients with coronary artery disease, hyperlipidaemia, hyperglycemia, hypertension, ionizing radiation-induced cardiotoxicity, and aging-related syndrome [24]. Endothelial dysfunction can be characterized by the following key features: visible changes in endothelial cell morphology, loss of CD31 receptor, redistribu-

tion of VE cadherin, elevated secretion of TNF-α, angiotensin II, VEGF, decreased in nitric oxide synthesis, and loss of antithrombic nature [2,25]. Therefore, in order to understand endothelial cell biology under normal physiological and different pathological conditions, reproducible isolation and culture procedures for pure populations of endothelial cells are essential.

Protocol for isolation of mouse cardiac endothelial cells

Isolation and culture of cardiac endothelial cells using an efficient protocol contributes to the success of numerous *in vitro* studies related to cellular and molecular aspects of cell physiology and the role in pathophysiology of different diseases. The following protocol for endothelial cell isolation used in our laboratory was prepared using several sources as cited in the text, most notably Lim and Luscinskas [26], Brigham and Women's Hospital/ Harvard Medical School Cell Biology Core Facility, and Invitrogen's Dynal Bead Separation procedures.

Materials and preparations

Gelatin-coated plates. To make gelatin-coated plates, prepare 0.1% gelatin solution by adding 500 mL deionized water in a bottle containing 0.5 g of gelatin powder. Mix and autoclave the solution for 30 minutes. Cool the 0.1% gelatin solution to room temperature. Gelatin solution can be stored at 4°C for up to 2 months. Coat plates with 1 mL of 0.1% gelatin, remove excess, and dry the gelatin-coated plate for 4 hours inside cell culture hood. Prepare one gelatin-coated plate per two mice and for each passage.

Cell Isolation Medium. Dulbecco's Modified Eagle Media (DMEM with 4.5 g/L glucose; Cellgro), 20% fetal bovine serum (Hyclone), 1× penicillin/ streptomycin/ amphotericin B mixture (Calbiochem, Cat# 516104).

Cell Culture Medium. DMEM (glucose 4.5 g/L) with fetal bovine serum (20%), heparin (100 μg/mL) (Sigma H-3933), endothelial cell growth supplement (ECGS) (100 μg/mL) (Biomedical Technologies #BT-203), HEPES (25 mM), L-glutamine (2 mM), 1× sodium pyruvate, 1× nonessential amino acids, and

1× penicillin/ streptomycin/ amphotericin B (Calbiochem).

Dissection tools and reagents. Hemostats (two), forceps (two), scissors (two), 70% ethanol, sterile gauze, 15-mL centrifuge tubes.

Tools for tissue dissociation. sterile Petri dishes, small forceps, fine scissors, 15-mL centrifuge tubes, 70 μm pore size cell strainer (Fisher #08-771-2), and 14-gauge metal cannula (Fisher #1482516N).

Matrix degrading enzyme. Type I collagenase (approximately 230 U/mg) (Worthington, Lakewood, NJ; Cat# S8B10315-A). Dissolve collagenase I (2 mg/mL) in warm Dulbecco's Phosphate Buffered Saline (DPBS) with Ca^{2+} and Mg^{2+} (37°C) and sterilize using 0.22 μm filter (prepare 10 mL/ two hearts).

Dynabeads® sheep anti-rat IgG (Invitrogen/Dynal #110.35). Concentration = 4×10^8 beads/mL.

Endothelial cell-specific antibodies. (i) Purified rat anti-mouse CD31 antibody (Pharmingen #553369): 0.5 mg/mL for first cell sorting; (ii) Purified rat anti-mouse CD102 antibody (Pharmingen #553325): 1 mg/mL for second selection of endothelial cells.

Magnetic separator/rack (Invitrogen).

Buffer 1. DPBS (without Ca^{2+} and Mg^{2+}) with 0.1% BSA and 2 mM EDTA, pH 7.4.

Trypsin (0.25%)–EDTA (2.21 mM). in HBSS without sodium bicarbonate, calcium, and magnesium (Cellgro, Cat # 25-053-Cl).

Sterile Class II Type A/B3 laminar flow hood.

Procedures
Dynabeads washing procedures and preparation of anti-mouse CD31 and CD102 coupled Dynabeads

1. Dynabeads sheep anti-rat IgG binds monoclonal rat IgG. Resuspend the Dynabeads (Dynabeads sheep anti-rat IgG in PBS pH 7.4 with 0.1% BSA and 0.02% NaN_3) and aliquot an appropriate amount (at least 200 μl) in a 1.5-mL microfuge tube.
2. Put tube on a magnetic separator and leave for 1 minute.

3. Pipette off and discard supernatant, add 1 mL of Buffer 1 to bead containing tube, mix well, place on magnetic separator for 1 minute. Repeat Steps 2–3 for three times.
4. Resuspend Dynabeads in 200 μL Buffer 1.
5. Add 10 μL of purified antibody for each 200 μL of beads and transfer to a 0.5-mL tube.
6. Incubate antibody containing bead solution overnight on a rotator at 4°C.
7. Place tube on magnetic separator and leave for 1 minute.
8. Pipette off and discard supernatant. Add 1 mL of Buffer 1 to the bead-containing tube, mix well, and place on a magnetic separator for 1 minute. Repeat Steps 7–8 for three times.
9. Resuspend beads in 200 μL Buffer 1 (this will maintain the original concentration of beads at 4×10^8 beads/mL)
10. Antibody-bound Dynabeads can be stored at 4°C and use within 2–3 weeks.

Collection of hearts
1. Anesthetize a young adult mouse with isoflurane (Baxter Healthcare Corp., IL) and kill by cervical dislocation.
2. Soak belly skin with 70% EtOH and wipe top surface.
3. Pick up the skin above the pubis with forceps and make a small incision with sterile fine scissors; deglove skin just below the neck.
4. With sterile scissors, cut open the anterior abdomen, take down the anterior diaphragm, and open up the chest cavity. Apply hemostats to both sides of the skin and open the chest cavity.
5. Grip the heart with sterile forceps, detach from the lungs and vessels using sterile scissors, and place the heart in a 10-cm sterile Petri dish.
6. Cut heart in half through the ventricle to drain remaining blood and place in 10 mL cold Cell Isolation Medium in a 15-mL sterile polypropylene centrifuge tube.
7. Repeat Steps 1–6 for a second mouse, combine the hearts, and gently agitate the tissue in the Cell Isolation Medium for 1–2 minutes to clean the heart tissues.

Cardiac tissue dissociation
1. In a sterile laminar flow hood, transfer the tissue from the Cell Isolation Medium to a new 10-cm sterile Petri dish.

2. Trim out any connective tissue surrounding heart and chop heart into small pieces with two sterile fine scissors for 1 minute (to avoid cell damage, do not chop the tissue for longer time).

3. Put chopped hearts in 10 mL of prewarmed (37°C) collagenase type I (2 mg/mL) in a 50-mL polypropylene tube.

4. Incubate minced tissue containing tube at 37°C with gentle shaking for 45–60 minutes.

5. Triturate the suspension 10 times using a sterile 30 mL syringe with cannula.

6. Allow undissociated heart tissue to settle at the bottom of the tube. Collect the suspension carefully and filter through a 70-μm cell strainer (Falcon #35 2350) into a 50-mL conical tube. Wash sieve with 5 mL of Buffer 1.

7. Transfer cell suspension to a sterile 15-mL polypropylene centrifuge tube and spin down at 1300 rpm for 10 minutes at 4°C.

8. Pipette off and discard supernatant. Resuspend the cell pellet in 1 mL of cold Buffer 1 and transfer to a sterile microfuge tube.

Antibody-based cardiac endothelial cell selection (first round)

1. Add anti-mouse CD31 Dynabeads (prepared as described earlier) to cell suspension (15 μl of beads/ mL of cell suspension) and then incubate the tube containing cell suspension and Dynal mix on a rotator at room temperature for 10 minutes.

2. Put the tube in the magnetic separator, and leave for 1 minute to attach the magnetic bead-bound endothelial cells to the wall of the tube.

3. Remove supernatant carefully without disturbing the pellet. Collect the supernatant in a new sterile tube. (*The supernatant can be used separately to positively select for fibroblasts.*)

4. Resuspend the bead-bound cells in 1 mL Cell Isolation Medium (pipetting up and down several times to break the cell clumps fully).

5. Put the tube in the magnetic separator for 1 minute.

6. Repeat Steps 3–5 for three times.

7. Resuspend the cell pellet in Growth Medium and plate Dynabead-bound cells in a gelatin-coated Petri dish (one dish/ two hearts).

8. After 24 hours, rinse the Petri dish twice with Cell Isolation Medium and add new Growth Medium. Feed the cells with Growth Medium every other day.

Allow cells to grow to confluence (generally, cultures reach to 80–90% confluence in 5–7 days after plating).

Second antibody-based selection of cardiac endothelial cells

1. Trypsinize to detach cells when confluence is reached: rinse once with 10 mL of Ca^{2+}/Mg^{2+}-free PBS, add 2 mL of trypsin:EDTA (0.25%:1 mM) to cover the cells; remove any excess trypsin:EDTA, and allow the cells to detach at 37°C (less than 5°minutes). (To avoid cell death, do not over trypsinize.)

2. After the cells detach and round up, resuspend cells in 10 mL of Cell Isolation Medium.

3. Transfer trypsin-treated cell suspension to a sterile 15-mL polypropylene tube and spin down at 1300 rpm for 10 minutes.

4. Pipette off supernatant carefully and discard; resuspend cell pellet in 1 mL Buffer 1.

5. Add CD102-coated Dynabeads to the cell suspension (15 μl CD102-coated Dynabeads/ mL cell suspension). Incubate for 10 minutes at room temperature on a rotator.

6. Put the tube containing mixture of cell suspension and antibody-coated Dynabeads on a magnetic separator and leave for 1 minute. Remove supernatant carefully without disturbing the pellet.

7. Wash the bead-bound cells gently four times in 1 mL of Isolation medium.

8. Resuspend the cell pellet in Cell Growth Medium and seed at a 1:3 split ratio on sterile gelatin-coated Petri dishes.

Cell culture and maintenance

Feed the cells with Growth Medium every other day and split cells 1:3 onto gelatin-coated Petri dishes when they reach 80–90% confluence. Do not allow cells to remain confluent for more than a day or two as small numbers of nonendothelial cells (fibroblasts, smooth muscle cells) will continue to divide and further contaminate the culture.

In subsequent passaging, it is important to determine the quality of endothelial cells based on their morphology, shape, and size. Generally, endothelial cells grow in clusters that later develop a cobblestone appearance and become a more uniform endothelial monolayer (Figure 15.1A).

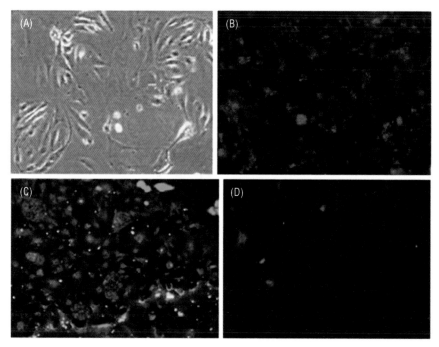

Figure 15.1 Mouse cardiac endothelial cells (MCEC) isolated and cultured following the primary protocol in this chapter: (A) light microscopy, (B) acetylated-LDL labelling, (C) CD31 positive, (D) α-SMA negative staining of purified mouse cardiac endothelial cells.

Cell viability count and replating. Resuspend the cell pellet in DMEM and count the viable cells using Countess Automated Cell Counter (Invitrogen; Catalog No. C10227) following manufacturer's instruction as follows.

1. Mix 10 µL of cell suspension with 10 µL of 0.4% trypan blue stain in an Eppendorf tube.

2. Add the mixture of cell suspension and trypan blue (10 µL) into the halfmoon-shaped chamber port on the Countess cell counting chamber slide.

3. Insert slide, sample side first, into the slide port of the instrument until a soft click sounds.

4. Optimize image following the manufacturer's instruction.

5. To count cells, press "count cells" button to obtain results.

6. Results will show the number of live and dead cells per mL of cell suspension.

Important notes

1. The purity of isolated cardiac endothelial cells can be identified using Dil-Ac-LDL (Biomedical Technologies #BT-902) and following the company's instructions for labeling as described here:

a. Dilute DiI-Ac-LDL (200 µg/mL; Biomedical Tech., Cat # BT-902) to 10 µg/mL in complete growth media.

b. Aspirate the media and add the diluted Dil-Ac-LDL to cell culture wells and incubate for 4 hours at 37°C in an incubator.

c. Remove media and wash with probe-free media.

d. Observe stained cells under a fluorescence microscope and photograph (Figure 15.1B).

The purity of the isolated cardiac endothelial cells can be further confirmed by FITC-tagged CD31 (positive) and α-SMA immunostaining (negative) as described here:

a. Culture isolated endothelial cells in six-chambered slides overnight.

b. Aspirate media and fix the cells with ice-cold methanol for 10 minutes at −20°C.

c. Remove fixative and wash with 1 × PBS and air dry.

d. Block with 1% fetal bovine serum (FBS) in PBS for 30 minutes and rinse once with 1 × PBS.

e. Incubate the cells with FITC-tagged CD31 or α-SMA (1 : 50 or appropriate dilution based on the concentration of the antibody) for 1 hour at room temperature.

f. Wash the cells twice in 1 × PBS; add a drop of mounting medium and place a cover slip on the mounting medium.

g. Observe under a fluorescence microscope and photograph (Figure 15.1C (CD31) and 15.1D (α-SMA)).

2. As high glucose has an influence on endothelial cell morphology and differentiation, avoid culture of primary endothelial cells in media containing high glucose for a longer period of time. Also, use low passages of primary culture of endothelial cells grown in low glucose and low fetal bovine serum for *in vitro* study such as TGF-β-induced endothelial to mesenchymal transition (EndMT).

Alternative approaches

Isolation and characterization of microvascular and macrovascular endothelial cells from human hearts was described by Gräfe and colleagues [27].

Isolation and culture procedure

1. Excise out the muscle segment around the distal left descending coronary artery and store immediately in Ringer solution (aqueous solution of NaCl, KCl, and CaCl$_2$, a physiological solution for bathing animal tissues) at 4°C (up to 4 hours)

2. Wash the surface of the muscle segment briefly with 70% ethanol.

3. Put the preparation in a modified Langendorff perfusion system.

4. Cannulate the coronary artery and perfuse the muscle segment with warm Krebs–Henseleit buffer (KHB, Cat # K3753, Sigma) with calcium (37°C) followed by calcium-free KHB (close the dissected vessels with small clamps in order to minimize the leakage at the edge of the tissue).

5. Perfuse (for 30 minutes at perfusion pressure 60 cmH$_2$O) the heart muscle with an enzyme solution containing 0.074% collagenase type II (digest triple-helical native collagen fibrils in connective tissue), 0.012% dispase (5000 U/mL) (digest fibronectin and collagen IV), 0.012% trypsin and 0.27% BSA dissolved in calcium-free KHB.

6. Digest the partially dissociated tissue in enzyme solution (as described in Step 5) for 20 minutes.

7. At the end of incubation, determine the dissociation level of the microvessels from the heart tissues.

8. Filter the tissue homogenates through a nylon mesh (200 μm) to separate the undissociated tissues.

9. Centrifuge the filtered tissue homogenates at low speed and resuspend the cell pellets in Culture Medium 199 containing 20% human serum, 10 mM HEPES buffer, 50 mg/mL heparin, 10 ng/mL endothelial cell growth factor and antibiotics (100 μg/mL streptomycin and 100 U/mL penicillin).

10. Seed the resuspended microvascular cell pellets in two or three gelatin-coated T-75 flasks and culture at 37°C incubator with 5% CO$_2$.

Isolation of macrovascular endothelial cells

1. Excise part of epicardial coronary arteries from explanted hearts and transfer immediately in cold Medium 199 (composition as described previously).

2. Clean the epicardial coronary artery (using sterile scissors and forceps) by removing the surrounding tissues.

3. Incubate the cleaned artery in 0.2% collagenase type II at 37°C for 30 minutes for tissue dissociation.

4. Flush out the detached cells by rinsing the vessels with Medium 199.

5. Spin down the cells and resuspend the pellet in fresh Medium 199 and seed on gelatin-coated T-25 flasks.

6. Culture the cells in a humidified 37°C incubator with 5% CO$_2$.

Selection of endothelial microvascular and macrovascular cells

1. Prepare lectin-linked Dynabeads by incubating Tosylactivated Dynabeads (4 × 108 beads/mL; M450 Dynal, Life Technologies) with the lectin *Ulex europaeus* agglutinin I (UEA-I, a glycoprotein, Sigma) in 0.5 M borate buffer (pH 9.5) for 24 hours.

2. Detach the primary culture of cells using trypsin-EDTA; centrifuge and wash the trypsinized cells once with 1 × PBS.

3. Incubate cells with lectin-coupled Dynabeads for 30 minutes in PBS (bead to cell ratio 10:1).

4. Separate the Dynabead-coupled endothelial cells using a magnetic separator (Dynal, Life Technologies) as described earlier in the first protocol and culture the cells in Medium 199.

Note. For cell count, viability test, and cell propagation follow the steps as described in the first primary protocol.

A novel protocol of endothelial cell isolation

The protocol is as described by Teng and colleagues [28].

1. Anesthetize mouse and soak the belly skin with 70% ethanol. Open the chest of the anesthetized mouse to expose the heart (for details follow the first protocol in this chapter).

2. Excise the heart with an intact aortic arch and immersed in ice cold Krebs–Henseleit (KH) solution containing 118 mM NaCl, 1.2 mM $MgSO_4$, 1.2 mM KH_2PO_4, 25 mM $NaHCO_3$, 2.5 mM $CaCl_2$, and 11 mM glucose) in a sterile Petri dish.

3. Trim out the surrounding connective tissue from the heart using sterile scissors and forceps (keep the aortic arch intact).

4. Transfer the cleaned heart with intact aorta to a fresh Krebs–Henseleit (KH) solution-containing sterile Petri dish.

5. Insert a 25-gauge needle filled with HBSS (5.0 mM KCl, 0.3 mM KH_2PO_4, 138 mM NaCl, 4.0 mM $NaHCO_3$, 0.3 mM $Na_2HPO_4 \cdot 7H_2O$, 5.6 mM D-glucose, and 10.0 mM HEPES, with 2% penicillin/ streptomycin antibiotics) into the aortic lumen opening (keep the whole heart in the ice-cold buffer solution).

6. Insert the needle deeply into the heart close to the aortic valve.

7. Tie the aorta with the needle very close to the base of the heart.

8. Start the infusion pump with a 20-mL syringe containing warm HBSS (37°C) through an intravenous extension set at a rate of 0.1 mL/minute

9. Collect the perfusion fluid in a sterile 15-mL centrifuge tube on ice and flush the heart for 15 minutes.

10. Next, flush (0.1 mL/minute) the heart with warm enzyme solution (1 mg/mL collagenase type I, 0.5 mg/mL soybean trypsin inhibitor, 3% BSA, and 2% antibiotic–antimycotic).

11. Collect the perfusion fluid at different time points (30, 60, and 90 minutes). At 90 minutes, cut the heart with scissor, and open the apex to flush out the cells accumulated inside the ventricle.

12. Centrifuge the fluid at 1000 rpm for 10 minutes, discard supernatant, and mix the cell-rich pellets with culture medium.

13. Culture the cells in 2% gelatin-coated six-well plates containing culture medium (Medium 199-F-12 Medium (1:1) with 10% FBS and 2% antibiotics) and incubate in humidified 37°C incubator with 5% CO_2.

14. Change the medium on day 3 after cell isolation and grow until the cells reach confluence.

Note. Follow the steps as described in the first primary protocol in this chapter for cell count, viability test, and cell propagation.

Conclusions

The study of endothelial function and dysfunction in response to cellular stresses in a complex *in vivo* system comprised of multiple cell types and matrices is difficult. In order to better understand endothelial cell function *in vitro*, a purer culture of endothelial cells is necessary. Here, we describe in detail the isolation and culture procedures to obtain cardiac endothelial cells. The isolation and *in vitro* culture of pure populations of endothelial cells using the described procedures are extremely useful for the study of: (i) cytokine cell signaling and global gene expression, including microRNAs; and (ii) regulation of endothelial cell physiology, morphology, growth, differentiation, senescence, and apoptosis. For example, recent studies from several laboratories suggest that endothelial cells may also differentiate to mesenchymal or fibroblast-like cells by a biological phenomenon called endothelial to mesenchymal transition (EndMT). EndMT is a normal physiological phenomenon during embryonic heart, lung, and other organ development. However, in adults, EndMT-derived fibroblast-like cells synthesize and secrete Type I collagen and other ECM proteins that may significantly contribute to pathogenesis of cardiac fibrosis [11,29–31]. In order to understand the exact molecular basis of EndMT *in vitro* and its contribution in cardiac profibrogenic signaling, very early passages of pure primary cultures of vascular endothelial cells with all the endothelial cell features are essential. Proper understanding of the normal and pathological behaviors of vascular endothelial cells *in vitro* will be very useful to design meaningful *in vivo* experimental strategies as well as to develop new therapeutic strategies for numerous endothelial-dysfunction-related cardiovascular diseases.

Acknowledgements

This work was supported by a NIH-NHLBI grant.

References

1 Gerritsen ME. Functional heterogeneity of vascular endothelial cells. *Biochem Pharmac* 1987; **36**: 2701–2711.

2 Stancu CS, Toma L, Sima AV. Dual role of lipoproteins in endothelial cell dysfunction in atherosclerosis. *Cell Tissue Res* 2012; **349**: 433–446.

3 Fu Y, Chang AC, Fournier M, Chang L, Niessen K, Karsan A, *et al.* RUNX3 maintains the mesenchymal phenotype after termination of the Notch signal. *J Biol Chem* 2011; **286**: 11803–11813.

4 Muñoz-Chápuli R, Carmona R, Guadix JA, Macías D, Pérez-Pomares JM. The origin of the endothelial cells: an evo-devo approach for the invertebrate/vertebrate transition of the circulatory system. *Evol Dev* 2005; **7**: 351–358.

5 Yee A, Sakurai Y, Eskin SG, McIntire LV. A validated system for simulating common carotid arterial flow in vitro: alteration of endothelial cell response. *Ann Biomed Eng* 2006; **34**: 593–604.

6 Yee A, Bosworth KA, Conway DE, Eskin SG, McIntire LV. Gene expression of endothelial cells under pulsatile non-reversing vs. steady shear stress; comparison of nitric oxide production. *Ann Biomed Eng* 2008; **36**: 571–579.

7 Conway DE, Sakurai Y, Weiss D, Vega JD, Taylor WR, Jo H, *et al.* Expression of CYP1A1 and CYP1B1 in human endothelial cells: regulation by fluid shear stress. *Cardiovasc Res* 2009; **81**: 669–677.

8 Conway DE, Williams MR, Eskin SG, McIntire LV. Endothelial cell responses to atheroprone flow are driven by two separate flow components: low time-average shear stress and fluid flow reversal. *Am J Physiol Heart Circ Physiol* 2010; **298**: H367–H374.

9 Sumpio BE, Riley JT, Dardik A. Cells in focus: endothelial cell. *Int J Biochem Cell Biol* 2002; **34**: 1508–1512.

10 Hirashima M, Bernstein A, Stanford WL, Rossant J. Gene-trap expression screening to identify endothelial-specific genes. *Blood* 2004; **104**: 711–718.

11 McCall MN, Kent OA, Yu J, Fox-Talbot K, Zaiman AL, Halushka MK, *et al.* MicroRNA profiling of diverse endothelial cell types. *BMC Med Genomics* 2011; **4**: 78.

12 Ingenito EF, Craig JM, Labesse J, Gautier M, Rutstein DD. Cells of human heart and aorta grown in tissue culture. *AMA Arch Pathol* 1958; **65**: 355–359.

13 Jaffe EA, Hoyer LW, Nachman RL. Synthesis of antihemophilic factor antigen by cultured human endothelial cells. *J Clin Invest* 1973; **52**: 2757–2764.

14 Jaffe EA, Nachman RL, Becker CG, Minick CR. Culture of human endothelial cells derived from umbilical veins. Identification by morphologic and immunologic criteria. *J Clin Invest* 1973; **52**: 2745–2756.

15 Gimbrone MA Jr, Cotran RS, Folkman J. Human vascular endothelial cells in culture. Growth and DNA synthesis. *J Cell Biol* 1974; **60**: 673–684.

16 Nachman RL, Jaffe EA. Endothelial cell culture: beginnings of modern vascular biology. *J Clin Invest* 2004; **114**: 1037–1040.

17 Olofsson B, Pajusola K, Kaipainen A, von Euler G, Joukov V, Saksela O, *et al.* Vascular endothelial growth factor B, a novel growth factor for endothelial cells. *Proc Natl Acad Sci USA* 1996; **93**: 2576–2581.

18 Mahmoud M, Upton PD, Arthur HM. Angiogenesis regulation by TGFβ signaling: clues from an inherited vascular disease. *Biochem Soc Trans* 2011; **39**: 1659–1666.

19 van Meeteren LA, ten Dijke P. Regulation of endothelial cell plasticity by TGF-β. *Cell Tissue Res* 2012; **347**: 177–186.

20 Hayashi M, Lee JD. Role of the BMK1/ERK5 signaling pathway: lessons from knockout mice. *J Mol Med (Berl)* 2004; **82**: 800–808.

21 Roberts OL, Holmes K, Müller J, Cross DA, Cross MJ. ERK5 and the regulation of endothelial cell function. *Biochem Soc Trans* 2009; **37**: 1254–1259.

22 Roberts OL, Holmes K, Müller J, Cross DA, Cross MJ. ERK5 is required for VEGF-mediated survival and tubular morphogenesis of primary human microvascular endothelial cells. *J Cell Sci* 2010; **123**: 3189–3200.

23 Ohnesorge N, Viemann D, Schmidt N, Czymai T, Spiering D, Schmolke M, *et al.* Erk5 activation elicits a vasoprotective endothelial phenotype via induction of Kruppel-like factor 4 (KLF4). *J Biol Chem* 2010; **285**: 26199–26210.

24 Endemann DH, Schiffrin EL. Endothelial dysfunction. *J Am Soc Nephrol* 2004; **15**: 1983–1992.

25 Jelonek K, Walaszczyk A, Gabryś D, Pietrowska M, Kanthou C, Widłak P, *et al.* Cardiac endothelial cells isolated from mouse heart – a novel model for radiobiology. *Acta Biochim Pol* 2011; **58**: 397–404.

26 Lim YC, Luscinkas FW. Isolation and culture of murine heart and lung endothelial cells for in vitro model systems. *Methods Mol Biol* 2006; **341**: 141–154.

27 Gräfe M, Auch-Schwelk W, Graf K, Terbeek D, Hertel H, Unkelbach M, *et al.* Isolation and characterization

of macrovascular and microvascular endothelial cells from human hearts. *Am J Physiol* 1994; **267**: H2138–2148.

28 Teng B, Ansari HR, Oldenburg PJ, Schnermann J, Mustafa SJ. Isolation and characterization of coronary endothelial and smooth muscle cells from A1 adenosine receptor-knockout mice. *Am J Physiol Heart Circ Physiol* 2006; **290**: H1713–1720.

29 Zeisberg EM, Tarnavski O, Zeisberg M, Dorfman AL, McMullen JR, Gustafsson E, *et al.* Endothelial-to-mesenchymal transition contributes to cardiac fibrosis. *Nat Med* 2007; **13**: 952–961.

30 Ghosh AK, Bradham WS, Gleaves LA, De Taeye B, Murphy SB, Covington JW, *et al.* Genetic deficiency of plasminogen activator inhibitor-1 promotes cardiac fibrosis in aged mice: involvement of constitutive transforming growth factor-beta signaling and endothelial-to-mesenchymal transition. *Circulation* 2010; **122**: 1200–1209.

31 Ghosh AK, Nagpal V, Covington JW, Michaels MA, Vaughan DE. Molecular basis of cardiac endothelial-to-mesenchymal transition (EndMT): differential expression of microRNAs during EndMT. *Cell Signal* 2012; **24**: 1031–1036.

16 Isolation and culture of cardiac fibroblasts

Asish K. Ghosh, Joseph W. Covington and Douglas E. Vaughan

Northwestern University Feinberg School of Medicine, Chicago, IL, USA

Introduction

Fibroblasts are spindle-shaped cells of mostly mesenchymal origin and the major cellular source of extracellular matrix protein production in a tissue-specific manner. Although, cardiomyocytes occupy the maximum area of the heart, fibroblasts are the most abundant (~95%) noncardiomyocyte and most abundant cell type (60%) in the heart [1]. Mesenchymal fibroblasts synthesize a variety of extracellular matrix proteins and growth factors which control the function and longevity of cardiomyocytes [2–4]. Using coculture system of cardiac fibroblasts and cardiomyocytes, Ieda et al. [5] reported that while embryonic cardiac fibroblasts induce cardiomyocyte proliferation, adult cardiac fibroblasts induce cardiomyocyte hypertrophy. Embryonic cardiac fibroblast-specific signals mediated by collagen, fibronectin, and epidermal growth factor (EGF)-like growth factor play important roles in cardiomyocyte proliferation, and cardiomyocyte expressed α1-integrin is essential for this proliferation. Fibroblasts express their signature marker genes such as Type I collagen, a major extracellular matrix (ECM) protein; S-100 super-family protein fibroblast specific protein-1 (FSP-1), a small Ca^{2+} binding protein; discoidin domain receptor2 (DDR2), a tyrosine kinase receptor; and cytoskeletal protein α-smooth muscle actin (α-SMA) (Table 16.1) [6].

Fibroblasts are the most abundant cell type in connective tissues. However, fibroblasts originating from different parts of the body posses common and unique features based on their gene expression profile. It is also documented that the gene expression profile of skin fibroblasts is different from lung and cardiac fibroblasts [7,8]. Recent studies demonstrated that cardiac fibroblasts are not only of mesenchymal origin but are also derived from epithelial or endothelial cells, or pericytes, or circulating monocytes during embryonic development, as well as under pathophysiological conditions in adults [9–11]. Fibroblasts play a significant role in cell–cell communication, wound healing, and tissue homeostasis. Wound healing is generally characterized by an immediate inflammatory phase followed by connective tissue formation and tissue remodeling [12,13]. Upon tissue injury such as myocardial infarction (MI), infiltrating mononuclear cells move to the wound site, protecting the wound area from pathogens, secreting cytokines and growth factors such as transforming growth factor-beta (TGF-β), connective tissue growth factor (CTGF), and platelet derived growth factor (PDGF), which induce fibroblast migration to the wound area and activate fibroblasts to proliferate or differentiate to myofibroblasts. Myofibroblasts synthesize high levels of extracellular matrix protein and help in tissue remodeling in the wound area [14–17]. The multifaceted cytokine TGF-β is known to induce the differentiation of fibroblasts to myofibroblasts [18], which may lead to a sustained excessive synthesis and accumulation of collagen and other ECM proteins. Thus prolonged profibrotic signaling by

Manual of Research Techniques in Cardiovascular Medicine, First Edition. Edited by Hossein Ardehali, Roberto Bolli, and Douglas W. Losordo.

TGF-β causes elevated synthesis and accumulation of collagen that disrupts the tissue homeostasis, the pathological manifestation of tissue fibrosis [19,20]. It is noteworthy that 45% of total disease-related deaths in developed countries are associated with abnormal proliferation and differentiation of fibroblasts, which affects the tissue homeostasis in almost every organ in the body [21]. Therefore, it is important to understand the biology of fibroblasts in response to different cytokines and growth factors, and under different pathological conditions. Reproducible isolation procedure and culture of a pure population of cardiac fibroblasts is necessary for a successful *in vitro* study of these aspects, including myofibroblasts differentiation, secretion of ECM proteins, senescence, and apoptosis of cardiac fibroblasts.

Cardiac fibroblasts isolation protocol

In our laboratory, we routinely isolate and culture mouse cardiac fibroblasts (Figure 16.1) following the initial common procedure for isolation of both mouse cardiac endothelial cells and cardiac fibroblasts (follow up to Step 3 as described under First round cell sorting in Chapter 15). Isolation of cardiac fibroblasts during Dynabead-captured endothelial cell sorting makes the fibroblast population almost free of endothelial cells. For the isolation of mouse cardiac fibroblasts only, in the following protocol proceed to Step 17 after Step 15 (i.e. skip Step 16, endothelial cell sorting using Dynabead-bound CD31).

Materials and preparations

Cell Isolation Medium. Dulbecco's Modified Eagle Media (DMEM), with 4.5 g/L glucose, 20% fetal bovine serum, penicillin/streptomycin/amphotericin B (Calbiochem).

Cell Culture Medium. Dulbecco's Modified Eagle Media (DMEM), with 1 g/L glucose, 10% fetal bovine serum (FBS), penicillin/ streptomycin/ amphotericin B (Calbiochem).

Table 16.1 Fibroblast signature genes

Type I collagen (COL1A1 and COL1A2): triple helix of two COL1A1 polypeptides and one COL1A2 polypeptide; the major extracellular matrix protein synthesized by fibroblasts
Type III collagen (COL3A1): triple helix of three COL3A1 polypeptides; second predominant collagen in ECM of many tissues
Fibroblast specific protein-1 (FSP-1): a S-100 superfamily protein; a cytoplasmic calcium binding protein; highly expressed in fibroblasts
Discoidin domain receptor2 (DDR2): a receptor tyrosine kinase; highly expressed in cardiac fibroblasts; binds to collagen as its ligand; plays a role in cell–cell communication
α-smooth muscle actin (α-SMA): a cytoskeletal protein; plays an important role in fibroblasts contractility
Fibronectin: a high molecular weight ECM glycoprotein; plays a role in cell adhesion, growth, migration
Fibrillin 1: an ECM protein; regulates the bioavailability of active TGF-β; interacts with other proteins in microfibrils

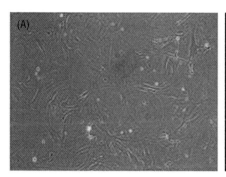 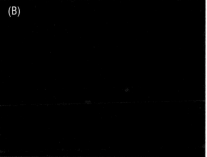

Figure 16.1 Mouse cardiac fibroblasts (MCF) isolated and cultured following the primary protocol. (A) Light microscopy; (B) Dil-acetylated-LDL negative labeling of isolated mouse cardiac fibroblasts.

Instruments/materials for animal dissection. Sterile scissors (two), sterile forceps (two), hemostats (two), 70% ethanol, sterile gauze, sterile 15-mL polypropylene centrifuge tubes.

Instruments for tissue dissociation. Autoclaved small forceps, fine scissors, sterile Petri dishes, sterile 15-mL polypropylene centrifuge tubes, 14-gauge metal cannula (Fisher #1482516N), and 70 μm pore size cell strainer (Fisher #08-771-2).

Type I collagenase. (230 U/mg; Worthington # S8b10315-A) Concentration: 2 mg/mL Dulbecco's Phosphate Buffered Saline (DPBS) with calcium and magnesium and 0.22 μm sterile filtered (prepare 10 mL/ two hearts).

Buffer 1. Dulbecco's Phosphate Buffered Saline (DPBS) (without Ca^{2+} and Mg^{2+}), 0.1% bovine serum albumin (BSA), 2 mM EDTA, pH 7.4.

Sterile Class II laminar flow hood.

Procedures for isolation of mouse cardiac fibroblasts

1. Anesthetize a young adult mouse (6–8 weeks old) with isoflurane and sacrifice by cervical dislocation.
2. Wet the belly skin with 70% ethanol.
3. Make a small incision in the skin above the pubis and deglove skin to just below the neck.
4. With a clean sterile scissor, cut open anterior abdomen, take down the anterior diaphragm, and open up the chest cavity. Apply hemostats to both sides of the skin and open the ribcage cavity.
5. Hold the heart with forceps and separate the heart from the lungs and vessels using sterile fine scissors; place the clean heart in a sterile 10-cm Petri dish.
6. Cut heart in half and place in 10 mL cold Cell Isolation Medium in a sterile 15-mL centrifuge tube.
7. Repeat Steps 1–6 for a second mouse, combine the hearts, and gently shake the tissue in the Cell Isolation Medium for 1 minute.
8. Transfer the tissue from the Cell Isolation Medium to a sterile 10-cm Petri dish placed in a sterile laminar flow hood.
9. Trim out attached connective tissue and chop the heart tissue fully with sterile fine scissors for 1 minute.

10. Transfer fully minced hearts in 10 mL of prewarmed (37°C) collagenase I (2 mg/mL) in a sterile 15-mL polypropylene tube.
11. Incubate at 37°C with gentle agitation for 60 minutes on a shaker.
12. Triturate the suspension 10 times using a 30 mL syringe attached to a cannula.
13. Allow undissociated tissue to settle at the bottom of the tube. Pipette out cell suspension and pass through a 70-μm disposable cell strainer (Falcon #35 2350) into a 50-mL conical tube. Wash sieve with 5 mL Buffer 1.
14. Transfer cell suspension to a sterile 15-mL centrifuge tube and spin down at 1300 rpm for 10 minutes at 4°C.
15. Resuspend the cell pellet in 1 mL of cold Buffer 1 and transfer to an Eppendorf microfuge tube.

(As described in Chapter 15, we use cell suspensions from this step for endothelial cell sorting: (i) Add anti-mouse CD31 Dynabeads to cell suspension at 15 μl of beads/ mL of cell suspension. (ii) Incubate on a rotator at room temperature for 10 minutes. (iii) Mount in the magnetic separator, and leave for 1 minute. While bead-bound cells are primarily endothelial cells, the supernatant is the enriched source of cardiac fibroblasts.)

Fibroblast culture:
16. Collect supernatant from CD31 Dynabead mediated endothelial cell sorting step. (The supernatant is relatively free of cardiomyocyte and endothelial cells and enriched in fibroblasts.) **OR**
17. Plate the cell suspension from Step 15 onto uncoated sterile cell culture dishes for 30 minutes. (This plating step allows the preferential attachment of fibroblasts to the bottom of the uncoated culture dish while other nonfibroblastic cells will still float in the culture media. In order to avoid contamination of nonfibroblast cells in the culture, do not allow the cell suspension to settle more than 30 minutes.)
18. Aspirate and remove unattached cells. Wash carefully once with cell culture media and add fresh medium (DMEM with 1 g/L glucose; Cellgro) supplemented with 10% FBS and antibiotics (penicillin, streptomycin, and amphotericin B mixture, Calbiochem) to the culture.

Cell propagation and maintenance

1. Change media every other day and grow the cells to confluence.

2. Split cells 1:3 onto uncoated plates when they reach 80–90% confluence. Aspirate the culture media and wash the cells once with 1×PBS and add trypsin-EDTA to detach the cells. Stop trypsinization by adding 10% FBS-containing DMEM. Centrifuge at 1300 rpm for 5 minutes and resuspend the pellet in cell culture medium. Incubate the cell cultures in a 37°C incubator with humidified atmosphere of 5% CO_2.

Cell viability count and replating. Resuspend the cell pellet in DMEM and count the viable cells using Countess Automated Cell Counter (Invitrogen; catalog no. C10227) following manufacturer's instruction as follows.

> **i.** Mix 10 μL of cell suspension with 10 μL of 0.4% trypan blue stain in an Eppendorf tube.
> **ii.** Add mixture of the cell suspension and trypan blue (10 μL) into the halfmoon-shaped chamber port on the Countess cell counting chamber slide.
> **iii.** Insert slide, sample side first into the slide port of the instrument until a soft click sound.
> **iv.** Optimize images following the manufacturer's instructions.
> **v.** To count cells, press "count cells" button to obtain results.
> **vi.** Results will show the number of live and dead cells per mL of cell suspension.

Notes. As primary cultures of cardiac fibroblasts in 10% FBS containing DMEM can also undergo differentiation when cultured for long periods of time (even in the absence of exogenous profibrotic cytokine TGF-β), it is important to use low passages of cells (up to six passages) in order to avoid mixed populations of fibroblasts and differentiated myofibroblasts in the characterization of fibroblast biology under different experimental conditions. It is also important to maintain fibroblast cultures in DMEM with normal glucose level (1 g/L) because high glucose also can induce fibroblast to myofibroblast differentiation.

Alternative approaches

Isolation and culture of cardiac ventricular fibroblasts from rats as described by Lijnen and colleagues [22].

Isolation of cardiac ventricular fibroblasts from rats

1. Weigh 7 to 8-week-old Wister rats.

2. Heparinize (625 units/100 g body weight) and anesthetize the rat intraperitoneally with Nembutal (50 mg/100 g body weight).

3. Soak the ventral skin with 70% ethanol and wipe with paper towel.

4. Open the chest with scissors and forceps as described in the previous protocol.

5. Remove the hearts and put in sterile Joklik's buffer (Sigma) in a sterile Petri dish.

6. Allow the heart to eject the residual blood and connect the aorta with a cannula. Flush out the residual blood with 10 mL of basic salt solution containing 130 mM NaCl, 3 mM KCl, 1.2 mM KH_2PO_4, 1 mM $MgSO_4$, 1.25 mM $CaCl_2$, 10 mM glucose, 10 mM HEPES, pH 7.2.

7. Perfuse the hearts via the ascending aorta according to the Langendorff method with Joklik's medium for 5 minutes.

8. Recirculate (flow rate: 5 mL/minute) Joklik's medium containing 0.02% collagenase A and 2% BSA for 35 minutes.

9. Remove the atria and vessels using sterile fine scissors and forceps and place the ventricular tissue in Joklik's medium containing 1% BSA and 0.01% collagenase A for an additional 10 minutes (37°C).

10. Chop the ventricular tissues into fine pieces with sterile scissors and filter through a 200-µm mesh net.

11. Allow the undissociated tissue to settle at the bottom of the tube for 15 minutes; collect the supernatant carefully and transfer to a new sterile tube.

12. To precipitate the cells, centrifuge the supernatant at 350 g for 10 minutes.

13. Resuspend the cell pellet in DMEM supplemented with 10% FBS and 1% penicillin/ streptomycin antibiotic solution.

14. Seed the resuspended cells in a sterile 80-cm^2 tissue culture flask.

15. Incubate the cell cultures at 37°C in humidified air with 5% CO_2 for 4 hours.

16. Aspirate the medium with unattached cells and add fresh DMEM, supplemented with 10% FBS and 1% penicillin/ streptomycin.

17. Feed the cells with fresh DMEM culture medium (with 10% FBS and 1% penicillin/ streptomycin) every other day and grow the cells to confluence and then passaged with trypsin-EDTA as described in the previous protocol.

Notes. Under the previously mentioned conditions of isolation, coronary smooth muscle and endothelial cells are rarely seen in the primary cultures; myocytes do not survive in this isolation procedure due to lack of oxygenation, as described by Lijnen *et al.* [22].

Conclusions

Pure populations of cultured cardiac fibroblasts are an essential component for *in vitro* study to enable a better understanding of the role of cardiac fibroblasts in fibrogenic processes in response to profibrotic cytokines and stresses. Isolated from mouse or rat, cardiac fibroblasts, the predominant noncardiomyocytic cells in the heart, are largely used for *in vitro* studies related to normal wound healing and pathological fibrosis. *In vitro* studies include: (1) cytokine response, (2) subcellular localization of a particular protein factor under physiological and pathological conditions, and (3) transfection of cultured cardiac fibroblasts with plasmid or viral expression vectors for overexpression or depletion of a particular factor, in order to determine the role of that factor on a particular signal transduction pathway in fibroblasts. For example, activated fibroblasts or differentiated myofibroblasts are the major source of collagen and other extracellular matrix proteins in heart and other tissues. Fibroblast to myofibroblast transition in response to profibrotic signaling such as TGF-β signaling is an essential step in the process of fibrogenesis. Although extensive studies have been performed to identify the mediators of fibroblast differentiation and to understand the origin of myofibroblasts from cardiac resident fibroblasts as well as other cell types [19,23–26], the exact molecular basis of myofibroblast differentiation during cardiac fibrogenesis is not well understood.

To delineate the molecular basis of myofibroblast differentiation and its contribution in physiological wound healing or pathological fibrosis, availability of a pure population of undifferentiated cardiac fibroblasts in culture is crucial. The outcome of such *in vitro* cell culture studies are required to design *in vivo* studies using animal models of wound healing and fibrosis.

References

1 Vliegen HW, van der Laarse A, Cornelisse CJ, Eulderink F. Myocardial changes in pressure overload-induced left ventricular hypertrophy. A study on tissue composition, polyploidization and multinucleation. *Eur Heart J* 1991; **12**: 488–494.

2 Eghbali M, Czaja MJ, Zeydel M Weiner FR, Zern MA, Seifter S, *et al.* Collagen chain mRNAs in isolated heart cells from young and adult rats. *J Mol Cell Cardiol* 1988; **20**: 267–276.

3 Eghbali M, Blumenfeld OO, Seifter S, Buttrick PM, Leinwand LA, Robinson TF, *et al.* Localization of types I, III and IV collagen mRNAs in rat heart cells by in situ hybridization. *J Mol Cell Cardiol* 1989; **21**: 103–113.

4 Eghbali M, Tomek R, Woods C, Bhambi B. Cardiac fibroblasts are predisposed to convert into myocyte phenotype: specific effect of transforming growth factor beta. *Proc Natl Acad Sci USA* 1991; **88**: 795–799.

5 Ieda M, Tsuchihashi T, Ivey KN, Ross RS, Hong TT, Shaw RM, *et al.* Cardiac fibroblasts regulate myocardial proliferation through beta1 integrin signaling. *Dev Cell* 2009; **16**: 233–244.

6 Smolenski A, Schultess J, Danielewski O, Garcia Arguinzonis MI, Thalheimer P, Kneitz S, *et al.* Quantitative analysis of the cardiac fibroblast transcriptome-implications for NO/cGMP signaling. *Genomics* 2004; **83**: 577–587.

7 Chang HY, Chi JT, Dudoit S, Bondre C, van de Rijn M, Botstein D, *et al.* Diversity, topographic differentiation, and positional memory in human fibroblasts. *Proc Natl Acad Sci USA* 2002; **99**: 12877–12882.

8 Rinn JL, Bondre C, Gladstone HB, Brown PO, Chang HY. Anatomic demarcation by positional variation in fibroblast gene expression programs. *PLoS Genet* 2006; **2**: e119.

9 Brown RD, Ambler SK, Mitchell MD, Long CS. The cardiac fibroblast: therapeutic target in myocardial remodeling and failure. *Annu Rev Pharmacol Toxicol* 2005; **45**: 657–687.

10 Baudino TA, Carver W, Giles W, Borg TK. Cardiac fibroblasts: friend or foe? *Am J Physiol Heart Circ Physiol* 2006; **291**: H1015–H1026.

11 Arciniegas E, Frid MG, Douglas IS, Stenmark KR. Perspectives on endothelial-to-mesenchymal transition: potential contribution to vascular remodeling in chronic pulmonary hypertension. *Am J Physiol Lung Cell Mol Physiol* 2007; **293**: L1–8.

12 Sun Y, Weber KT. Infarct scar: a dynamic tissue. *Cardiovasc Res* 2000; **46**: 250–256.

13 Weber KT, Sun Y, Katwa LC. Myofibroblasts and local angiotensin II in rat cardiac tissue repair. *Int J Biochem Cell Biol* 1997; **29**: 31–42.

14 Tuuminen R, Nykänen A, Keränen MA, Krebs R, Alitalo K, Koskinen PK, *et al.* The effect of platelet-derived growth factor ligands in rat cardiac allograft vasculopathy and fibrosis. *Transplant Proc* 2006; **38**: 3271–3273.

15 Bujak M, Frangogiannis NG. The role of TGF-beta signaling in myocardial infarction and cardiac remodeling. *Cardiovasc Res* 2007; **74**: 184–195.

16 Booth AJ, Csencsits-Smith K, Wood SC, Lu G, Lipson KE, Bishop DK, *et al.* Connective tissue growth factor promotes fibrosis downstream of TGFbeta and IL-6 in chronic cardiac allograft rejection. *Am J Transplant* 2010; **10**: 220–230.

17 Daniels A, van Bilsen M, Goldschmeding R, Van Der Vusse GJ, Van Nieuwenhoven FA. Connective tissue growth factor and cardiac fibrosis. *Acta Physiol* 2009; **195**: 321–338.

18 Petrov VV, Fagard RH, Lijnen PJ. Stimulation of collagen production by transforming growth factor-beta1 during differentiation of cardiac fibroblasts to myofibroblasts. *Hypertension* 2002; **39**: 258–263.

19 Ghosh AK, Bradham WS, Gleaves LA, De Taeye B, Murphy SB, Covington JW, *et al.* Genetic deficiency of plasminogen activator inhibitor-1 promotes cardiac fibrosis in aged mice: involvement of constitutive transforming growth factor-beta signaling and endothelial-to-mesenchymal transition. *Circulation* 2010; **122**: 1200–1209.

20 Ghosh AK, Vaughan DE. Fibrosis: is it a coactivator disease? *Front Biosci (Elite Ed)* 2012; **4**: 1556–1570.

21 Bitterman PB, Henke CA. Fibroproliferative disorders. *Chest* 1991; **99**: 81S–84S.

22 Lijnen PJ, Petrov VV, Fagard RH. Angiotensin II-induced stimulation of collagen secretion and production in cardiac fibroblasts is mediated via angiotensin II subtype 1 receptors. *J Renin Angiotensin Aldosterone Syst* 2001; **2**: 117–122.

23 Petrov VV, Fagard RH, Lijnen PJ. Transforming growth factor-beta (1) induces angiotensin-converting enzyme synthesis in rat cardiac fibroblasts during their differentiation to myofibroblasts. *J Renin Angiotensin Aldosterone Syst* 2000; **1**: 342–352.

24 Kis K, Liu X, Hagood JS. Myofibroblast differentiation and survival in fibrotic disease. *Expert Rev Mol Med* 2011; **13**: e27.

25 Zeisberg EM, Kalluri R. Origins of cardiac fibroblasts. *Circ Res* 2010; **107**: 1304–1312.

26 Ghosh AK, Nagpal V, Covington JW, Michaels MA, Vaughan DE. Molecular basis of cardiac endothelial-to-mesenchymal transition (EndMT): differential expression of microRNAs during EndMT. *Cell Signal* 2012; **24**: 1031–1036.

17 Murine bone marrow transplantation model

Prasanna Krishnamurthy, Suresh Kumar Verma, and Raj Kishore

Northwestern University Feinberg School of Medicine, Chicago, IL, USA

Introduction

Animal studies and clinical trials have demonstrated the therapeutic potential of bone marrow (BM)-derived endothelial progenitor cells in neovascularization during wound healing, limb ischemia and postmyocardial infarction. These cells also play a critical role in endothelialization of vascular grafts, atherosclerosis, retinal and lymphoid organ neovascularization, and vascularization during tumor growth [1–9]. Therefore, studies designed to understand the contribution of BM-derived cells to neovascularization and tissue repair is crucial. However, it is important to overcome the challenges of identifying BM-derived cells *in situ*. Bone marrow transplantation (BMT) models allow us to distinguish BM cells from tissue-specific cells by using genetically marked donor BM cells from either transgenic mice or viral-transduction of a marker gene.

Materials

Donor mice:
- Age 8–10 weeks.
- Male, if planning to detect Y chromosome.
- One donor mouse is sufficient to transplant into three recipient mice.
- Donor BM can be from transgenic mouse with either a ubiquitously expressed marker gene (e.g. ACTbEGFP) or a marker gene driven by an endothelial cell-specific promoter (e.g. Tie2/GFP).

- Mice background: C57BL/6-Tg (ACTbEGFP), eGFP mice; Flk-1/LacZ mice (B6.129); B6.129-*Gt(ROSA)26Sor^{tm1Joe}*/J; B6.Cg-Tg(TIE2GFP)287Sato/1J; FVB/N-Tg(TIE2-lacZ)182Sato/J [10–13].

Recipient mice:
- Age 6–8 weeks.
- Female, if planning to detect donor Y chromosome.
- Background of the mice should be the same as donor mice (syngeneic).

Reagents/equipment:
Phosphate-buffered saline with 5 mM EDTA (PBS-E)
Lysis buffer (ACK lysis buffer)
Histopaque-1083
Petri dishes
15-mL conical tubes
1-mL tuberculin syringe
5-mL syringe
Needles: 27 G, 18 G
Cell strainer (70 µm)
Scissor, scalpel, forceps
Sterile pipette
Mouse pie cage
Irradiator
Restrainer

Procedure

Irradiation of recipient mice:
1. Place the mice in a mouse pie cage (Braintree Scientific, Inc. MA) with a continuous airflow

Manual of Research Techniques in Cardiovascular Medicine, First Edition. Edited by Hossein Ardehali, Roberto Bolli, and Douglas W. Losordo.

between two opposing ^{137}Cs-ray sources (Gamma cell 40; Nordion International, Kanata, Ontario, Canada). Irradiate the mice with two fractionated doses of 4.5 Gy each with a 4-hour interval (one before beginning to isolate donor BM and another before injecting the BM cells).

Bone marrow isolation:
2. Sacrifice the donor mice by CO_2 asphyxiation and cervical dislocation; spray mice with 70% EtOH and harvest the femurs and tibias into cold PBS-E on ice.

Note. The rest of the isolation procedures should be carried out under a hood to maintain aseptic conditions.

3. Thoroughly scrape the tibia and femur of fascia, muscle, and connective tissue. Carefully clip the ends of the bones. Flush out the BM with PBS-E into a conical tube using a 27-guage needle until the red marrow is completely removed from inside the bone.
4. Carefully lay the BM cell suspension (12 mL) onto histopaque-1083 (3 mL, brought to room temperature prior to laying cells) in a 15-mL conical tube.
5. Centrifuge at 900 g for 20 minutes at room temperature without brakes.
6. After discarding the upper layer (opaque) with a Pasteur pipette, carefully collect the middle, mononuclear cells (MNCs)-rich layer into a new 15-mL conical tube using a 5-mL syringe with an 18-G needle and suspend the cells in PBS-E for washing.
7. Centrifuge at 1200 g for 5 minutes at 4°C.
8. Aspirate PBS-E, resuspend cell pellet in 10°mL ACK buffer and set on ice for 15 minutes.
9. Wash cells with cold PBS-E again, centrifuge, and resuspend pellet in 1 mL PBS.
10. Filter MNCs through a 70-μm cell strainer and count using trypan blue method and prepare 2×10^6 cells in 100 μL PBS for injection into recipient mice.

Transplantation:
11. After the second dose of irradiation, anesthetize the mice with Avertin (2,2,2 tribromoethanol) (125 mg/kg IP) and inject 2×10^6 MNCs in 100 μL PBS through the lateral tail vein using a 27-G needle. Allow the mice to recover on a warm heating pad.
12. Allow 4–6 weeks for BM reconstitution.

Confirmation of BM reconstitution:
13. After 6 weeks of BM reconstitution, cells from peripheral blood or BM are subjected to flow-cytometry analysis and real-time (quantitative) PCR analysis of genomic DNA [14]. Furthermore, tissue homing/ recruitment can be confirmed by histological staining for eGFP (anti-GFP antibodies), lacZ (X-gal staining), or Y chromosome *in situ* hybridization.

Animal husbandry

Recipient mice are given acidified water (pH 1.3–2.0) containing antibiotics, 1–2 weeks prior to transplantation. The mice are kept on acidic, antibiotic water for 2 weeks after irradiation and then switched to acidic water without antibiotics for the rest of their lives. Recipients are housed in sterile cages post-transplant for an additional 2 weeks. After that they can be moved to regular cages. Transplanted mice undergo a 5 to 10-day irradiation sickness period from which they generally recover within 14 days [15]. A mortality rate of 10–15% can be expected as a result of radiation necrosis during the first week after transplantation. Sudden death of recipient mice after donor cell injection might result from pulmonary embolization due to injection of cell aggregates (gently tapping the syringe prior to injection might help).

Alternative approaches

Treosulfan- or busulfan-treatment possesses both myeloablative and immunosuppressive properties and can be used as an alternative to irradiation-induced myeloabalation [16]. However, toxicity of the chemo agents and its effect on mortality and morbidity in mice should be considered.

Weaknesses and strengths of the method

Irradiation is effective to myeloabalate rapidly proliferating immunocompetent cells particularly T cells, and hematopoietic progenitor cells in the recipients. However, it is warranted to consider fractionated low-dose irradiation over single dose, as it is more effective and has been shown to reduce morbidity and mortality [17]. Further it is also important to note that irradiation dose vary with different strains of mice. B6 mice strains tolerate higher irradiation doses, BALB/c tolerate lesser doses and SCID mice are profoundly sensitive to irradiation. Therefore, researchers should consider the strain, total dose and dosing schedule for their experiments. If difficulties in detecting donor cell GFP signals are encountered, the signals might be amplified by anti-GFP antibody and confocal microscopy.

References

1 Kalka C, Masuda H, Takahashi T, Kalka-Moll WM, Silver M, Kearney M, et al. Transplantation of ex vivo expanded endothelial progenitor cells for therapeutic neovascularization. Proc Natl Acad Sci U S A. 2000; 97(7): 3422–3427.

2 Jung SY, Choi JH, Kwon SM, Masuda H, Asahara T, Lee YM, et al. Decursin inhibits vasculogenesis in early tumor progression by suppression of endothelial progenitor cell differentiation and function. J Cell Biochem. 2012.

3 Orlic D, Kajstura J, Chimenti S, Bodine DM, Leri A, Anversa P, et al. Transplanted adult bone marrow cells repair myocardial infarcts in mice. Ann N Y Acad Sci. 2001; 938: 221–229; discussion 229-230.

4 Losordo DW, Schatz RA, White CJ, Udelson JE, Veereshwarayya V, Durgin M, et al. Intramyocardial transplantation of autologous CD34+ stem cells for intractable angina: a phase I/IIa double-blind, randomized controlled trial. Circulation. 2007; 115(17562958): 3165–3172.

5 Asai J, Takenaka H, Kusano KF, Ii M, Luedemann C, Curry C, et al. Topical sonic hedgehog gene therapy accelerates wound healing in diabetes by enhancing endothelial progenitor cell-mediated microvascular remodeling. Circulation. 2006; 113(20): 2413–2424.

6 Krishnamurthy P, Thal M, Verma S, Hoxha E, Lambers E, Ramirez V, et al. Interleukin-10 deficiency impairs bone marrow-derived endothelial progenitor cell survival and function in ischemic myocardium. Circ Res. 2011; 109(11): 1280–1289.

7 Jameel MN, Li Q, Mansoor A, Qiang X, Sarver A, Wang X, et al. Long-term functional improvement and

gene expression changes after bone marrow-derived multipotent progenitor cell transplantation in myocardial infarction. Am J Physiol Heart Circ Physiol. 2010; 298(5): H1348–1356.

8 Kaushal S, Amiel GE, Guleserian KJ, Shapira OM, Perry T, Sutherland FW, et al. Functional small-diameter neovessels created using endothelial progenitor cells expanded ex vivo. Nat Med. 2001; 7(9): 1035–1040.

9 Sata M, Saiura A, Kunisato A, Tojo A, Okada S, Tokuhisa T, et al. Hematopoietic stem cells differentiate into vascular cells that participate in the pathogenesis of atherosclerosis. Nat Med. 2002; 8(4): 403–409.

10 Yang J, Ii M, Kamei N, Alev C, Kwon SM, Kawamoto A, et al. CD34+ cells represent highly functional endothelial progenitor cells in murine bone marrow. PLoS One. 2011; 6(5): e20219.

11 Oshima RG, Lesperance J, Munoz V, Hebbard L, Ranscht B, Sharan N, et al. Angiogenic acceleration of Neu induced mammary tumor progression and metastasis. Cancer Res. 2004; 64(1): 169–179.

12 Soriano P. Generalized lacZ expression with the ROSA26 Cre reporter strain. Nat Genet. 1999; 21(1): 70–71.

13 Schlaeger TM, Bartunkova S, Lawitts JA, Teichmann G, Risau W, Deutsch U, et al. Uniform vascular-endothelial-cell-specific gene expression in both embryonic and adult transgenic mice. Proc Natl Acad Sci U S A. 1997; 94(7): 3058–3063.

14 Sun Z, Zhang Y, Brunt KR, Wu J, Li SH, Fazel S, et al. An adult uterine hemangioblast: evidence for extramedullary self-renewal and clonal bilineage potential. Blood. 2010; 116(16): 2932–2941.

15 Duran-Struuck R, Dysko RC. Principles of bone marrow transplantation (BMT): providing optimal veterinary and husbandry care to irradiated mice in BMT studies. J Am Assoc Lab Anim Sci. 2009; 48(1): 11–22.

16 Sjoo F, Hassan Z, Abedi-Valugerdi M, Griskevicius L, Nilsson C, Remberger M, et al. Myeloablative and immunosuppressive properties of treosulfan in mice. Exp Hematol. 2006; 34(1): 115–121.

17 Cui YZ, Hisha H, Yang GX, Fan TX, Jin T, Li Q, et al. Optimal protocol for total body irradiation for allogeneic bone marrow transplantation in mice. Bone Marrow Transplant. 2002; 30(12): 843–849.

In vitro differentiation and expansion of vascular endothelial cells derived from mouse embryonic stem cells

Anees Fatima, Carey Nassano-Miller, and Tsutomu Kume

Northwestern University Feinberg School of Medicine, Chicago, IL, USA

Introduction

Vascular endothelium plays a vital role in blood vessel formation, vascular homeostasis, permeability, and regulation of inflammation [1]. Endothelial cells (EC) provide specific functional requirements to assure delivery of blood containing nutrients and oxygen to the tissue and remove the metabolic wastes. EC prevent thrombosis and regulate arterial reactivity through synthesis and release of vasoactive molecules [2]. EC clearly have more interesting and active roles than just acting as passive channels of blood circulation. They can promote stem-cell development and organ formation by acting as sources of paracrine signals to surrounding cells [3]. Additionally, vascular EC or endothelial progenitor cells derived from stem cells could potentially lead to a variety of clinically relevant applications. EC are required for tissue engineered vascular grafts [4]. Since EC can release proteins directly into the bloodstream, they are ideal candidates for use in gene therapy.

During embryogenesis, the formation of the vascular network is a highly complex event, controlled on multiple levels in a spatiotemporal manner. Initially the vascular network is formed by "vasculogenesis" wherein a primitive vasculature is formed *de novo* by mesodermal endothelial progenitor cells known as angioblasts. Following these events, subsequent remodeling and expansion of primitive network occurs by "angiogenesis" [5]. Once vascular progenitors have been generated, they undergo specification to arterial, venous, and lymphatic EC. This specification is influenced by a combination of genetic programming and extrinsic factors like hemodynamic flow [6,7]. In recent years, we have begun to understand the genetic control of normal process of vascular development and remodeling [8]. However, there still exists a large gap in understanding of the mechanisms that regulate EC specification and differentiation. Looking into the potential therapeutic applications of EC and a pressing need to further understand the underlying mechanisms, it becomes imperative to develop *in vitro* culture models of EC.

Embryonic stem cells (ES-cells) serve as an excellent source to develop such models. We know from prior studies that it is possible to isolate from mouse ES-cells a subpopulation of angioblast precursors expressing Flk-1 [9]. The Flk-1[+] mesodermal cells will eventually give rise to mature endothelium that is capable of mimicking the process of vascularization *in vitro* [10]. Furthermore, Flk-1[+]cells also generate cells of hematopoietic lineage, smooth muscle cells, and cardiomyocytes [10]. In this chapter we describe a technique of harvesting ES-cell derived Flk-1[+]cells and their differentiation into EC. We used mouse ES line

Manual of Research Techniques in Cardiovascular Medicine, First Edition. Edited by Hossein Ardehali, Roberto Bolli, and Douglas W. Losordo.

PRX-129/s6 derived from the inner mass of blastocysts of 129SvEv strain mice. ES-cells derived from 129SvEv mice have in the past successfully differentiated to EC [11].

Materials

Tissue culture
- PRX-129/s6 ES-cells (a generous gift from Dr. Lynn Doglio)
- Irradiated primary mouse embryonic fibroblasts (MEFs) (Stem Cell Core Facility, Northwestern University)
- Dulbecco's phosphate-buffered saline (DPBS) (Cellgro, Cat. No: 21-030-CM)
- Gelatin (Sigma Cat. No: G2500-100G)
- Trypsin (Hyclone Cat. No: SH30236.01)
- Cell Stripper (Cellgro, Cat. No: 25-056-Cl)
- 15-mL sterile centrifuge tubes (Corning, Cat. No: 430790)
- Six-well tissue culture plate (Becton-Dickinson, Cat. No: 35-3045)
- 100-mm² cell culture dishes (Corning, Cat. No: 439167)
- Collagen-IV Biocoat-Cellware (Becton-Dikinson, Cat. No: 354459)
- Nalgene 0.75 mm Filter Unit, 500 mL (Nalge-Nunc International)
- Nalgene cryogenic vials (Nalge-Nunc International, Cat. No: 5000-0020)
- Nalgene Cryo 1°-freezing containers (Nalge-Nunc, Cat. No: 5100-0001)

Media
- High-glucose Dulbecco's modified Eagle's medium (DMEM) (Gibco, Cat. No: 11965-092)
- Iscove's modified Dulbecco's medium (IMDM) (Gibco Cat. No: 12440-053)
- Fetal bovine serum (FBS) (Hyclone Cat. No: SH30070.03)
- Penicillin–streptomycin (Cellgro, Cat. No: 30-0020-CI)
- L-Glutamine (Hyclone, Cat. No: SH30034.01)
- Nonessential amino acids (Cellgro, Cat. No: 25-025-Cl)
- Transferrin (Roche, Cat. No: 10652202001)
- L-ascorbic acid (Sigma-Aldrich, Cat. No: A4544-100G)

- Monothioglycerol (Sigma-Aldrich Cat. No: M6145-25ML)
- LIF (Millipore, Cat. No: ESG1106)
- HEPES buffer (Sigma-Aldrich, Cat. No: H0887)
- β-mercaptoethanol (Sigma Cat. No: M6250-250ML)
- Dimethyl sulfoxide (DMSO) (Sigma-Aldrich Cat. No: D5879-500ML)
- ES-cell media: to prepare 250 mL medium, combine 205 mL DMEM, 35 mL FBS (14%), 2.5 mL (100 μM) each of L-glutamine, HEPES, nonessential amino acids, penicillin–streptomycin (1000 U/L), 25 μL LIF (1000 U/mL), and 3.4 μL (5×10^{-5} M) β-mercaptoethanol.
- Freezing medium (FM): to prepare 10 mL freezing medium, combine 9 mL ES cell media and 1 mL (10%) sterile DMSO.
- ES-cell differentiation medium: to prepare 500 mL media combine 425 mL IMDM, 75 mL FBS (15%), 5 mL L-glutamine (1%), 500 μL penicillin–streptomycin (100 U/mL), 167 μL transferrin (200 μg/mL), 0.044 g L-ascorbic acid (0.5 mM), 22.5 μL monothioglycerol (4.5×10^{-4} M).

FACS purification of Flk-1$^+$ cells
- Accutase (Millipore, Cat. No: SCR005)
- DPBS (Cellgro Cat. No: 21-030-CM)
- Phycoerythrin (PE) conjugated rat anti-mouse Flk-1 antibody (clone: AVAS 12α1) (BD-Pharmingen, Cat. No: 555308)
- 5-mL sterile round-bottom tubes (Becton-Dikinson, Cat. No: 352235)
- Recombinant human VEGF-165aa (Miltenyi Biotec, Cat. No: 130-094-031)

General equipment
- Water bath at 37°C
- Hemocytometer for cell counting
- Phase-contrast microscope (4×, 10× objectives)
- Humidified incubator (37°C, 5% CO$_2$)
- Laminar air-flow hood
- Micropipettes and tips (10, 20, 100, 200, 1000 μL)
- Glass Pasteur pipettes
- Disposable pipettes
- Refrigerator (4°C) and freezers (−20 and −80°C)
- Tabletop centrifuge
- Cell sorter: Beckman Coulter Mo Flo

Methods

ES-cell culture (see Notes 1 and 2)

Freezing of ES-cells

1. Wash cells with 1 mL DPBS (see Note 3).
2. Trypsinize the ES-cells growing on MEFs.
3. For cells on a six-well plate add 0.5–1 mL of 0.05% trypsin.
4. Incubate cells in the incubator for 5 minutes (see Note 4).
5. Pellet the cells by centrifugation (1000 rpm, 5 minutes).
6. Remove the supernatant.
7. Resuspend the pellet by adding cell FM dropwise. Shake the cell suspension for even distribution of FM.
8. Distribute the cells in FM to cryovials, 1 mL/ cryovial (see Note 5).
9. Immediately transfer the cryovials to a Cryo 1°C freezing container and place it in −70°C/ −80°C for 24 hours.
10. Next day transfer the vials to liquid nitrogen (see Note 6).

Thawing of ES-cells

1. Thaw the cells in a 37°C water bath, until a small ice droplet remains (see Note 6).
2. While the vial is thawing, add 4 mL ES-cell media to a 15-mL centrifuge tube.
3. Transfer thawed cells to the centrifuge tube containing ES-cell media.
4. Pellet the cells by centrifugation (1000 rpm, 5 minutes).
5. Gently resuspend the cells in fresh media.
6. Transfer cells to culture dish with MEFs (see Notes 7 and 8) and place in the incubator.
7. Replace media the next day.

Culture of ES-cells

1. Thaw the ES-cells as described in section Thawing of ES-cells.
2. Plate 1–5×10^5 cells/ MEF coated well of a six-well plate containing 3 mL ES-cell medium.
3. Replace media the next day.
4. Subculture the ES-cells before colonies begin to touch (see Note 9). With the cell density as stated earlier, cells should be ready on day 2 for subculture (Figure 18.1A).

ES-cell subculture (see Note 10)

1. Remove media and rinse cells with 1 mL PBS.
2. Add 0.5–1 mL trypsin/ well of a six-well plate.
3. Incubate cells in incubator for 3–4 minutes.
4. To disaggregate cells, gently pipette up and down two times.
5. Add 4 mL media to a 15-mL centrifuge tube, and transfer trypsinized cells to this tube.
6. Centrifuge at 1000 rpm for 5 minutes.
7. Remove supernatant.
8. Resuspend the pellet in 3 mL media and replate cells (1–5×10^5) on 3-MEF coated wells.

Differentiation of ES-cells to Flk-1$^+$ progenitors

The ES-cells are subcultured on 0.1% gelatin for two passages (4 days) before switching to differentiation. This minimizes the number of MEFs in culture while allowing the ES-cells to expand.

Gelatin coating procedure for culture dishes

1. Prepare 0.1% gelatin in ultrapure distilled water.
2. Autoclave and store at room temperature.
3. To coat add 10 mL 0.1% gelatin to the 100-mm culture dishes.
4. Leave the dishes at 37°C (see Note 11).
5. Aspirate the gelatin thoroughly before seeding the cells.

Weaning of ES-cells from MEFs (see Note 12)

1. For ES-cell dissociation, remove media from the well, wash cells with PBS, and add 1 mL cell stripper/ well of a six-well plate.
2. Incubate at 37°C for 30–45 minutes.
3. Collect the cell stripper solution from the well (see Note 13) and add to a 15-mL tube containing 4 mL ES-cell media. Centrifuge at 1000 rpm for 5 minutes.
4. Remove the supernatant.
5. Resuspend cells in 1 mL ES-cell media.
6. Seed cells 5×10^5 cells/100-mm dish (Figure 18.1B).
7. Repeat the steps 1–6 for another passage (see Note 14).

Differentiation of ES-cells to Flk-1$^+$ progenitors

1. Wash ES-cells with 5 mL DPBS.
2. Dissociate weaned ES-cells with trypsin (3 mL/100-mm dish).
3. Incubate at 37°C for 5 minutes.

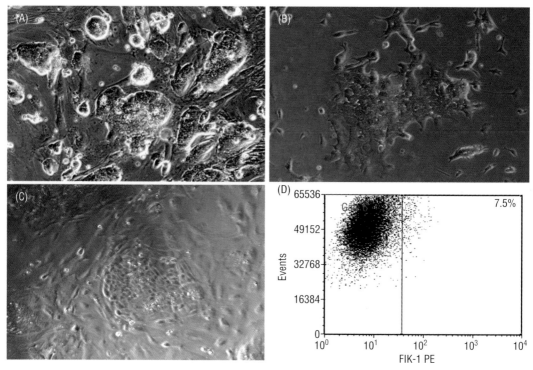

Figure 18.1 ES-to-Flk-1 differentiation: (A) PRX-129/s6 cells on MEFs; (B) weaned ES-cells on gelatin; (C) differentiating ES-cells 4-day on CollV; (D) dot-plot of sorted Flk-1+ cells.

4. Collect cell suspension from the well and add to 15-mL tube containing 4 mL ES differentiation media. Centrifuge at 1000 rpm for 5 minutes.

5. Remove the supernatant.

6. Resuspend cells in 1 mL ES differentiation media.

7. Count cells on hemocytometer.

8. Plate 30,000 cells on 35-mm collagen-IV plates.

9. Grow the cells in an incubator for 4–4.5 days. Do not change media during these 4 days (Figure 18.1C).

Purification of Flk-1+ cells

Following 4 days of growth on collagen-IV the ES-cells would now have a heterogeneous population of cells, including a subpopulation of Flk-1+vascular progenitor cells [9]. These Flk-1+cells are then sorted/ purified by flow cytometry (see Note 15).

1. Remove culture medium and wash cells with 3 mL DPBS.

2. Dissociate cells using 3 mL Accutase, incubate at 37°C for 30–40 minutes (see Note 16).

3. Gently pipette cells up and down two to three times. In case some cells remain adhered to the bottom, pipette up and down a few more times.

4. Transfer cells to 15-mL tube containing 4 mL media with FBS.

5. Centrifuge at 1000 rpm for 5 minutes.

6. Wash cells in 3 mL cold DPBS two times.

7. Count the cells using a hemocytometer.

8. Take 50 μL of cell suspension for control "cells-only".

9. To the remaining cells add PE-conjugated anti-Flk-1 antibody (0.2 μg/100,000 cells/100 μL PBS).

10. Incubate at 4°C 30 minutes.

11. Wash cells in 3 mL cold DPBS three times.

12. Resuspend cells in 0.5–1 mL fresh cold DPBS, and pass the suspension through a 40-μm cell strainer and transfer cells to a 5-mL round bottomed polystyrene FACS tube.

13. Fill a 15-mL centrifuge tube with 5 mL ES differentiation media, and use this as a collecting tube.

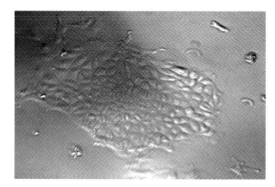

Figure 18.2 Differentiation of Flk-1⁺ cells to EC showing cobblestone morphology.

14. Sort the cells for Flk-1⁺population (Figure 18.1D) (see Note 17).

Expansion/differentiation of Flk-1⁺ cells

1. After sorting, centrifuge the collecting tube containing Flk-1⁺cells 1000 rpm, 3 minutes.

2. Remove supernatant and resuspend cells into 1 mL fresh ES-cell differentiation media.

3. Plate cells at a density of 50,000–60,000 cells/ 35-mm collagen-IV dish (see Note 18).

4. Fill each dish with 2 mL ES differentiation media.

5. Add VEGF-165 (50 ng/mL).

6. Incubate cells for 4 days in the incubator. Do not disturb the dish for 4 days.

7. Observe for growth of EC at the end of 4 days (Figure 18.2).

8. EC differentiation can be confirmed by testing for expression of EC cell markers by qPCR, flow cytometry, or immunostaining (see Note 18).

Notes

1. The cells should be sterile throughout passaging and differentiation.

2. Warm up solutions and media to 37°C before use.

3. Before trypsinization, wash cells with DPBS containing antibiotics to remove residual FBS/FCS.

4. During trypsinization do not exceed incubation time above 5 minutes. Add media to neutralize trypsin.

5. The cells should be frozen in 1-mL cryovials, at a density of 5–10×10⁶.

6. Freeze cells slowly and thaw quickly. Cells are stored in liquid nitrogen for long-term use.

7. To maintain ES-cells in an undifferentiated state, they are grown on MEFs. Make sure to prepare the MEFs at least 4–6 hours prior to seeding the cells.

8. Irradiated MEFs can be used for up to 10 days.

9. ES-cells should be subcultured before the colonies touch, which may cause differentiation.

10. The PRX-129/s6 ES-cells can be passaged for up to 25 passages.

11. Gelatin coating should be carried out at least for 45 minutes at room temperature.

12. For weaning, use a nonenzymatic method of cell dissociation.

13. Gently tap the tube with index finger to obtain a single-cell suspension.

14. On weaning, ES-cells lose the typical colony morphology and start to grow like a monolayer (Figure 18.1B).

15. During cell sorting, take special care to keep cells sterile.

16. For FACS, use a gentle form of cell-dissociation solution, Accutase.

17. The subpopulation of Flk-1⁺cells will range anywhere between 10 and 30%. We were able to get up to 10% Flk-1⁺ cells. Considering you get at least 10% Flk-1⁺ cells, it will take 2–3 hours of cell sorting to obtain a population of 5–6×10⁴ cells.

18. Due to the FACS procedures, expect a lot of cells to die.

19. We tested the differentiation of EC by quantifying the expression of EC markers such as CD31 and Tie-2 by qPCR.

Acknowledgements

We thank Dr. Changwon Park, Assistant Professor at University of Illinois at Chicago for his valuable input for the Flk-1 cell-sorting. Dr. Lynn Doglio, Core Director/ Research Associate Professor at Transgenic and Targeted Mutagenesis Core, Northwestern University-Chicago for sharing the PRX-129/s6 cells. This work was supported by National Institutes of Health grants HL074121 and EY019484 to T.K.

References

1 Aird WC. Phenotypic heterogeneity of the endothelium: I. Structure, function, and mechanisms. *Circ Res* 2007; **100**: 158–173.

2 Michiels C. Endothelial cell functions. *J Cell Physiol* 2003; **196**: 430–443.

3 Coultas L, Chawengsaksophak K, Rossant J. Endothelial cells and VEGF in vascular development. *Nature* 2005; **438**: 937–945.

4 Stegemann JP, Kaszuba SN, Rowe LS. Review: advances in vascular tissue engineering using protein-based biomaterials. *Tissue Eng* 2007; **13**: 2601–2613.

5 Carmeliet P. Angiogenesis in health and disease. *Nat Med* 2003; **9**: 653–660.

6 Kume T. Specification of arterial, venous, and lymphatic endothelial cells during embryonic development. *Histol Histopathol* 2010; **25**: 637–646.

7 Le Noble F, Moyon D, Pardanaud L, Yuan L, Djonov V, Matthijsen R, *et al.* Flow regulates arterial-venous differentiation in the chick embryo yolk sac. *Development* 2004; **131**: 361–375.

8 Herbert SP, Stainier YRD. Molecular cell behavior during blood vessel morphogenesis. *Nat Rev Mol Cell Biol* 2011; **12**: 551–564.

9 Yamashita J, Itoh H, Hirashima M, Ogawa M, Nishikawa S, Yurugi T, *et al.* Flk1-positive cells derived from embryonic stem cells serve as vascular progenitors. *Nature* 2000; **408**: 92–96.

10 Kattman SJ, Huber TL, Keller GM. Multipotent flk-1+ cardiovascular progenitor cells give rise to the cardiomyocyte, endothelial, and vascular smooth muscle lineages. *Dev Cell* 2006; **11**: 723–732.

11 Gualandris A, Annes JP, Arese M, Noguera I, Jurukovski V, Rifkin DB, *et al.* The latent transforming growth factor-b– binding protein-1 promotes in-vitro differentiation of embryonic stem cells into endothelium. *Mol Biol Cell* 2000; **11**: 4295–4308.

Part 3

Manipulation of the Heart and Vessels *in Vivo* and *ex Vivo*

Coronary ligation

Alexander R. Mackie and Hossein Ardehali

Northwestern University Feinberg School of Medicine, Chicago, IL, USA

Introduction

Although the long-term consequences of coronary heart disease in the human population are well established, the mechanisms that facilitate the accompanying pathophysiological processes are still being investigated. To effectively study the cardio-vascular impact of coronary heart disease or to develop successful therapeutics against it, a strong and reproducible model system is required. Fortunately, the murine model of left anterior coronary artery ligation (CAL) is capable of mimicking both the short- and long-term consequences of coronary artery blockade in humans. Additionally, the CAL procedure is probably the most widely used model for inducing heart failure in mice given the efficacy by which a large infarct decreases left ventricular function [1].

The following protocol focuses on one specific method commonly used to induce permanent CAL in mice, which requires both intubation and mechanical ventilation. Given the widespread and historical use of the CAL model, several other excellent resources [2–5] exist to help scientists achieve efficiency and consistency with this model. With that in mind, someone expecting to become extremely proficient with this technique can expect to do so in 1 to 3 months, depending on the level of commitment. Since the full development of the infarct is generally complete within 4 weeks after CAL and that assessment of infarct size will necessitate histological analysis of practice hearts, it is reasonable to assume that multiple practice cycles will be required. One should also plan on initially using only normal control mice to practice this procedure in order to ensure technique proficiency prior to testing genetic models that may inherently suffer far worse mortality than their wild-type controls.

Although the protocol described here may vary slightly from other available protocols, the key to producing high-quality data with any surgical protocol is to maintain consistency between test subjects. By following the protocol in the following text, along with engaging in a fair amount of practice, this protocol should yield reproducible infarct size while limiting postsurgical mortality.

Protocol

Note. Please see the accompanying video associated with this chapter in the online supplemental material for this text (Video clip 19.1).

1. Assemble and prepare all surgical equipment, tools and supplies (Tables 19.1 and 19.2) at an appropriate surgical station (Figure 19.1). Turn the bead sterilizer on and ensure that all instruments have been appropriately sterilized for aseptic survival surgery.

Manual of Research Techniques in Cardiovascular Medicine, First Edition. Edited by Hossein Ardehali, Roberto Bolli, and Douglas W. Losordo.

Table 19.1 Required surgical equipment

Fiber-optic surgical lamp
Dissecting microscope
Small animal ventilator
Thermostatic heating pad
Hair clippers
Surgical bead sterilizer
Surgical cauterizer

Table 19.2 Required surgical tools and supplies

2 10" lengths of 4-0 braided suture	Sterile field drapes
6-0 monofilament polypropylene suture (general suture)	Cotton-tipped swabs
8-0 monofilament polypropylene suture (ligation suture)	Surgical tape
1 22 G × 1″ i.v. catheter (chest tube)	Surgical board
2 Graefe forceps (FST 11051-10)	Topical antibiotic ointment
2 Halsted Mosquito Hemostat (FST 13009-12)	15 mg/mL Tribromoethanol
1 Fine scissors (FST 14090-09)	Buprenorphine
1 Superfine Vannas scissors (WPI 501778)	Meloxicam
2 S&T forceps (FST 00649-11)	Betadine
1 or 2 Microsuture holder with lock (Miltex 17-1020)	Sterile saline
i.v. intubation catheter 22 G × 1″	Nair
1 mL 25 G 5/8″ syringes	Alcohol wipes
1″ × 1″ gauze	Paper towels

2. Adult mice (ideally 8–10 weeks of age) are anesthetized with tribromoethanol (dose: 250 mg/kg of 15 mg/mL tribromoethanol stock) via a single intraperitoneal injection. Please keep in mind that significant age [6], sex [7,8], and strain [9,10] differences have been noted for the CAL procedure and that special attention should be placed on understanding how these variables will impact your study. Additionally, both body temperature and pH balance [11] have also been implicated in influencing

infarct size. Therefore, care should be taken to avoid fluctuations in these parameters.

3. After a standard toe pinch fails to elicit a response, the chest hair is removed with hair clippers. Any remaining hair is removed with the use of a depilatory, which is then washed away with warm water. Disinfect the skin area with Betadine and 70% ethanol.

4. Placed the mouse on a surgical board overlying a thermostatically controlled water heating pad. A looped suture thread secured to one end of the board is placed horizontally under the top teeth of the mouse to hold the upper jaw in place. Gently extract the tongue and lay it to one side of the mouth. Use a small absorbent tip to remove any oral secretions prior to intubation.

5. Visualize the trachea via transesophageal illumination. Intubate the mouse by inserting a 24G i.v. tube catheter into the trachea. Confirm proper intubation by visualizing synchronous chest movements once the catheter is connected to the ventilator. Fully immobilize the limbs and the intubation catheter using surgical tape (Figure 19.2), although avoid applying so much force as to cause unwanted constriction of the chest. The right hind and front legs are gently pulled downward while the left front leg is pulled upward, which will allow the ribs to be more easily separated.

6. Using Graefe forceps, lift the skin away from the chest and use small scissors to make a 1.0-cm incision in the skin perpendicular to the sternum directly overlying the 4th intercostal space. Perform a blunt dissection to separate the skin from the underlying muscle and fat. Any fat overlying the chest muscles can also be cut away.

7. Using S&T forceps, undermine and lift the pectoralis muscles (both the major and minor muscles) away from the ribs. Once isolated, they are then severed using small scissors. Place the free muscle ends under the skin flaps to prevent them from drying out.

Note. Surgical cauterization should be used to prevent bleeding, although sparingly, since excessive use will cause scarring that may influence the quality of postsurgical echocardiographic assessments.

8. Prior to opening the thoracic cavity, attach the ventilation tubing to the intubation catheter and

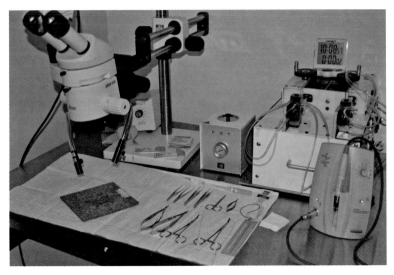

Figure 19.1 Depiction of a typical surgical station with the required equipment and surgical tools.

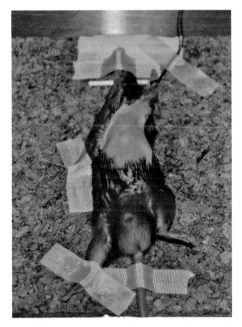

Figure 19.2 Optimal placement of the mouse on the surgical board.

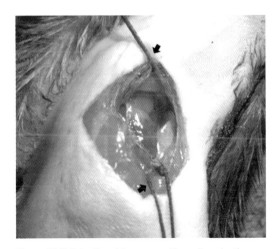

Figure 19.3 Retraction of the upper and lower ribs using the suture line retractors.

9. Using S&T forceps, grab and lift the 4th rib away from the underlying organs. Cut through the muscles of the 4th intercostal space using cauterization if necessary. Avoid cutting too close to the sternum to prevent damaging the nonvisible internal mammary artery. Cut the intercostal muscles laterally to create a 10–12-mm opening.

10. Use the braided suture retractors to retract both the 4th and 5th ribs to reveal a better view of the heart (Figure 19.3). Secure the retractor sutures to the surgical board with tape.

secure the connection to the surgical board with tape. Both ventilation rate and volume vary with mouse strain, gender, and age, although for adult 25-g male mice, 110 breaths/minute with a tidal volume of 0.5 mL is appropriate.

11. Using S&T forceps, rupture the pericardium being careful to avoid damaging any blood vessels encapsulated within it. A portion of the pericardium can be draped over the left lung to protect it from inadvertent trauma.

12. Using the left atrium as a landmark, locate the left anterior descending artery (LAD) where it runs down the anterior wall of the left ventricle. If

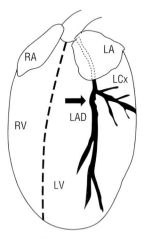

Figure 19.4 Drawing of the approximate location of the left anterior descending artery (LAD).

visualization is difficult, the left atrium can be lifted up to reveal the LAD branching off of the circumflex artery (Figure 19.4).

Note. The LAD is best visualized immediately after opening the thoracic cavity. The longer the heart is exposed to the cool room air, the harder the LAD will be to visualize.

Typically, the ligation site is ~2 mm below the left atrium. Using a needle holder, insert the 8-0 polyethylene suture needle into the heart, carefully undermine the LAD (see the white arrow in Figure 19.5A), and exit the surface of the heart on the other side of the LAD. Using a double surgeon's knot followed by two single knots in opposing directions, tighten the suture against the artery to permanently occlude blood flow distal to the ligation site. Refrain from over-tightening the knot and try to include as little cardiac tissue in your knot as possible.

Note. If an ischemia/reperfusion (I/R) injury is being induced, place a 3-mm long piece of PE10 tubing inside the suture knot prior to tightening. Tying the knot around the tubing causes temporary artery occlusion but allows for the subsequent removal of the ligation following an appropriate

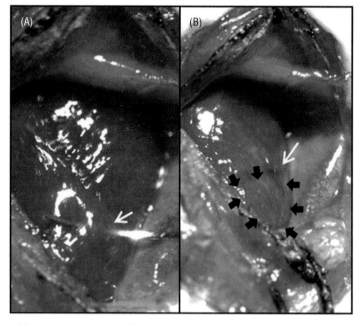

Figure 19.5 Placement of the suture needle under the left anterior descending artery. The white arrows indicate the LAD resting on top of the suture needle in (A) and the knotted suture following ligation in (B). The black arrows in panel B denote the epicardial blanching that occurs following ligation of the LAD.

ischemic period. Reperfusion of the ischemic area is achieved by removing the occluding suture and tubing from the heart.

13. After ligation, evaluate the cardiac tissue distal to the ligation point – clear blanching of the anterior wall epicardium should be visible (see area denoted by the black arrows in Figure 19.5B). Cut the suture as close to the knot as possible to avoid irritation of the surrounding tissue. If possible, drape the pericardium back over the heart.

14. Remove the rib retractors and then insert a chest tube into the thoracic cavity. Run the tube under the skin of the abdomen and then secondly under the chest muscle layers before entering the open thoracic cavity. The open end of the catheter tube should rest between the heart and the left lung (Figure 19.6). Ensure that the lungs are inflated and pink. Re-inflation can be promoted by temporarily occluding the exhalation tube on the ventilator, being extremely careful to avoid causing a pnuemothorax.

15. Using a single 6.0 suture knot, pull the 4th and 5th ribs back together. Ensure that the alignment of the ribs is anatomically correct since misalignment will compromise postsurgical breathing.

16. Re-attach the cut ends of the pectoralis major and minor muscles with a single 6.0 suture knot being careful to avoid over-tightening since the suture could tear the delicate muscles.

17. Using a running stitch, suture the outer skin, being sure to avoid over-tightening. The top and bottom skin flaps should re-meet at their original location.

18. Attach a 5-mL syringe to the chest tube needle hub. While drawing back on the syringe plunger (to re-establish negative pleural pressure), extract the tube from the chest. A small amount of fluid/blood may be sucked out of the chest cavity. Coat the skin incision with antibiotic ointment.

19. Remove the tape securing the mouse to the surgical board and carefully de-attach the intubation tubing from the intubation catheter. The animal should initiate independent breathing after a few seconds, at which point, subcutaneous administration of pain (i.e. 0.05 mg/kg buprenorphine) and anti-inflammatory medication (i.e. 1 mg/kg meloxicam) should be administered. With the intubation tube still in place, place the mouse on a thermostatically controlled heating pad. Once the mouse is breathing well, extubation can be performed. Upon recovering full mobility (usually within 1 hour), they can be returned to a clean cage and their normal housing conditions. Food pellets should be placed on the cage floor to prevent unneeded stretching of the incision site. Additional administration of anti-inflammatory medication should follow IACUC guidelines. Postoperative care also includes daily monitoring for the first week to verify adequate mobility, grooming, and eating habits.

20. Surgical instruments should be cleaned with 70% ethanol and re-sterilized in the bead sterilizer prior to the next surgery. The estimated time for this procedure, if performed by an experienced surgeon, should be between 15 and 20 minutes.

21. Postsurgical assessment of cardiac function and tissue harvesting should be completed using appropriate protocols and occur at time points based on the experimental goals.

Alternative approaches

Although we describe the use of tribromoethanol as the anesthetic agent, other options for achieving effective surgical plane anesthesia are available and include: (1) the inhaled anesthetics isoflurane, halothane, and sevoflurane; (2) ketamine/ xylazine compounds; and (3) sodium pentobarbital. Additionally, other postsurgical pharmacological

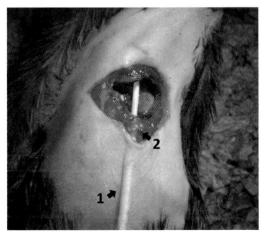

Figure 19.6 Proper insertion of the chest tube into the thoracic cavity.

options for analgesia control are also available. The common standard regimen includes buprenorphine for pain management combined with an NSAID anti-inflammatory such as meloxicam or carprofen. With these available options, the choice of the most appropriate anesthetic/ analgesic agents will require critical evaluation of your individual surgical procedure and must also fall in line with the IACUC recommendations at your institution.

Considering both the invasive nature of the ligation procedure and the current impossibility of performing intravascular coronary occlusion in the mouse, very few alternative methods are currently available. The coronary ligation model presented here remains a standard procedure for modeling acute myocardial infarction. As mentioned, it is possible to avoid permanent ligation of the artery by performing what is commonly referred to as the ischemia–reperfusion (I/R) model. Considering that manual revascularization of occluded coronary arteries is common practice in humans, the I/R model more closely reflects the current clinical situation.

Additionally, a newer method that performs CAL in a far shorter time period [12] than the conventional method was recently published. Although this alternative procedure is effective for evaluating the impact of CAL in genetic models, the absence of intubation and ventilation may limit the execution of additional surgical procedures such as the intracardiac administration of therapeutic agents. Lastly, another method has utilized a cryoinjury technique [13] to permanently occlude the LAD that produces similar functional deficits seen following CAL, although it does require some specialized cryoequipment.

Weaknesses and strengths of the method

A major weakness of the CAL model relates to the observed variability of the infarct size within treatment groups. Despite consistent surgical methodology, some of the variability in infarct size can be attributed to architectural differences in the coronary vasculatures between mice [14]. Aside from intragroup differences in infarct size, there are also differences in the abilities of various mouse strains to tolerate CAL. This fact can be seen more clearly in the observation of divergent mortality rates in genetically modified and

immunocompromised mice subjected to CAL as compared to control mice. In addition, published reports indicate that CAL in female mice will result in ~10% mortality while age-matched males can display upwards of 30% mortality at 4 weeks post-CAL [8]. A plethora of evidence has indicated that female sex hormones, such as estrogen, are cardioprotective [15] and this helps to explain the observed differences in mortality between gender. In wild-type C57 background mice, the occurrence of one to three deaths per ten mice subjected to CAL is generally accepted as a successful outcome.

Improvement of postsurgical survival in more sensitive strains (i.e. some gene knockout or immune-compromised mice) can necessitate the reduction of the infarct size. Although infarct sizes can be reduced by ligation of the LAD at lower branch points, it also inevitably increases infarct size variability within a study population independent of other study variables. These are factors that must be addressed if experiments involving CAL require use of these types of mice.

The major strength of this procedure lies in its clear relevance to the human condition by mimicking the pathological processes observed in human patients who have suffered an acute myocardial infarction (AMI). Additionally, the use of this small animal model allows for the rapid assessment of the long-term consequences of AMI in a relatively short period of time.

Conclusions

In conclusion, this highly effective and relatively simple surgical protocol has been used extensively to induce CAL in mice with reproducible results.

Acknowledgments
The authors would like to thank Masaaki Ii, MD, PhD, Department of Pharmacology, Faculty of Medicine, Osaka Medical College, Osaka, Japan and Haruki Sekiguchi MD, PhD, Cardiology, Aoyama Hospital, Tokyo Women's Medical University for lending their surgical expertise in Video 19.1.

References

1 Zaragoza C, Gomez-Guerrero C, Martin-Ventura JL, Blanco-Colio L, Lavin B, Mallavia B, *et al.* Animal Models

of Cardiovascular Diseases. *J Biomed Biotechnol* 2011; **2011**: 497841.

2 Virag JA, Lust RM. Coronary artery ligation and intramyocardial injection in a murine model of infarction. *J Vis Exp* 2011; (**52**). pii: 2581.

3 Borst O, Ochmann C, Schonberger T, Jacoby C, Stellos K, Seizer P, et al. Methods employed for induction and analysis of experimental myocardial infarction in mice. *Cell Physiol Biochem* 2011; **28**: 1–12.

4 Klocke R, Tian W, Kuhlmann MT, Nikol S. Surgical animal models of heart failure related to coronary heart disease. *Cardiovasc Res* 2007; **74**: 29–38.

5 Redel A, Jazbutyte V, Smul TM, Lange M, Eckle T, Eltzschig H, et al. Impact of ischemia and reperfusion times on myocardial infarct size in mice in vivo. *Exp Biol Med (Maywood)* 2008; **233**: 84–93.

6 Yang Y, Ma Y, Han W, Li J, Xiang Y, Liu F, et al. Age-related differences in postinfarct left ventricular rupture and remodeling. *Am J Physiol Heart Circ Physiol* 2008; **294**: H1815–1822.

7 Fang L, Gao XM, Moore XL, Kiriazis H, Su Y, Ming Z, et al. Differences in inflammation, MMP activation and collagen damage account for gender difference in murine cardiac rupture following myocardial infarction. *J Mol Cell Cardiol* 2007; **43**: 535–544.

8 Cavasin MA, Tao Z, Menon S, Yang XP. Gender differences in cardiac function during early remodeling after acute myocardial infarction in mice. *Life Sci* 2004; **75**: 2181–2192.

9 Gorog DA, Tanno M, Kabir AM, Kanaganayagam GS, Bassi R, Fisher SG, et al. Varying susceptibility to myocardial infarction among C57BL/6 mice of different genetic background. *J Mol Cell Cardiol* 2003; **35**: 705–708.

10 Gao XM, Ming Z, Su Y, Fang L, Kiriazis H, Xu Q, et al. Infarct size and post-infarct inflammation determine the risk of cardiac rupture in mice. *Int J Cardiol* 2010; **143**: 20–28.

11 Guo Y, Flaherty MP, Wu WJ, Tan W, Zhu X, Li Q, et al. Genetic background, gender, age, body temperature, and arterial blood pH have a major impact on myocardial infarct size in the mouse and need to be carefully measured and/or taken into account: results of a comprehensive analysis of determinants of infarct size in 1,074 mice. *Basic Res Cardiol* 2012; **107**: 288.

12 Gao E, Lei YH, Shang X, Huang ZM, Zuo L, Boucher M, et al. A novel and efficient model of coronary artery ligation and myocardial infarction in the mouse. *Circ Res* 2010; **107**: 1445–1453.

13 van den Bos EJ, Mees BM, de Waard MC, de Crom R, Duncker DJ. A novel model of cryoinjury-induced myocardial infarction in the mouse: a comparison with coronary artery ligation. *Am J Physiol Heart Circ Physiol* 2005; **289**: H1291 1300.

14 Salto-Tellez M, Yung Lim S, El-Oakley RM, Tang TP, ALmsherqi ZA, Lim SK, et al. Myocardial infarction in the C57BL/6J mouse: a quantifiable and highly reproducible experimental model. *Cardiovasc Pathol* 2004; **13**: 91–97.

15 Cavasin MA, Sankey SS, Yu AL, Menon S, Yang XP. Estrogen and testosterone have opposing effects on chronic cardiac remodeling and function in mice with myocardial infarction. *Am J Physiol Heart Circ Physiol* 2003; **284**: H1560–1569.

Transverse aortic constriction: a model to study heart failure in small animals

Suresh Kumar Verma, Prasanna Krishnamurthy, and Raj Kishore

Northwestern University Feinberg School of Medicine, Chicago, IL, USA

Introduction

Heart diseases are the major cause of death in United States and other developing and developed countries; therefore, understanding the mechanisms of these diseases will help in developing potential therapeutic drugs to treat these diseases. The cultured cells model is important to identify underlying mechanisms at the molecular level. However, for therapeutic applications, it is important to understand the complexity as well as mechanisms of these diseases in the animal model. Recently, mouse models that mimic human diseases have been developed as important tools for investigating underlying mechanisms in many disease states, including cardiovascular diseases [1]. It is now clear that very similar pathways regulate the development of the heart and vasculature in mice and humans [2]. Furthermore, the mouse genome has been extensively characterized and gene-targeted deletion (i.e. knockout) and transgenic overexpression experiments are more commonly performed using mice rather than rats and other large animals [3].

Aortic banding (constriction) is an established method to induce left ventricular hypertrophy in mice [4–6]. The condition develops from the elevated blood pressure in the left ventricular chamber and mimics similar syndromes in humans, which occur in aortic stenosis or as a consequence of chronic systemic hypertension. Depending on the experimental requirement, aortic constriction can be made at three different locations on the aorta: (1) ascending, (2) transverse, and (3) descending [1]. Aortic constriction has been used for many years to develop pressure-overload-induced hypertrophy in small mammals, such as rodents, thus allowing researchers to study the causes of congenital heart failure [2,4]. In this procedure, a constricting band is placed between the branches of the right and left carotid arteries (Figure 20.1). Aortic ligation is achieved by tying a 7-0 silk suture ligature around the aorta and an accompanying blunt needle, which acts as a spacer to determine the scope of the constriction. When the needle is pulled out from within the suture loop, only the aorta remains within the constricting band. The result is that the aorta may be narrowed, for example in mice the aorta is often constricted to about 0.4 mm in diameter, to produce a transverse aortic constriction (TAC) of 65–70% [2]. TAC initially (2 weeks) leads to compensated hypertrophy of the heart, which often is associated with a temporary enhancement of cardiac contractility. Over time, however, the response to the chronic hemodynamic overload becomes maladaptive, resulting in cardiac dilatation and heart failure (4–6 weeks). As compared to other experimental models of heart failure, TAC provides a more reproducible model of cardiac hypertrophy and a more gradual time course in the development of heart failure [2]. Researchers are usually exposed to brief descriptions of the procedures in scientific journals, which they then attempt to reproduce by

Manual of Research Techniques in Cardiovascular Medicine, First Edition. Edited by Hossein Ardehali, Roberto Bolli, and Douglas W. Losordo.

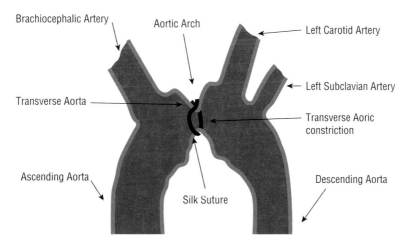

Figure 20.1 Location of aortic ligation during transverse aortic surgery. The constriction is made at the aortic arch with 7-0 silk suture under the guidance of a 27G needle to provide a 0.4-mm diameter passage.

trial and error. This often leads to a number of mistakes and unnecessary loss of animals. Therefore, in this chapter, we describe a step-by-step procedure to perform surgical TAC in mice.

Material

Mice. A number of recent reports show a significant correlation between development of hypertrophy and race or ethnic background, suggesting the presence of genetic modifiers conferring differential susceptibility to the pressure overload-induced left ventricular remodeling and hypertrophy [7,8]. In addition, because many studies use genetically engineered mouse models maintained on out-bred and mixed-bred backgrounds, genetic variability may contribute to observed phenotypic differences, including cardiac response to TAC [9]. In general, C57BL/6J and 129S1/svImJ (129S1) inbred strains are most widely used to generate genetically engineered mice but many studies are also done on B6 and 129S1 mixed background [10]. Since these two strains of mice have different baseline cardiac phenotype [11], it is likely divergent cardiac responses to chronic pressure overload in mixed background will occur [9]. It is also reported that the B6 mice are more susceptible to developing left ventricular abnormalities after pressure-overload compared to 129S1 and B6129F1 (F1) mice [9]. Overall, mice of any background can be used for this

surgery provided an appropriate control (for example, wild type littermates of the same genetic background if studying a gene knock-out model) is included.

Surgical procedures may be performed on transgenic, knock-out, and wild-type mice but extra precaution should be taken in immunosuppressive transgenic mice. Adult, male mice at 10–12 weeks of age are preferred because the developmental growth of the heart is complete at this time. The weight of mice could range between 25 and 28 g. Female mice can also be used, but are not preferred as many articles suggested that females are less susceptible for heart diseases.

Surgical tools. The following basic surgical tools are necessary during the operative procedure.

1. Curved forceps (Roboz, Cat. no. RS-5228) (the angle is slightly increased to 45%).
2. Slightly curved forceps (Roboz, Cat. no. RS-5136).
3. Foerster curved forceps (Roboz, Cat. no. RS-5101), curvature is increased to 90%.
4. Spring scissor with ball tip to prevent piercing of underlying tissues (FST, Cat. no. 15033-09).
5. Fine scissor to cut the skin (FST, Cat. no. 14090-09).
6. Blunt chest retractor (FST, Cat. no. 18200-10) with Elastomers (FST, Cat. no. 18200-07).
7. Needle holder (FST, Cat. no. 12060-02).

Occasionally some other tools are needed; these are described further in the text.

Sutures and needles (from Ethicon).

1. 6-0 Silk suture for the chest cavity and skin closure.
2. 4-0 Silk or absorbable suture for ribcage.
3. 7-0 Silk for aorta banding.

Respiratory support, heating systems.

1. Mouse volume-controlled ventilator 687 series (Harvard Apparatus).
2. Gaymar circulating water pump to maintain the animal body temperature in the physiological range during surgery.
3. A regular pharmacy heating pad at a low setting to maintain the body temperature at recovery.

Illumination. Power light with flexible horns.

Hair removal. Animal hair clipper to shave the chest.

Hot bead sterilizers. To sterilize tools between surgeries.

Procedure

Preparation of the operative field

The operation room must be controlled under negative pressure. Before surgery the operating area is disinfected with 70% ethyl alcohol. It is important to make sure that the heating pad is on and at the right temperature. A recommended system for operation is a small metallic procedure table equipped with temperature controller and heart rate recorder. Alternatively, a Gaymar circulating water pump connected to a therapy pad that is maintained at 37°C ± 1°C can be used. It is important to maintain normal body temperature during surgery to avoid a rapid decrease in heart rate. Preautoclaved surgical tools are sterilized in a hot bead sterilizer before and during the surgical procedure. Rinse the tools with autoclaved saline during the surgery. It is always advisable to have autoclaved sterile cotton applicators in case of bleeding.

Anesthesia, intubation, and ventilation

Since the surgical procedure is relatively short, it is not necessary to withhold food and water from mice

Table 20.1 Different settings of tidal volume and breath rates on Harward mini ventilator

Animal's weight (grams)	Tidal volume (μL)	Breath rate (per minutes)
21	120	146
22	130	145
23	140	143
24	140	141
25	150	140
26	160	138
27	160	137
28	170	136
29	170	135
30	180	133
31	190	132
32	190	131
33	200	130
34	200	129
35	210	128

prior to surgery. Pentobarbital sodium at 70 mg/kg (intraperitoneal, i.p.) is the anesthetic of choice because it provides an adequate depth of anesthesia for 30–40 minutes. Alternatively, 2% isoflurane mixed with 100% O_2 (0.5–1.0 L/min) may also be used to anesthetized mice. Shave the chest from the neck with the hair clipper.

Position the animal on the surgical stage for the subsequent intubation, thread 3-0 silk behind the front incisors, pull taut, and fix with tape. Using curved forceps in one hand, the tongue is gently manipulated to the side. With the other hand, endotracheal intubation is performed using a 20 G catheter, attached to the extender. The endotracheal tube is then connected to a Harvard volume-cycled rodent ventilator, cycling at 125–150 breaths/minute and a tidal volume of 0.1–0.3 mL (depends on the weight of the mouse, Table 20.1). During the surgical procedure, anesthesia is maintained at 1.5–2% isoflurane with 0.5–1.0 L/min 100% O_2. The correct level of anesthesia is verified by applying pressure on the mouse nail bed (toe-pinch reflex). The surgical field is disinfected with 70% alcohol. To prevent contamination of the surgical field during the operation, a sterile drape is placed over the mouse leaving only the operation field exposed. As narcotic analgesic (such as buprenorphine) reduces the animals respiratory rate, it is not recommended to administer analgesic dose before the surgery [2].

Aortic banding (constriction of transverse aorta)

A small midline skin cut is made just above the sternum of the mice and muscles are gently separated until trachea is visible. Partial left-side thoracotomy to the second rib is performed with blunt-ended spring scissors and the sternum should be retracted using a chest retractor. Blunt-tip 45° angled forceps are used to gently separate the two lobes of thymus and to clean fat tissue from the aortic arch. The tracheal tube may be used as a landmark to track the aortic arch. With blunted curved forceps, create a passageway underneath the aortic arch (just above the trachea). Following the creation of a clear passageway, a small piece of a 7-0 silk suture (presoaked in sterile saline) is placed between the innominate and left carotid arteries (Figure 20.1) using a 90° curved forceps. Two loose knots are tied around the transverse aorta and a small piece of a 27 G blunt needle placed parallel to the transverse aorta. The first knot is quickly tied against the needle, followed by the second and the needle promptly removed in order to yield a constriction of 0.4 mm in diameter [12]. During this procedure there is a prominent increase in blood flow in the right carotid artery. The chest retractor is removed and all the tissues, including thymus, are placed in their original position. The ribcage is closed using a 4-0 silk/ absorbable suture with a single interrupted suture. The skin is closed using a 6-0 prolene suture with a continuous suture pattern. To avoid infection at suture sites, Betadine solution should be applied.

Postoperative care

Postoperative care for most of the cardiac surgeries is fairly universal. The measures taken are directed to alleviate pain, provide supplementary heat to prevent hypothermia, control respiratory depression, and sometimes a dose of saline to compensate water loss. Administer the first dose of analgesic, Buprenex 0.1 mg/kg (Reckitt Benckiser Healthcare (UK) Ltd.), intraperitoneally immediately at the completion of the surgery. Move the mice to another ventilator in a designated recovery area with 100% oxygen loosely connected to its inflow. Keep the mouse on a heating pad until it fully recovers. Once the mouse makes an attempt to breathe spontaneously (normally after 15–20 minutes), disconnect the intubation tube from the ventilator. Keep the intubation tube in the trachea for another 10–15 minutes until the mouse resumes a normal breathing pattern. Give the mouse supplementary oxygen (the mouse is placed next to the source of oxygen).

Notes

• The tidal volume and ventilation rate are calculated using formulas provided by the manufacturer of the ventilator:

$$\text{Tidal volume} = 0.0062 \times (\text{animal weight in grams})^{1.01}$$

$$\text{Ventilation rate (min}^{-1}) = 53.5 \times (\text{animal's mass})^{-0.26}$$

Details of tidal volumes and rates for particular body weights are shown in Table 20.1.

• Inappropriate ventilation is one of the major causes of surgical loss during TAC surgery. After intubation the operator/ surgeon should visually confirm rhythmic movements of the chest synchronized to the ventilator. Always try to avoid excessive dead space in ventilation tubes.

• Animals should be securely taped to the surgical platform. Small movements might damage the trachea of mice.

• In incidence of any bleeding, use of sterile cotton applicators with low pressure should reduce the blood loss.

• Extra care should be taken during thoracotomy. The internal thoracic artery is invisible and small mistakes will cause excessive bleeding and loss of animals.

• An important control for aortic banding is sham surgery. During sham surgery all the steps are same except making a ligature.

• Analgesia (buprenorphine) should be continued every 24 hours for the next 48 hours.

Limitations

A limitation of this particular example of a constriction protocol is that it causes a breach of the pleural space and necessitates mechanical ventilation of the mammal. The use of mechanical ventilation requires additional time, expertise, and equipment.

Moreover, inflammatory reactions within the chest may complicate the analyses of cardiac function and pathology.

Confirmation of constriction

The best approach used to confirm the ligation is to monitor blood flow rates in right and left carotid arteries using a computer-based Doppler signal processor (Indus instrument, Houston Texas). For a perfect TAC, the flow ratio of right and left carotid arteries should be about 1:6 to 1:8. But if constriction is tighter this ratio may be over 1:8 [12,13]. An alternate approach via a echocardiography technique can also be used to confirm the position of the suture. It is important to get a visual presence of the suture on the aorta at the end of study during removal of the heart.

Expected outcomes

For an accurate result of aortic constriction, it is important to have a consistent constriction between animals and during the course of a study as well. To validate the response of aortic constriction, it is important to measure cardiac functions in these animals before surgery (baseline) and 7, 14, 21, and 28 days after surgery. During early phase of stress, the heart tries to compensate the excessive pressure by increasing in size, which is known as adaptive hypertrophy. During the adaptive hypertrophic phase, heart function is normal but its wall becomes thicker and the size increases. The length of the compensatory phase is usually 2–3 weeks after surgery. The compensatory phase slowly proceeds to the remodeling of the heart and ultimately leads to heart failure. The failure phase usually occurs from the 4th to 6th week after surgery, depending on the tightness of the constriction. During the failure phase, the ventricular functions are severely worsened, which can be measured by echocardiography. The left ventricle (LV) becomes dilated, and LV mass is also significantly increased. As we mentioned earlier, remodeling starts from 3–4 weeks after surgery, accompanied by substantial fibrosis, visualized easily in post-mortem heart sections. Recently, a new MRI-based technique, called diffusion spectrum magnetic resonance imaging (DSI) tractography, has been used to determine myoarchitectural disarray in models of cardiomyopathy. This technique gives details of myofilament expression, cardiac fiber alignment, and torsional rotation in the setting of congenital hypertrophic cardiomyopathy [14].

Alternative approaches

Chemical infusion methods can also be used to induce cardiac hypertrophy and associated heart failure in small animals. The chemicals most commonly use to induce hypertension-induced hypertrophy and heart failure include endothelin, isoproterenol and angiotensin II. These chemicals can be delivered using miniosmotic pumps that are available with various specifications to deliver at constant rate in small animals. However, due to their indirect and off target effects, recently very few investigators like to use this method. In addition, complete occlusion of the left anterior descending (LAD) coronary artery can also be used to induce heart failure in small animals. Please see chapter 19 for details.

Weaknesses and strengths of the method

Although TAC is most acceptable method available till date to induce left ventricular hypertrophy and associated heart failure, it has conceptual and methodological limitations. The major limitation is the consistency and extent of constriction on the aorta using suture materials. A small difference between animals will show major differences on disease outcome. The strain and sex differences are another issue with this surgery. Some strains are more susceptible for aortic constriction however some are less. Because of this issue use of mixed background animals might complicate the outcome. Therefore selection of appropriate strain is also important during the experiment. Overall, compared to other available experimental models of heart failure, such as LAD coronary artery ligation and chemical-induced hypertrophy models, TAC provides a more reproducible method to induce cardiac hypertrophy and allows gradual development of heart failure without any off target effects.

Conclusions

Use of *in vitro* cell model is an invaluable tool for studying cardiac function, regulation, and pathology at the autonomous cellular level. Although, these cells are widely used to study the electrophysiology, intracellular calcium fluxes, immunohistochemistry, contractile mechanics, etc., the presence of different kinds of signaling network in the organ system limit the use of *in vitro* system at the translational level; therefore, animal models have been actively used as a cutting-edge technique in recent years. TAC, which mimics human aortic stenosis, is a common method to induce cardiac hypertrophy and heart failure in mice. Alternative sites for aortic constriction include the ascending and abdominal aorta. Transverse aortic constriction is the preferred model to induced hypertrophy and heart failure in mice as this provides a moderate pressure overload on left ventricle as compare to other two aortic constriction models, that is ascending aortic constriction (which provides an extreme and more rapid overload) and abdominal aortic constriction (which does not provide extreme overload) [1]. Although this procedure can be technically challenging, with practice we have achieved a survival rate of 75–80% in wild-type mice. The age of mice as well as tightness of the transverse aortic constriction determines the degree of hypertrophy development and the time-frame in which cardiac failure and dilatation develops. Older mice (>12 months of age) take longer to develop an adaptive response of the carotid arteries to TAC, and are likely to develop dilated cardiomyopathy faster than younger mice (3–4 months of age). Use of less than 2-month-old mice are not advisable as they are still in their growth stage [12,13].

References

1 Tarnavski O, McMullen JR, Schinke M, Nie Q, Kong S, Izumo S, *et al.* Mouse cardiac surgery: Comprehensive techniques for the generation of mouse models of human diseases and their application for genomic studies. *Physiol Genomics* 2004; **16**: 349–360.

2 Tarnavski O. Mouse surgical models in cardiovascular research. *Methods Mol Biol* 2009; **573**: 115–137.

3 Lin MC, Rockman HA, Chien KR. Heart and lung disease in engineered mice. *Nat Med* 1995; **1**: 749–751.

4 Rockman HA, Ross RS, Harris AN, Knowlton KU, Steinhelper ME, Field LJ, *et al.* Segregation of atrial-specific and inducible expression of an atrial natriuretic factor transgene in an in vivo murine model of cardiac hypertrophy. *Proc Nat Acad Sci USA* 1991; **88**: 8277–8281.

5 Ding B, Price RL, Borg TK, Weinberg EO, Halloran PF, Lorell BH, *et al.* Pressure overload induces severe hypertrophy in mice treated with cyclosporine, an inhibitor of calcineurin. *Circ Res* 1999; **84**: 729–734.

6 van Berlo JH, Elrod JW, Aronow BJ, Pu WT, Molkentin JD. Serine 105 phosphorylation of transcription factor gata4 is necessary for stress-induced cardiac hypertrophy in vivo. *Proc Nat Acad Sci USA* 2011; **108**: 12331–12336.

7 Cooper-DeHoff RM, Handberg EM, Cohen J, Kowey P, Messerli FH, Mancia G, *et al.* Characteristics of contemporary patients with hypertension and coronary artery disease. *Clin Cardiol* 2004; **27**: 571–576.

8 Okin PM, Kjeldsen SE, Dahlof B, Devereux RB. Racial differences in incident heart failure during antihypertensive therapy. *Circ Cardiovasc Qual Outcomes* 2011; **4**: 157–164.

9 Barrick CJ, Rojas M, Schoonhoven R, Smyth SS, Threadgill DW. Cardiac response to pressure overload in 129s1/svimj and c57bl/6j mice: Temporal- and background-dependent development of concentric left ventricular hypertrophy. *Am J Physiol Heart Circ Physiol* 2007; **292**: H2119–2130.

10 Auerbach W, Dunmore JH, Fairchild-Huntress V, Fang Q, Auerbach AB, Huszar D, *et al.* Establishment and chimera analysis of 129/svev- and c57bl/6-derived mouse embryonic stem cell lines. *BioTechniques* 2000; **29**: 1024–1028, 1030, 1032.

11 Deschepper CF, Olson JL, Otis M, Gallo-Payet N. Characterization of blood pressure and morphological traits in cardiovascular-related organs in 13 different inbred mouse strains. *J Appl Physiol* 2004; **97**: 369–376.

12 deAlmeida AC, van Oort RJ, Wehrens XH. Transverse aortic constriction in mice. *J Vis Exp* 2010; (**38**). pii: 1729.

13 Li YH, Reddy AK, Ochoa LN, Pham TT, Hartley CJ, Michael LH, *et al.* Effect of age on peripheral vascular response to transverse aortic banding in mice. *J Gerontol A Biol Sci Med Sci* 2003; **58**: B895–899.

14 Wang TT, Kwon HS, Dai G, Wang R, Mijailovich SM, Moss RL, *et al.* Resolving myoarchitectural disarray in the mouse ventricular wall with diffusion spectrum magnetic resonance imaging. *Ann Biom Eng* 2010; **38**: 2841–2850.

21 Pharmacological models of hypertrophy and failure

Angela C. deAlmeida, Tariq Hamid, and Sumanth D. Prabhu

University of Alabama at Birmingham, Birmingham, AL, USA

Overview

The pathogenesis of heart failure (HF) is complex, involving multiple pathophysiological responses following an index injury, such as mechanical stress, neurohormonal activation, hemodynamic alterations, and left ventricular dysfunction and dilatation [1,2]. Animal models of HF have been invaluable for understanding the underlying mechanisms and developing new therapeutic strategies [2–4]. Large and small animal HF models are primarily generated using surgical or electrophysiological techniques to induce myocardial infarction, augment hemodynamic load (pressure and/or volume overload), or produce sustained tachycardia in an effort to mimic human disease [2–4]. While these models lend invaluable insights regarding integrated pathophysiological mechanisms, if specific causal connections are being isolated, alternative models may be required. Moreover, the surgical route may be particularly challenging in view of the technical skill level required and the mortality rates associated with the invasive procedure.

Pharmacological models of left ventricular (LV) hypertrophy and/or dysfunction are less complex to generate and can be used to isolate causal connections related to the activation of specific neurohumoral pathways (or the effects of specific cardiotoxins), and complement the information derived from surgical models. The availability of a variety of pharmacological agents, together with advances in osmotic drug delivery systems, have facilitated opportunities to study hypertrophy and HF in a less invasive and more reproducible fashion that recapitulates key mechanistic events in human disease.

Osmotic minipumps (currently manufactured by Alzet®, DURECT Corp.) were developed in the 1970s and have been used in laboratory animals to deliver a wide variety of compounds (Figure 21.1) [5–8]. These pumps are governed by osmotic displacement – the osmotic pressure differential between tissue interstitial fluid and the hyperosmotic outer layer of the pump forces preloaded solution out of the central pump reservoir at a constant rate, thereby delivering drugs in a controlled and steady-state manner. The pumps may be implanted subcutaneously or intraperitoneally for systemic drug administration, or attached to a catheter for targeted drug delivery to a tissue or organ. Alternative delivery approaches include direct injection (via the intraperitoneal or subcutaneous routes) and the more recently developed implantable microelectromechanical systems (MEMS) [9]. Although osmotic pumps and bolus injection are most often employed experimentally, newer MEMS approaches have been suggested to offer more tissue-selective and targeted drug delivery.

The administration of isoproterenol and angiotensin II, either via osmotic minipumps or direct injection, are particularly well-established

Manual of Research Techniques in Cardiovascular Medicine, First Edition. Edited by Hossein Ardehali, Roberto Bolli, and Douglas W. Losordo.
© 2014 John Wiley & Sons, Ltd. Published 2014 by John Wiley & Sons, Ltd.

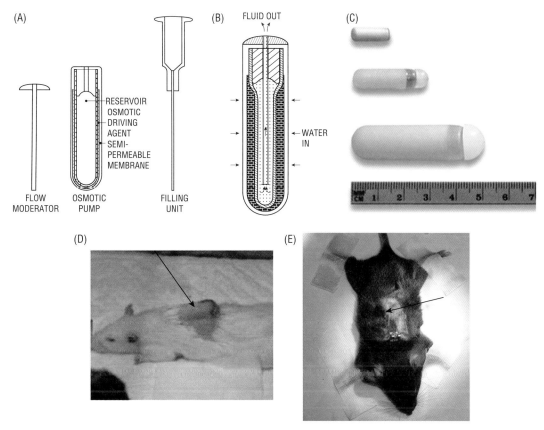

Figure 21.1 Osmotic minipumps as a mode of drug delivery. (A) The components of the miniaturized osmotic pump include the flow moderator, the cylindrical pump comprised of an impermeable collapsible reservoir surrounded by a hyperosmotic layer under a semipermeable membrane cover. The reservoir is filled with solution using the filling unit and syringe. (B) Schematic of a fully assembled and filled pump that, when placed in the body, draws water to the hyperosmotic layer impinging the reservoir and thereby pumping fluid out of the flow moderator at a controlled rate. (C) Physical sizes for assembled 100, 200, and 2000-μL reservoir Alzet® osmotic minipumps. (D) 100-μL pump freshly implanted subcutaneously between the scapulae (arrow) in a mouse. (E) Well-healed 100-μL pump implant (arrow) in a mouse 7 days after surgery. (Source: (A and B) Theeuwes F 1976 [6]. Reproduced with permission from Springer. (C) www.alzet.com with permission from DURECT Corporation).

pharmacological models of cardiac dysfunction (Table 21.1). The cardiac phenotypes induced upon administration of the beta-adrenergic receptor agonist isoproterenol is both dose and duration dependent, and range from cardiac hypertrophy and fibrosis without systolic dysfunction at lower cumulative doses (in mice and rats 0.3–3 mg/kg/day for 1 week) [10–12], cardiac hypertrophy with mild to moderate systolic dysfunction at intermediate doses (e.g. 9–15 mg/kg/day for 1 week) [13,14], to severe ventricular dilatation and dysfunction at higher doses (e.g. 30 mg/kg/day for 4–8 weeks) [15]. Direct isoproterenol injection also carries dose- and time-dependent effects. In rats, 2 weeks after two subcutaneous doses of isoproterenol, rats receiving >170 mg/kg exhibited significant ventricular dilatation and dysfunction, whereas rats receiving lower doses did not [16].

The octapeptide vasopressor, angiotensin II, plays a central role in mediating the progression of pathological remodeling in HF [1]. Continuous infusion of angiotensin II via osmotic minipumps (or intermittent serial bolus injection) in rodents can induce cardiac hypertrophy, dysfunction, oxidative stress, and fibrosis in as little as 1–2 weeks over a range of doses, including low doses that do

Table 21.1 Neurohumoral models of cardiac hypertrophy and failure in rodents

Agent	Delivery mode	Dose	Phenotype	Animal [references]
Isoproterenol	Osmotic pump	0.3–3 mg/kg/day × 7 days	Cardiac hypertrophy, fibrosis, oxidative stress	mice [10], rats [11,12]
		8.7–15 mg/kg/day × 7 days	Above with mild to moderate systolic ventricular dysfunction	mice [13,14]
		30 mg/kg/day × >4 weeks	Above with severe ventricular dilatation and systolic dysfunction	mice [15]
	sc injection	170–340 mg/kg/day × 2 days	Severe ventricular dilatation and dysfunction after 2 weeks	rats [16]
Angiotensin II	Osmotic pump	0.1–0.3 mg/kg/day × 2 weeks	Cardiac hypertrophy, systolic dysfunction, oxidative stress, and fibrosis without significant blood pressure elevation	mice [17,18], rats [19]
		≥ 0.4 mg/kg/day × 1–2 weeks	Cardiac hypertrophy and dysfunction as above with blood pressure elevation	mice [13], rats [19,21]
	sc injection	0.5 mg/kg sc every 2 day for 2 weeks	Remote cardiac hypertrophy and fibrosis observed months after angiotensin II	mice [20]
Phenylephrine	Osmotic pump	75 mg/kg/day × 2 weeks	Cardiac hypertrophy with systemic hypertension	mice [13]

not raise blood pressure (e.g. 0.1–0.3 mg/kg/day pump infusion or 0.5 mg/kg/day s.c. every 2 days for 2 weeks) [17–20], and higher doses (>0.4 mg/kg/day infusion for 1–2 weeks) that will also raise blood pressure (Table 21.1) [13,19,21]. Late detrimental effects in the heart (hypertrophy, systolic dysfunction, fibrosis) are also observed at remote time points after angiotensin II administration in the absence of residual vasopressor effects [20]. In lieu of angiotensin II, continuous infusion of the α-adrenergic receptor agonist phenylephrine (e.g. 75 mg/kg/day) can also be used to induce both hypertension and cardiac hypertrophy [13]. The dose chosen and whether elevation in blood pressure is a desirable or confounding variable will necessarily depend on the particular study design and objectives. Taken together, pharmacological models of hypertrophy and heart failure by continuous drug infusion offer a powerful tool to investigate underlying mechanisms in HF progression and test novel therapies related to specific neurohumoral pathways.

As alluded to previously, surgical models commonly used to produce hypertrophy and/or HF include nonreperfused or reperfused myocardial infarction (to induce postinfarction remodeling) and transverse (or ascending) aortic banding (to induce pressure overload). As compared with pharmacological models, surgical models usually induce integrated and often severe cardiac phenotypes that are analogous to similar pathologies seen in humans. With sufficient time following the surgical intervention, significant myocyte/ chamber hypertrophy, fibrosis, cell loss, chamber dilatation, and mechanical dysfunction are evident. In contrast, pharmacological approaches offer a more graded or "tunable" response in the heart, ranging from mild to severe and fulminant, that is directly dependent on the drug type, drug dose, and duration of exposure. Indeed, pharmacological models can be controlled to exhibit tissue-level pathological responses in the heart (e.g. fibrosis, myocyte hypertrophy, oxidant stress) in the absence of (or disconnected from) marked systolic dysfunction at the chamber level (Table 21.1). Such distinctions in cardiac responses need to be carefully considered by the investigator when formulating the experimental design.

Protocols

Preparation and surgical implantation of osmotic minipumps in mice and rats. The animal size, agent to be delivered, as well as delivery duration and volume should be carefully considered when choosing the appropriate pump model. Aseptic technique should be used when filling, priming, and performing surgical implantation of osmotic minipumps. Freely available DURECT (ALZET®) corporate resources (www.alzet.com) provide useful information regarding minipump selection, experimental protocols, and citations of osmotic minipump usage. Depending on the fill volume and mean pumping rate of the specific pump model, pharmacological agents can be delivered continuously for durations ranging from 1 day to 6 weeks with a single minipump. Longer durations can be accomplished by serial pump implantation. As a general guide, the following steps should be followed for osmotic pump delivery in rodents.

Filling pumps. It is important to completely fill each pump and to avoid introducing bubbles into the pump reservoir as this could result in pumping rate fluctuations.

1. Filter the solution to be delivered into a sterile tube, using a syringe and a 0.22-μm syringe-filter.
2. Draw the solution into a 1.0-mL syringe and attach the blunt-tipped, 27-gauge filling tube provided with the pump.
3. Hold the pump in an upright position and place the filling tube inside the pump. Slowly load the filter-sterilized solution into the pump, taking care not to introduce bubbles.
4. Insert the flow moderator until the rim is flush with the top of the pump and wipe off the excess solution.

Priming pumps. This step is imperative when the study requires immediate pumping, a catheter is attached to the pump, or a viscous solution is being administered.

1. Immerse the prefilled pumps in 0.9% saline for 4–6 hours at 37°C before implantation (overnight is preferable if time permits).
2. Remove the pumps from saline and promptly implant.

Subcutaneous implantation. This is the least-invasive implantation procedure and is more often used in mice. The pump is generally placed on the back of the mouse between the scapulae (Figure 21.1) [10].

1. Sterilize the surgical instruments in a glass bead sterilizer heated to 250°C and sanitize the surgical area with 70% ethanol. Repeat this procedure three times.
2. Anesthetize the mouse in an induction chamber with 2% isoflurane mixed with 0.5–1.0 L/min 100% O₂.
3. Use hair clippers to shave the back of the mouse near the scapulae.
4. Place the mouse in the prone position and disinfect the skin at the surgical site with Betadine solution followed by 70% ethanol. Cover the mouse with a sterile drape.
5. Make a 1-cm skin incision in the dorsal neck region perpendicular to the tail.
6. Create a pocket by using blunt-tipped scissors to separate subcutaneous tissue from the skin atraumatically.
7. Insert the minipump into the pocket, with the flow moderator side first, and pinch the skin to position the pump toward the lower back.
8. Close the skin incision with 5-0 prolene sutures. Sterile wound clips may also be used to close the incision.
9. Administer buprenorphine (0.1–2.5 mg/kg s.c.) for pain relief.
10. Allow the mouse to recover in a separate cage atop a heating pad.

Intraperitoneal implantation. This procedure, which is more common in rats, is more invasive than s.c. implantation but generally well tolerated [12]. Due to greater invasiveness, the animal will require a minimum postoperative recovery period of 48 hours prior to further manipulation.

1. Sterilize the surgical instruments in a glass bead sterilizer heated to 250°C and sanitize the surgical area with 70% ethanol. Repeat this procedure three times.
2. Anesthetize the rat in an induction chamber with 3% isoflurane mixed with 0.5–1.0 L/min 100% O_2.
3. Use hair clippers to shave the abdominal area.
4. Place the rat in the supine position and disinfect the skin at the surgical site with Betadine solution followed by 70% ethanol. Repeat this procedure three times. Apply an appropriate-size sterile drape to the surgical field.
5. Make a small, vertical midline incision in the skin overlying the lower abdomen.
6. Make a second vertical midline incision in the abdominal muscle (proceed with caution here as to not puncture the bowel).
7. Insert the minipump into the peritoneal cavity, with the flow modulator side first.
8. Use continuous 5-0 absorbable sutures to close the abdominal muscle.
9. Close the skin incision using 5-0 prolene sutures or sterile wound clips.
10. Administer buprenorphine (0.1–2.5 mg/kg s.c.) for pain relief.
11. Allow the rat to recover in a separate cage atop a heating pad.

Explantation procedure. Pumps should be removed promptly after their "expiration" and may not be reused. However, if longer drug infusion time is needed, minipumps can be serially implanted.

1. Sterilize surgical tools and sanitize the surgical area as described earlier.
2. Anesthetize the animal and prepare, disinfect, and aseptically isolate the surgical site accordingly.
3. Make a small incision at the implantation site and remove the spent pump while maintaining aseptic technique. Use forceps if necessary to tease away the surrounding connective tissue.
4. Close the incision with either 5-0 prolene sutures or sterile wound clips.
5. Allow the animal to recover in a separate cage atop a heating pad.

Postoperative care and troubleshooting.

1. Continuously monitor animals for the first 2 hours, and then daily for the subsequent 7 days.
2. If signs of redness occur, continue to monitor closely for necrosis, ulceration, or infection.
3. Carefully inspect the incision site for signs of dehiscence. If an incision requires additional sutures or wound clips, or if a pump seems to be placing pressure on the skin, perform the necessary corrections immediately.
4. If an animal does not properly recover from any of the aforementioned adverse effects, it may be necessary to exclude the animal from the study due to possible confounding factors as well as animal distress.
5. Remove sutures or wound clips 14 days postoperatively.

Alternative approaches

As alluded to previously, bolus injections offer an alternative to osmotic pump infusion and have been used in several studies for the pharmacological agents discussed earlier [16,20]. This method is particularly advantageous when investigating rapidly occurring *in vivo* processes or when a single dose is required. Furthermore, direct injection is technically simple, relatively inexpensive, and does not require a surgical procedure. In contrast, disadvantages relate to the lack of precise control of the rate and pattern of absorption, and drug concentration at the target site; this may lead to higher long-term costs due to the need for additional drugs and animals [7,8]. Also, repeated animal handling is required for serial injections, which may increase stress levels and skew results. Intracoronary and intravenous injection of the cardiotoxic antineoplastic drug doxorubicin has been used to induce HF (toxic cardiomyopathy) in a variety of animal species, including rodents, dogs, sheep, and cows, but can be expensive owing to repeated injections and limited by variable LV dysfunction and drug-related systemic toxicity [2,4,22]. A recent study used serial administration of doxorubicin in cows to induce a HF model that could be used to study the effects of LV assist devices [22]. Similarly, intravenous injection of imipramine (7.5 mg/kg), an antidepressant medication known to impair cardiac function, has been used to create a model of short-term reversible HF in canines [23]. Although these toxic models have inherent limitations, they nonetheless may be useful to evaluate specific cardiac interventions and pathologies.

Strengths and weaknesses of the method

The strength of the osmotic minipump infusion model rests on its level of fine control, relative nonintrusive nature, and continuous drug delivery. Osmotic minipumps are particularly well suited for administering agents with a short half-life [24]. There are various sizes of pumps available with a wide range of delivery duration and flow rates, and if longer infusion time is needed, pumps may be sequentially implanted without adverse effects. Additionally, simultaneous manipulations can be performed on the animal without affecting the dose of the infused drug. Finally, the osmotic minipump infusion model is cost-effective, particularly when the benefits from relative low animal stress, due to decreased handling, and high reproducibility of the delivery regimens, are considered.

Although the advantages of miniaturized osmotic pumps are considerable, several limitations should also be considered. For example, some drugs are too labile to be delivered by a pump. Moreover, although osmotic minipump implantation is relatively simple, surgical complications can occur. Hence, as previously mentioned, particular care must be taken when implanting the pump and choosing the suture material to avoid outcomes such as infection and tissue necrosis, which can produce pain and discomfort to the animal and variability in the experimental data.

Conclusions

Pharmacological models of cardiac hypertrophy and HF, particularly those that utilize continuous drug infusion via osmotic minipumps, provide a valuable research tool and have played a major role in furthering our understanding of underlying pathophysiological mechanisms. Continuous drug infusion is being increasingly utilized in a broad range of research fields and advances in drug delivery systems are ongoing. Hence, used alone or in combination with surgical approaches to recapitulate the complexities of human disease, the use of pharmacological models is expected to become increasingly prevalent in preclinical studies.

References

1 Jessup M, Brozena S. Heart failure. *New Engl J Med*. 2003; **348**: 2007–2018.

2 Houser SR, Margulies KB, Murphy AM, Spinale FG, Francis GS, Prabhu SD, *et al*. Animal models of heart failure: A scientific statement from the American Heart Association. *Circ Res* 2012; **111**: 131–150.

3 Patten RD, Hall-Porter MR. Small animal models of heart failure: Development of novel therapies, past and present. *Circ Heart Fail* 2009; **2**: 138–144.

4 Hasenfuss G. Animal models of human cardiovascular disease, heart failure and hypertrophy. *Cardiovasc Res* 1998; **39**: 60–76.

5 Amsden BG. Delivery approaches for angiogenic growth factors in the treatment of ischemic conditions. *Expert Opin Drug Deliv* 2011; **8**: 873–890.

6 Theeuwes F, Yum SI. Principles of the design and operation of generic osmotic pumps for the delivery of semisolid or liquid drug formulations. *Ann Biomed Eng* 1976; **4**: 343–353.

7 Herrlich S, Spieth S, Messner S, Zengerle R. Osmotic micropumps for drug delivery. *Adv Drug Deliv Rev* 2012; **64**: 1617–1627.

8 Verma RK, Arora S, Garg S. Osmotic pumps in drug delivery. *Crit Rev Ther Drug Carrier Syst* 2004; **21**: 477–520.

9 Meng E, Li PY, Lo R, Sheybani R, Gutierrez C. Implantable MEMS drug delivery pumps for small animal research. *Conf Proc IEEE Eng Med Biol Soc* 2009; **2009**: 6696–6698.

10 Garlie JB, Hamid T, Gu Y, Ismahil MA, Chandrasekar B, Prabhu SD, *et al*. Tumor necrosis factor receptor 2 signaling limits beta-adrenergic receptor-mediated cardiac hypertrophy in vivo. *Basic Res Cardiol* 2011; **106**: 1193–1205.

11 Murray DR, Prabhu SD, Chandrasekar B. Chronic beta-adrenergic stimulation induces myocardial proinflammatory cytokine expression. *Circulation* 2000; **101**: 2338–2341.

12 Srivastava S, Chandrasekar B, Gu Y, Luo J, Hamid T, Hill BG, *et al*. Downregulation of CuZn-superoxide dismutase contributes to beta-adrenergic receptor-mediated oxidative stress in the heart. *Cardiovasc Res* 2007; **74**: 445–455.

13 Sundaresan NR, Gupta M, Kim G, Rajamohan SB, Isbatan A, Gupta MP, *et al*. Sirt3 blocks the cardiac hypertrophic response by augmenting Foxo3a-dependent antioxidant defense mechanisms in mice. *J Clin Invest* 2009; **119**: 2758–2771.

14 Oudit GY, Crackower MA, Eriksson U, Sarao R, Kozieradzki I, Sasaki T, *et al*. Phosphoinositide 3-kinase gamma-deficient mice are protected from isoproterenol-induced heart failure. *Circulation* 2003; **108**: 2147–2152.

15 Shan J, Kushnir A, Betzenhauser MJ, Reiken S, Li J, Lehnart SE, *et al*. Phosphorylation of the ryanodine receptor mediates the cardiac fight or flight response in mice. *J Clin Invest* 2010; **120**: 4388–4398.

16 Teerlink JR, Pfeffer JM, Pfeffer MA. Progressive ventricular remodeling in response to diffuse isoproterenol-induced myocardial necrosis in rats. *Circ Res* 1994; **75**: 105–113.

17 Pillai JB, Gupta M, Rajamohan SB, Lang R, Raman J, Gupta MP, *et al*. Poly(ADP-ribose) polymerase-1-deficient mice are protected from angiotensin II-induced cardiac hypertrophy. *Am J Physiol Heart Circ Physiol* 2006; **291**: H1545–1553.

18 Bendall JK, Cave AC, Heymes C, Gall N, Shah AM. Pivotal role of a gp91phox-containing NADPH oxidase in angiotensin II-induced cardiac hypertrophy in mice. *Circulation* 2002; **105**: 293–296.

19 Mokni W, Keravis T, Etienne-Selloum N, Walter A, Kane MO, Schini-Kerth VB, *et al*. Concerted regulation of cGMP and cAMP phosphodiesterases in early cardiac hypertrophy induced by angiotensin II. *PloS One* 2010; **5**: e14227.

20 Zhou G, Li X, Hein DW, Xiang X, Marshall JP, Prabhu SD, *et al*. Metallothionein suppresses angiotensin II-induced nicotinamide adenine dinucleotide phosphate oxidase activation, nitrosative stress, apoptosis, and pathological remodeling in the diabetic heart. *J Am Coll Cardiol* 2008; **52**: 655–666.

21 Shanmugam P, Valente AJ, Prabhu SD, Venkatesan B, Yoshida T, Delafontaine P, *et al*. Angiotensin-II type 1 receptor and NOX2 mediate TCF/LEF and CREB dependent WISP1 induction and cardiomyocyte hypertrophy. *J Mol Cell Cardiol* 2011; **50**: 928–938.

22 Bartoli CR, Brittian KR, Giridharan GA, Koenig SC, Hamid T, Prabhu SD, *et al*. Bovine model of doxorubicin-induced cardiomyopathy. *J Biomed Biotechnol* 2011; **2011**: 758736.

23 Lucas CM, Cheriex EC, van der Veen FH, Habets J, van der Nagel T, Penn OC, *et al*. Imipramine induced heart failure in the dog: A model to study the effect of cardiac assist devices. *Cardiovasc Res* 1992; **26**: 804–809.

24 Perkins L, Peer C, Murphey-Hackley P. The use of mini-osmotic pumps in continuous infusion studies. In: Smith D, Healing G, eds. *Handbook of Pre-clinical Continuous Intravenous Infusion*. London: Taylor and Francis, 2000, p. 330.

Hindlimb ischemia

Jerry C. Lee, Ngan F. Huang, and John P. Cooke

Stanford University School of Medicine, Stanford, CA, USA

Introduction

Peripheral arterial disease (PAD) is typically due to atherosclerosis, affecting the aortoiliac, femoral, and/or infrapopliteal arteries, and impairing blood flow to the legs. The disease afflicts about 8 million Americans [1] with a prevalence of 4% in individuals over 50 [2], though some estimates are as high as 29% in individuals over the age of 70, as well as smokers or diabetics over the age of 55 [3]. Despite this high prevalence, recognition of PAD is poor [4] and physicians often fail to optimally manage PAD. Patients with PAD may present with calf, thigh, and/or buttock pain during ambulation, which is relieved by rest (intermittent claudication). More severe arterial disease may lead to pain at rest, gangrene, and amputation [5]. In addition to causing severe morbidity, PAD is also a consistent and powerful predictor of mortality from coronary artery and cerebrovascular disease [6]. Therapy for PAD includes modification of risk factors (e.g. treatment of hypercholesterolemia, hypertension, and diabetes), an effective approach to reduce major adverse cardiovascular events. Supervised exercise programs substantially increase walking distance, however, the benefit of drug therapy to improve functional capacity (e.g. cilostazol) is modest. New therapies to relieve intermittent claudication and increase walking distance are needed.

Potential therapies to treat PAD are often tested in the murine model of hindlimb ischemia due to its reproducibility and relative ease. Other advantages of the hindlimb ischemia model include the ease of preclinical imaging, using laser Doppler to confirm ischemia and follow the course of its resolution. One can also employ bioluminescence in this small animal model so as to noninvasively track cell therapies [7]. In addition, it is relatively easy to assess capillary density and arteriolar size by immunohistochemistry, so as to quantify changes with angiogenic or vasodilator therapies.

These attributes have made the murine hindlimb ischemia model a favored approach to test angiogenic, vasodilator, or metabolic therapies, in the form of small molecules, gene therapy, angiogenic growth factors, or cell therapy. However, many potential therapies that have been effective in this mouse model, have failed in man. This may be due to certain deficiencies of the model, as it does not replicate all of the pathobiology of PAD. The acute surgical ligation in the C57Bl6 mouse creates acute ischemia, whereas PAD is due to slowly developing intrinsic vascular disease, in the setting of aging, tobacco exposure, diabetes mellitus, and other metabolic perturbations. Accordingly, it may be possible to improve the model by adding metabolic perturbations, as with apoE hyperlipidemic mice or streptozotocin-treated diabetic mice, for example [8]. The Balb C mouse is much more susceptible to femoral artery ligation, developing signs of critical limb ischemia, that is gangrene and limb loss [9]. The choice of experimental manipulation should

Manual of Research Techniques in Cardiovascular Medicine, First Edition. Edited by Hossein Ardehali, Roberto Bolli, and Douglas W. Losordo.

be carefully considered when accounting for the presumed mechanism of drug action. With these caveats, the hindlimb ischemia model can be a useful methodology for testing new therapies for PAD and other ischemic syndromes.

Protocol

We describe a standard protocol for a murine model of unilateral hindlimb ischemia by femoral artery ligation and excision. This method reliably reduces limb blood flow to 10–20% of normal perfusion levels, as assessed by laser Doppler. As with the case for all animal experiments, please first consult your organization's veterinary care facility for detailed information regarding animal handling and anesthesia, and obtain institutional approval for these procedures.

Induction of anesthesia

1. To prepare the animal for depilation and surgery, we favor the use of an inhalational anesthetic. The advantages over injectable agents include easier animal handling and control, larger margin of safety, and quicker recovery times. For inhalational anesthesia, we use an isoflurane vaporizer, oxygen supply and regulator, oxygen flow meter, induction chamber, and tubing/valves with a switch system that can divert gas between the induction chamber and an open-air nose cone.

2. Place the mouse into the induction chamber, receiving oxygen with 1–3% isoflurane at a flow rate of 1–2 L/min. Actual dosage and flow rate depends on the number of animals in the chamber, their age, and strain. To assess for sufficient anesthesia, animals should be unresponsive to toe pinch while maintaining a regular breathing rate. Animals breathing too quickly (over 120 breaths/min.) require more isoflurane; animals with shallow or sharp breaths need more oxygen or less isoflurane. Deep, steady breathing is optimal.

Hair removal prior to surgery

1. Hair must be removed from animal at the site of incision, as well as those regions to be assessed by laser Doppler. Once anesthetized, transfer the mouse from the induction chamber to nosecone, which

should deliver oxygen with 1–3% isoflurane at a flow rate sufficient to maintain anesthesia. Laying the mouse in the supine position, remove all hair from the anterior region inferior to the sternum, as well as hair on the posterior hindlimb. Use an electric clipper, razor, depilatory cream, or tweezers for plucking, if the hair is minimal. Because an electric clipper or razor may not shave close enough to the skin, we recommend using a gentle depilatory cream (Nads or Nair). These creams can result in burns, especially because they are not designed for small animal use, so they should only be used for short periods of time (<1 min). Lather the body with the cream, gently mixing it into the hair by rubbing together folds of the skin.

2. After leaving the cream on the hair for about 30 seconds, wipe away the cream with either a paper towel or with the handle of forceps. Take care to do this gently, as skin abrasions can be induced otherwise. The hair should come off easily. After the cream is largely removed, wash the mouse in a warm water bath, making sure to thoroughly rinse off any remaining cream. Dry with a paper towel and place the mouse into a cage. Use a heat lamp to warm the animal; you may need to direct the lamp slightly away from the mouse to avoid overheating.

3. If an electric clipper is used, collect all loose hair and dander with a vacuum or an adhesive (i.e. tape or lint remover).

Surgery preparation

1. Prepare the surgery station as shown in Figure 22.1. Note the circulating water blanket underneath the absorbent drape; this is important in preventing hypothermia. A metal base plate is used to secure the nosecone and the magnetized animal retractor. Three small basins contain solutions of 70% ethanol, Phosphate buffered saline (PBS), and sterile PBS. The ethanol is used for cooling and cleaning tools after sterilization, PBS for wetting cotton swabs, and sterile PBS to replenish lost fluids if there is substantial blood loss. An adjustable microscope stage and lights are necessary. Wear a mask, sterile gloves, and clean lab coat/scrubs. The surgery space should be free of clutter and traffic.

2. After induction of general anesthesia, place a lubricating ophthalmic ointment on the animal's eyes to protect the cornea from desiccation. Secure all limbs of the animal with tape, in the supine

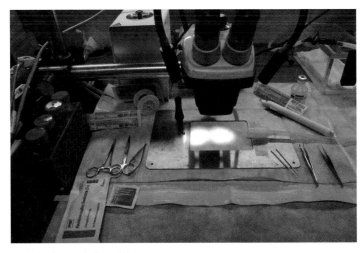

Figure 22.1 Surgical setup, showing required materials.

position. The animal should be positioned horizontally, with the hindlimb extended 90° from primary axis of the body. It is very important that the hindlimbs are secured and taut. Cover the animal with a sterile drape, leaving the surgical site uncovered.

3. The surgical instruments needed for the operation are listed in Table 22.1. Sterilize these prior to surgery using a hot bead sterilizer or autoclave. If using a hot bead sterilizer, place the tips of the instruments in the sterilizer for 10 seconds at the maximum temperature and cool them afterward by submerging them in 70% ethanol.

4. Confirm the animal is anesthetized by toe pinch for unresponsiveness. Remove any excess hair or dander from the medial surface of the hindlimb. Aseptically prepare the surgical site (entire thigh region, proximal calf, and the groin/ abdomen area) with three alternating Betadine (povidone–iodine) and alcohol scrubs. Cleanse the area first with the alcohol wipes, starting from the thigh and wiping outward in a circular fashion. Do the same with the Betadine swabs. After letting the Betadine dry for a few seconds, wipe the area again with the alcohol pad.

Femoral artery ligation

1. The femoral artery/ vein can be easily visualized directly underneath the skin in a properly shaved mouse. By holding the skin taut in the inguinal region, one can locate the femoral artery and vein, which are in the neurovascular bundle enclosed by the femoral sheath. The neurovascular bundle should be apparent closer to the calf. At the thigh region, the neurovascular bundle disappears underneath adipose tissue. Using sterile surgical scissors, start the skin incision just distal from where the neurovascular bundle starts to disappear. Make a 1-cm longitudinal incision, stopping just proximal to where the abdominal wall starts to appear.

2. Use PBS-moistened fine-pointed cotton swabs to gently separate the subcutaneous fat tissue surrounding the thigh muscle. Once the entire fat pad can be visualized, use the curved forceps to pierce underneath the fat pad, isolating it from the surrounding tissue. Lift up the forceps and open/ close them a few times, loosening up the tissue. Then using the cautery, transversely burn through the entire fat pad. The underlying femoral AV bundle should be revealed. There should be some vessels running through the fat pad, and at this point there may be some minor bleeding. Use the cotton-tipped applicators to remove any excess serum or blood.

3. Use the retractor to open the incision and properly visualize the neurovascular bundle. Securing the fixator on the base plate and the retractor on the retractor wire, place the retractor at the proximal incision point such that it retracts the abdominal wall. Fix the retractor wire into the fixator. At this

Table 22.1 List of materials

Material/Tool	Type	Recommended
Depilatory cream	Hair removal cream	Nads Sensitive Hair Removal Crème
Fine angled forceps	Surgical instrument	Roboz Inox 5/45 RS-5005
Curved forceps	Surgical instrument	Roboz Dumostar 7 RS-4982
Spring scissors	Surgical instrument	Roboz McPherson-Vannas RS-5631
Fine scissors	Surgical instrument	FST CeramaCut 14958-11
Needle holder/scissors	Surgical instrument	Roboz Olsen-Hegar RS-7880
Retractor set (base plate, fixator, wire, retractor)	Surgical instrument	FST (18200-03, 18200-01 or 18200-02, 18200-09, 18200-05)
Cautery	Surgical equipment	Bovie Change-A-Tip DEL1
Hot bead sterilizer	Surgical equipment	FST 18000-45
Dissecting microscope	Surgical equipment	
Light source	Surgical equipment	Dolan Jenner Fiber-Lite, PL-750
Warming blanket	Surgical equipment	Gaymar pump with pad (TPP622)
Pointed cotton swabs	Surgical tool	Constix SC-7
Cotton-tipped applicators	Surgical tool	Puritan 25-803-2WC
Tape	Surgical tool	3M Transpore Medical Tape
6-0 non-absorbable suture	Surgical tool	Braided silk suture, spool
5-0 absorbable suture	Surgical tool	Polysorb/Vicryl braided
Syringe	Surgical tool	BD insulin syringe
Ophthalmic ointment	Reagent	Lacri-Lube
Povidone-iodine swab sticks	Reagent	PDI S41125
Alcohol prep pads	Reagent	Dynarex 1104
Phosphate buffered saline (PBS)	Reagent	Invitrogen
Lidocaine	Reagent	
Temperature monitor/probe	Doppler equipment	Physitemp TCAT-2LV and RET-3
Heating plate	Doppler equipment	Physitemp HP-1M
Non-reflective material	Doppler equipment	Black T-shirt
Laser Doppler	Doppler equipment	Perimed PeriScan PIM3 system

point, use the dissection microscope at 10× or 20× magnification to obtain a better field of view. The inguinal ligament should appear as a white band running along the abdominal wall.

4. A membranous, translucent femoral sheath should cover the neurovascular bundle. Remove this with the curved forceps and fine-pointed cotton swab. At any point during the surgery, use the cotton swabs in concert with the curved forceps to gently separate and remove any unwanted fascia.

5. The femoral vein is larger than the artery and the color is darker. The artery is immediately lateral to the vein and is attached to the vein by a thin layer of connective tissue (Figure 22.2). Use the cotton swabs

to separate the artery from the vein as much as possible without damaging the vessels. The first ligation site is just distal to the inguinal ligament (Figure 22.3). At this site, there should be a small space in which the connective tissue between the artery and vein is weak and easily loosened. Prepare a 1-cm strand of 6-0 (or smaller) silk suture and pass it underneath the artery at this location, and through the connective tissue between the artery and vein, using the fine angled forceps. Use caution not to pierce the femoral vein with the forceps. Then occlude the artery using double knots.

6. Continue to dissect free the femoral artery from the vein along its length. Find the distal ligation site.

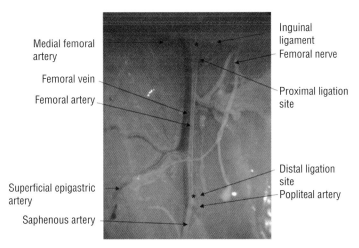

Figure 22.2 Anatomy of the hindlimb vasculature. Asterisks indicate the locations of ligation. (Source: Niiyama H 2009 [28]).

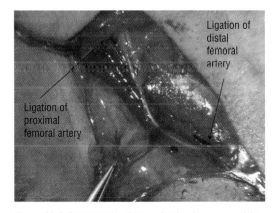

Figure 22.3 Representative diagram showing the anatomy of the hindlimb after ligation of the femoral artery at the proximal and distal ligation sites. (Source: Niiyama H 2009 [28]).

This area should be distal to the superficial epigastric artery (which can be seen with connective tissue as it arises from the superficial femoral artery), and immediately proximal to where the femoral artery branches into the popliteal and saphenous arteries. Again, separate the femoral artery from the vein at this site, and then occlude the distal femoral artery with a double knot.

7. For gripping purposes, tie another knot immediately proximal to the distal ligature. This knot will be useful later as a marker of the distal femoral artery and a means to manipulate the vessel.

8. Cut the distal femoral artery using the spring scissors. The location of the transection is between the two distal ligatures. There should be slight bleeding from the residual blood inside the femoral artery.

9. Excise the femoral artery between the proximal and distal ligatures. There will be collateral vessels along the length of the femoral artery that will need to be cut with the spring scissors, and compressed for approximately 1 minute to obtain hemostasis. With the more proximal distal ligature in one forceps, gently pull the artery away from the vein, separating the vessels from each other at the same time with the cotton swabs. The most challenging region is immediately proximal to the distal ligation site, where the superficial epigastric artery meets the femoral artery. Use considerable caution not to pierce the femoral vein at this location, or damage the femoral nerve that also traverses this region. Take care to remove as much of the connective tissue as possible. Once the superficial epigastric artery is separated from the femoral artery with the spring scissors, there will be a considerable amount of bleeding. Stop the bleeding using the cotton tipped applicators. Often, to continue separating the femoral artery from the vein proximally, the femoral artery must be carefully teased away from the connective tissue and nerves of this area.

10. There are more proximal collateral vessels, but these can be transected without much bleeding or damage to the surrounding tissue. Once the femoral artery has been completely separated, make a final cut immediately distal to the proximal ligature to fully excise and remove this section of the femoral artery.

11. Remove the retractor and close the incision using 5-0 synthetic (Vicryl or Polysorb) sutures. Tie discontinuous sutures. These sutures will dissolve over time, so they do not need to be removed later. Surgical staples could also be used, but these are bulkier and may prevent the animal from walking effectively.

12. For analgesia, inject 1–2% lidocaine (2–4 mg/kg) into the surgical site. The onset of this analgesic will be 5–10 minutes and its effects will persist for 1–2 hours. Place the animal in a cage without bedding, heated with a heat lamp or pad. Monitor continuously for 1 hour. After the animal has recovered, proceed with laser Doppler perfusion to confirm ischemia.

13. Because animals tend to bite on the sutures, check daily to determine if the wound has dehisced. It may be necessary to resuture the wound; a needle holder with an attached scissors is ideal for this procedure.

Laser Doppler

1. Anesthetize the mouse as described earlier. Shave the entire anterior lower half of the animal if not shaved already. Remove the hair on the back of the hindlimbs as well.

2. Turn on the laser Doppler imager and the acquisition software. Our images are acquired with Perimed's PeriScan PIM 3 System, but other companies like Moor Instruments also manufacture laser Doppler imagers. Specify the field of view (70 × 70 mm image width/ height should suffice). Use a user-defined perfusion color scale of 0 to 1000 to better compare succeeding images, instead of using a relative scale.

3. Place the animal prone on a heated surface under a continuous flow of isoflurane. Checking with a rectal temperature probe, heat the animal until the body temperature reaches 37°C. After surgery, the operated limb will typically be stiff, but be sure to gently tuck both hindlimbs underneath the animal for appropriate heating.

4. Once the animal reaches 37°C, place the animal supine on a non-reflective light-absorbing material, such as matte paper or black cloth. Underneath

this material, place another heated surface such that the animal will maintain heat as the Doppler is being conducted. Extend the hindlimbs to ensure that they are not blocking any part of the animal from being imaged. Movement of the animal due to breathing should be minimized during the imaging process.

5. Open a new file in the imager program. Click "mark area." Looking at the animal, a laser-bound square should incorporate the entire inferior region of the animal. Adjust the Doppler position and resolution if necessary. Close the "mark area" window on the computer and press "start" to begin acquiring. Do not move the animal or Doppler at any point. Once the imager detects the distance of the Doppler to the mouse, click "ok." Typically, it will take approximately 3 minutes to acquire the image at high spatial resolution.

6. After acquisition, the image will show, in a range of colors, the tissue perfusion in the imaged region. The ischemic leg should appear black or dark blue, and the contralateral, unoperated leg should appear yellow or red. Save the file. Return the animal to the recovery cage and monitor continuously until awake.

7. To calculate perfusion ratios, open the appropriate file. Set the threshold intensity to 0.2. Using the circle or rectangle tool, select two regions of interest (ROIs) that cover each of the hindlimbs. To be consistent, use the same anatomical landmark to standardize the ROI (each ROI should cover the same region in each animal). Typically, our ROIs incorporate the entire hindlimb distal to the pelvis. After creating the ROIs, a box should appear, indicating the size of the ROI and the mean perfusion in that ROI. After confirming that the sizes of the ROIs are similar, a perfusion ratio between the ischemic limb and the control limb can be easily determined.

8. The perfusion ratio is measured as the ratio of the mean perfusion of the ischemic leg divided by the mean perfusion of the control leg. The perfusion ratio of a representative animal is shown in Figure 22.4, over 28 days post-ischemia. Laser Doppler images assessing tissue perfusion in a pre- and postoperative animal are shown in Figure 22.5.

Alternative methods

Barring any complications, an experienced technician can complete a hindlimb ischemia model in 30 minutes. A variety of shortcuts can reduce

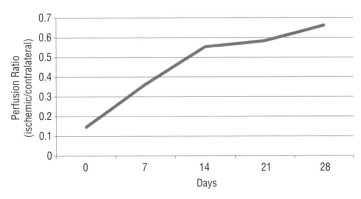

Figure 22.4 Representative graph showing tissue perfusion as assessed by laser Doppler over 28 days after induction of hindlimb ischemia.

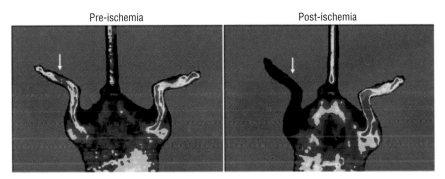

Figure 22.5 Representative laser Doppler images showing tissue perfusion before and after the induction of hindlimb ischemia to the left hindlimb (indicated by the arrow). (Source: Niiyama H 2009 [28]).

surgery time to 20 minutes. First, the second distal ligature, used for gripping purposes, is optional if the operator grips the free end of the femoral artery directly, after the distal incision is made. In this way, the artery can be manipulated with the forceps without the need for another ligature to serve as a marker and grip. The caveat is that the artery can easily disappear under connective tissue due to the loss of tension in the vessel, or can be difficult to identify from the surrounding fascia, especially if there is bleeding. Second, separating the femoral artery from the vein can be done fairly quickly just by manipulating the free end of the artery after the distal incision. By applying the appropriate amount of tension, one could carefully pull on the loose end of the artery to free it away from the vein. This requires a fair amount of experience, knowing how much tension to apply and where the collateral vessels are, because there is a high risk of tearing the femoral vein. Third, an experienced operator can use

the two forceps and the spring scissors to finish the entire ligation/excision procedure without the need for the fine-pointed cotton swabs. The cotton swabs serve as a wetting device and a blunt instrument to reduce the risk of accidental punctures when dissecting the vessels, but a skilled operator can use the forceps alone. Although wetting the area is helpful in visualizing the anatomy, the area should be adequately hydrated during the short, 20-minute surgeries.

Therapeutics could also be delivered intra-arterially or intravenously directly to the site of ischemia by injecting through the femoral artery, vein, or any of its numerous side branches [10].

Common considerations

General
• Exposure to isoflurane may cause adverse health effects, including cognitive impairment, reproductive,

or hepatotoxic effects [11–17]. Therefore, it is important that when working with isoflurane, personnel exposure is reduced by ensuring the following:

– Reduce exposure to isoflurane by working in a fume hood or using vacuum lines, or passive scavenging of isoflurane using a precision vaporizer with charcoal filtration.

– Inspect, seal, and clean nose cones, gas lines, and induction chambers immediately before and after use to ensure a proper fit.

– Ensure a tight seal around the animal's face and use an anesthetic mask.

• As for all animal procedures, proper maintenance of body temperature and length of isoflurane exposure are extremely important. Low body temperatures and long isoflurane exposure may increase morbidity and mortality of the animals.

• Animal age greatly contribute to the variability of these procedures. Younger C57Bl mice generally recover quickly, and therefore we suggest using older mice (15+ weeks) to obtain a more sustained ischemia. It may be preferable to use younger animals if one is assessing antiangiogenic factors [18].

• Each animal strain has particular idiosyncrasies that affect the response to the techniques described here. Immunodeficient mice (SCID, nude) tend to ulcerate more easily from the depilatory cream, have less perivascular connective tissue, and more fragile vessel walls. C57Bl/6tend to become obese at old age and have much more connective tissue, making the excision of the femoral artery more difficult. BALB/c mice develop a more profound ischemia and higher frequency of necrosis than other strains [9].

Hair removal

• Ulceration caused by overuse of depilatory cream is a common problem. Since laser Doppler assesses superficial microvessels, ulcers create "dead zones" – dark spots showing zero perfusion – which can produce highly inaccurate perfusion readings. Depilatory cream should be thoroughly lathered into the hair, but skin should not be exposed for more than 1 minute to minimize ulcerative damage.

• Ideally, hair needs to be removed the day before the surgical procedure to reduce anesthesia exposure time in the course of one day. If performing multiple experiments throughout the week, shaving twice a week should be sufficient to keep the skin glabrous.

Femoral artery ligation

• The severity of ischemia, strain, and age of animal, and extent of postsurgical injury (self-inflicted or by other animals) are the largest contributors to limb necrosis. The hindlimb ischemia model described here does not typically result in necrosis in C57Bl/6 mice, although a minority do manifest toe necrosis. More severe models, in which the epigastric and other collaterals are ligated, result in greater limb loss [19,20]. Increased age of animal also increases the risk of limb loss, but housing animals in separate cages can mitigate some of that, especially for male mice.

• Animals in pain will more likely bite and remove their sutures, causing ulcerations that may lead to necrosis. Some animals will remove their sutures immediately after the procedure, so animals will need to be monitored a few hours after surgery and daily afterwards for 1 week.

• Appropriate analgesics, as determined by the Institutional Animal Care and Use Committee (IACUC), are to be administered for these animals. One consideration is that certain analgesics may interfere with angiogenesis. Opioids have been shown to modulate angiogenesis [21–23], as do non-steroidal anti-inflammatory drugs [24–27]. Consult IACUC for the most appropriate analgesic to use. At the minimum, we recommend injecting lidocaine as a local anesthetic.

Laser Doppler

• The greatest cause of the variation seen in laser Doppler perfusion imaging is the animal's body temperature. Even slight temperature changes of less than 0.5°C will cause large fluctuations in perfusion of the limb. Use an accurate temperature probe. It is critically important that all animals be imaged at precisely the same temperature.

• Heat loss during the imaging itself also needs to be minimized. The addition of a second heating pad applied during imaging mitigates some loss of heat, but there is individual variation as to how quickly and how much heat is lost over time.

• Similarly, there is individual variation as to how quickly each animal reaches the predetermined body temperature for imaging (recommended: 37°C or 38°C). Ideally, the core body temperature of an anesthetized animal should start below 35°C, at which point, steady warm heat should be applied over the course of several minutes until the appropriate temperature is achieved. Be careful not to overheat the animal, which can cause morbidity or death.

• The expected perfusion ratio by this model on day 0 should be 10–20%. Without treatment, we find perfusion to naturally increase to up to 60–70% of the unoperated limb within 28 days after induction of hindlimb ischemia in older mice (15+ weeks) (Figure 22.4). Younger C57Bl/6 mice may reach almost normal levels of perfusion after 4 weeks, making it difficult to observe any effect of an angiogenic agent.

Acknowledgements

This work was supported by grants from National Institutes of Health to J.P.C. (U01HL100397, RC2HL103400) and N.F.H. (K99HL098688).

References

1 Selvin E, Erlinger TP. Prevalence of and risk factors for peripheral arterial disease in the United States: results from the National Health and Nutrition Examination Survey, 1999–2000. *Circulation* 2004; **110**: 738–743.

2 Ostchega Y, Paulose-Ram R, Dillon CF, Gu Q, Hughes JP. Prevalence of peripheral arterial disease and risk factors in persons aged 60 and older: data from the National Health and Nutrition Examination Survey 1999–2004. *J Am Geriatr Soc* 2007; **55**: 583–589.

3 Hirsch AT, Criqui MH, Treat-Jacobson D, Regensteiner JG, Creager MA, Olin JW, *et al*. Peripheral arterial disease detection, awareness, and treatment in primary care. *JAMA* 2001; **286**: 1317–1324.

4 Hirsch AT, Murphy TP, Lovell MB, Twillman G, Treat-Jacobson D, Harwood EM, *et al*. Gaps in public knowledge of peripheral arterial disease: the first national PAD public awareness survey. *Circulation* 2007; **116**: 2086–2094.

5 Cooke JP. Critical determinants of limb ischemia. *J Am Coll Cardiol* 2008; **52**: 394–396.

6 Golomb BA, Dang TT, Criqui MH. Peripheral arterial disease: morbidity and mortality implications. *Circulation* 2006; **114**: 688–699.

7 Huang NF, Niiyama H, De A, Gambhir SS, Cooke JP. Embryonic stem cell-derived endothelial cells for treatment of hindlimb ischemia. *J Vis Exp* 2009; (**23**). pii: 1034.

8 Waters RE, Terjung RL, Peters KG, Annex BH. Preclinical models of human peripheral arterial occlusive disease: implications for investigation of therapeutic agents. *J Appl Physiol* 2004; **97**: 773–780.

9 Dokun AO, Keum S, Hazarika S, Li Y, Lamonte GM, Wheeler F, *et al*. A quantitative trait locus (LSq-1) on mouse chromosome 7 is linked to the absence of tissue loss after surgical hindlimb ischemia. *Circulation* 2008; **117**: 1207–1215.

10 Huang NF, Niiyama H, Peter C, De A, Natkunam Y, Fleissner F, *et al*. Embryonic stem cell-derived endothelial cells engraft into the ischemic hindlimb and restore perfusion. *Arterioscler Thromb Vasc Biol* 2010; **30**: 984–991.

11 Lin D, Zuo Z. Isoflurane induces hippocampal cell injury and cognitive impairments in adult rats. *Neuropharmacology* 2011; **61**: 1354–1359.

12 Xie Z, Dong Y, Maeda U, Moir RD, Xia W, Culley DJ, *et al*. The inhalation anesthetic isoflurane induces a vicious cycle of apoptosis and amyloid beta-protein accumulation. *J Neurosci* 2007; **27**: 1247–1254.

13 Kuehn BM. Anesthesia-Alzheimer disease link probed. *JAMA* 2007; **297**: 1760.

14 Sinha A, Clatch RJ, Stuck G, Blumenthal SA, Patel SA. Isoflurane hepatotoxicity: a case report and review of the literature. *Am J Gastroenterol* 1996; **91**: 2406–2409.

15 Brown BR, Jr. Hepatotoxicity and inhalation anesthetics: views in the era of isoflurane. *J Clin Anesth* 1989; **1**: 368–376.

16 Eger EI, 2nd. Isoflurane: a review. *Anesthesiology* 1981; **55**: 559–576.

17 Cohen EN. Toxicity of inhalation anaesthetic agents. *Br J Anaesth* 1978; **50**: 665–675.

18 Niiyama H, Kai H, Yamamoto T, Shimada T, Sasaki K, Murohara T, *et al*. Roles of endogenous monocyte chemoattractant protein-1 in ischemia-induced neovascularization. *J Am Coll Cardiol* 2004; **44**: 661–666.

19 Saqib A, Prasad KM, Katwal AB, Sanders JM, Lye RJ, French BA, *et al*. Adeno-associated virus serotype 9-mediated overexpression of extracellular superoxide dismutase improves recovery from surgical hind-limb ischemia in BALB/c mice. *J Vasc Surg* 2011; **54**: 810–818.

20 Xie D, Li Y, Reed EA, Odronic SI, Kontos CD, Annex BH, *et al*. An engineered vascular endothelial growth factor-activating transcription factor induces therapeutic angiogenesis in ApoE knockout mice with hindlimb ischemia. *J Vasc Surg* 2006; **44**: 166–175.

21 Leo S, Nuydens R, Meert TF. Opioid-induced proliferation of vascular endothelial cells. *J Pain Res* 2009; **2**: 59–66.

22 Blebea J, Mazo JE, Kihara TK, Vu JH, McLaughlin PJ, Atnip RG, *et al*. Opioid growth factor modulates angiogenesis. *J Vasc Surg* 2000; **32**: 364–373.

23 Pasi A, Qu BX, Steiner R, Senn HJ, Bar W, Messiha FS, *et al*. Angiogenesis: modulation with opioids. *Gen Pharmacol* 1991; **22**: 1077–1079.

24 Monnier Y, Zaric J, Ruegg C. Inhibition of angiogenesis by non-steroidal anti-inflammatory drugs: from the

bench to the bedside and back. *Curr Drug Targets Inflamm Allergy* 2005; **4**: 31–38.

25 Tarnawski AS, Jones MK. Inhibition of angiogenesis by NSAIDs: molecular mechanisms and clinical implications. *J Mol Med (Berl)* 2003; **81**: 627–636.

26 Dermond O, Ruegg C. Inhibition of tumor angiogenesis by non-steroidal anti-inflammatory drugs: emerging mechanisms and therapeutic perspectives. *Drug Resist Updat* 2001; **4**: 314–321.

27 Jones MK, Wang H, Peskar BM, Levin E, Itani RM, Sarfeh IJ, *et al*. Inhibition of angiogenesis by nonsteroidal anti-inflammatory drugs: insight into mechanisms and implications for cancer growth and ulcer healing. *Nat Med* 1999; **5**: 1418–1423.

28 Niiyama H, Huang NF, Rollins MD, Cooke JP. Murine model of hindlimb ischemia. *J Vis Exp* 2009; (**23**). pii: 1035.

23 The Langendorff preparation

Hugh Clements-Jewery[1] and Michael J. Curtis[2]

[1] West Virginia School of Osteopathic Medicine, Lewisburg, WV, USA

[2] Kings College London, London, UK

Introduction

The Langendorff preparation was first described by Oskar Langendorff in 1895 [1]. In his experiment, Langendorff observed that it was possible to revive an excised mammalian heart that had ceased to contract by connecting the aorta of the heart to a reservoir of blood. This was possible because the pressure of blood in the aorta closed the aortic valve, directing blood through the coronary ostia into the coronary vasculature. Langendorff observed that the ensuing contractile activity could thereafter be maintained for hours. The preparation has evolved over the decades such that with appropriate equipment and preparation an experiment can be conducted with a high success rate [2].

The fundamental properties of the preparation are as follows. Cannulation of the aorta allows perfusion solution to enter the coronary arteries. The entire coronary vasculature is then perfused under control of the experimenter. This can be achieved by constant flow or constant pressure (allowing measurement of coronary vascular resistance or coronary flow, respectively). The heart rate is regulated by the sinoatrial node, which is either perfused or superfused by coronary effluent depending on the species [3]. The difference between baseline heart rate of hearts perfused using the Langendorff method and heart rate *in vivo* varies between species (as do many other aspects of the preparation). Thus, in rats, heart rate in the conscious animal (~400 beats/min) [4–6] compares with a value of ~300 beats/min in the Langendorff preparation [2,7–11]. Yet in mice the conscious animal rate of ~600 beats/min [12] falls to ~300 beat/min in the Langendorff preparation under similar experimental conditions [13] whereas, in contrast, in the rabbit the heart rate in the Langendorff preparation of ~200 beats/min [14,15] is well maintained compared with the rate in the conscious animal which is also ~200 beats/min [16]. The reasons for this species-dependent variation are unknown but presumably reflect species-dependent difference in dominance in the baseline sympathetic/parasympathetic tone. In this vein, the removal of the sympathetic influence in the Langendorff preparation has a lesser outcome in species in which baseline heart rate is not under strong sympathetic control.

There are certain misconceptions about the preparation that should be dispelled. First, it is commonly perceived that the preparation's vasculature is "maximally dilated." It is certainly true that coronary flow is much lower in the blood-perfused Langendorff preparation [17] compared with the crystalloid-perfused equivalent [18]. However, if the Langendorff preparation were maximally dilated then vasodilator drugs would be without effect. This is clearly not the case, since in the rat Langendorff preparation the L-type calcium antagonist verapamil [19], the nitric oxide precursor L-arginine [20], the phosphodiesterase-V inhibitor zaprinast [21], the PAF antagonist BN-50739 [22], epinephrine and norepinephrine [18], nitrate [23], the K_{ATP} activator cromakalim [24], and other agents all cause sustained vasodilatation. There are fewer data sets from other species but coronary flow has been shown to be elevated by serotonin and several related agonists in the guinea pig Langendorff preparation [25,26], and by epinephrine and norepinephrine in the mouse Langendorff preparation [13].

There are several very important technical issues that can render the Langendorff preparation fit or unfit for purpose. These include the manner of cardiac excision and cannulation, preparation and constituents of the perfusion solution, thermoregulation, choice of the method of solution delivery (constant pressure versus flow), and method of recording of readout such as left ventricular pressure. These aspects are addressed in the following section.

Protocol

In order to ensure the Langendorff preparation is fit for purpose, certain procedures and approaches should be adopted. In many instances the evolution and validation of the approaches are not documented in the peer-reviewed literature so the approaches we offer here are in many instances based on personal experience. The effectiveness of the approaches, however, is evident from published research.

Cannulation of the aorta

The first stage of experimentation involves cardiac excision and cannulation of the aorta. In our experience, the quality of the preparation is maximized by limiting the interval between the moment when the thorax is opened (representing the moment of termination of lung inflation and the start of hypoxic circulation) and the onset of heart perfusion. However, anecdotal experience suggests that provided the heart is arrested in cold (<6°C) solution there is no need to rush. We have conducted experiments, as part of undergraduate teaching, in which rat hearts were subjected to 30 minutes global ischemia at room temperature (20°C) and found that during reperfusion the diastolic and systolic left ventricular pressures fully recovered to their preischemic values. That cooling can preserve function is not a surprise; cold cardioplegia is a

standard method for preserving human hearts during sustained heart surgery [27]. Thus, once a heart has been arrested in cold perfusion solution the next stage of experimentation may be undertaken at a more leisurely pace.

Another technique that has not been validated by direct experiment is administration of heparin prior to cardiac excision. However, earlier experiments in which heparin was not used yielded poor coronary flow values [28]. This may be explained by clot formation in the ventricular lumen in the absence of heparin that gives rise to microemboli in the coronary vasculature if dislodged during perfusion. For convenience heparin can be injected intraperitoneally (i.p.) together with anesthetic [29]; alternatively, heparin can be injected into the femoral vein when the animal is fully anesthetized prior to cardiac excision [30].

Cardiac excision should be performed carefully to ensure the entire aortic arch remains attached to the heart. This can be achieved by removing the lungs with the heart, using round-tipped scissors. Careful manipulation can allow this to be undertaken without fingers touching the heart itself, which should be avoided.

Cannulation of the aorta is simple to achieve. First, the lungs and thymus should be cut away from the heart, keeping the heart in the cold perfusion solution as much as possible to ensure it is kept cool and arrested. It will then be possible to visualize the aortic arch together with the first three arterial branches emanating from the aorta. The aortic arch should then be cut at an angle down to the first vessel branching from the ascending aorta, the brachiocephalic artery. This will provide a large amount of aorta to manipulate onto the cannula, which should be fixed, pointing downwards as part of the perfusion apparatus. It is most convenient to manufacture a cannula with an external diameter that exceeds the internal diameter of the aorta by 1–2 mm. This will vary for different species and different animal age. For rats of 200–300 g, a cannula with an external diameter of ~3 mm allows the aorta to attach without the heart slipping off the cannula before it is secured using black silk thread (3-0). If the cannula is made of stainless steel it can be machined to possess fine grooves, which may facilitate the attachment. Some investigators use an artery clip to hold the aorta on the cannula before the thread is attached and tied. We find this unnecessary when using a cannula of 3 mm external diameter, although it may be necessary if using a cannula of smaller external diameter. The cannulation of the aorta is best achieved using small curved serrated forceps. First, one pair of forceps should be used to grip the aorta on one side. The heart may then be brought close to the cannula. When in place, the second pair of forceps may be taken in hand and the other side of the aorta gripped. This is preferable to gripping the aorta with both pairs of forceps before taking the heart to the cannula as slight careless movement can rip the aorta. Some investigators allow a small amount of solution to flow from the cannula during heart attachment, either by partially obstructing the perfusate supply with a clamp or by switching on a constant flow device at a low rate. However, we do not advocate this since it mandates use of an artery clip to secure the heart as it is attached, and it initiates a heart beat before full flow can be achieved. Instead we ensure there is no air introduced into the aortic arch by allowing one drip of solution to hang from the cannula tip as we attach the heart. When attaching the heart to the cannula, it is convenient to rest the wrists on the edge of a perfusion trough for added stability. When attaching the heart it is important to not pull the aorta too far up the cannula or the tip of the cannula may pass through the aortic valve. This is why one should seek to maximize the amount of aorta available by avoiding cutting the aorta much (<1 mm) beyond the first arterial junction in the direction of the heart itself. An incompetent aortic valve is easy to identify once the perfusion solution is switched on; the left ventricle bulges as it inflates with perfusate and paradoxically the coronary flow (under constant pressure perfusion) can be rather low since the cannula may occlude the coronary ostia. If this occurs the heart must be pushed down the cannula. This is tricky with the aorta tightly tied to the cannula, and is best avoided. There are marked species differences in our experience. The guinea pig heart has a rather short length of aorta between the heart and the brachiocephalic artery and during cardiac excision it is common to find that there is too little aorta present to avoid passing the cannula through the aortic valve, meaning that extra care is required during dissection.

Perfusion solution constituents, thermoregulation, and mode of delivery

The preparation and constituents of the perfusion solution are trivial yet vitally important aspects of Langendorff perfusion. First, we recommend filtration of perfusion solution prior to use. We use 5-μm pore filters to exclude particulate contaminants. We have no objective evidence that this has value but anecdotally our average baseline coronary flow values exceed by more than 50% the values we encountered before we used this approach. The most common solution used for heart perfusion is Krebs–Henseleit buffer. The problem with this solution is that it contains 5.9 mM potassium, a concentration that far exceeds normal plasma potassium values [31]. The reason for this is historical – in the past, estimates of blood potassium concentration tended to be overestimates owing to the influence of hemolysis or hypoxia, both of which can greatly elevate free potassium in a blood sample. The hyperkalemia of standard Krebs solution likely explains why prior to 1989, despite decades of experimentation with the Langendorff preparation, there had been almost no work done with it to examine ischemia-induced arrhythmias. We now know that standard Krebs, containing 5.9 mM potassium, prevents ischemia-induced ventricular fibrillation (VF) [8], explaining the absence of ischemia-induced VF in earlier studies using standard Krebs [32]. As a consequence, we now use 3 mM potassium for arrhythmia studies, which guarantees a high incidence of VF in control Langendorff perfused rat hearts [8]. This modification paved the way to allow protective drugs to be examined [14,15,33–36]. However, use of an intraventricular balloon to measure contractile function (see Section Recording of left ventricular pressure, ECG, and coronary flow) can evoke artifact arrhythmias; these can be prevented by slightly elevating the potassium concentration in the perfusion solution to 4 mM [6]. Thus for contractile function studies, Krebs solution containing 4 mM potassium is typically used (e.g. [37]). Calcium concentration may also affect arrhythmia susceptibility; an elevation from 1.4 mM to 2.8 mM appears to facilitate reperfusion-induced VF in relatively resistant species such as rabbit [14,15]. Finally, Krebs may be supplemented with other biochemicals to produce desirable hemodynamic or electrical properties of the preparation. For example, addition of norepinephrine (313 nM) and epinephrine (75 nM) to perfusion solutions has been used in the rat and mouse Langendorff preparation to restore heart rate to a level equivalent to that found in the conscious animal [13,18]. In the mouse this has the advantage of converting an ischemia-induced VF-resistant preparation to a susceptible preparation [13].

Thermoregulation is critically important. Among the many flaws introduced into early Langendorff studies was poor temperature control, which affects susceptibility to ischemia/reperfusion injury, hemodynamic performance, and the actions of drugs. In the rat heart, poor temperature control is easily evident from the values of heart rate. Cardiac cooling can result from inadequate insulation of Krebs solution or from low coronary flow, since this allows more time for heat loss from warmed perfusion solution before it enters the heart. If the temperature of the heart is dependent on flow rate,

it may be necessary to exclude the hearts in which the coronary flow is sufficiently outside the acceptable range to make the heart too warm (38°C) or too cold (35°C). To achieve good thermoregulation we use water-jacketed reservoirs to hold the perfusion solution and deliver it under gravity to the heart via a small manifold. A water-jacketed junction block or cannula can also be used to ensure the solution is at the desired temperature at the point it enters the heart to prevent fluctuation of temperature with variations in coronary flow (Figure 23.1). It is important to validate the set up by measuring the temperature of the solution leaving the cannula over a range of simulated coronary flows. In our system, values remain constant at the desired 37°C provided flow exceeds 1 mL/min (far lower than any encountered in rat or even mouse studies) [13].

The choice of whether to deliver perfusion solutions using constant pressure or constant flow is influenced by the nature of the experiment. Although we prefer constant pressure perfusion (gravity fed)

Cannulation, coronary ligature and regional ischemia

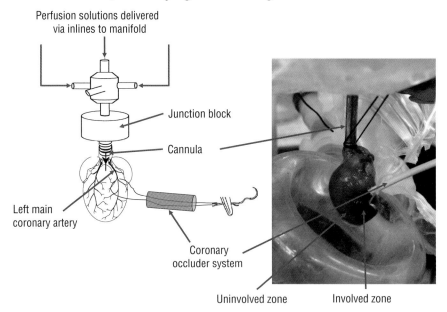

Figure 23.1 Cannulation of a Langendorff perfused heart, showing location of cannula in relation to perfusion solutions (from reservoirs, not shown) and the placement of a coronary ligature for regional ischemia studies. The photo is of a Langendorff perfused rat heart with regional ischemia, demarcated by disulfine blue entrapment in the involved region. Rat, rabbit, and mouse hearts are collateral-deficient meaning a vascular marker such as disulfine blue is trapped by coronary ligation, revealed when the solution is switch to wash out the marker from the uninvolved zone as shown.

we accept that constant flow perfusion may have an advantage in certain circumstances. One example is when it is impractical or unfeasible to load a large reservoir with a solution containing a drug and gas and warm the solution prior to delivery; this problem can be circumvented by delivering warmed and gassed Krebs solution using constant flow and infusing the drug into the Krebs solution at a known rate immediately prior to the solution entering the heart.

It is important to note that perfusion of hearts with Krebs buffer requires prior gassing of the solution with a mixture of oxygen and carbon dioxide. With the correct ratio of CO_2 to bicarbonate concentration, the solution will be amply oxygenated and will have a pH of 7.4. However, Krebs solution should be warmed at the same time it is gassed. This is because oxygen and carbon dioxide are more readily soluble in cold water, and subsequent warming of pregassed solution can result in formation of small bubbles in the perfusion lines, which can cause obstructive emboli if they enter the coronary vasculature. Bubble formation can be a particular problem in constant flow perfusion because the plumbing is usually not entirely arranged "top down" (unlike gravity-driven constant pressure perfusion).

Recording of left ventricular pressure, ECG, and coronary flow

ECG (or more precisely, electrogram) recording is easily achieved by impaling the ventricle with a needle electrode, with an electrode attached to the aortic cannula as the reference electrode [8], or by pressing a blunted needle cannula against the anterior surface of the left ventricle to minimize injury in smaller hearts [13]. The filtering settings for ECG recording and the possibility of recording from atria and apposing ventricles are described in more detail elsewhere [38]. Electrical noise can be a problem because common recording platforms, such as AD Instrument's PowerLab, require users to modify their ECG electrodes for use *in vitro*. Noise may be minimized by two techniques. The first is to ensure clean connections. Perfusion solution can leave insulating deposits and cause corrosion of electrodes. The regular inspection of leads and the avoidance of residual wetness after cleaning the apparatus are recommended. The latter can be

achieved by using boiling water in the final clean, or by rinsing or spraying with concentrated ethanol. The second is to ensure that the recording leads are kept well apart from mains electrical leads and any badly earthed electrical equipment.

Processing the ECG readout can be challenging. We are one of the few groups who have attempted to measure all major ECG intervals in the Langendorff preparation. The QT interval can be hard to determine, especially in mouse and rat hearts in which the T wave is superimposed in the QRS complex, which itself has a relatively long tail, meaning there can be substantial imprecision in locating exactly the point of 100% repolarization [13–15,35]. Our approach is to measure QT at 90% repolarization [18,34]. Processing arrhythmias can also be vexing. Further details can be found in a review [39].

Global ischemia can be induced simply by blocking supply of Krebs through the aortic cannula, and reperfusion occurs when flow is restored. Regional ischemia may be induced using a suture and fine tubing to fashion an occluder (Figure 23.1) to evoke ventricular arrhythmias [39]. The involved region of ischemia and/or reperfusion can be evaluated by dye exclusion (Figures 23.1 and 23.2). There are two ways in which this can be performed. Our preferred method involves perfusing the whole heart (involved and uninvolved zones) with blue disulfine dye, then reoccluding, to trap dye in the involved region, and restoring perfusion with normal Krebs solution to wash out the dye in the uninvolved tissue. Once the perfusate exiting from the heart becomes clear, perfusion can be stopped, and the involved (stained) and uninvolved (unstained) tissue are then separated carefully using fine scissors (Figure 23.2). A disadvantage of this method is that it will interfere with determination of how much of the involved zone is infarcted using triphenyltetrazolium chloride staining. In addition, stained involved tissue will also interfere with subsequent measurement of biochemical mediators in the involved tissue by photometric methods. Therefore an alternative method is to reocclude, and inject blue dye only into the uninvolved tissue. The involved tissue will remain unstained, and can then be used for infarct determination or photometric assay.

Contractile function may be measured using an intraventricular balloon. The requirements are that

Dissection of involved region

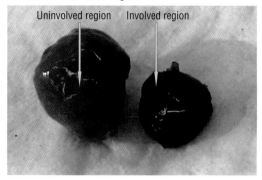

Figure 23.2 In a collateral deficient heart (rat shown here, rabbit or mouse) the involved zone is transmural and may be dissected from the uninvolved zone after demarcation with disulfine blue vascular marker entrapment.

the balloon be made of thin, compliant material that does not contribute to the values recorded, and which is oversized so the balloon itself is never inflated to a point that it generates a pressure over the range of inflation required in the experiment [28], as shown in Figure 23.3A. In our experience the best material to use to construct a balloon is plastic food wrap. It is important to validate the balloon by showing that added volume over the experimental range does not generate a pressure in the balloon (tested with the balloon attached to the recording device but not inserted into the heart). The longevity of the balloon is extended by keeping it soaked in liquid between use, and by filling it with liquid that is resistant to fungal growth. Saline serves for both these purposes. Balloon insertion can be tricky. The approach is to first wash the balloon in coronary effluent (as it drips from the heart), ensure it is fully deflated, and fashioned into a spear shape. The balloon should then be carefully inserted through the mitral valve into the left ventricle after a scissor snip is made in the left atrium or after the left atrium is completely excised (Figure 23.3B). A small inflation of the balloon (less than $10\,\mu L$ for a rat heart) will cause the pressure readout to lurch from negative to positive. If a graduated syringe is used for this purpose, the arbitrary value on the syringe is noted as the "zero volume", and the Starling curve may be generated by adding volumes from this value [19]. A typical Starling curve in a rat

Langendorff preparation will have a slope of added volume versus developed pressure that is much steeper than the slope for added volume versus diastolic pressure, and will obtain >70% of maximum developed pressure before the diastolic pressure has reached 10 mmHg (Figure 23.3C). However, following ischemia and reperfusion, severe injury is manifested by the added volume versus diastolic pressure slope exceeding the added volume versus developed pressure slope (Figure 23.3D).

Coronary flow may be measured simply by timed collection of coronary effluent since all effluent that exits the cut pulmonary artery must first pass through the coronary circulation [2,8]. The most accurate method for achieving this is to collect flow over a minute and weigh it, since 1 mL of water-based effluent weighs 1 g. In studies with regional ischemia, the rat heart, which is collateral deficient, generates a readout that allows calculation of flow recovery and hyperemia during reperfusion [20]. Also, provided constant pressure perfusion is used, shear stress is not altered by coronary vasodilatation meaning that shear-stress-independent effects of drugs and disease may be examined [40]. Likewise, provided that constant pressure perfusion is used, coronary flow in the uninvolved region is not altered by regional ischemia caused by adjacent coronary ligation or (during reperfusion) by coronary steal [2].

Alternative approaches

Excluding consideration of *in vivo* methodology, which is beyond the scope of this chapter, there are other modes of heart perfusion that may be considered. The most well known is the "working" heart preparation of Neely [41]. Here the left atrium is cannulated and the heart ejects perfusate from the aorta against a set afterload. The advantages of this preparation are that cardiac output may be measured directly. Disadvantages are noted in the following text.

A modification of the Langendorff preparation known as the Dual Perfusion model [42] is a technically more demanding preparation with certain advantages. Here a dual lumen catheter is inserted into the aorta allowing independent perfusion of the left and right coronary beds. This is

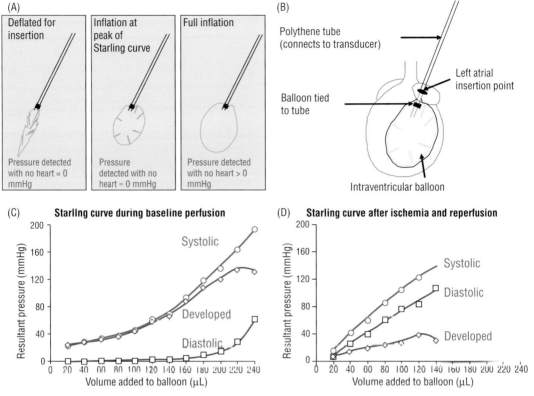

Figure 23.3 (A) Left ventricular pressure recording is achieved in the Langendorff preparation using a home-made balloon from thin kitchen food wrap available in the USA, Europe, and elsewhere. The requirements are that the balloon is sufficiently small that it may be inserted deflated into the left ventricle and remain in position as it is inflated, and sufficiently large that it would not be fully inflated and therefore would not itself generate any pressure when inflated inside the left ventricle to generate peak developed pressure (peak of the Starling curve). This means that when fully inflated (to generate a pressure from its own inflation) its volume would exceed that of the ventricular lumen (impossible without causing an unphysiological elevation of diastolic pressure). (B) Left ventricular pressure recording in a Langendorff heart, showing (in cutaway) an appropriately proportioned balloon partially inflated sufficient to generate peak pressure development. (C) A Starling curve generated by balloon inflation in a Langendorff perfused rat heart. Developed pressure reaches 70% maximum before diastolic pressure reaches 10 mmHg in a healthy heart. (D) A Starling curve generated by balloon inflation in a Langendorff perfused rat heart subjected to 30-minute normothermic global ischemia and 30-minute normothermic reperfusion. Developed pressure is severely attenuated at all added balloon volumes (impaired inotropy), while diastolic pressure rises steeply with added volume, indicating impaired relaxation (impaired lusitropy and/or stiffness). Crossover of the diastolic and developed pressure curves indicates severe diastolic and systolic dysfunction. Systolic pressure values are not in themselves useful indices of healthy function (compare readout with the trace shown in (C)).

useful in species that are coronary collateral deficient, such as the rat and mouse. The difficulty is the process of alignment of the holes in the cannula with the coronary ostia. This requires training and practice. However the preparation has the advantage that it allows bioassay of putative arrhythmogenic mediators, and determination of the site of action (and hence the mechanism of action) of test agents [22,43–46].

Weaknesses and strengths of the method

The Langendorff preparation will allow assessment of any available readout with obvious limitations. Often the limitations are perceived rather than validated. For example the preparation is often described in rather pejorative terms as "retrograde perfused." This is a misconception since the coronary vessels are orthograde perfused in the Langendorff preparation. The only part of the perfusion that is retrograde is that in the aortic arch, and this is not relevant (and indeed the blood that enters the coronaries *in vivo* is ejected from the left ventricle and therefore must enter the coronary ostia "retrogradely" in relation to the prevailing direction of aortic flow). True weaknesses of the preparation are those validated to represent flaws that generate data that misleads. There are examples.

Coronary flow in the crystalloid-perfused Langendorff preparation is approximately fivefold more than that in equivalent hearts *in vivo*. Use of blood instead of crystalloid solution rectifies this [17], but brings additional difficulties that offset the benefit. The crystalloid-perfused heart has the advantage that drug concentrations are easily set by adding known amounts to the perfusion solution. There is no need to sample the solution leaving the cannula and assay the drug content unless there is reason to suspect the drug binds to the apparatus (whether it be made of glass or plastic). Certainly, one should consider this possibility. However in blood-perfused hearts measurement of free drug content is mandatory in order to account for plasma protein binding. The blood-perfused model is also flawed owing to the activation of platelets and the binding of white blood cells to components of the recirculation processes (including the support animal) [17].

Poor recovery of flow upon reperfusion may be problematic since it may extend the duration of ischemia and make the beneficial effects of a drug hard to detect. There is a greater likelihood of this being a problem in the reperfused globally ischemic heart, because beating of the heart assists the flow of solution through the coronary vasculature. However, in our experience we typically observe hyperemia rather than hypoperfusion upon reperfusion, although the extent of flow recovery does depend on the duration of the preceding ischemic period [47]. In addition, poor recovery of flow is likely to reflect the intrinsic biology of the preparation rather than being a limitation of the model, because in the constant pressure perfusion mode that mimics the *in vivo* situation, flow is dependent only on vascular resistance, which is an independent property. Thus while regional hypercontracture that might result in poor recovery of flow might be important clinically it is not a limitation of the isolated perfused heart preparation per se.

Compared with the working heart preparation, it is not possible to measure cardiac output directly. Instead one relies upon measurement of contractility under isovolumic conditions. This is not physiological. However the "working" aspect (the hemodynamic expense of external work) of the "working" heart preparation has theoretical rather than practical advantages over the Langendorff preparation. The Langendorff preparation allows generation of Starling curves and assessment of systolic and diastolic function rather easily by inflating the intraventricular balloon [36,37]. By comparison, in the working heart, although it is possible to alter preload, it is not possible to regulate end diastolic pressure as precisely as achievable in the Langendorff preparation.

Conclusions

The Langendorff preparation is simple to use, versatile, and robust. There are some methodological quirks that differ between species, and provided care is taken the model can generate a range of valuable readouts.

References

1 Langendorff O. Untersuchen am uberlebenden Saugethierherzen. *Pflugers Arch* 1895; **66**: 291–332.

2 Ctis MJ, Hearse DJ. Reperfusion-induced arrhythmias are critically dependent upon occluded zone size: relevance to the mechanism of arrhythmogenesis. *J Mol Cell Cardiol* 1989; **21**: 625–637.

3 Johns TNP, Olson BJ. Experimental myocardial infarction. 1. A method of coronary occlusion in small animals. *Ann Surg* 1954; **140**: 675–682.

4 Curtis MJ, Johnston KM, Macleod BA, Walker MJ. The actions of felodipine on arrhythmias and other responses to myocardial ischaemia in conscious rats. *Eur J Pharmacol* 1985; **117**: 169–178.

5 Curtis MJ, Macleod BA, Walker MJ. Models for the study of arrhythmias in myocardial ischaemia and infarction: the use of the rat. *J Mol Cell Cardiol* 1987; **19**: 399–419.

6 Curtis MJ, Walker MJ. The mechanism of action of the optical enantiomers of verapamil against ischaemia-induced arrhythmias in the conscious rat. *Br J Pharmacol* 1986; **89**: 137–147.

7 Bernier M, Curtis MJ, Hearse DJ. Ischemia-induced and reperfusion-induced arrhythmias: importance of heart rate. *Am J Physiol* 1989; **256**: H21–31.

8 Curtis MJ, Hearse DJ. Ischaemia-induced and reperfusion-induced arrhythmias differ in their sensitivity to potassium: implications for mechanisms of initiation and maintenance of ventricular fibrillation. *J Mol Cell Cardiol* 1989; **21**: 21–40.

9 Nakata T, Hearse DJ, Curtis MJ. Are reperfusion-induced arrhythmias caused by disinhibition of an arrhythmogenic component of ischemia? *J Mol Cell Cardiol* 1990; **22**: 843–858.

10 Farkas A, Curtis MJ. Limited antifibrillatory effectiveness of clinically relevant concentrations of class I antiarrhythmics in isolated perfused rat hearts. *J Cardiovasc Pharmacol* 2002; **39**: 412–424.

11 Yamada M, Hearse DJ, Curtis MJ. Reperfusion and readmission of oxygen. Pathophysiological relevance of oxygen-derived free radicals to arrhythmogenesis. *Circ Res* 1990; **67**: 1211–1224.

12 Mitchell GF, Jeron A, Koren G. Measurement of heart rate and Q-T interval in the conscious mouse. *Am J Physiol* 1998; **274**: H747–751.

13 Stables CL, Curtis MJ. Development and characterization of a mouse in vitro model of ischaemia-induced ventricular fibrillation. *Cardiovas Res* 2009; **83**: 397–404.

14 Rees SA, Curtis MJ. Specific IK1 blockade: a new antiarrhythmic mechanism? Effect of RP58866 on ventricular arrhythmias in rat, rabbit, and primate. *Circulation* 1993; **87**: 1979–1989.

15 Rees SA, Curtis MJ. Selective IK blockade as an antiarrhythmic mechanism: effects of UK66,914 on ischaemia and reperfusion arrhythmias in rat and rabbit hearts. *Br J Pharmacol* 1993; **108**: 139–145.

16 Murakami H, Liu JL, Zucker IH. Blockade of AT1 receptors enhances baroreflex control of heart rate in conscious rabbits with heart failure. *Am J Physiol* 1996; **271**: R303–309.

17 Clements-Jewery H, Hearse DJ, Curtis MJ. The isolated blood-perfused rat heart: an inappropriate model for the study of ischaemia- and infarction-related ventricular fibrillation. *Br J Pharmacol* 2002; **137**: 1089–1099.

18 Clements-Jewery H, Hearse DJ, Curtis MJ. Independent contribution of catecholamines to arrhythmogenesis during evolving infarction in the isolated rat heart. *Br J Pharmacol* 2002; **135**: 807–815.

19 Farkas A, Qureshi A, Curtis MJ. Inadequate ischaemia-selectivity limits the antiarrhythmic efficacy of mibefradil during regional ischaemia and reperfusion in the rat isolated perfused heart. *Br J Pharmacol* 1999; **128**: 41–50.

20 Pabla R, Curtis MJ. Effects of NO modulation on cardiac arrhythmias in the rat isolated heart. *Circ Res* 1995; **77**: 984–992.

21 Pabla R, Bland-Ward P, Moore PK, Curtis MJ. An endogenous protectant effect of cardiac cyclic GMP against reperfusion-induced ventricular fibrillation in the rat heart. *Br J Pharmacol* 1995; **116**: 2923–2930.

22 Baker KE, Curtis MJ. Protection against ventricular fibrillation by the PAF antagonist, BN- 50739, involves an ischaemia-selective mechanism. *J Cardiovasc Pharmacol* 1999; **34**: 394–401.

23 Ridley PD, Yacoub MH, Curtis MJ. A modified model of global ischaemia: application to the study of syncytial mechanisms of arrhythmogenesis. *Cardiovasc Res* 1992; **26**: 309–315.

24 Rees SA, Tsuchihashi K, Hearse DJ, Curtis MJ. Combined administration of an IK(ATP) activator and Ito blocker increases coronary flow independently of effects on heart rate, QT interval, and ischaemia-induced ventricular fibrillation in rats. *J Cardiovasc Pharmacol* 1993; **22**: 343–349.

25 Ellwood AJ, Curtis MJ. Mechanism of 5-hydroxytryptamine-induced coronary vasodilation assessed by direct detection of nitric oxide production in guinea-pig isolated heart. *Br J Pharmacol* 1996; **119**: 721–729.

26 Ellwood AJ, Curtis MJ. Mechanism of actions of sumatriptan on coronary flow before and after endothelial dysfunction in guinea-pig isolated heart. *Br J Pharmacol* 1997; **120**: 1039–1048.

27 Karthik S, Grayson AD, Oo AY, Fabri BM. A survey of current myocardial protection practices during coronary artery bypass grafting. *Ann R Coll Surg Engl* 2004; **86**: 413–415.

28 Curtis MJ, Macleod BA, Tabrizchi R, Walker MJ. An improved perfusion apparatus for small animal hearts. *J Pharmacol Methods* 1986; **15**: 87–94.

29 Farkas A, Curtis MJ. Does QT widening in the Langendorff-perfused rat heart represent the effect of repolarization delay or conduction slowing? *J Cardiovasc Pharmacol* 2003; **42**: 612–621.

30 Hatcher AS, Alderson JM, Clements-Jewery H. Mitochondrial uncoupling agents trigger ventricular fibrillation in isolated rat hearts. *J Cardiovasc Pharmacol* 2011; **57**: 439–446.

31 Nordrehaug JE, von der Lippe G. Hypokalaemia and ventricular fibrillation in acute myocardial infarction. *Br Heart J* 1983; **50**: 525–529.

32 Curtis MJ, Macleod BA, Walker MJ. The effects of ablations in the central nervous system on arrhythmias induced by coronary occlusion in the rat. *Br J Pharmacol* 1985; **86**: 663–670.

33 Tsuchihashi K, Curtis MJ. Influence of tedisamil on the initiation and maintenance of ventricular fibrillation: chemical defibrillation by Ito blockade? *J Cardiovasc Pharmacol* 1991; **18**: 445–456.

34 Ridley PD, Curtis MJ. Anion manipulation: a new antiarrhythmic approach. Action of substitution of

chloride with nitrate on ischemia- and reperfusion-induced ventricular fibrillation and contractile function. *Circ Res* 1992; **70**: 617–632.

35 Rees SA, Curtis MJ. Tacrine inhibits ventricular fibrillation induced by ischaemia and reperfusion and widens QT interval in rat. *Cardiovasc Res* 1993; **27**: 453–458.

36 Curtis MJ, Garlick PB, Ridley PD. Anion manipulation, a novel antiarrhythmic approach: mechanism of action. *J Mol Cell Cardiol* 1993; **25**: 417–436.

37 Pabla R, Curtis MJ. Effect of endogenous nitric oxide on cardiac systolic and diastolic function during ischemia and reperfusion in the rat isolated perfused heart. *J Mol Cell Cardiol* 1996; **28**: 2111–2121.

38 Curtis MJ, Baczko I, Baker KE. The ECG in man and laboratory animals: recording methods, analysis and interpretation. In: Walker MJA, Pugsley MK, eds. *Methods in Cardiac Electrophysiology*. Basel, Switzerland: CRC Press, 1997, pp. 105–130.

39 Curtis MJ. Characterisation, utilisation and clinical relevance of isolated perfused heart models of ischaemia-induced ventricular fibrillation. *Cardiovasc Res* 1998; **39**: 194–215.

40 Ellwood AJ, Curtis MJ. The role of shear stress-independent release of nitric oxide in mediating drug-induced coronary vasodilatation can be assessed in the Langendorff constant pressure perfusion preparation. *Med Sci Res* 1998; **26**: 79–81.

41 Rovetto MJ, Whitmer JT, Neely JR. Comparison of the effects of anoxia and whole heart ischemia on carbohydrate utilization in isolated working rat hearts. *Circ Res* 1973; **32**: 699–711.

42 Avkiran M, Curtis MJ. Independent dual perfusion of left and right coronary arteries in isolated rat hearts. *Am J Physiol Heart Circ Physiol* 1991; **261**: H2082–2090.

43 Baker KE, Curtis MJ. Left regional cardiac perfusion in vitro with platelet-activating factor, norepinephrine and K+ reveals that ischaemic arrhythmias are caused by independent effects of endogenous "mediators" facilitated by interactions, and moderated by paradoxical antagonism. *Br J Pharmacol* 2004; **142**: 352–366.

44 Curtis MJ. The rabbit dual coronary perfusion model: a new method for assessing the pathological relevance of individual products of the ischaemic milieu: role of potassium in arrhythmogenesis. *Circ Res* 1991; **25**: 1010–1022.

45 Rees SA, Curtis MJ. Further investigations into the mechanism of antifibrillatory action of the specific IK1 blocker, RP58866, assessed using the rat dual coronary perfusion model. *J Mol Cell Cardiol* 1995; **27**: 2595–2606.

46 Baker KE, Wood LM, Whittaker M, Curtis MJ. Nupafant, a PAF-antagonist prototype for suppression of ventricular fibrillation without liability for QT prolongation? *Br J Pharmacol* 2006; **149**: 269–276.

47 Ravingerova T, Tribulova N, Slezak J, Curtis MJ. Brief, intermediate and prolonged ischemia in the isolated crystalloid perfused rat heart: relationship between susceptibility to arrhythmias and degree of ultrastructural injury. *J Mol Cell Cardiol* 1995; **27**: 1937–1951.

24 Myocarditis and other immunological models of cardiac disease

Daniela Čiháková and Noel R. Rose

Johns Hopkins University, Baltimore, MD, USA

Introduction

Myocarditis is an important cause of heart disease, predominantly among children and young adults. Most people with viral myocarditis recover, but about one-third may progress to dilated cardiomyopathy [1,2]. The most common virus associated with human myocarditis in the United States is Coxsackievirus B3 (CVB3), which can lead to autoimmune myocarditis in genetically predisposed individuals [3,4]. Similar dependence on genetic susceptibility can be observed in the murine model of CVB3-induced myocarditis, where all mice develop acute viral myocarditis, but only susceptible strains develop chronic, autoimmune myocarditis [5]. We identified mouse cardiac myosin heavy chain as the major antigen associated with viral myocarditis and we were able to induce experimental autoimmune myocarditis (EAM) in mice by immunization with cardiac myosin purified from murine hearts and adjuvant [6,7]. In some mouse strains (A/J, BALB/c), the cardiac α-myosin heavy chain peptide sequences that are able to induce EAM have been identified [8–10]. To produce EAM, complete Freund's adjuvant (CFA) is injected with the antigen (myosin or myocarditogenic peptide) twice, 7 days apart. Inflammation in the heart appears about 14 days after the first injection, peaks around day 21 and then gradually declines, although, in some mice can persist to day 60 or later. At later time points, inflammation is reduced and fibrosis is evident in the heart.

Only certain mouse strains are susceptible to EAM. Usually, susceptible mice have an "A" background, such as A/J, A.CA, and A.SW. Moderate responders are BALB/c mice, while C57BL/10 and C57BL/6 are resistant to EAM [7].

Protocol

Induction of EAM

The following describes our standard protocol for induction of EAM with myosin or α-cardiac myosin heavy chain peptide. We have previously published the procedure for the preparation of murine cardiac myosin [9].

Material and equipment

1. Cardiac myosin, or α-cardiac myosin heavy chain peptide (henceforth peptide), is used for EAM induction. For A/J mice, the myocarditogenic peptide is mc-myhc-α position 334–352 with the amino acid sequence, DSAFDVLSFTAEEKAGVYK [10]. For BALB/c mice, it is the peptide position 614–643 with the sequence, Ac-SLKLMATLFSTYASADTGDSGKGKGGKKKG [11]. Recently, a shorter version of this peptide (myhc-α 614–629) was reported, Ac-SLKLMATLFSTYASAD-OH) [8].

Manual of Research Techniques in Cardiovascular Medicine, First Edition. Edited by Hossein Ardehali, Roberto Bolli, and Douglas W. Losordo.

2. CFA (Sigma, St. Louis, MO, USA) supplemented with 4 mg/mL of heat-killed *Mycobacterium tuberculosis* strain H37Ra (Difco, Detroit, MI, USA).

3. *Bordetella pertussis* toxin (List Biological Laboratories): prepare 50 µg/100mL stock dilution in sterile double-distilled water (ddH₂O).

4. Phosphate buffer saline (PBS) 1%, sterile. (Biofluids).

5. 2 × 1-mL glass syringes with slots (Hamilton, Nevada).

6. stopcock.

7. Sterile needles 25 G.

8. 1-mL plastic syringes.

9. Susceptible mouse strain, sex matched, aged matched, typically 6–10 weeks old.

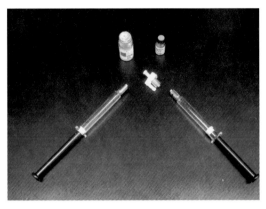

Figure 24.1 Material needed for emulsion preparation: two glass syringes, stopcock reconstituted peptide, and supplemented CFA.

Day 1

To induce disease using peptide, choose the correct peptide based on the mouse strain selected (BALB/c or A/J) and proceed with Step 1A. To immunize mice with cardiac myosin, proceed to Step 1B.

1A. Peptide reconstitution: for one mouse, 100 nmol of peptide is needed, but allow for additional 10–20% for loss in the syringes. Dilute the peptide in 1% PBS to a concentration of 100 nmol of peptide per 50 µL (the dose for one mouse). Leave the peptide at room temperature for 30 minutes to dissolve completely.

1B. Cardiac myosin is dissolved in 1×PBS 100–250 µg/50 µL (the dose for one mouse), depending on the degree of disease that you wish to achieve. Similar to Step 1A, add 10–20% for losses. The final emulsion will be diluted 1:1 with CFA; so the final myosin concentration should be 100–250 µg/100 µL.

2. Prepare two glass syringes with slots, coupler, reconstituted peptide or myosin, and supplemented CFA (Figure 24.1). The volume of the glass syringe should be more than twice the volume of the myosin or peptide solution that is used.

3. Draw all the peptide or myosin solution in the first syringe and remove the needle. Gently advance the plunger to push the air bubbles out and have the solution at the tip of the syringe.

4. Mix CFA and transfer an equal volume immediately into a second glass syringe. Connect the stopcock to the CFA syringe; push CFA in the stopcock until it is visible in the opposite orifice. Now attach the first syringe with the peptide or myosin to the stopcock.

5. Push CFA very slowly into the syringe with myosin/ peptide. During the process, rotate both syringes so that the oily CFA mixes with the watery myosin or peptide. Repeat very slowly, mixing the content by pushing it back and forth from one syringe to the other. Continue until the fluid in the syringes is homogenous.

6. Start to mix faster, while ensuring that the stopcock is tight and the emulsion is not leaking. The process of mixing can take about 45–60 minutes or even longer (Video clip 24.1). The key is to make a thick and stable emulsion. When there is resistance while mixing, test the thickness of the emulsion by placing a drop on a surface of water in small beaker. The drop should remain intact rather than dispersing (Figure 24.2).

7. Dilute pertussis toxin from stock (concentration 50 µg/100 µL) to 1:100 in sterile 1% PBS (final concentration 500 ng/100 µL). The dose for one mouse is 500 ng in 100 µL. Draw the final dilution of toxin in a 1-mL plastic syringe.

8. Anesthetize the mouse.

9. Inject 0.1 mL of emulsion subcutaneously in the posterior axillary area. If the emulsion is thick and well prepared the emulsion deposit will be visible under the skin and will not leak out.

10. Inject 0.1 mL of the pertussis toxin intraperitoneally (the dose should be 500 ng/mouse).

Day 7: Boost

Repeat the Steps 1–8 from day 0, but do not use pertussis toxin. Inject the emulsion into the side opposite to the one used on day 0.

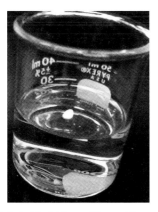

Figure 24.2 Test of the thickness of the emulsion on water surface in a small beaker. The emulsion drop should remain intact rather than dispersing.

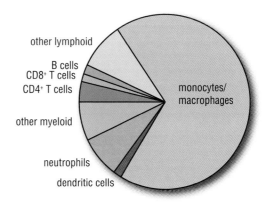

Figure 24.3 Example of cells infiltrating the heart as found in the WT Balb/c mice heart on day 21 of EAM by flow cytometry.

Day 21: Sacrifice day and assessment of myocarditis

Anesthetize the mice and weigh them. Remove their hearts. Gently squeeze blood from the hearts. Weigh the hearts. Fix each heart in 10% formalin or SafeFix (Fisher Scientific). Have the tissues embedded longitudinally, and 5-μm serial sections cut and stained with hematoxylin and eosin. To obtain additional information about the cellular composition of the infiltrate, identify heart-infiltrating leukocytes by flow cytometry. We have published a protocol previously [12]. In short, the heart is perfused through the aorta for 3 minutes with $1 \times$ PBS + 0.5% FBS, and digested in GentleMACS C Tubes according to manufacturer's instructions (Miltenyi Biotec). Prior to surface staining, viability is determined by LIVE/DEAD staining according to manufacturer's instructions (Molecular Probes). Cells are washed and FcγRII/III blocked with αCD16/32 (eBiosciences). Surface markers are stained with fluorochrome-conjugated mAbs (eBiosciences, BD Pharmingen, BioLegend). The cardiac infiltrate consist mostly of monocytes/macrophages (up to 75% of CD45+ cells in the heart). Neutrophils, CD4+ T cells, CD8+ T cells, NK cells, B cells, γδ T cells, mast cells, and eosinophils can also identified in the infiltrate (Figure 24.3).

Histology assessment of EAM

Measure the percentage of myocardium infiltrated with lymphocytes and fibrosis under a microscope,

Table 24.1 EAM severity grading for histology scoring

Score	Percent of inflammation in the heart
1	less than 10%
2	10–30%
3	30–50%
4	50–90%
5	more than 90%

using the scoring system in Table 24.1. A grid in the microscope is helpful for the calculation. Examples of mild and severe disease are shown in Figure 24.4. Grading should be performed by a minimum of two independent, blinded investigators and scores averaged.

Notes

• BALB/c short peptide is very difficult to dissolve, necessitating addition of dimethyl sulfoxide (DMSO) to maximal final concentration of 2%. A/J peptide usually does not require DMSO to dissolve.

• Dissolved peptide could be kept in +4°C for about a week. It can be also frozen and used for a few months.

• CFA contains dead *Mycobacterium tuberculosis* which can not cause infection, but may be considered immunogenic. Therefore, caution is necessary while working with CFA. Wear an eye protection, mask, and gloves.

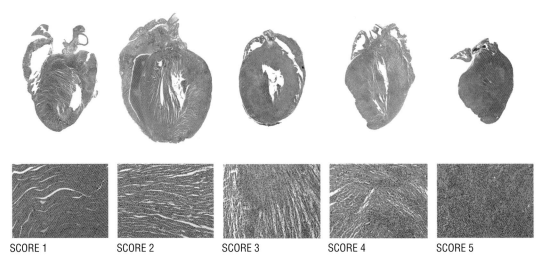

SCORE 1   SCORE 2   SCORE 3   SCORE 4   SCORE 5

Figure 24.4 Example of EAM severity grading for histology scoring: score 1, infiltrating cells are present in less than 10% of heart section; score 2, 10–30%; score 3, 30–50%; score 4, 50–90%; score 5, more than 90%.

• Pertussis toxin is a biological toxin and many institutions will allow only registered users to work with it. Make all necessary steps to assure compliance with biosafety requirements of your institution.

• When working with pertussis toxin, use a mask in addition to lab coat and gloves and work in a hood. It is best to reconstitute the toxin through the rubber cap without opening the bottle to minimize the possible exposure.

• A thick, stable emulsion is critical for EAM induction. The most important step is slow mixing in the first phase of emulsification. Use only a ratio of CFA to peptide solution of 1:1.

• The use of supplemented CFA is needed on both days 0 and 7. Efforts to replace at least one CFA immunization with different adjuvant such as incomplete Freund adjuvant led to failure to induce myocarditis (Cihakova *et al.*, manuscript in preparation).

• In our experience, pertussis toxin is not essential for EAM induction. However, mice injected with the pertussis toxin on day 0 have more severe myocarditis. Two injections of pertussis toxin (on day 0 and day 7) are not advisable, since they do not increase disease severity.

• If the emulsion remains fluid despite being mixed for over 1 hour, it is possible that the emulsion is too warm. Placing both syringes with stopcock on ice for

about 30 minutes should help in making the emulsion more stable.

• It is critical that each mouse in an experiment receive the same amount of antigen. To make sure that the same amount of the emulsion is injected to each mouse, bubbles must be removed from the emulsion. Be careful when removing the needle from the mouse skin so that the emulsion does not leak out.

Alternative approaches

Other myocarditis models can be used as alternatives to EAM. Coxsackie B3 virus induced myocarditis has two stages of heart inflammation. All mice strains develop acute viral myocarditis, but only susceptible strains will develop chronic, autoimmune myocarditis [5]. The susceptibility of mouse strains, immune responses, and the histological changes in the chronic stage of CVB3-induced myocarditis closely resemble EAM. CVB3-myocarditis murine models have an advantage in providing the opportunity to study both stages of heart infiltration, i.e. viral and autoimmune; however, the presence of the virus comes with challenges in interpreting the results. Use of knockout mice that do not produce certain inflammatory cytokines might interfere with the mouse's ability to clear the virus during the first stage of the disease. The myosin-induced model enables an investigator to examine the autoimmune form of heart disease without concern for the viral clearance. Another advantage of EAM is lower requirement for equipment, laboratory space, and trained personnel since working with live CVB3 virus is strictly regulated. On the other hand, if viral myocarditis is the focus of the research, CVB3-myocarditis is preferred to EAM. Another myocarditis model available to investigators is troponin I myocarditis, which is induced by immunization with troponin I and CFA [13]. A CFA-free model of myocarditis induction using activated and self-antigen loaded dendritic cells transfer has also been described [14].

Strength and weaknesses of the method

EAM is a well-defined and widely studied model of myocarditis. The model enables the researcher to examine processes involved in inflammatory heart disease and events responsible for cardiac remodeling, fibrosis, and failure. Given that about 75% of the infiltrate are cells of monocytic lineage, EAM closely resembles giant cell myocarditis in humans [12]. The availability of α-cardiac myosin heavy chain peptide for A/J and BALB/c mice allows a relatively convenient use of this model without tedious preparation of cardiac myosin. The fact that the susceptible mice are white strains such as A/J and BALB/c mice, limits the use of more widely available genetically modified black strains. Induction of the EAM model is dependent on flawless preparation of the emulsion.

Conclusions

In this chapter, we have described the induction of EAM in a susceptible strain of mice using myosin or α-cardiac myosin heavy chain peptide emulsified in CFA. We have emphasized the necessary steps for a successful preparation of the emulsion, which is a key factor in a successful implementation of the EAM model.

Acknowledgement

The authors would like to thank SuFey Ong for help with Figure 24.4, Jobert Barin for providing Figure 24.3 and Lei Wu for help with the demonstration of emulsion preparation in the video clip. This work was supported by NIH/NHLBI grants R01 HL67290, R01 HL113008, and a Grant-in-Aid from the American Heart Association (to Noel Rose). Daniela Cihakova was supported by the Michel Mirowski MD Discovery Foundation; the W.W. Smith Charitable Trust, heart research grant H1103, and the Children's Cardiomyopathy Foundation.

References

1 Rose NR, Hill SL. Autoimmune myocarditis. *In J Cardiol* 1996; **54**: 171–175.

2 Rose NR, Afanasyeva M. From infection to autoimmunity: the adjuvant effect. *ASM News* 2003; **69**: 132–137.

3 Rose NR, Neumann DA, Herkowitz A. Coxsackievirus myocarditis. In: Stollerman GH, LaMont JT, Leonard JJ, Siperstein MD, eds. *Advances in Internal Medicine*. St. Louis, Missouri: Mosby Year Book, 1992, 411–429.

4 Rose NR, Wolfgram LJ, Herkowitz A, Beisel KW. Postinfectious autoimmunity: two distinct phases of Coxsackievirus B3-induced myocarditis. *Ann New York Acad Sci* 1986; **475**: 146–156.

5 Fairweather D, Kaya Z, Shellam GR, Lawson CM, Rose NR. From infection to autoimmunity. *J Autoimmun* 2001; **16**: 175–186.

6 Neu N, Beisel KW, Traystman MD, Rose NR, Craig SW. Autoantibodies specific for the cardiac myosin isoform are found in mice susceptible to Coxsackievirus B3-induced myocarditis. *J Immunol* 1987; **138**: 2488–2492.

7 Neu N, Rose NR, Beisel KW, Herskowitz A, Gurri-Glass G, Craig SW, *et al*. Cardiac myosin induces myocarditis in genetically predisposed mice. *J Immunol* 1987; **139**: 3630–3636.

8 Eriksson U, Kurrer MO, Sonderegger I, Iezzi G, Tafuri A, Hunziker L, *et al*. Activation of dendritic cells through the interleukin 1 receptor 1 is critical for the induction of autoimmune myocarditis. *J Exp Med* 2003; **197**: 323–331.

9 Cihákova D, Sharma RB, Fairweather D, Afanasyeva M, Rose NR. Animal models for autoimmune myocarditis and autoimmune thyroiditis. *Methods Mol Med* 2004; **102**: 175–193.

10 Donermeyer DL, Beisel KW, Allen PM, Smith SC. Myocarditis-inducing epitope of myosin binds constitutively and stably to I-Ak on antigen-presenting cells in the heart. *J Exp Med* 1995; **182**: 1291–1300.

11 Pummerer CL, Luze K, Grassl G, Bachmaier K, Offner F, Burrell SK, *et al*. Identification of cardiac myosin peptides capable of inducing autoimmune myocarditis in BALB/c mice. *J Clin Invest* 1996; **97**: 2057–2062.

12 Afanasyeva M, Georgakopoulos D, Belardi DF, Ramsundar AC, Barin JG, Kass DA, *et al.* Quantitative analysis of myocardial inflammation by flow cytometry in murine autoimmune myocarditis: correlation with cardiac function. *Am J Pathol* 2004; **164**: 807.

13 Göser S, Andrassy M, Buss SJ, Leuschner F, Volz CH, Ottl R, *et al.* Cardiac troponin I but not cardiac troponin T induces severe autoimmune inflammation in the myocardium. *Circulation* 2006; **114**: 1693–1702.

14 Eriksson U, Ricci R, Hunziker L, Kurrer MO, Oudit GY, Watts TH, *et al.* Dendritic cell-induced autoimmune heart failure requires cooperation between adaptive and innate immunity. *Nat Med* 2003; **9**: 1484–1490.

Models of pacing-induced heart failure

James A. Shuman, Rupak Mukherjee, and Francis G. Spinale

University of South Carolina School of Medicine, Columbia, SC and Medical University of South Carolina, Charleston, SC, USA

Introduction

Congestive heart failure (CHF) is a constellation of signs and symptoms, which include shortness of breath and exercise intolerance. While the precipitating events and etiologies for the initiation of CHF are diverse, the primary underlying defect is the inability of the left ventricle (LV) to maintain an adequate forward stroke volume. Accordingly, significant research efforts have focused upon the fundamental mechanisms that contribute to the initiation and progressive changes in LV pump function that occurs with CHF. One important cause of CHF is the dilated cardiomyopathies (DCMs) that comprise a family of intrinsic myocardial disease states. While the originating stimuli for the initiation and progression of DCM can be diverse, there is uniformity in key changes that occur with respect to LV geometry, function, and neurohormonal systems. Specifically, DCM is characterized by remodeling the LV myocardium in such a manner as to cause LV chamber dilation without a parallel growth in wall thickness, resulting in significantly increased wall stress. This amplified LV wall stress places an additional load upon the myocardium, in which there is a significant and inherent impairment of the contractile performance of the cardiac myocytes. As a consequence, all indices of LV ejection performance are severely reduced and thereby forward stroke volume and systemic perfusion become compromised. The increased LV volumes with reduced ejection performance result in high venous and capillary hydrostatic pressures and cause peripheral and pulmonary edema. The reduction in systemic perfusion in turn provokes compensatory neurohormonal and renal mechanisms, such as increased catecholamine synthesis and release, activation of the renin–angiotensin–aldosterone system (RAAS), and increased expression and production of bioactive peptides, such as endothelin and natriuretic factors. These changes in LV geometry, function, and neurohormonal pathways give rise to the constellation of signs and symptoms of CHF. Since clinical presentation of DCM is often in accompaniment with CHF, it is often difficult to determine the natural history and pathogenesis of this process. Moreover, mechanistic studies that could identify underlying cellular and molecular pathways contributing to DCM can be problematic in the clinical context. Thus, the identification of contributory mechanisms and potential therapeutic targets for DCM would require the use of an animal model that would properly recapitulate the clinical phenotype of DCM and progression to CHF.

The DCM phenotype can be achieved in rodent models through using genetic constructs, infectious, or toxin-based approaches, which are presented in other sections of this text. However, one large animal model that fulfills the criteria in terms of the clinical

Manual of Research Techniques in Cardiovascular Medicine, First Edition. Edited by Hossein Ardehali, Roberto Bolli, and Douglas W. Losordo.

phenotype of DCM and progression to CHF is that of chronic rapid pacing. This rapid pacing model was initially characterized by Wipple and colleagues in the early 1960s [1]. Since that time, this rapid pacing model has been utilized for a number of mechanistic and interventional studies, and a recent National Library of Medicine search (PubMed; Feb 2012) revealed over 1500 publications using this animal model. The scope of this chapter will be to address several fundamental issues regarding this animal model:

1. describe the generalized techniques, approaches, and technical considerations of the rapid pacing model;
2. examine the progression of changes in LV geometry and function that reflect the DCM morphology with chronic rapid pacing;
3. identify common neurohormonal pathways activated in this rapid pacing model as well as relevant receptor transduction pathways with a particular focus on those likely to hold relevance or parallel clinical DCM;
4. demonstrate how this rapid pacing model has been utilized to examine cellular and molecular pathways during the initiation and progression of DCM;
5. explore potential substrates in terms of electrophysiology relevant to arrhythmogenicity with chronic rapid pacing;
6. provide examples of how this rapid pacing model has been utilized in pharmacology and device studies;
7. provide a decision template for when this rapid pacing model of DCM may be of utility.

Rapid pacing models – protocols

There is an inverse relationship between organism size and heart rate, and therefore, the model of rapid pacing to produce DCM and CHF has been mainly performed in large animal models with an intrinsically low ambient resting heart rate. Accordingly, this review will focus upon those studies and approaches that have utilized chronic rapid pacing in dogs, pigs, and sheep. There are some advantages and disadvantages of these animal models with respect to regulatory and husbandry considerations that extend beyond the scope of this

review. However, in terms of inducing chronic pacing, all of these species have been successfully used to recapitulate the DCM phenotype and the manifestations of CHF [2–9].

The majority of past studies have utilized epicardial or endocardial pacing leads and a modified unipolar pacemaker. Transvenous lead placement allows for the stimulation electrode to be placed in the right atrium or ventricle. However, caution should be exercised with transvenous lead placement as the significant contraction rates and progressive myocardial remodeling that occurs may cause alterations in lead placement and dislodgement. It is strongly recommended that when performing the initial lead placement, the stimulation characteristics, such as amplitude and duration, are carefully programmed, and clear electromechanical capture is achieved. The optimal approach is to simultaneously obtain an electrocardiogram (ECG) and an echocardiogram to ensure that there is both electrical and mechanical synchrony at the high stimulation rates. The choice of location of the stimulation electrode is based upon species and instrumentation considerations. In dogs, the significant atrioventricular delay can prevent conduction of high atrial stimulation rates [10–13]. Thus, in the canine model, the most common location for the stimulation electrode is in the right ventricle (RV) [3–7,14–30]. However, the location of the pacing electrode in the RV is also of important consideration, whereby the placement of the stimulation electrode in the infundibular (outflow tract) of the RV produces a more progressive and consistent DCM phenotype [14–30]. There have been a number of studies that have utilized rapid LV pacing, but this tends to produce a more rapid progression to CHF in the absence of significant LV dilation and remodeling [2,12,13]. This is probably due to the fact that rapid LV electrical stimulation causes acute heterogeneous depolarization patterns and dyssynchrony of myocardial contractions. Both atrial and ventricular pacing can be achieved in the pig model [2,3,7,31–34]. This laboratory established the rapid atrial pacing DCM model in pigs through the use of epicardial lead placement on the left atrium [7,32,33,35–38]. The rationale for this approach was twofold. First, the atrioventricular conduction of the adult pig allowed for 1:1 atrial–ventricular capture with atrial pacing rates of

220–240 bpm, and therefore, provided a more uniform ventricular depolarization and contraction pattern. Second, placement of an epicardial atrial lead allowed for future unimpeded vascular and ventricular access. In general, the chronic rapid pacing rates utilized ranges from 180–250 bpm, and the duration of the pacing protocols are from 7–28 days depending upon the protocol and the desired endpoint. The DCM phenotype that is characterized by significant LV dilation and dysfunction, accompanied by neurohormonal activation and signs of CHF, usually occur by 21–28 days of continuous rapid pacing. Longer periods of sustained, chronic rapid pacing are not well-tolerated due to the development of severe CHF.

Functional and hemodynamic expectations

There have been a number of studies that have characterized LV function and hemodynamics during the progression of pacing-induced DCM [3,4,7,24,26,27–30,36,37]. During the first 7 days of rapid pacing, LV dilation occurs with a fall in ejection performance. This early remodeling phase is not associated with a significant compromise in systemic perfusion pressures and cardiac output. However, by 14 days of rapid pacing, the usual presentation is one of significant LV dilation, uniform reductions in all indices of LV ejection performances, and changes in systemic hemodynamics, which include higher central venous pressure, pulmonary artery pressure, and increased systemic vascular resistance [2–12,27–30,39]. By 21 days of persistent chronic rapid pacing in dogs, pigs, or sheep, signs and symptoms of CHF become manifest and include ascites, dyspnea, and peripheral edema. The summarized example of the progressive changes in LV volumes and ejection fraction with rapid pacing are shown in Figure 25.1. In general, there is a sharp rise in LV end-diastolic volume that tends to plateau by the final weeks of rapid pacing. By the third week of chronic rapid pacing, a significant fall in LV developed pressure and forward stroke volume occurs, ultimately resulting in reduced systemic arterial pressure, peripheral underperfusion, and vasoconstriction.

While the LV dilation and increased central venous pressures that occur early with chronic rapid pacing are likely adaptive, sustained rapid pacing causes a significant fall in load–ejection relationships. In order to more carefully examine whether changes in the Frank–Starling mechanism occur with pacing-induced CHF, Komamura and colleagues performed a series of LV volume loading experiments in conscious dogs in the control state and following 3 weeks of rapid pacing [17]. While a linear increase in LV stroke work was observed with increased preload in normal dogs, the slope of this relationship was significantly depressed in these same animals following 3 weeks of chronic pacing (Figure 25.1). Thus, LV dilation and pump dysfunction with chronic rapid pacing is associated with exhaustion of the Frank–Starling mechanism. The progressively increased LV volumes without a substantial increase in wall thickness with chronic rapid pacing results in time-dependent and significantly increased LV wall stress patterns [4,15,16,40,41]. The relationship between LV systolic wall stress and ejection performance was examined in normal pigs and in pigs with pacing-induced DCM [41]. A linear relationship existed between changes in LV fractional shortening and increases in LV end-systolic wall stress induced by phenylephrine infusion. However, with the development of pacing-induced DCM, the relationship between LV end-systolic wall stress and LV fractional shortening fell far below the normal range. These findings suggest that the significant reduction in LV pump function with pacing-induced CHF is not simply due to alterations in loading conditions, but inherent abnormalities in LV contractile function.

Several indices of LV contractile function have been examined with the development of pacing-induced DCM [4,14,15,31,42]. In order to more carefully examine load-independent indices of LV contractile performance, LV pressure–volume loops have been constructed in chronically instrumented animals at baseline and following the development of pacing-induced DCM [15,43]. For example, Cheng *et al.* demonstrated a significant shift to the right in the LV pressure–volume relationship both at rest and with exercise in dogs with pacing-induced DCM [43]. Shannon *et al.* determined the slope of the LV end-systolic stress–volume relationship, or LV end-systolic elastance, in conscious dogs before and after the development of pacing-induced CHF [15]. In this past report, a 44% decline in LV

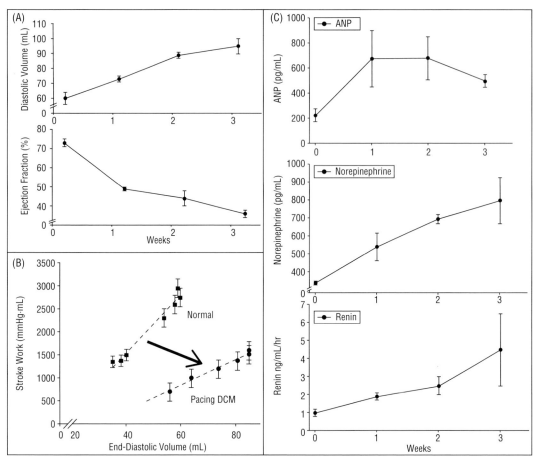

Figure 25.1 (A)Time-dependent changes in LV geometry and function with chronic rapid pacing. An abrupt increase in LV volumes occurs with rapid pacing which plateaus with longer durations of pacing. A decline in LV ejection performance occurs, which by 3 weeks causes a significant compromise in LV forward stroke volume and systemic perfusion. Plotted data extrapolated from reference [40].
(B) The Frank-Starling relationship was developed in conscious dogs by volume loading and measuring indices of LV ejection performance. In these studies, a significant shift downward and to the right occurred following 3 weeks of chronic rapid pacing (arrow). These findings demonstrated that a significant shift in this relationship occurred and would be indicative of intrinsic myocardial dysfunction. Results extrapolated from reference [17].(C) Neurohormonal activation is a key feature of the chronic rapid pacing model. An early and robust increase in the natriuretic peptides occurs by 7 days of rapid pacing, but plateaus with longer durations of pacing. In some studies, it has been identified that natriuretic peptide levels may actually fall with longer pacing durations. Plasma catecholamines increase as a function of the pacing duration, and with longer pacing durations and the manifestation of CHF, activation of the renin–angiotensin–aldosterone system occurs as evidenced by increased plasma renin activity. (Source: Data from Moe GW 1989 [27]).

end-systolic elastance was observed following the development of pacing-induced DCM. Taken together, these studies clearly demonstrate that chronic rapid pacing causes significant LV dilation, reduced ejection performance, and fundamental defects in myocardial contractile function.

One of the consequences of the significant and progressive LV dilation that occurs with rapid pacing, which is not dissimilar to the clinical phenotype of DCM, is mitral regurgitation (MR) [8,9,43–45]. The onset and relative magnitude of MR in the chronic pacing model is dependent upon the site of pacing, the degree of LV dilation, and the imaging approaches utilized. Nevertheless, uniform findings with respect to the MR induced by chronic rapid pacing is dilation of the mitral annulus, failure of full coaptation of the mitral leaflets, and a robust regurgitant jet into the left atrium [8,9,43–45]. It is likely that this MR contributes to the significant left atrial dilation that occurs with chronic rapid pacing, and in turn may contribute to the atrial arrhythmogenicity of this pacing-induced DCM model [34,46–50], which is discussed in a subsequent section. It is now well recognized that MR in and of itself can contribute to the progression of CHF secondary to clinical forms of DCM. Thus, the invariable and time-dependent occurrence of MR with rapid pacing-induced DCM may serve as a useful response variable in terms of evaluating therapeutic devices.

Neurohormonal aspects and expectations

One of the predominant features of the rapid pacing model is the predictable and time-dependent changes in neurohormonal pathways and the synthesis and release of bioactive peptides. Moreover, the temporal relationship of these neurohormonal pathways to the progression to CHF in the pacing DCM model allows for the proposed natural history of these events, which may not be possible in the clinical context of DCM. Thus, one of the clear strengths of this rapid pacing model is a reproducible pattern of neurohormonal and bioactive signaling that is amenable to pharmacological targeting, a subject of a subsequent section. The rapid pacing model has been utilized to establish a clear relationship between the synthesis, release, and subsequent receptor activation of the natriuretic peptides [19,20,26]. For example, Moe *et al.* reported that a threefold increase in both plasma atrial natriuretic peptide (ANP) and brain natriuretic peptide (BNP) occurred in 7 days of chronic rapid pacing, and was accompanied by the initial LV and atrial dilation [20]. With longer periods of rapid pacing, both ANP and BNP tend to plateau and can actually fall with the development of pacing-induced DCM and CHF. This is likely due to several contributory mechanisms including exhaustion of the ANP/BNP synthesis as well as receptor desensitization [19,20,26]. Consistent with the clinical phenotype of DCM, chronic rapid pacing is associated with significant activation of the sympathetic autonomic pathway and also causes

spillover of norepinephrine into the systemic vasculature [24–26]. With the progressive development of pacing-induced DCM and elaboration of CHF, the RAAS system becomes activated, reflected by increased plasma renin and angiotensin II levels [27–30]. A generalized summary of these changes in neurohormonal profiles is shown in Figure 25.1. Other bioactive peptides that mediate vasoconstriction as well as the effects on myocyte contractility become altered with persistent rapid pacing [21,22,35,39,51]. For example, a time-dependent increase in the local synthesis and release of endothelin occurs as a function of rapid pacing duration [21,22]. The increased synthesis and subsequent binding of endothelin to the type-A receptor results in pulmonary and systemic vasoconstriction. While mediators of vasoconstriction are robustly expressed with rapid pacing-induced DCM, the vasodilator response, such as nitric oxide, becomes impaired [39,51]. In light of the significant changes in neurohormonal pathways and bioactive signaling cascades that occur with pacing-induced DCM, this model has been significantly utilized in the research and development of pharmacological agents targeted at these systems and pathways. Some examples of this application are presented in a subsequent section.

Cellular and biochemical considerations to chronic rapid pacing

In the normal state, an acute increase in heart rate causes increased intracellular Ca^{+2} availability to the myofilaments. The increased intracellular Ca^{+2} with increased stimulation frequency is due to a reduced period of time for Ca^{+2} efflux from the cell, which is mediated primarily by the Na^+/Ca^{+2} exchanger. This results in an increased uptake of Ca^{+2} within the sarcoplasmic reticulum, which will then be discharged into the cytosol with the subsequent depolarization. Therefore under normal conditions, with stepped increases in frequency of contraction, a progressive rise in contractile performance occurs. In a study by Eising and colleagues, this force–frequency relation was examined in pigs before and after the development of pacing-induced CHF [31]. Increasing heart rate in the normal state caused a linear increase in LV peak developed pressure.

However, following the development of pacing-induced DCM, the slope of the heart rate LV dP/dt relation was significantly reduced. These results suggest that a significant abnormality in intracellular Ca^{+2} handling and/or myofilament response to Ca^{+2} had occurred with the development of pacing-induced DCM. For example, Perreault *et al.* observed a prolongation of the Ca^{+2} transient in papillary muscles taken from dogs with pacing-induced CHF [42]. Cory and colleagues reported a reduction in Ca^{+2} cycling activity in LV myocardial membranes with the development of pacing-induced CHF [52]. Vatner and colleagues reported a reduction in the density of the sarcoplasmic reticulum calcium release channel with pacing-induced LV failure [53]. Other investigations have revealed defects in multiple aspects of the excitation–contraction coupling process which includes the voltage-sensitive Ca^{+2} channel, the sarcolemmal sodium–potassium ATPase, and transverse tubule formation and function [37,38,54]. The summation of these changes in the excitation–contraction coupling process with pacing-induced DCM results in significant defects in absolute myocyte contractile function and inotropic responsiveness [35,36,40,55]. Specifically, in isolated myocyte preparations, intrinsic defects in the rate and extent of shortening as well as defects in the rate of relaxation have been identified with the development and progression of pacing-induced DCM [40,55]. Moreover, the effects of inotropic stimulation with either extracellular calcium or a beta-adrenergic agonist is blunted in terms of myocyte contractile response with pacing-induced DCM [36,37,40].

In addition to fundamental defects in myocyte contractile processes, changes in cellular growth and viability occur as a result of pacing-induced DCM [56–58]. For example, chronic rapid pacing appears to induce a number of proapoptotic cascades [56–58]. In addition, the LV dilation with pacing-induced DCM is not associated with a significant increase in LV mass; thus, in addition to an apparent loss in the absolute number of cardiac myocytes, significant cellular remodeling occurs [36]. This remodeling without a hypertrophic response may be due to a failure of the myocardial growth "gene program" [59,60]. Therefore, the pacing model of DCM and progression to CHF is accompanied by myocyte remodeling, apoptosis, and a failure of an adaptive growth response, despite significantly elevated wall stress patterns. These cellular and subcellular changes parallel findings that can be observed in clinical forms of idiopathic DCM.

Matrix remodeling and chronic rapid pacing

While significant remodeling occurs within the cellular compartment with pacing-induced DCM, robust changes occur within the extracellular matrix as well [55,61–65]. Specifically, a loss of normal fibrillar collagen content and distribution occurs with pacing-induced DCM [61,62], which in turn would cause alterations in myocyte support and alignment within the LV myocardial wall. In addition, the capacity of the myocytes to bind to critical components of the extracellular matrix is diminished in pacing DCM [63], suggesting that abnormalities in the matrix–integrin interface has occurred. Finally, increased matrix metalloproteinase (MMP) activity and expression has been identified with the development of pacing-induced DCM and progression to CHF [64,65]. The activation of these MMPs occurs early with rapid pacing and actually precedes significant defects in myocyte contractile function [65]. These findings would suggest that an early contributory event and likely mechanism for the LV remodeling and progression of pacing DCM is a loss of normal myocardial extracellular matrix structure, composition, and function.

Electrophysiology and arrhythmogenesis in chronic rapid pacing

Arrhythmias, both ventricular and atrial, commonly occur in the setting of DCM. The pacing-induced DCM model has been demonstrated to develop an arrhythmia-susceptible substrate [34,46–50]. For example, Balaji *et al.* reported a higher incidence of inducibility of ventricular arrhythmias and increased mortality due to refractory ventricular fibrillation in pigs with pacing DCM [34]. Animals subjected to rapid pacing, either from the atria or the ventricles, are also susceptible to atrial fibrillation (AF) [46–50]. Most commonly, rapid atrial pacing, with or without ventricular rate control, has been used to induce structural and electrical remodeling within the atria. AF with pacing DCM recapitulates a number of characteristics of AF in patients, which include increased fibrous content in the atrial myocardium, mitral regurgitation, and electrophysiological changes, including reduced effective refractory periods [47,48,50]. Mechanisms for arrhythmogenesis in pacing DCM include changes in action potential characteristics [34,37], which are associated with abnormalities in ion channel function [48]. Specific changes in action potential morphology that occur with pacing DCM include a more depolarized resting membrane potential, alterations in rapid depolarization, and altered action potential duration [37]. Concomitantly, changes in functioning of the L-type calcium channel, the sodium–calcium exchanger, calcium resequestration, and repolarizing potassium currents have all been reported with pacing DCM [37,48,53,54]. Therefore, the pacing DCM model provides opportunities to target specific ionic and molecular processes, contributing to arrhythmogenesis and developing novel therapeutic and/or device-based antiarrhythmic modalities.

Chronic rapid pacing-induced heart failure: the issue of reversibility

Unlike other models of CHF that are described in this text, the pacing-induced DCM model is not stable. That is, with persistent rapid pacing, LV remodeling and dysfunction is progressive and further necessities the termination of the pacing protocol within 3 to 4 weeks due to severe CHF. With termination of the pacing protocol after the manifestation of DCM, significant changes in LV geometry, function, and neurohormonal pathways occur [40,41,55,66,67]. For example, LV volumes will progress towards normal values and LV systolic performance will return to within normal limits by 7 to 14 days following cessation of rapid pacing [40,41,67]. However, this does not imply that LV structure and function has returned to the normal state. Specifically, unlike the progression to pacing-induced DCM, the regression from this process results in LV hypertrophy and fibrillar collagen accumulation, giving rise to abnormalities in diastolic function [41,66]. At the cellular level, isolated myocyte hypertrophy occurs as evidenced by increased myocyte cross-sectional area [40,55]. Thus, the regression from pacing-induced DCM is

not a true normalization and reversibility, but rather a transition to another form of LV remodeling and dysfunction. These are important considerations for this pacing model in terms of repeated rapid pacing episodes and the timing of studies. For example, a remarkably rapid resolution of the symptoms of CHF can be achieved with the cessation of the pacing stimulus (~24 hours) without significant changes in LV geometry or function. However, longer periods following pacing cessation (>72 hours) will result in changes in LV geometry and function that may no longer recapitulate the DCM phenotype. Therefore, careful consideration must be given to the time elapsed from the cessation of rapid pacing to the end-point measurements to be obtained.

Chronic pacing model for therapeutic research and development: technical considerations and limitations

In light of the predictable and time-dependent changes in LV function and geometry with chronic rapid pacing and the relatively short time span at which these changes occur, this model has been extensively used for pharmacological discovery and proof-of-concept studies [26,68–79]. Angiotensin converting enzyme inhibition (ACEI) has been utilized in this rapid pacing model and uniformly demonstrated as an attenuation in the extent of LV remodeling and dysfunction, which was paralleled by reduced neurohormonal system activation. ACEI instituted at the time of the initiation of the rapid pacing stimulus resulted in a significant improvement in LV ejection performance. The rapid pacing model has been utilized to examine the effects of specific receptor transduction pathways, such as endothelin through the use of selective endothelin receptor antagonists [68,73]. The rapid pacing model has been employed to examine the effects of hormonal supplementation, such as thyroid hormone and glucagon [72,76], as well as the potential of inotropic agents, such as levosimendan [78]. In general terms, the rapid pacing model is amenable to pharmacological studies and has yielded concordant results across laboratories and classes of pharmacological agents.

Another area of potential utility for the pacing-induced DCM model is that of therapeutic devices, particularly surgical devices whereby the indication is a reduction in LV remodeling [80–84]. These devices can be placed at the time pacing DCM has become manifest, or at earlier time points during the development of this process [80–84]. However, it should be pointed out that with the development of pacing-induced DCM and progression to CHF, significant hemodynamic instability and an arrhythmogenic substrate can be encountered. Nevertheless, due to the significant uniformity of the LV remodeling process and the clear recapitulation of the DCM phenotype, the pacing model can be utilized to examine the acute effects of myocardial restraint devices [80,83]. Furthermore, as described in an earlier section, pacing-induced DCM is associated with significant MR, and therefore the use of these passive restraint devices to evaluate the effects on this response variable is possible [8,83,84].

Summary

There are strengths and limitations to any animal model in terms of properly representing the cardiovascular disease state of interest, and the pacing model of DCM and progression to CHF is certainly no exception. The strengths of this model include the following: (1) instrumentation for inducing rapid pacing is straightforward, and modified pacing stimulators are readily available; (2) a predictable and uniform time course of progression

to DCM and ultimately to CHF, which thereby provides for reasonable sample size estimates and experimental designs; (3) recapitulates LV geometry, function, and neurohormonal pathways that can be encountered in clinical forms of DCM and CHF; and (4) readily amenable to pharmacological/therapeutic treatment studies. The limitations of this rapid pacing model include the following: (1) not stable in terms of reaching a steady-state period of LV remodeling and dysfunction; (2) the model is rapidly progressive, requiring end-point studies or pacing deactivation; and (3) termination of pacing does not result in complete reversal and total normalization of LV geometry, structure, and function. A streamlined algorithm for the potential utility of the chronic rapid pacing model is shown in Figure 25.2. The key considerations are that this model of DCM is of a nonischemic etiology and does not result in a robust hypertrophic response and therefore will not recapitulate ischemic or hypertensive heart disease, respectively. However, this pacing model is ideally suited for drug discovery, feasibility, and translational studies in the context of rapidly evolving LV remodeling and dysfunction.

Acknowledgements

This work was supported by the National Institute of Health grants HL057952 and HL095608 and a

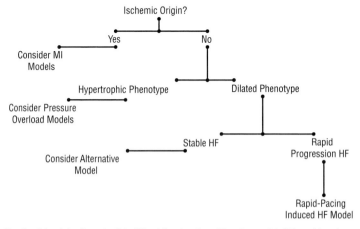

Figure 25.2 An algorithm for determining the potential utility of the chronic rapid pacing model. This rapid pacing model recapitulates the clinical phenotype of dilated cardiomyopathy in terms of LV remodeling, dysfunction, and neurohormonal activation.

Merit Award from the Veterans' Affairs Health Administration.

References

1 Whipple GH, Sheffield LT, Woodman EG, Thoephilis C, Friedman S. Reversible congestive heart failure due to rapid stimulation of the normal heart. *Proc New Eng Cardiovasc Soc* 1961–1962; **20**: 39–40.

2 Helmer GA, McKirnan MD, Shabetai R, Boss GR, Ross J Jr, Hammond HK, *et al.* Regional deficits of myocardial blood flow and function in left ventricular pacing-induced heart failure. *Circulation* 1996; **94**: 2260–2267.

3 Chow E, Woodard JC, Farrar DJ. Rapid ventricular pacing in pigs: an experimental model of congestive heart failure. *Am J Physiol* 1990; **258**: H1603–1605.

4 Moe GW, Angus C, Howard RJ, Parker TG, Armstrong PW. Evaluation of indices of left ventricular contractility and relaxation in evolving canine experimental heart failure. *Cardiovasc Res* 1992; **26**: 362–366.

5 Armstrong PW, Stopps TP, Ford SE, DeBold AJ. Rapid ventricular pacing in the dog: pathophysiologic studies of heart failure. *Circulation* 1986; **74**: 1075–1084.

6 Wilson JR, Douglas P, Hickey WF, Lanoce V, Ferraro N, Muhammad A, Reicheck N, *et al.* Experimental congestive heart failure produced by rapid ventricular pacing the dog: cardiac effects. *Circulation* 1987; **75**: 857–867.

7 Spinale FG, Hendrick DA, Crawford FA, Smith AC, Hamada Y, Carabello BA, *et al.* Chronic supraventricular tachycardia causes ventricular dysfunction and subendocardial injury in swim. *Am J Physiol* 1990; **259**: H218–H229,

8 Byrne MJ, Kaye DM, Mathis M, Reuter DG, Alferness CA, Power JM, *et al.* Percutaneous mitral annular reduction provides continued benefit in an ovine model of dilated cardiomyopathy. *Circulation* 2004; **110**: 3088–3092.

9 Timek TA, Dagum P, Lai DT, Liang D, Daughters GT, Tibayan F, *et al.* Tachycardia-induced cardiomyopathy in the ovine heart: mitral annular dynamic three dimensional geometry. *J Thorac Cardiovasc Surg* 2003; **125**: 315–324.

10 Hettrick DA, Mittelstadt JR, Kehl F, Kress TT, Tessmer JP, Krolikowski JG, *et al.* Atrial pacing lead location alters the hemodynamic effects of atrial ventricular delay in dogs with pacing induced cardiomyopathy. *Pacing Clin Electrophysiol* 2003; **26**: 853–861.

11 Prinzen FW, Augustijn CH, Allessie MA, Arts T, Delhaas T, Reneman RS, *et al.* The time sequence of electrical and mechanical activation during spontaneous beath and ectopic stimulation. *Eur Heart J* 1992; **13**: 535–543.

12 Badke FR, Bionay P, Cvell JW. Effects of ventricular pacing on regional left ventricular performance in the dog. *Am J Physiol* 1980; **238**: H858–867,.

13 Dzemali O, Bakhtiary F, Wittlinger T, Dogan S, Ackermann H, Pitschner HF, *et al.* Hemodynamic effects of left ventricular pacing site in an animal model of heart failure. *Thorac Cardiovasc Surg* 2007; **55**: 481–484.

14 Chen X, Sala-Mercado JA, Hammond RL, Ichinose M, Soltani S, Mukkamala R, *et al.* Dynamic control of maximal ventricular elastance via the baroreflex and force-frequency relation in awake dogs before and after pacing-induced heart failure. *Am J Physiol Heart Circ Physiol* 2010; **299**: H62–69.

15 Shannon RP, Komamura K, Stambler BS, Bigaud M, Manders WT, Vatner SF, *et al.* Alterations in myocardial contractility in conscious dogs with dilated cardiomyopathy. *Am J Physiol* 1991; **260**: H1903–1911.

16 Tibayan FA, Lai DT, Timek TA, Dagum P, Liang D, Daughters GT, *et al.* Alterations in left ventricular torsion in tachycardia-induced dilated cardiomyopathy. *J Thorac Cardiovasc Surg* 2002; **124**: 43–49.

17 Komamura K, Shannon RP, Ihara T, Shen YT, Mirsky I, Bishop SP, *et al.* Exhaustion of Frank-Starling mechanism in conscious dogs with heart failure. *Am J Physiol* 1993; **265**: H119.

18 Komamura K, Shannon RP, Pasipoularides A, Ihara T, Lader AS, Patrick TA, *et al.* Alterations in left ventricular diastolic function in conscious dogs with pacing induced heart failure. *J Clin Invest* 1992; **89**: 1825–1838.

19 Moe GW, Grima EA, Wong NL, Howard RJ, Armstrong PW. Dual natriuretic peptide system in experimental heart failure. *J Am Coll Cardiol* 1993; **22**: 891–898.

20 Moe GW, Grima EA, Wong NL, Howard RJ, Armstrong PW. Plasma and cardiac tissue atrial and brain natriuretic peptides in experimental heart failure. *J Am Coll Cardiol* 1996; **27**: 720–727.

21 Cavero PG, Miller WL, Heublein DM, Margulies KB, Burnett JC Jr. Endothelin in experimental congestive heart failure in the anesthetized dog. *Am J Physiol* 1990; **259**: F312–317.

22 Margulies KB, Hildebrand FL Jr, Lerman A, Perrella MA, Burnett JC Jr. Increased endothelin in experimental heart failure. *Circulation* 1990; **82**: 2226–2230.

23 Huntington K, Picard P, Moe G, Stewart DJ, Albernaz A, Monge JC, *et al.* Increased cardiac and pulmonary endothelin-1 mRNA expression in canine pacing-induced heart failure. *J Cardiovasc Pharmacol* 1998; **31** (**Suppl 1**): S424–426.

24 Spinale FG, Holzgrefe HH, Mukherjee R, Hird RB, Walker JD, Arnim-Barker A, *et al.* Angiotensin-converting enzyme inhibition and the progression of congestive cardiomyopathy. Effects on left ventricular and myocyte structure and function. *Circulation* 1995; **92**: 562–578.

25 Piccirillo G, Magrì D, Ogawa M, Song J, Chong VJ, Han S, *et al.* Autonomic nervous system activity measured directly and QT interval variability in normal and

pacing-induced tachycardia heart failure dogs. *J Am Coll Cardiol* 2009; **54**: 840–850.

26 Riegger GA, Elsner D, Kromer EP, Daffner C, Forssmann WG, Muders F, *et al*. Atrial natriuretic peptide in congestive heart failure in the dog: plasma levels, cyclic guanosine monophosphate, ultrastructure of atrial myoendocrine cells, and hemodynamic, hormonal, and renal effects. *Circulation* 1988; **77**: 398–406.

27 Moe GW, Stopps TP, Angus C, Forster C, De Bold AJ, Armstrong PW, *et al*. Alterations in serum sodium in relation to atrial natriuretic factor and other neuroendocrine variables in experimental pacing-induced heart failure. *J Am Coll Cardiol* 1989; **13**: 173–179.

28 McCurley JM, Hanlon SU, Wei SK, Wedam EF, Michalski M, Haigney MC, *et al*. Furosemide and the progression of left ventricular dysfunction in experimental heart failure. *J Am Coll Cardiol* 2004; **44**: 1301–1307.

29 Osorio JC, Xu X, Vogel T, Ochoa M, Laycock S, Hintze TH, *et al*. Plasma nitrate accumulation during the development of pacing-induced dilated cardiac myopathy in conscious dogs is due to renal impairment. *Nitric Oxide* 2001; **5**: 7–17.

30 Riegger GA, Liebau G, Holzschuh M, Witkowski D, Steilner H, Kochsiek K, *et al*. Role of the renin-angiotensin system in the development of congestive heart failure in the dog as assessed by chronic converting-enzyme blockade. *Am J Cardiol* 1984; **53**: 614–618.

31 Eising GP, Hammond JK, Helmer GA, Gilpin E, Ross J. Force frequency relations during heart failure in pigs. *Am J Physiol* 1994; **367**: H2516–H2522.

32 Spinale FG, Grine RC, Tempel GE, Crawford FA, Zile MR. Alterations in the myocardial capillary vasculature accompany tachycardia-induced cardiomyopathy. *Basic Res Cardiol* 1992; **87**: 65–79.

33 Mukherjee R, Hewett KW, Spinale FG. Myocyte electrophysiological properties following the development of supraventricular tachycardia induced cardiomyopathy. *J Mol Cell Cardiol* 1995; **27**: 1333–1348.

34 Balaji S, Hewett KW, Krombach RS, Clair MJ, Ye X, Spinale FG, *et al*. Inducible lethal ventricular arrhythmias in swine with pacing-induced heart failure. *Basic Res Cardiol* 1999; **94**: 496–503.

35 Thomas PB, Liu EC, Webb ML, Mukherjee R, Hebbar L, Spinale FG, *et al*. Exogenous effects and endogenous production of endothelin in cardiac myocytes: potential significance in heart failure. *Am J Physiol* 1996; **271**: H2629–2637.

36 Spinale FG, Fulbright BM, Mukherjee R, Tanaka R, Hu J, Crawford FA, *et al*. Relationship between ventricular and myocyte function with tachycardia induced cardiomyopathy. *Circ Res* 1992; **71**: 174–187.

37 Mukherjee R, Hewett KW, Walker JD, Basler CG, Spinale FG. Changes in L-type calcium channel abundance and function during the transition to pacing-induced congestive heart failure. *Cardiovasc Res* 1998; **37**: 432–444.

38 Spinale FG, Clayton C, Tanaka R, Fulbright BM, Mukherjee R, Schulte BA, *et al*. Myocardial Na+,K(+)-ATPase in tachycardia induced cardiomyopathy. *J Mol Cell Cardiol* 1992; **24**: 277–294.

39 Sun D, Huang A, Zhao G, Bernstein R, Forfia P, Xu X, *et al*. Reduced NO-dependent arteriolar dilation during the development of cardiomyopathy. *Am J Physiol Heart Circ Physiol* 2000; **278**: H461–468.

40 Spinale FG, Holzgrefe HH, Mukherjee R, Arthur SA, Child MJ, Powell JR, *et al*. Left ventricular and myocyte structure and function with recovery from tachycardia induced cardiomyopathy. *Am J Physiol* 1995; **268**: H836–H847.

41 Tomita M, Spinale FG, Crawford FA, Zile MR. Changes in left ventricular volume, mass, and function during the development and regression of supraventricular tachycardia-induced cardiomyopathy. Disparity between recovery of systolic versus diastolic function. *Circulation* 1991; **83**: 635–644.

42 Perreault CL, Shannon RP, Komamura K, Vatner SF, Morgan JP. Abnormalities in intracellular calcium regulation and contractile function in myocardium from dogs with pacing-induced heart failure. *J Clin Invest* 1992; **89**: 932–938.

43 Cheng CP, Noda T, Nozawa T, Little WC. Effect of heart failure on the mechanism exercise induced augmentation of mitral valve flow. *Circulation* 1994; **89**: 2241–2250.

44 Howard RJ, Moe GW, Armstrong PW. Sequential echocardiographic-Doppler assessment of left ventricular remodelling and mitral regurgitation during evolving experimental heart failure. *Cardiovasc Res* 1991; **25**: 468–474.

45 Timek TA, Dagum P, Lai DT, Liang D, Daughters GT, Ingels NB Jr, *et al*. Pathogenesis of mitral regurgitation in tachycardia-induced cardiomyopathy. *Circulation* 2001; **104 (Suppl 1)**: I47–153.

46 Power JM, Beacom GA, Alferness CA, Raman J, Farish SJ, Tonkin AM, *et al*. Effects of left atrial dilatation on the endocardial atrial defibrillation threshold: a study in an ovine model of pacing induced dilated cardiomyopathy. *Pacing Clin Electrophysiol* 1998; **21**: 1595–1600.

47 Laurent G, Moe G, Hu X, Leong-Poi H, Connelly KA, So PP, *et al*. Experimental studies of atrial fibrillation: a comparison of two pacing models. *Am J Physiol Heart Circ Physiol* 2008; **294**: H1206–1215.

48 Sridhar A, Nishijima Y, Terentyev D, Khan M, Terentyeva R, Hamlin RL, *et al*. Chronic heart failure and the substrate for atrial fibrillation. *Cardiovasc Res* 2009; **84**: 227–236.

49 Power JM, Beacom GA, Alferness CA, Raman J, Wijffels M, Farish SJ, et al. Susceptibility to atrial fibrillation: a study in an ovine model of pacing-induced early heart failure. J Cardiovasc Electrophysiol 1998; 9: 423–435.

50 Li D, Fareh S, Leung TK, Nattel S. Promotion of atrial fibrillation by heart failure in dogs: atrial remodeling of a different sort. Circulation 1999; 100: 87–95.

51 Recchia FA, McConnell PI, Bernstein RD, Vogel TR, Xu X, Hintze TH, et al. Reduced nitric oxide production and altered myocardial metabolism during the decompensation of pacing-induced heart failure in the conscious dog. Circ Res 1998; 83: 969–979.

52 Cory CR, McCutcheon LJ, O'Grady M, Pang AW, Geiger JD, O'Brien PJ, et al. Compensatory downregulation of myocardial Ca channel in SR from dogs with heart failure. Am J Physiol 1993; 264: H926–937.

53 Vatner DE, Sato N, Kiuchi K, Shannon RP, Vatner SF. Decrease in myocardial ryanodine receptors and altered excitation-contraction coupling early in the development of heart failure. Circulation 1994; 90: 1423–1430.

54 Balijepalli RC, Lokuta AJ, Maertz NA, Buck JM, Haworth RA, Valdivia HH, et al. Depletion of T tubules and specific subcellular changes in sarcolemmal proteins in tachycardia-induced heart failure. Cardiovasc Res 2003; 59: 67–77.

55 Spinale FG, Zellner JL, Johnson WS, Eble DM, Munyer PD. Cellular and extracellular remodeling with the development and recovery from tachycardia-induced cardiomyopathy: changes in fibrillar collagen, myocyte adhesion capacity and proteoglycans. J Mol Cell Cardiol 1996; 28: 1591–1608.

56 Kajstura J, Zhang X, Liu Y, Szoke E, Cheng W, Olivetti G, et al. The cellular basis of pacing-induced dilated cardiomyopathy. Myocyte cell loss and myocyte cellular reactive hypertrophy. Circulation 1995; 92: 2306–2317.

57 Cesselli D, Jakoniuk I, Barlucchi L, Beltrami AP, Hintze TH, Nadal-Ginard B, et al. Oxidative stress-mediated cardiac cell death is a major determinant of ventricular dysfunction and failure in dog dilated cardiomyopathy. Circ Res 2001; 89: 279–286.

58 Liu Y, Cigola E, Cheng W, Kajstura J, Olivetti G, Hintze TH, Anversa P, et al. Myocyte nuclear mitotic division and programmed myocyte cell death characterize the cardiac myopathy induced by rapid ventricular pacing in dogs. Lab Invest 1995; 73: 771–787.

59 Ojaimi C, Qanud K, Hintze TH, Recchia FA. Altered expression of a limited number of genes contributes to cardiac decompensation during chronic ventricular tachypacing in dogs. Physiol Genomics 2007; 29: 76–83.

60 Smith CJ, Huang R, Sun D, Ricketts S, Hoegler C, Ding JZ, et al. Development of decompensated dilated cardiomyopathy is associated with decreased gene expression and activity of the milrinone sensitive cAMP phosphodiesterase PDE3A. Circulation 1997; 96: 3116–3123.

61 Spinale FG, Tomita M, Zellner JL, Cook JC, Crawford FA, Zile MR, et al. Collagen remodeling and changes in LV function during development and recovery from supraventricular tachycardia. Am J Physiol 1991; 261: H308–318.

62 Weber KT, Pick R, Silver MA, Moe GW, Janicki JS, Zucker IH, et al. Fibrillar collagen and remodeling of dilated canine left ventricle. Circulation 1990; 82: 1387–1401.

63 Zellner JL, Spinale FG, Eble DM, Hewett KW, Crawford FA Jr. Alterations in myocyte shape and basement membrane attachment with tachycardia-induced heart failure. Circ Res 1991; 69: 590–600.

64 Coker ML, Thomas CV, Clair MJ, Hendrick JW, Krombach RS, Galis ZS, et al. Myocardial matrix metalloproteinase activity and abundance with congestive heart failure. Am J Physiol 1998; 274: H1516–1523.

65 Spinale FG, Coker ML, Thomas CV, Walker JD, Mukherjee R, Hebbar L, et al. Time-dependent changes in matrix metalloproteinase activity and expression during the progression of congestive heart failure: relation to ventricular and myocyte function. Circ Res 1998; 82: 482–495.

66 Moe GW, Stopps TP, Howard RJ, Armstrong PW. Early recovery from heart failure: insights into the pathogenesis of experimental chronic pacing-induced heart failure. J Lab Clin Med 1988; 112: 426–432.

67 Moe GW, Grima EA, Howard RJ, Seth R, Armstrong PW. Left ventricular remodelling and disparate changes in contractility and relaxation during the development of and recovery from experimental heart failure. Cardiovasc Res 1994; 28: 66–71.

68 Spinale FG, Mukherjee R, Krombach RS, Clair MJ, Hendrick JW, Houck WV, et al. Chronic amlodipine treatment during the development of heart failure. Circulation 1998; 98: 1666–1674.

69 Spinale FG, de Gasparo M, Whitebread S, Hebbar L, Clair MJ, Melton DM, et al. Modulation of the renin-angiotensin pathway through enzyme inhibition and specific receptor blockade in pacing-induced heart failure: I. Effects on left ventricular performance and neurohormonal systems. Circulation 1997; 96: 2385–2396.

70 Spinale FG, Mukherjee R, Iannini JP, Whitebread S, Hebbar L, Clair MJ, et al. Modulation of the renin-angiotensin pathway through enzyme inhibition and specific receptor blockade in pacing-induced heart failure: II. Effects on myocyte contractile processes. Circulation 1997; 96: 2397–2406.

71 Nikolaidis LA, Doverspike A, Huerbin R, Hentosz T, Shannon RP. Angiotensin-converting enzyme inhibitors

improve coronary flow reserve in dilated cardiomyopathy by a bradykinin-mediated, nitric oxide-dependent mechanism. *Circulation* 2002; **105**: 2785–2790.

72 Walker JD, Crawford FA, Kato S, Spinale FG. The novel effects of 3,5,3′-triiodo-L-thyronine on myocyte contractile function and beta-adrenergic responsiveness in dilated cardiomyopathy. *J Thorac Cardiovasc Surg* 1994; **108**: 672–679.

73 McConnell PI, Olson CE, Patel KP, Blank DU, Olivari MT, Gallagher KP, *et al.* Chronic endothelin blockade in dogs with pacing-induced heart failure: possible modulation of sympathoexcitation. *J Card Fail* 2000; **6**: 56–65.

74 Nikolaidis LA, Poornima I, Parikh P, Magovern M, Shen YT, Shannon RP, *et al.* The effects of combined versus selective adrenergic blockade on left ventricular and systemic hemodynamics, myocardial substrate preference, and regional perfusion in conscious dogs with dilated cardiomyopathy. *J Am Coll Cardiol* 2006; **47**: 1871–1881.

75 Margulies KB, Perrella MA, McKinley LJ, Burnett JC Jr. Angiotensin inhibition potentiates the renal responses to neutral endopeptidase inhibition in dogs with congestive heart failure. *J Clin Invest* 1991; **88**: 1636–1642.

76 Nikolaidis LA, Elahi D, Hentosz T, Doverspike A, Huerbin R, Zourelias L, *et al.* Recombinant glucagon-like peptide-1 increases myocardial glucose uptake and improves left ventricular performance in conscious dogs with pacing-induced dilated cardiomyopathy. *Circulation* 2004; **110**: 955–961.

77 Rademaker MT, Charles CJ, Nicholls MG, Richards AM. Hemodynamic, hormonal, and renal actions of adrenomedullin 2 in experimental heart failure. *Circ Heart Fail* 2008; **1**: 134–142.

78 Pagel PS, McGough MF, Hettrick DA, Lowe D, Tessmer JP, Jamali IN, *et al.* Levosimendan enhances left ventricular systolic and diastolic function in conscious dogs with pacing-induced cardiomyopathy. *J Cardiovasc Pharmacol* 1997; **29**: 563–573.

79 Trochu JN, Mital S, Zhang X, Xu X, Ochoa M, Liao JK, *et al.* Preservation of NO production by statins in the treatment of heart failure. *Cardiovasc Res* 2003; **60**: 250–258.

80 Dixon JA, Goodman AM, Gaillard WF 2nd, Rivers WT, McKinney RA, Mukherjee R, *et al.* Hemodynamics and myocardial blood flow patterns after placement of a cardiac passive restraint device in a model of dilated cardiomyopathy. *J Thorac Cardiovasc Surg* 2011; **142**: 1038–1045.

81 Kashem A, Kashem S, Santamore WP, Crabbe DL, Margulies KB, Melvin DB, *et al.* Early and late results of left ventricular reshaping by passive cardiac-support device in canine heart failure. *J Heart Lung Transplant* 2003; **22**: 1046–1053.

82 Lee KF, Dignan RJ, Parmar JM, Dyke CM, Benton G, Yeh T Jr, *et al.* Effects of dynamic cardiomyoplasty on left ventricular performance and myocardial mechanics in dilated cardiomyopathy. *J Thorac Cardiovasc Surg* 1991; **102**: 124–131.

83 Kashem A, Santamore WP, Hassan S, Melvin DB, Crabbe DL, Margulies KB, *et al.* CardioClasp changes left ventricular shape acutely in enlarged canine heart. *J Card Surg* 2003; **18** (**Suppl 2**): S49–60.

84 Raman JS, Byrne MJ, Power JM, Alferness CA. Ventricular constraint in severe heart failure halts decline in cardiovascular function associated with experimental dilated cardiomyopathy. *Ann Thorac Surg* 2003; **76**: 141–147.

26 Porcine myocardial ischemia models

Xian-Liang Tang and Roberto Bolli
University of Louisville, Louisville, KY, USA

Introduction

The pig model of regional myocardial ischemia and reperfusion plays an increasingly important role in translational medicine. The pig has the cardiac size required for surgical instrumentation, along with cardiac anatomy and great vessels which are close to those in humans. An ischemic/reperfused myocardial region can be compared to a control region remote from the ischemic zone in the same individual [1]. Beside the size and morphologic characteristics, there are physiological similarities in the areas of coronary blood flow and growth of the cardiovascular system [2]. The coronary circulation of the pig has few subepicardial collateral anastomoses, similar to 90% of the human population, and the circulation to the conduction system is predominantly right-side dominant from the posterior septal artery. Consequently, the temporal and spatial development of myocardial infarction resembles that seen in humans [3–6]. Conceptually, all cardioprotective phenomena, including hibernation [7], ischemic preconditioning [8], pharmacological preconditioning [9], ischemic postconditioning, and remote conditioning, have been demonstrated in pig hearts. In addition, pigs can be easily bred, are reasonably inexpensive, and easy to keep. In this chapter, we describe two techniques for producing regional ischemia and myocardial infarction, that is an anesthetized closed-chest model with an intraluminal angioplasty balloon occlusion and a conscious model with a surgically placed extravascular balloon occlusion.

Methods

Anesthetized pig model with an angioplasty balloon-induced ocolusion
Surgical procedure
Experimental myocardial infarction is performed in castrated male domestic pigs weighing 30–40 kg. The animals are acclimatized for at least 1 week prior to the experiment and assigned randomly to control or ischemic preconditioning (IPC) group. Pigs are fasted for at least 12 hours prior to sedation for the closed chest myocardial infarct procedure. On the day of the coronary artery occlusion, pigs are premedicated with an intramuscular injection of a solution containing ketamine hydrochloride (20 mg/kg) and xylazine (2 mg/kg). An intravenous catheter is placed in a marginal ear vein for the administration of fluids and drugs. Diazepam (1 mg/kg, i.v.) is administered to allow for endotracheal intubation. An appropriately sized endotracheal tube is inserted for mechanical ventilation. The pig is then moved to the cath-lab and placed on a heating blanket to maintain rectal temperature between 37.4 and 38.9°C. The pig is ventilated on 50/50 oxygen/air at 15–20 breaths per minute and 10–12 mL/kg tidal volume. General anesthesia is maintained with continuous infusion of methohexital sodium (5–10 mg/kg/h, i.v.), which is started once the pig is

Manual of Research Techniques in Cardiovascular Medicine, First Edition. Edited by Hossein Ardehali, Roberto Bolli, and Douglas W. Losordo.

on ventilation. The purpose to use methohexital sodium as the anesthetic agent is that this relatively short-acting anesthetic does not modify myocardial infarct size and does not interfere with the cardioprotective effects of ischemic preconditioning as volatile anesthetics do [10,11]. Normal physiological ranges of pH (7.35–7.45) and P_{CO_2} (30–40 mmHg) are ensured by repeated analysis of arterial blood values and adjustment in ventilation as necessary. Fluid status is maintained by i.v. infusion of 0.9% sodium chloride solution at a rate of 10 mL/kg/h. Animals are anticoagulated with heparin (300 units/kg, i.v.) and medicated with aspirin (300 mg, i.v.), cefazolin (30 mg/kg, i.v.), and gentamicin (0.7 mg/kg, i.v.) prior to the experiment. External defibrillator pads are placed on the pig's chest for "hands-free" cardioversion if ventricular fibrillation occurs. Surface EKG leads (limb lead II) are placed to provide continuous electrocardiographic data. All surgical procedures are carried out using standard sterile technique. All instruments and devices to be utilized in the procedure are sterilized beforehand.

A left femoral cut-down is performed and a 7F fast-cath sheath is introduced and a 5F pigtail catheter is advanced with a 0.038″ guide wire to the left ventricle. This catheter is used to inject microspheres for measurement of regional myocardial blood flow (RMBF) and the first injection is done after placement of the catheter. Next, a right femoral artery cut-down is performed and an 8F fast-cath sheath is introduced. The side arm of the 8F sheath is connected to a fluid filled pressure transducer to measure arterial blood pressure. A 7F hockey-stick catheter over a 0.038″ guide wire is inserted through the 8F sheath and advanced under fluoroscopic guidance and the ostium of the left coronary artery (LAD) is selectively engaged. The guide wire is then removed. Next, a bolus of contrast dye is injected to obtain a coronary cineangiogram for determining the site of balloon placement and the size of balloon catheter. After angiographic measurement of the mid-LAD diameter at the site of occlusion, a 0.014″ guide wire is advanced into the distal LAD and an appropriately sized (2.5-mm to 3.5-mm) balloon-tipped angioplasty catheter is telescoped over the wire and positioned at the mid-LAD distal to the second diagonal terminal branch. Position of the balloon placement is verified

by intracoronary contrast injection, and documented by cineangiogram prior to inflation. In our experience, occlusion of the mid-LAD coronary artery distal to the second diagonal branch would create a targeted area-at-risk at approximately 35% of the left ventricular mass.

Myocardial ischemia/ reperfusion

Following the instrumentation described earlier, the pig is stabilized for 5 minutes. Baseline hemodynamics and blood sample for cardiac troponin I (cTnI) are collected following stabilization and baseline microsphere dose (Samarium, isotope #1) is given. A prophylactic dose of amiodarone (2 mg/kg, i.v.) is administered slowly over 10 minutes and an intravenous amiodarone drip is followed at a rate of 2.4 mg/kg/h, until 30 minutes after reperfusion to prevent arrhythmias or incidence of ventricular fibrillation often observed during the ischemic period or at onset of reperfusion. Additionally, a lidocaine bolus (2 mg/kg, i.v.) is given followed by a lidocaine drip at a rate of 3.0 mg/kg/h.

The angioplasty balloon is inflated at an appropriate pressure to occlude the coronary artery completely and induce nil-flow myocardial ischemia. After balloon inflation, a cineangiographic images are obtained by contrast injection through the hockey-stick guiding catheter to confirm the balloon position and complete occlusion of the distal LAD. In control pigs, the LAD occlusion is maintained for 60 minutes as an index ischemia, targeting an infarct size of approximately 50–55% of the area-at-risk. Inflation and position of the balloon are confirmed by contrast angiogram again at the end of ischemia. If ventricular fibrillation occurs, defibrillation at 360 Joules direct current shocks is applied through the fixed skin electrodes. At 45 minutes into occlusion, a second microsphere dose (Europium, isotope #2) is given to quantify collateral blood flow to the area at risk, which is used as a covariate of infarct size. In pigs undergoing ischemic preconditioning (IPC), three 5-minute LAD occlusion/10-minute reperfusion cycles are performed prior to the 60-minute index ischemia. After the 60-minute ischemic period, the intracoronary balloon is deflated to initiate reperfusion and the balloon catheter is withdrawn. After the balloon withdrawal, an additional cineangiogram is obtained to verify vessel patency. The 7F hocky-stick catheter is then withdrawn after confirming the lack of coronary spasm. Another microsphere dose (Lutetium, isotope #3) is injected at 15 minutes time point from reperfusion to confirm vessel patency and early reperfusion. After the third microsphere dose, the pigtail catheter is withdrawn and the femoral sheaths are removed. The groin incisions are closed in three layers using 3-0 Vicryl for internal stitches and 3-0 PDS for the final subcutaneous layer. After closing the groin, the pig is turned on his left side to scrub the neck for a cut-down on the right external jugular vein. A 7F Hydrocoatf polyurethane catheter (Access Technologies) is implanted, secured and tunneled to the back of the neck for serial blood samples to measure cTnI levels at the postoperative time points. Buprenorphine is given for postprocedural analgesia at an initial dose of 0.01 mg/kg, i.v., 15 minutes after reperfusion and, 2 to 3 hours later, followed by a subsequent dose of 0.05–0.10 mg/kg s.c. b.i.d. for at least 48 hours. The initial low dose of buprenorphine is to avoid delays in weaning the animal from mechanical ventilation due to potential adverse effect of higher doses. The pig is weaned from anesthesia and extubated when the animal begins to chew on the endotracheal tube and exhibits a gag reflex. Blood samples are collected for cTnI analyses at 2, 4, 6, 24, and 48 hours after reperfusion.

At 72 hours after reperfusion, the pig is reanesthetized and intubated as described earlier, and transported to the cath lab for final data collection. In the cath lab, the right carotid artery cut-down is performed and a 6F pig-tail catheter is advanced into the left ventricle for injection of the 72-hour microsphere dose (Lanthanum, isotope #4) to determine RMBF in the postinfarcted myocardium. The pig is heparinized (100 units/kg, i.v.) and euthanized with injection of saturated KCl (2 mL/kg) through the pig-tail catheter. After cessation of vital signs, the chest is opened through a left thoracotomy and the heart is harvested for postmortem staining and sectioning.

Conscious pig model with an extravascular balloon-induced occlusion

Surgical instrumentation

Castrated male domestic pigs weighing 30–40 kg are used. Pigs are fasted for at least 12 hours prior to sedation for surgical instrumentation. Pigs are premedicated with an intramuscular injection of a solution containing ketamine hydrochloride (20 mg/kg) and xylazine (2 mg/kg). After establishment of a venous access by placing a 20-gauge angiocatheter on a marginal ear vein, diazepam (1 mg/kg, i.v.) is administered to allow for endotracheal intubation. Then, the pig is transported to the surgical suite and ventilated on oxygen-enriched room air at 15–20 breaths per minute and 10–12 mL/kg tidal volume. Ventilation pressure is maintained between 18 and 22 cmH₂O. Anesthesia is maintained with isoflurane (1.5–3.0% with 50/50 oxygen/air). Body temperature is monitored continuously with a rectal probe attached to a thermocouple and maintained between 37.4 and 38.9°C using a hot air veterinary blanket (Bear Hugger warmer).

ECG is monitored using surface ECG leads. The pigs are shaved and the surgical area washed three times, alternating Hibiclens and isopropyl alcohol. After the skin surface has dried, Betadine is applied with sterile gauze to the surgical area and allowed to dry. A transparent, sterile, adhesive drape (3M) is used as a barrier on the surgical site. All instruments and devices to be utilized in the procedure are sterilized beforehand.

A midline sternotomy is performed using a scalpel for the initial skin incision and an electrocautery cutting blade to continue the incision down to the sternum, sparing the manubrium. The use of the midline sternotomy to expose the heart in the interpleural space without breaking plural membrane is an effort to reduce the incidence of postsurgical pulmonary complications. Thus, extra care is taken to keep the pleural membrane intact during the opening of the mediastinum. In case of pleural membrane brakeage, effort is made to close the tear by reapproximation of pleural membrane with 6-0 Prolene and to reestablish a negative pressure in the pleural cavity using a withdrawal tube with a purse-string closure. After the chest is open, the pericardium is cut vertically and the heart is exposed and suspended in a pericardial cradle. After sprinkling a few drops of lidocaine on the heart surface, the LAD coronary artery distal to the second diagonal branch is carefully dissected free for about 1.0 to 1.5 cm long with a vessel loop. A lubricated umbilical tape is tunneled underneath and a brief occlusion of the LAD is performed to macroscopically examine the size of area-at-risk by pulling the umbilical tape against a cotton-tip applicator. An extravascular balloon cuff (Vascular Occluder, Cat. no. OC-3 to OC-4, Access Technologies, USA. http://www.norfolkaccess.com) is used to encircle the freed LAD segment and is anchored in place with 6-0 Prolene. The position of the occluder placement is determined according to the visual estimation in an effort to make a targeted area-at-risk at ~25% (neither less than 15% nor greater than 35%) of the LV. In our previous studies with a 60-minute coronary occlusion, 20 out of the 26 instrumented pigs (23% exclusion rate) successfully completed the study and the area-at-risk was 24.6 ± 6.1% of LV (Figures 26.1 and 26.2). A 7F Hydrocoatf polyurethane catheter (Access Technologies) is placed in the left atrium (for administration of microspheres) and two more are placed in the left internal thoracic artery (for arterial pressure measurement and blood sample collection) and left internal thoracic vein (ancillary line, drug administration). The pericardium is then approximated. The vascular occluder and the catheters are tunneled under the skin and exteriorized through a small incision on the back. Before closing the chest, sterile, warm normal saline (approximately 500 mL) is used to flush the thoracic cavity and antibiotic (gentamicin) solution is sprinkled in the chest cavity. This flush is suctioned out prior to closing. A single mediastinal tube (8-gauge Tygon tubing) connected to a three-way stopcock and a 60-mL syringe is used to evacuate any remaining fluids around the heart and to reestablish negative intrapleural pressure in case of a tear in the pleural membrane. The sternum is closed with 22-gauge stainless steel suture. The chest is closed in layers (0 PDS II suture for the muscle and 2-0 PDS II suture for the skin subcutaneously). The mediastinal tube is removed after no visible air leak or blood accumulation is noticed. A purse-string suture (2-0 PDS II) is used to ensure an airtight seal. The skin incision is then glued with Vetbond adhesive. The inhaled anesthetic is then turned off, the animal extubated when appropriate, and allowed to recover. A fentanyl transdermal patch (25–50 µg/h) is placed on the back immediately after closing the chest. Pigs received chewable form of carprofen (2–4 mg/kg, p.o.) every 24 hours for the first 48 hours after surgery. Cefazolin (30 mg/kg b.i.d.) and gentamicin (0.7 mg/kg b.i.d.) are administered i.v. before surgery

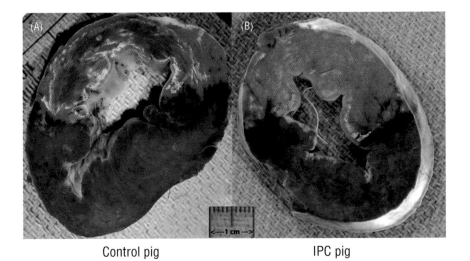

Control pig   IPC pig

Figure 26.1 Representative transverse LV section in a control pig (A) and in a ischemic preconditioned pig (B). Surgically instrumented pigs underwent a 60-minute coronary occlusion and 72-hour reperfusion in conscious state. IPC pig was preconditioned by two cycles of 5-minute occlusion/10-minute reperfusion prior to the 60-minute occlusion. Hearts were postmortem perfused with phthalo blue dye to stain the nonischemic myocardium and TTC to stain the area-at-risk. The dark blue tissue is the nonischemic myocardium; the fresh red (TTC-positive) tissue is the surviving myocardium after ischemia/ reperfusion; the white/ yellow/ brown (TTC-negative) tissue is the infarcted myocardium. Note the crisp demarcation of the area-at-risk in both cases. In the control pig the infarct is confluent and hemorrhagic; in the preconditioned pig the infarct is patchy and much smaller.

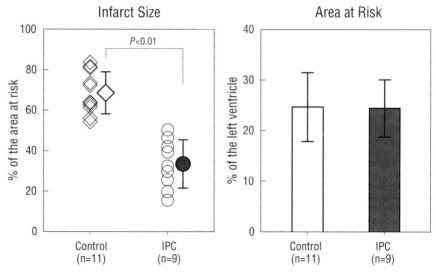

Figure 26.2 Infarct size and the area-at-risk in surgically instrumented pigs after a 60-minute coronary occlusion followed by 72-hour reperfusion in conscious state without (control) or with (IPC) an antecedent ischemic preconditioning (2 cycles of 5-minute occlusion/10-minute repertusion). Note that placement of occluder cuff on LAD coronary artery distal to the second diagonal branch created an area-at-risk at about 25% of the left ventricle. A protocol of 60-minute coronary occlusion/ 72-hour reperfusion in the conscious pig model resulted in an infarction in about 70% of the area-at-risk. Ischemic preconditioning significantly reduced infarct size. Data are mean ± SD.

and daily thereafter for 3 days. Pigs are allowed to recover for a minimum of 7 days after surgery and are trained for at least 3 days to lie quietly in a specially designed cage before the conscious studies.

Myocardial ischemia/ reperfusion in conscious state

On the day of coronary occlusion/ reperfusion, pigs are studied as they lie quietly in a cage in a quiet, dimly lit room. Food is provided *ad libitum*. Ketoprofen (3.0 mg/kg s.c.) is given 2 hours before LAD occlusion. Diazepam is given intravenously starting 10 minutes before LAD occlusion at an initial dose of 1 mg/kg with additional doses up to 4 mg/kg as needed, until the pig lies quietly in the cage. Heparin (50 units/kg, i.v.) is given before occlusion for prophylactic treatment of coronary arterial thrombosis. Aortic pressure and surface ECG are monitored continuously starting before LAD occlusion until 1 hour after reperfusion. External defibrillator pads are placed on the pig's chest for "hands-free" cardioversion if ventricular fibrillation occurs. To prevent arrhythmias, pigs are given lidocaine (2 mg/kg i.v. bolus, then 3.0 mg/kg/h

drip) and amiodarone (4 mg/kg i.v. over 10 minutes, then 2.4 mg/kg/h) starting 10 minutes before LAD occlusion and ending 30 minutes after reperfusion.

Pigs are randomly assigned to control or IPC group. After baseline blood sample for cTnI is collected and microsphere dose (Samarium, isotope #1) is given, control pigs are occluded for 60-minute as the index ischemia by inflating the surgically positioned vascular occluder, whereas pigs undergoing IPC are subjected to two cycles of 5-minute occlusion/10-minute reperfusion prior to the 60-minute ischemia. Second microsphere dose (Europium, isotope #2) is given at 45 minutes time point into the 60-minute occlusion. At the end of 60-minute occlusion, reperfusion is initiated by deflating the vascular occluder. Another microsphere dose (Lutetium, isotope #3) is given at 15 minutes after reperfusion. If ventricular fibrillation occurs, defibrillation is performed immediately (360 Joules). Sodium bicarbonate (initial dose 1.0 mEq/kg i.v. bolus, subsequently 0.5–1.0 mEq/kg/h i.v. injections until an arterial pH to ~7.40) is administered as needed after defibrillation to counteract acidosis as indicated by blood gases. Blood samples are collected for cTnI analyses at 2, 4, 6, 24, and 48 hours after reperfusion.

At 72 hours after reperfusion, the pig is reanesthetized and intubated as described earlier. Anesthesia is maintained with 1.5–3.0% isoflurane. After final hemodynamic data are collected, the 72-hour microsphere dose (Lanthanum, isotope #4) is given to determine no-reflow phenomenon in the infarcted myocardium. The pig is heparinized (100 units/kg, i.v.) and euthanized with injection of saturated KCl (2 mL/kg) through the left atrial line. After cessation of vital signs, the chest is opened through a left thoracotomy and the heart is harvested for postmortem staining and sectioning. Because strong adhesions may have formed between the heart and the sternum from the open-chest surgical procedure, extra care should be taken to free the heart from the sternum without tearing the epicardial surface when dissecting the scar tissue.

Postmortem perfusion

The heart is mounted onto a dual perfusion system. The LAD at the site of the previous occlusion is cannulated to perfuse the ischemic/ reperfused myocardium (referred to as the "area-at-risk" or the "risk region" as it is at risk of infarction) while the aortic root is cannulated to retrogradely perfuse the nonischemic myocardium. After perfusion with Krebs–Henseleit solution at 37°C (to remove any blood), the LAD cannula is perfused with a solution of 1% (w/v) triphenyl tetrazolium chloride (TTC) in phosphate buffer at 37°C and the aortic cannula with a 5% (v/v) solution of phthalo blue dye (Cat. no..#14-2097, Quantum Ink Company, Louisville, KY. http://quantumink.com/) in normal saline. The driving pressure is maintained at approximate 80 mmHg for both cannulas. After perfusion for about 15 minutes and when a deep red color is seen in the epicardial surface of the risk zone, the perfusion is stopped. The heart is then sectioned, from apex to base, into six or seven transverse slices, each ~1 cm thick. The LV slices are fixed in 10% neutral buffered formalin for 4 to 24 hours. This dual perfusion stains the nonischemic myocardium in dark blue, the surviving tissue (TTC-positive region) in fresh red, and the infarcted tissue (TTC-negative region) in white/ yellow/ pale tan color (Figure 26.1). In the reperfused MI model, infarcted tissue is often hemorrhagic but the blood in the tissue is difficult to differentiate from the TTC-stained surviving tissue, the formaldehyde turns the blood into a brown color making the infarct much easier to see (Figure 26.1). After formalin fixation, the atrial and RV tissue are removed, the LV slices are numbered from apex to base as 1 through 6 or 7, weighed, and photographed together with a ruler. From the digital images of each LV cross-section, the sizes of the nonischemic, ischemic/ reperfused, and infarcted areas are measured by means of the planimetry method using the NIH ImageJ software. The values measured from the apical and basal side of the corresponding area are averaged for each LV section and multiplied by that section's weight. The individual values from each LV section are then summed to give the weight of the corresponding areas for the entire heart. The size of area-at-risk is expressed as a percentage of the total LV and the size of infarction is expressed as a percentage of the area-at-risk (Figure 26.2).

Measurement of RMBF distribution using microspheres

For measurement of RMBF, BioPAL stable-isotope neutron-activated microspheres (15 ± 5 μm, BioPhysics Assay Laboratory, Inc., Worcester, MA) are used as described [12,13]. Microspheres are injected at four time points: baseline, during coronary occlusion (15 minutes before reperfusion), and 15 minutes and 72 hours after reperfusion. At each time point, a total of 5×10^6 microspheres labeled with samarium, europium, lutetium, or lanthanum are injected over a 30-second duration into the LV cavity through the pigtail catheter (anesthetized pig model) or into the left atrium (conscious pig model) while reference blood samples are simultaneously drawn from the side arm of the 7F sheath (anesthetized model) or the mammary arterial line (conscious model) using a syringer withdrawal pump (Harvard Apparatus, Millis, MA) for calculation of absolute myocardial blood flow. The withdrawal rate is set at 7 mL/min for a 90-second duration.

At the close of the experiment, four transmural tissue blocks (~1 g) are obtained from both the ischemic/ reperfused and the nonischemic regions (to avoid admixture of ischemic and nonischemic tissue, ischemic specimens are obtained at least 1 cm inside the boundaries of the occluded bed). Each specimen is divided into endocardial and epicardial halves, rinsed in a saline-free buffer, placed in tissue sample vials, and weighed. Tissue and reference blood samples are processed according to BioPAL's *General Protocol For Blood Flow Experiments* and are sent to BioPAL for analysis, which uses neutron activation technology for the measurement of microsphere content [13]. Absolute RMBF is computed in each sample with the formula: RMBF = (counts in tissue sample × reference blood sample withdrawal rate) / (counts in reference blood sample × tissue weight in grams) and expressed as mL/min/g (Table 26.1).

Measurement of cardiac troponin I as a noninvasive index of myocardial infarction

cTnI is a specific biomarker for cardiac tissue and is detected in the serum only if myocardial injury has occurred [14–16]. The troponin assay is able to detect small amounts of cardiomyocyte necrosis and therefore quantifies myocardial infarction [17]. cTnI has been shown to be a more sensitive indicator of myocardial cell injury than CK-MB [18,19]. By 6 hours after symptom onset, detection of cTnI is correlated to 95–99% of patients who are ultimately shown to have a myocardial infarction [16,20]. Thus, cTnI is a highly specific and highly sensitive biomarker to quantitatively evaluate acute myocardial infarction in pig model [21,22], and provides a noninvasive measure to estimate infarct size. In the

Table 26.1 Regional myocardial blood flow (mL/min/g)

	Control (n = 9)	IPC (n = 8)
Baseline		
Nonischemic endocardium	1.34 ± 0.49	1.23 ± 0.39
Nonischemic epicardium	1.12 ± 0.32	1.17 ± 0.26
Ischemic/ reperfused endocardium	1.04 ± 0.44	1.04 ± 0.33
Ischemic/ reperfused epicardium	0.96 ± 0.50	0.96 ± 0.32
45 minute Occlusion		
Nonischemic endocardium	1.33 ± 0.42	1.21 ± 0.54
Nonischemic epicardium	1.28 ± 0.47	1.12 ± 0.39
Ischemic/ reperfused endocardium	0.06 ± 0.10[a]	0.06 ± 0.08[a]
Ischemic/ reperfused epicardium	0.01 ± 0.02[a]	0.03 ± 0.03[a]
15 minute Reperfusion		
Nonischemic endocardium	1.87 ± 1.20	1.38 ± 0.79
Nonischemic epicardium	1.72 ± 1.14	1.36 ± 0.91
Ischemic/ reperfused endocardium	1.29 ± 1.04	1.74 ± 1.61
Ischemic/ reperfused epicardium	1.87 ± 0.54	1.68 ± 1.41
72 hour Reperfusion		
Nonischemic endocardium	1.46 ± 1.62	1.14 ± 0.54
Nonischemic epicardium	1.30 ± 1.44	0.94 ± 0.40
Ischemic/ reperfused endocardium	0.27 ± 0.42[a]	0.92 ± 0.60*
Ischemic/ reperfused epicardium	0.35 ± 0.53[a]	0.78 ± 0.59

Regional myocardial blood flow was measured using neutron-activated microspheres in conscious pigs. RMBF during occlusion was near zero in the area-at-risk of both groups, suggesting complete ischemia during LAD occlusion. RMBF at 72 hour reperfusion was significantly reduced in control pigs, suggesting the no-reflow phenomenon occurred in the infarcted myocardium. Note that ischemic preconditioning prevented the occurrence of the no-reflow phenomenon. Data are ± SD;
[a]$P < 0.01$ vs. baseline;
*$P < 0.05$ vs. control group.

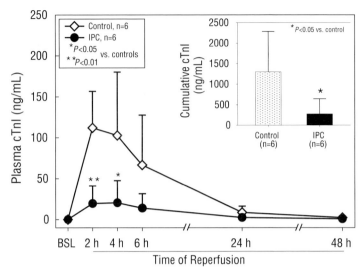

Figure 26.3 Plasma cTnI in conscious pigs undergoing a 60-minute coronary occlusion/72-hour reperfusion without (Control) or with an antecedent ischemic preconditioning (IPC). In IPC pigs, both peak cTnI levels and total cumulative cTnI release (area-under-the-curve, inset) were profoundly reduced, indicating that plasma cTnI enables detection of a cardioprotective effect in the pig model. Data are mean ± SD.

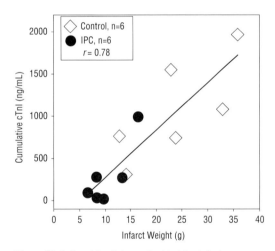

Figure 26.4 Correlation between absolute infarct size by tetrazolium (expressed in grams of tissue weight) and total cumulative cTnI release (area-under-the-curve) in conscious pigs. A high correlation was observed, supporting the use of cTnI as a noninvasive index of infarct size.

pig model, 1 mL of blood sample is collected at each time point: baseline, 2, 4, 6, 24, and 48 hours after reperfusion to determine the time course of cTnI release (Figure 26.3). Plasma cTnI levels peak at 2–3 hours and readily detect the infarct-sparing effects of ischemic PC (Figure 26.3), in high correlation to the TTC-based histological measurements of infarct size (Figure 26.4).

Conclusion

Pigs have been extensively used as animal models of myocardial infarction for the following reasons. First, pigs have cardiac size, baseline heart rate, and blood pressure closer to those in humans than small rodents. Second, the paucity of collateral vessels in the porcine heart [11,23,24] eliminates the variability in collateral flow that is inherent in canine models. Since collateral flow is the major determinant of the severity of myocardial injury, the elimination of this variable ought to result in more reproducible results among different animals. Although dogs are also a good species to study myocardial ischemia/ reperfusion, dogs have a well-developed innate collateral circulation [10]. Third, pigs are relatively inexpensive, can be easily bred, and are easy to keep. In most countries, it is now more difficult and expensive to do studies in dogs than in pigs. Finally, the temporal and spatial development of myocardial infarction in pigs also closely resembles that observed in humans. The conscious pig model, though relatively laborious, may be more clinically relevant because the results are less influenced by potential confounding factors, such as anesthesia, surgical trauma, fluctuations in body temperature, abnormal hemodynamic conditions, and cytokine release. The angioplasty balloon based model is similar to clinical procedure of angioplasty and therefore can be easily translated into clinical application if a novel cardioprotective regimen is discovered.

In conclusion, the pig model of myocardial infarction is of pivotal translational value for future cardiovascular research. From a pragmatic point of view, rodent heart models may be better suited to target novel mechanisms, whereas the confirmation of such novel mechanisms in the pig model of regional myocardial ischemia/ reperfusion appears mandatory for translation to clinical practice.

Acknowledgements

This work was supported in part by NIH grants U24HL-094373 and HL-74351.

References

1 Heusch G, Skyschally A, Schulz R. The in-situ pig heart with regional ischemia/reperfusion – ready for translation. *J Mol Cell Cardiol* 2011; **50**: 951–963.

2 Swindle MM. *Swine in the Laboratory: Surgery, Anesthesia, Imaging, and Experimental Techniques*, 2nd edn, 2007. Boca Raton: CRC Press.

3 Bloor CM, White FC, Lammers RJ. Cardiac ischemia and coronary blood flow in swine. In: Stanton HC and Mersmann HJ, eds. *Swine in Cardiovascular Research*. Boca Raton, FL: CRC Press, 1986, pp. 87–119.

4 Bloor CM, White FC, Roth DM. The pig as a model of myocardial ischemia and gradual coronary occlusion. In: Swindle MM, eds. *Swine as Models in Biomedical Research*. Ames, IA: Iowa State University Press, 1992, pp. 163–175.

5 White FC, Roth DM, Bloor CM. The pig as a model for myocardial ischemia and exercise. *Lab Anim Sci* 1986; **36**: 351–356.

6 Verdouw PD, van den Doel MA, de Zeeuw S, Duncker DJ. Animal models in the study of myocardial ischaemia and ischaemic syndromes. *Cardiovasc Res* 1998; **39**: 121–135.

7 St Louis JD, Hughes GC, Kypson AP, DeGrado TR, Donovan CL, Coleman RE, *et al.* An experimental model of chronic myocardial hibernation. *Ann Thorac Surg* 2000; **69**: 1351–1357.

8 Schulz R, Gres P, Heusch G. Activation of ATP-dependent potassium channels is a trigger but not a mediator of ischaemic preconditioning in pigs. *Br J Pharmacol* 2003; **139**: 65–72.

9 Louttit JB, Hunt AA, Maxwell MP, Drew GM. The time course of cardioprotection induced by GR79236, a selective adenosine A1-receptor agonist, in myocardial ischaemia-reperfusion injury in the pig. *J Cardiovasc Pharmacol* 1999; **33**: 285–291.

10 Kersten JR, Schmeling TJ, Pagel PS, Gross GJ, Warltier DC. Isoflurane mimics ischemic preconditioning via activation of K(ATP) channels: reduction of myocardial infarct size with an acute memory phase. *Anesthesiology* 1997; **87**: 361–370.

11 Cason BA, Gamperl AK, Slocum RE, Hickey RF. Anesthetic-induced preconditioning: previous administration of isoflurane decreases myocardial infarct size in rabbits. *Anesthesiology* 1997; **87**: 1182–1190.

12 Boodhwani M, Nakai Y, Mieno S, Voisine P, Bianchi C, Araujo EG, *et al.* Hypercholesterolemia impairs the myocardial angiogenic response in a swine model of chronic ischemia. role of endostatin and oxidative stress. *Ann Thorac Surg* 2006; **81**: 634–641.

13 Reinhardt CP, Dalhberg S, Tries MA, Marcel R, Leppo JA. Stable labeled microspheres to measure perfusion: validation of a neutron activation assay technique. *Am J Physiol Heart Circ Physiol* 2001; **280**: H108–116.

14 Adams JE 3rd, Bodor GS, Davila-Roman VG, Ladenson JH, Jaffe AS. Cardiac troponin I. A marker with high specificity for cardiac injury. *Circulation* 1993; **88**: 101–106.

15 Adams JE, 3rd, Schechtman KB, Landt Y, Ladenson JH, Jaffe AS. Comparable detection of acute myocardial infarction by creatine kinase MB isoenzyme and cardiac troponin I. *Clin Chem* 1994; **40**: 1291–1295.

16 Adams JE, 3rd, Sicard GA, Allen BT, Bridwell KH, Lenke LG, Dávila-Román VG, *et al.* Diagnosis of perioperative myocardial infarction with measurement of cardiac troponin I. *N Engl J Med* 1994; **330**: 670–674.

17 Twerenbold R, Reichlin T, Reiter M, Müller C. High-sensitive cardiac troponin: friend or foe? *Swiss Med Wkly* 2011; **141**: w13202.

18 Hamm CW, Ravkilde J, Gerhardt W, Jørgensen P, Peheim E, Ljungdahl L, *et al.* The prognostic value of serum troponin T in unstable angina. *N Engl J Med* 1992; **327**: 146–150.

19 Mair J, Wagner I, Puschendorf B, Mair P, Lechleitner P, Dienstl F, *et al.* Cardiac troponin I to diagnose myocardial injury. *Lancet* 1993; **341**: 838–839.

20 Mair J, Wagner I, Jakob G, Lechleitner P, Dienstl F, Puschendorf B, *et al.* Different time courses of cardiac contractile proteins after acute myocardial infarction. *Clin Chim Acta* 1994; **231**: 47–60.

21 Feng YJ, Chen C, Fallon JT, Lai T, Chen L, Knibbs DR, *et al.* Comparison of cardiac troponin I, creatine kinase-MB, and myoglobin for detection of acute ischemic myocardial injury in a swine model. *Am J Clin Pathol* 1998; **110**: 70–77.

22 Wu M, Bogaert J, D'Hooge J, Sipido K, Maes F, Dymarkowski S, *et al.* Closed-chest animal model of chronic coronary artery stenosis. Assessment with magnetic resonance imaging. *Int J Cardiovasc Imaging* 2010; **26**: 299–308.

23 Bolli R, Marban E. Molecular and cellular mechanisms of myocardial stunning. *Physiol Rev* 1999; **79**: 609–634.

24 Bergey JL, Wendt RL, Nocella K, McCallum JD, *et al.* Acute coronary artery occlusion-reperfusion arrhythmias in pigs: antiarrhythmic and antifibrillatory evaluation of verapamil, nifedipine, prenylamine and propranolol. *Eur J Pharmacol* 1984; **97**: 95–103.

Angiogenesis assays

Susmita Sahoo[1] and Douglas W. Losordo[2]

[1] Northwestern University Feinberg School of Medicine, Chicago, IL, USA
[2] Baxter Healthcare Corporation, Deerfield, IL, USA

Introduction

Angiogenesis, the process of growing new blood vessels from pre-existing vessels, has emerged as an important area of study in cardiovascular medicine at both clinical and fundamental scientific levels. For a comprehensive assessment of cellular and physiological triggers of angiogenesis, whole-animal assays are required, which provide the most quantitative information [1]. Assessment of cellular and physiological triggers of angiogenesis and understanding the rationale and limitations of the *in vivo* methods are important for interpreting the results of interventions that alter angiogenesis. Further, there is a need to adopt technically simple and reproducible methodologies for easy quantification of neoangiogenesis to enhance our understanding and ability to develop treatment methods. In the past few years two angiogenic assays that have gained prominence are the Matrigel plug assay and the corneal angiogenesis assay – the Matrigel plug assay for its simplicity and the ease of execution, and the corneal assay for being the gold standard angiogenic assay in which neovessels growing in an avascular corneal tissue are easily visualized [2]. In this chapter we outline both these methods and provide an overview on the choice of the assay suitable for cardiovascular therapies from our experience as scientists in vascular biology and angiogenesis research [3].

In vivo Matrigel plug assay

Definitive tests for angiogenesis require an *in vivo* assay, and the Matrigel plug assay has become a method of choice for many studies involving *in vivo* testing for angiogenesis. One of the advantages of the *in vivo* Matrigel assay is its ease of use without the need for highly technical surgical intervention. In the assay, both inhibitors and activators of angiogenesis can be tested by direct inclusion of the compounds within the injected Matrigel or, by systemic delivery, the activator/ inhibitor can be directly placed within the Matrigel plug after solidification. It must be noted, however, that Matrigel does not necessarily replicate physiologic or pathological neovascularization, processes that may depend intimately on a specific local tissue environment. Nevertheless, it serves a useful purpose to assess specific factors in a controlled environment.

In this assay, test angiogenesis-inducing compounds such as basic fibroblast growth factor (bFGF) [4,5] or tumor cells [6] are introduced into cold liquid Matrigel which, after subcutaneous injection, solidifies and permits penetration by host cells and the formation of new blood vessels. Assessment of angiogenesis in the Matrigel plug is achieved either by measuring hemoglobin or by scoring selected regions of histological sections for vascular density [6]. We now describe a modification of the Matrigel plug assay data analysis using flow cytometry [7],

Manual of Research Techniques in Cardiovascular Medicine, First Edition. Edited by Hossein Ardehali, Roberto Bolli, and Douglas W. Losordo.
© 2014 John Wiley & Sons, Ltd. Published 2014 by John Wiley & Sons, Ltd.

which permits a more precise quantification of the endothelial cells that migrate into the Matrigel plug in a process that mimics angiogenesis. This combination of fluorescence-activated cell sorting (FACS) analysis with the traditional Matrigel assay improves the ability to quantify *in vivo* angiogenesis rate, provides directional information, requires no histological analysis, and lends itself to photographic documentation and image analysis protocols [3,7].

Preparation of reagents and animals

• Mice (C57BL6/J, or athymic nu/nu, or SCID mice, Jackson Laboratory, 6–8 weeks of age).
• Cold sterile phosphate-buffered saline (PBS, Gibco 14040-117).
• Ice-cold liquid growth factor reduced Matrigel (BD Biosciences 356231), thaw overnight at 4°C and kept on ice.
• DMEM cell culture medium (Gibco), and, in the case of assaying cells, specific culture medium used for the cell type used.
• Fibroblast growth Factor-2 (R&D systems, to be used as a positive control for the assay), reconstitute in PBS (1 mg/mL stock), prepare aliquots and store at −20°C. Dilute to 100 µg/mL before the assay.
• Heparin (Gibco), prepare the stock by reconstituting to 1 mg/mL with PBS.
• 70 % Ethanol.
• 3-mL syringes, 21-gauge needles (keep on ice before the injections).
• Isoflurane (2–4%).

Reagents for quantification of angiogenesis

• Collagenase–dispase (F. Hoffmann-La Roche) 0.1% in 10 mM $MgCl_2$ and 200 units/mL DNase I (F. Hoffmann-La Roche) in 10% fetal calf serum/PBS for digestion of the plug.
• 70-mm filter (BD Biosciences).
• Phycoerythrin-conjugated rat anti-mouse-CD31 antibodies (BD Biosciences).
• Phycoerythrin-conjugated rat immunoglobulin G2a isotype (Invitrogen).
• FACS buffer (2 mM EDTA, 2% FBS in PBS, filtered with 0.22-µm filter).
• DAPI solution, 1 mg/mL (BD Pharmingen, I 51-900768).
• Ice-cold methanol for fixing, 100% ethanol, 90% ethanol and xylene solution for washing.
• Masson Trichrome Stain Kit (Richard Allan, 87019).

• Biotinylated GS lectin I (isolectin B4) (Vector Laboratories Inc, Burlingame, CA, USA, B-1205, used in 1:100 dilution).
• HRP-streptavidin (Vector Laboratories Inc, Burlingame, CA, USA, SA-5704), used in 1:100 dilution.
• DAB (Vetor Laboratories Inc, Burlingame, CA, USA, SK-4100).
• Hematoxylin (Poly Scientific, S212A) to stain the nuclei.

Equipment

• Electric clipper to shave hair.
• Rotary microtome HM 325 (Richard Allan).
• Bright field microscope (Olympus, Vanox).
• Flow cytometer FACScan (BD).
• FlowJo software (Tree Star).

Matrigel mixtures and injections

1. Prepare 4 mL of Matrigel angiogenic mixture for five injections for each condition. Mix equal volume (2 mL) of ice-cold DMEM (or 2–5 × 10^6 cells or exosomes from equal number of cells) and Matrigel in an ice-cold Eppendroff tube under laminar hood (we used peripheral blood derived human CD34⁺ stem cells or CD34⁺ cell-depleted total mononuclear cells and exosomes derived from them in our assays). Add 4 µL heparin from the stock (bFGF is effective when coupled to heparin).

2. Add 12 µL from the bFGF (FGF-2) stock to be used as a positive control (~300 ng/mL final concentration), or 12 µL of ice-cold PBS to be used as a negative experimental control; mix thoroughly, keep the mixtures on ice.

3. Anesthetize the mice with inhaled isoflurane (2–4%).

4. Inject 0.5 mL of the Matrigel-growth factors/ cells/ exosome/ PBS mixture subcutaneously. We have best results when the Matrigel is injected to the dorsal side flanks of the mice just above the hips, keeping a distance of at least 0.5 cm between the injected Matrigel plugs of either side.

Matrigel harvest and analysis

1. Sacrifice the mice after 1 or 2 weeks. If the lump from Matrigel injection is prominent, and has not changed much after injection, it is better to harvest the Matrigel after 2 weeks.

2. Wipe the flanks with 70% ethanol.

3. Excise the plug including a little bit of the skin from the perimeter. Wash the tissue with PBS.

4. The plug is cleaned (Figure 27.1A,B) and cut into two halves: fix one half in methanol and prepare the other half for flow cytometry analysis for quantification.

5. Histological analysis of the Matrigel plug:

a. To visualize vessel-like endothelial structures, fix the plug in methanol, embedded into paraffin blocks, and sectioned in to 6-μm slices. De-paraffinize with xylene wash, 3 × 5 minutes, 100% ethanol, 2 × 2 minutes, 90% ethanol 2 × 2 minutes, dH$_2$O 3 minutes.

b. To visualize the live incorporated cells in the Matrigel plug, stain the section with Masson Trichrome; follow the instructions in the kit and acquire images using an Olympus Vanox bright microscope (Figure 27.1C,D).

c. To specifically visualize the incorporation of endothelial cells, block the de-paraffinized section with 10% donkey serum for 30 minutes, stained with biotinylated isolectinB4 for 2 hours at 37°C, wash with PBS, conjugate with HRP-streptavidin for 30 minutes, wash 3× with PBS, DAB staining for 5 minutes, washing with dH$_2$O; stain the nuclei with hematoxylin, washed with dH$_2$O.

d. Acquire the images with an Olympus Vanox bright microscope (Figure 27.1E,F).

6. Quantification of incorporated endothelial cells by flow cytometry analysis:

a. Digest the other half of the plug with 0.1% collagenase/ dispase solution for 1 hour at 37°C.

b. Disperse the cells 4–5 times with a 21-g needle, pass through a 70-μm filter to remove debris.

c. Stain the CD31$^+$ cells with the PE-conjugated antibody or isotype control for 30 minutes on ice in the dark; wash off the unconjugated antibodies and re-suspend in FACS buffer.

d. Add 1 μL of DAPI solution per sample, incubate 2 minutes in the dark.

e. Acquire the data with the flow cytometer, analyze for the percentage of CD31$^+$ cells in total live single cell population using the FlowJo software (Figure 27.1G,H).

Notes

1. Histological staining to identify endothelial cells in the Matrigel can be done with CD31 antibodies;

however, in our experience, isolectin B4 staining was stronger.

2. Hemoglobin analysis can supplement or substitute the flow-cytometry analysis of endothelial cell migration to evaluate angiogenesis. In our assays, the hemoglobin assay was less sensitive in detecting angiogenesis.

Mouse corneal micropocket angiogenesis assay

The cornea is the only avascular transparent tissue in the body, so any vessel grown in the cornea is newly formed and readily visible and quantifiable. Moreover, the cornea is a "privileged site," protected from circulating cells, rapid immune reactions, and many serum constituents [2]. Therefore, corneal neovascularization is a useful model for quantitative investigation of angiogenesis and evaluation of substances with potential pro- and antiangiogenic properties. The other major advantage of using the corneal angiogenesis model is that it allows for continuous monitoring of angiogenesis *in vivo* [8,9]

The corneal assay was originally developed using rabbit cornea, which offers a surgically easier model with a larger implantation area [8]. However, rat and mouse models are more economical; moreover, transgenic and knockout mouse models allow for evaluation of unique environments and genes [1]. Here, we describe the corneal angiogenesis assay in a mouse model. The cornea has an avascular stroma and basal limbal venules. Implantation of a solid pellet containing proangiogenic regulator into a micropocket created in the corneal stroma induces vascular outgrowth from the peripherally located vascular limbus towards the implanted proangiogenic stimulus. Many methods regarding the induction and scoring of corneal angiogenesis have been developed. The micropocket assay, described here, uses implantation of a slow-release polymer pellet containing a known angiogenic factor, or testing reagent, and offers more flexibility and easy quantitation.

Preparation of reagents and animals

• Mice (C57BL6/J, or athymic nu/nu, or SCID mice, Jackson Laboratory, between 8 and 10 weeks of age; we used nude mice in our experiments with exosomes from human stem cells).

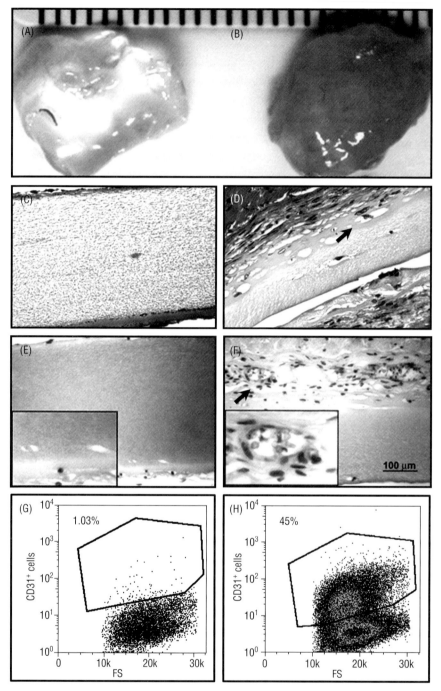

Figure 27.1 Matrigel plug assay. Matrigel plugs ((A) mixed with PBS and (B) with FGF) harvested after 7days; sections from the plug stained with Mason-Trichrome ((C) PBS and (D) FGF) to identify migrated live cells (arrows), and with isolectin to identify vessel-like endothelial structures ((E)PBS and (F) CD34+ exosomes, arrows and inset); quantification of CD31+ endothelial cells in the Matrigel plug by flow cytometry ((G) PBS and (H) FGF). (Source: Modified from Sahoo S 2011 [3]. Reproduced with permission from Wolters Kluwer Health).

• Sucrose octasulfate–aluminum complex (Sucralfate, Sigma S0652).
• Hydron (we used Hydron from HydroMed Sciences; however, it is no longer available). Poly-HEMA (Sigma P3932) [1] and Elvax-40 (Augustin) have been used successfully as a replacement for Hydron in corneal assays.
• Recombinant bFGF (R&D Systems, USA); prepare a stock solution of 1 mg/mL with PBS.
• Fluorescein-conjugated BS1-Lectin I (Vector Laboratories).
• 6-cm Petri dishes.
• 1% Paraformaldehyde.
• Absolute ethanol.
• Proparacaine hydrochloride ophthalmic solution 0.5% (wt/vol; Falcon, 6131401601).
• Avertin (tribromoethanol; Fisher, AC42143-0100).
• Triple antibiotic eye ointment (bacitracin, neomycin, and polymyxin).

Equipment
• Sterile surgical room.
• Surgical tools: sterile forceps, spatula, microspatula, disposable scalpel for microsurgery (no 10/11, Aesculap), jewelers forceps.
• 300-μm nylon mesh (Sefar America Inc., Depew, NY, USA, 03-300/51).
• Surgical binocular operating microscope (Zeiss).
• Surgical instruments (scissors and forceps) and glass slides for harvesting and mounting the corneas.
• Slit lamp stereomicroscope equipped with a digital camera.
• Fluorescence microscope (Zeiss).

Preparation of controlled slow-release pellet
1. Autoclave spatula and mesh before the experiment.
2. Make 12% Hydron in 100% ethanol. Hydron is very difficult to dissolve; therefore we routinely place it on a rotor overnight at room temperature.
3. Under a laminar hood, add 25 μL of bFGF from stock and 10 mg of Sucralfate (this will make about 80 pellets with about 100 ng of bFGF/pellet); mix well; add 10 μL of Hydron solution to the mixture. For control pellets, instead of bFGF solution, use 25 μL sterile water. For pellets with nonliving biological substance, such as conditioned media or exosomes isolated from the conditioned media, the Hydron/Sucralfate mixture is semidried, and the conditioned media or exosomes are in 20–50 μL

volume. If necessary, concentrate the conditioned media using an Amicon Ultracel concentrator with 3-kDa cutoff (Millipore, UFC800308 or UFC500324). Cell suspensions could be used for testing in corneal assay; prepare $2–4 \times 10^6$ cells in 50 μL in the medium, preferably without serum.
4. Immediately transfer the paste from the tube using a bent spatula to spread evenly onto a mesh in a sterile dish. Air-dry for about 20–30 minutes.
5. Release the pellets by pulling apart the fibers of the mesh carefully over a sterile Petri dish. Select the uniform, solid cubes under a microscope.

Surgical procedure
Successful and reproducible micropocket assay implantation requires meticulous surgical skills and practice to obtain a precise incision at the proper depth and distance of the micropocket to the limbus.

1. Anesthetize the mouse with intraperitoneal avertin.
2. Anesthetize the eye with one drop of proparacaine. Wait for 20–30 seconds.
3. Proptose the eye with the dull forceps by gripping the basal skin between the forceps and the eye.
4. Use the microknife to make a partial-thickness incision in the mid-cornea. The incision should be approximately 1 mm from the limbus (Figure 27.2A; note the distance of the pellet visible in the image from the basal limbus of the cornea). Insert the microspatula under the incision and push it towards the inferior limbus to lengthen the micropocket perpendicular to the incision. A small amount of the aqueous humor can be drained using an insulin syringe to reduce the corneal tension.
5. Moisten the pellet and implant it in the micropocket; push it inside the micropocket to make it secure. Ideally, we use one eye each for the stimulus and the control pellet: 5 μL of the suspended cells can be introduced in to the micropocket using a micropipette or an insulin syringe.
6. Apply antibiotic ointment to the eye daily.

Monitoring and quantification of angiogenesis
1. Anesthetize the mice with intraperitoneal avertin, monitor the pellets daily after day 3 using a slit lamp stereomicroscope. Prequantification can be carried out from the images using ImageJ software.
2. One week after implantation, inject the mice with 50 μL of fluorescein-conjugated BS1-LectinI intravenously and sacrifice 15 minutes later.

3. Harvest the eyes and fix with 1% paraformaldehyde.
4. Excise the corneas, clean thoroughly, cut at the sides to flatten them, and mount on a glass slide.
5. Take fluorescence photographs of the corneas (Figure 27.2A,B) and evaluate angiogenesis via BS-1Lectin fluorescence; quantify the length/ area of vessel growth in the cornea using ImageJ software (Figure 27.2C–E).

Although corneal angiogenesis assay is one of the cleanest and most useful assays, it is a technically demanding surgical procedure. Other technical factors such as the length of the assay and lack of automated quantification of vessel growth limit its application in large-scale screening.

Weaknesses and strengths

The Matrigel plug assay is a relatively easy assay, which involves a simple injection less painful to the animals; it may be suitable for carrying out multiple tests and large screenings. However, this assay should be used with caution as Matrigel is a complex mixture of proteins and its composition can vary from lot to lot. Unlike the Matrigel assay, the corneal assay is done under physiologic conditions in which neovessels growing in an avascular corneal tissue are easily visualized. However, the surgery for this method is demanding, requires considerable technical skill, and is not suitable for rapid evaluation

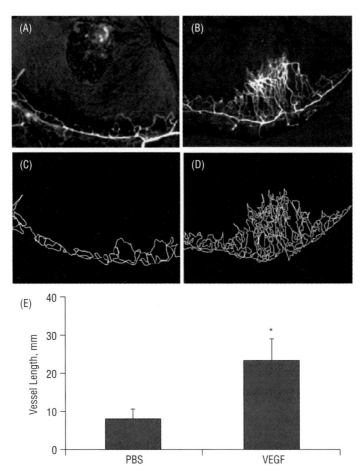

Figure 27.2 Corneal angiogenesis assay. Fluorescent images of mouse corneas implanted with pellets containing PBS (A,C) or VEGF (B,D), and stained with fluorescein-conjugated lectin. To quantify the vessel length, the vessels are traced with ImageJ software (C,D) and quantification of the total length of the vessels (E); n = 4–5; *P < 0.05. (Source: Modified from Sahoo S 2011 [3]. Reproduced with permission from Wolters Kluwer Health).

of test substances. Moreover, the test substance used in the corneal assay is processed as a hard pellet (using ethanol) to be implanted in the cornea; therefore, test of live cells is challenging using this assay.

Alternative approaches

In vitro chick chorioallantoic membrane (CAM) assay model exists to test the angiogenic potential of materials; however, the tests are done on chick cells and one major concern is the embryonic status of the CAM, due to which it undergoes rapid changes both morphologically and in the rate of endothelial cell proliferation, which makes it less suitable for our use.

Discussion and conclusion

In many of the drug-development applications for cardiovascular diseases, it is important to investigate angiogenic mechanisms of the stimulus in the target tissue. Under physiologic or pathological conditions one must determine the degree of remodeling, tissue damage, apoptosis, inflammation, mobilization of bone marrow cells, secretion of growth factors and a changing composition of the extracellular matrix etc. Because of the dynamic nature of the tissue influencing angiogenesis, it is difficult to assess angiogenesis in disease conditions within the tissue of interest. The most common ways of evaluating an angiogenic stimulus under these conditions are in small animal hind limb ischemia or myocardial infarction models. The angiogenic response under tissue ischemia can be easily assessed by quantification of capillaries within the hind limb or cardiac tissue. Typically, these studies involve assessment of the number of capillaries per muscle fiber or per nuclei, or the number of capillaries per area measured from the immunohistochemical examinations or quantification of blood flow using microspheres.

Moving forward, the ongoing challenge in the study of angiogenesis in cardiovascular medicine will be to determine how to link properties of angiogenic blood vessels identified in preclinical assays to those in human disease. Better understanding of the process of angiogenesis and properties of newly formed blood vessels will lead to even more informative assays and biomarkers. These in turn will help in screening and evaluating new, more efficacious drugs and other novel tools in vascular biology. Together, these advances will further the exploitation of vascular abnormalities as targets for drug delivery and the control of blood vessel growth and regression in health and disease.

Acknowledgement

We thank Dr. Delara Montlagh and Amy Cohen of Baxter Healthcare for providing the human CD34$^+$ cells used in this study, Sol Misener for assistance in corneal surgeries, Dr. Aiko Ito for histological analyses and Dr. W. Kevin Meisner for the editorial assistance. This work was supported by AHA-SDG-The Davee Foundation, Baxter-NU, and NeoStem.

References

1 Rogers MS, Birsner AE, D'Amato RJ. The mouse cornea micropocket angiogenesis assay. *Nat Protoc* 2007; **2**: 2545–2550.

2 Auerbach R. An overview of current angiogenesis assays: Choice of assay, precautions in interpretation, future requirements and direction. In: Staton CA, Lewis C, Bicknell R, eds. *Angiogenesis Assays: A Critical Appraisal of Current Techniques*. Wiley, 2006, pp. 361–374.

3 Sahoo S, Klychko E, Thorne T, Misener S, Schultz KM, Millay M, et al. Exosomes from human CD34+ stem cells mediate their proangiogenic paracrine activity. *Circ Res* 2011; **109**: 724–728.

4 Phillips GD, Stone AM, Jones BD, Schultz JC, Whitehead RA, Knighton DR, et al. Vascular endothelial growth factor (rhVEGF165) stimulates direct angiogenesis in the rabbit cornea. *In Vivo* 1994; **8**: 961–965.

5 Kano MR, Morishita Y, Iwata C, Iwasaka S, Watabe T, Ouchi Y, et al. VEGF-A and FGF-2 synergistically promote neoangiogenesis through enhancement of endogenous PDGF-B-PDGFRbeta signaling. *J Cell Sci* 2005; **118**: 3759–3768.

6 Passaniti T, Vitolo MI. In vivo Matrigel angiogenesis assays. In: Augustin HG, ed. *Methods in Endothelial Cell Biology* Berlin Heidelberg: Springer-Verlag, 2004, pp. 207–222.

7 Adini A, Fainaru O, Udagawa T, Connor KM, Folkman J, D'Amato RJ, et al. Matrigel cytometry: a novel method for quantifying angiogenesis in vivo. *J Immunol Methods* 2009; **342**: 78–81.

8 Siqing S, Dewhirst MW. Corneal angiogenesis assay. In: Staton CA, Lewis C, Bicknell R, eds. *Angiogenesis Assays: A Critical Appraisal of Current Techniques*. Wiley, 2006, pp. 203–228.

9 Morbidelli L, Cantara S, Ziche M. Corneal angiogenesis assay. In: Augustin HG, ed. *Methods in Endothelial Cell Biology*. Berlin, Heidelberg: Springer-Verlag, 2004, pp. 263–272.

Immunohistochemical analysis of cardiac tissue

Barbara Ogórek, Donato Cappetta, and Jan Kajstura

Brigham and Women's Hospital, Harvard Medical School, Boston, MA, USA

Introduction

The objective of immunohistochemistry is to identify antigens, usually proteins, in thin sections of normal or diseased tissues. This technique takes advantage of the ability of antibodies to bind with high specificity to their respective targets, that is epitopes, which constitute a unique part of the structure of antigens [1]. The interaction of the antibody with its epitope occurs via hydrogen, ionic, and hydrophobic bonds, as well as van der Waals forces. Each of these interactions is extremely weak in comparison with a covalent bond, but, if present in a large number, they can provide sufficient force to hold antibody and antigen together. This large number of weak bonds necessitates a precise structural match between two molecules, providing the basis for the high specificity of antigen–antibody reactions. And high specificity is the most attractive aspect of immunohistochemistry protocols.

The antibody–antigen interaction can be visualized in a number of ways. Most commonly, particularly in diagnostic clinical practice, the antibody is conjugated to an enzyme, which catalyzes a reaction yielding a colored product. Here, we will discuss applications employing antibodies tagged with a fluorophore, such as fluorescein or rhodamine. Although detection of fluorescent molecules requires complex and expensive instrumentation, the use of these markers has several advantages, including a precisely delineated localization of the antigen

at the site of immunoreaction, the well-defined stoichiometry of the reaction, and the possibility of multicolor imaging. These aspects make immunolabeling and microscopic analysis better suited to analytical approaches in basic research. However, working with fluorescent dyes imposes on the investigator several additional challenges, which are not encountered with the enzyme-based techniques. These problems can be successfully addressed, as discussed in the protocols listed in this chapter.

Direct and indirect immunofluorescence

There are two alternative approaches to immunofluorescence: direct and indirect. With direct fluorescence, the antibody itself is conjugated with the fluorochrome. With indirect fluorescence, the antibody is not modified, but a secondary anti-antibody, which is coupled with a fluorescent dye, is used. The major advantage of direct fluorescence is the simplification of multicolor labeling; the experimenter is not limited by the possible undesired interactions of secondary antibodies with nonrelevant primary antibodies. Essentially, with direct immunofluorescence the number of antibodies and colors is limited only by the optical setup of microscope to be used for the analysis. However, the major problem with this technique is the limited number of directly tagged

Manual of Research Techniques in Cardiovascular Medicine, First Edition. Edited by Hossein Ardehali, Roberto Bolli, and Douglas W. Losordo.
© 2014 John Wiley & Sons, Ltd. Published 2014 by John Wiley & Sons, Ltd.

antibodies that are commercially available. Conversely, a vast array of fluorescently labeled antibodies designed for flow cytometry can be purchased, but they perform poorly on formalin-fixed material. This problem can be overcome by performing fluorescent labeling of primary antibodies. An example of the protocol is listed.

Protocol 1: labeling of primary antibody

This protocol uses mouse monoclonal α-smooth muscle actin antibody (clone 1A4, Sigma, catalog number A5228) and Alexa Fluor® 488 antibody labeling kit (Invitrogen, catalog number A20181). Other types of antibodies, including polyclonal, and different fluorochromes can by easily implemented.

1. Verify the concentration of the antibody; it can be found in the Certificate of Analysis provided with the antibody. Dilute the antibody with PBS to reach the concentration of 1 mg/mL.
2. Take a 100 μL aliquot of the antibody and mix with 10 μL 1 M NaHCO₃.
3. Transfer the entire antibody solution to tube containing AlexaFluor 488 reactive dye (labeled as Component A by the manufacturer).
4. Dissolve the dye by inverting the tube several times. As always when working with antibodies, avoid violent stirring, e.g. vortexing.
5. Incubate the solution for 1 hour at room temperature, gently mixing from time to time.
6. Prepare the purification column as described by the manufacturer.
7. Apply the mixture of antibody and the dye on top of the purification column. Place the column in an empty tube (collection tube).
8. Centrifuge the tube with the column inside for 5 minutes at $1000 g$ in a swinging bucket rotor.
9. Discard the purification column; it contains now only the unbound dye. The labeled antibody is present at the bottom of the collection tube.

Frozen or paraffin sections

Frequently, frozen sections are preferred for immunohistochemistry because the antigen structure is preserved better than in formalin-fixed, paraffin embedded material. However, the latter offers several advantages, including a dramatically superior preservation of tissue structure, the

possibility to analyze larger sections, and ease in the storage of the samples. Unfortunately, fixation of tissue by formalin results in cross-linking of intra- and extracellular proteins. Formaldehyde binds to several amino acids: lysine, arginine, tyrosine, asparagine, histidine, glutamine, and serine. These reactions confer mechanical rigidity to the tissue and render it less prone to biodegradation, but they also have the undesired effect of restricting the penetration of the antibody in the tissue sections and hindering the antibody–antigen reaction.

In 1991, immunostaining on formalin-fixed, paraffin-embedded sections was made possible by the introduction of heat-mediated retrieval of immunoreactivity [2]. This method is now widely used and applies to the detection of the overwhelming majority of antigens, with few exceptions for which enzymatic retrieval is required [3]. The most popular antigen retrieval procedures include microwaving in citrate buffer and the pressure-cooker technique. The citrate-based solution is designed to break the protein crosslinks, and therefore unmask the epitopes in formalin fixed tissue sections, thus enhancing the staining intensity of antibodies. An example of this protocol is provided.

Protocol 2: antigen retrieval by microwaving

1. Prepare 10 mM citrate buffer, pH 6.0 (dissolve 2.4 g sodium citrate and 0.35 g citric acid in 1 L of water).
2. Fill two plastic Coplin jars with citrate buffer. Glass Coplin jars cannot be used for this purpose since they break when exposed to microwaves.
3. Insert deparaffinized and rehydrated slides into one of the Coplin jars.
4. Place jars in the microwave oven. Do not cover them tightly.

Several types of microwave ovens designed specifically for microwave antigen retrieval are commercially available. However, equally good results can be obtained with equipment designed for household use. The most important factor that has to be considered when using household equipment is the uniform distribution of heat inside the oven. Power of the oven should be 1–1.2 kW.

5. Turn on the oven, bring the buffer to boiling.
6. Set the oven timer for 10 minutes.

7. When the volume of the buffer in the jar containing the slides decreases, stop the oven. Using protective gloves, refill the jar with the hot citrate buffer from the other container. Usually this step has to be repeated every 2–3 minutes.

8. Continue the process until the 10-minute period passes by.

9. Remove the jars from the oven; use protective gloves.

10. Let the container with the slides cool down at room temperature for 30 minutes.

11. Wash in Ca/Mg-free PBS. The slides are now ready for staining.

Ah, those colorful images

One of the major advantages of fluorescence microscopy is the possibility of multicolor imaging. This approach provides an enormous advantage when co-localization of multiple proteins is the objective of analysis. The protocol summarized in the following text combines staining for α-sarcomeric actin, α-smooth muscle actin, and von Willebrand factor. It allows simultaneous visualization of the three main cellular compartments of the myocardium. This strategy involves AlexaFluor 488-labeled anti-α-smooth muscle actin, prepared, as described in Protocol 1. It is performed on 4-μm thin sections obtained from a mouse heart perfusion-fixed with 10% formalin. The sections are collected on poly-L-lysine-coated slides (Poly-Prep, Sigma, catalog number P0425).

Protocol 3: multicolor labeling of formalin-fixed, paraffin embedded myocardial sections

1. Deparaffinize and rehydrate slides by placing them for 30 minutes in an oven preheated to 70°C, and sequentially immersing in two changes of xylenes, 5 minutes each, two changes of 96% ethanol, 5 minutes each, and 90%, 80%, and 70% ethanol, 3 minutes each.

2. Rinse the slides in distilled water, place in Coplin jar filled with citric buffer and proceed with microwave antigen retrieval as detailed in Protocol 2.

3. Holding the slide horizontally, remove the excess PBS with absorbent paper towel. Leave a small amount of PBS on and around the section. This amount should be just enough to prevent drying of PBS around the specimen.

4. Apply anti-α-sarcomeric actin (mouse monoclonal, Sigma, catalog number A2172) diluted 1:500 in Ca/Mg-free PBS. The amount to be applied varies with the size of the section. As a rule of thumb, use 1 μl of antibody solution per 1 mm^2 of the sample.

5. Incubate in a moist chamber for 2 hours at 37°C.

6. Wash the slides in five changes of Ca/Mg-free PBS for a total of 10 minutes. Remove the excess of PBS as in Step 3.

7. Apply donkey TRITC-labeled anti-mouse IgM (Jackson ImmunoResearch, catalog number 715-025-140) diluted 1:40 in Ca/Mg-free PBS. Incubate in a moist chamber for 1 hour at 37°C.

8. Wash the slides in five changes of Ca/Mg-free PBS for a total of 10 minutes.

9. Immerse the slides in 4% solution of paraformaldehyde (Electron Microscopy Science, catalog number 15713) for 10 minutes. Wash the slides in five changes of Ca/Mg-free PBS for a total of 10 minutes. Paraformaldehyde cross-links the primary and secondary antibody, preventing their dissociation, which could interfere with antibodies used in the next steps.

10. Remove excess of PBS, apply AlexaFluor 488-labeled anti-α-smooth muscle actin (see Protocol 1). Incubate in a moist chamber for 1 hour at 37°C.

11. Wash the slides in five changes of Ca/Mg-free PBS for a total of 10 minutes. Remove the excess of PBS.

12. Apply anti-von Willebrand antibody (rabbit polyclonal, Dako, catalog number A0082) diluted 1:100 in Dako's Antibody Diluent (catalog number S0809) for 1 hour at 37°C.

13. Wash the slides in five changes of Ca/Mg-free PBS for a total of 10 minutes. Remove the excess of PBS.

14. Apply donkey Cy5-labeled anti-mouse IgG (Jackson ImmunoResearch, catalog number 715-175-150) diluted 1:40 in Ca/Mg-free PBS. Incubate in a moist chamber for 1 hour at 37°C.

15. Wash the slides in five changes of Ca/Mg-free PBS for a total of 10 minutes.

16. Incubate with DAPI (4′,6-diamidino-2-phenylindole, Sigma, catalog number D9564),

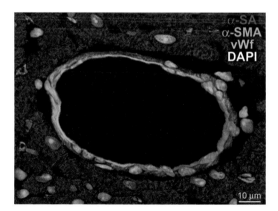

Figure 28.1 Coronary arteriole in the mouse heart. α-sarcomeric actin (α-SA, red), α-smooth muscle actin (α-SMA, green), von Willebrand factor (vWf, bright blue), and DAPI (white) identify, respectively, cardiomyocytes, smooth muscle cells, endothelial cells, and cell nuclei. Confocal microscopy, 60× lens with numerical aperture 1.42.

diluted at 100 ng/mL of Ca/Mg-free PBS, for 15 minutes at room temperature.

17. Wash the slides in five changes of Ca/Mg-free PBS for a total of 10 minutes.

18. Remove carefully PBS from the slide. Apply a small aliquot of Vectashield (Vector Laboratories, catalog number H1000) close to the center of the stained specimen. Use 8 and 14 μL of Vectashield for a 24 × 24 mm and 24 × 40 mm coverglass, respectively. Apply gently the coverglass, wait approximately 1 minute to allow Vectashield to spread uniformly.

The resulting four-color preparation requires a confocal microscope equipped with UV laser or blue diode laser. Similar protocols have been used in many of our works (for a review see references [4] and [5]). An example is illustrated in Figure 28.1.

Do your controls

An issue of paramount importance is the proper use of controls to ensure the specificity of the staining. Positive controls document that the antibody does interact with the appropriate epitope. The optimal strategy, although not always feasible, should include biological controls, that is tissues that are known to express the antigen of interest. They should be

processed together with the samples under examination. In the case of monoclonal antibodies, an excellent positive control is represented by a monoclonal antibody against an alternative epitope located on the same antigen. In this case, both antibodies should generate an identical signal. Negative controls serve to ascertain that the antibody does not react with irrelevant epitopes. Again, a biological control that is known not to express the target of interest constitutes an excellent material. A very elegant negative control consists of the use of a ligand-blocked antibody, in which the binding domains in the antibody are saturated by the antigen before the reagent is used for immunolabeling. An example of this procedure for laminin antibody is given in the following text.

Protocol 4: ligand-blocking of an antibody

1. Prepare solution of rabbit polyclonal anti-laminin (Sigma, catalog number L9393) at concentration twofold higher than that typically used in the staining, 1:50 in PBS. Calculate concentration of the antibody (in this case, 27.6 μg/mL), and molar concentration (molecular weight of IgG is 160,000 Da, therefore the solution is 0.17 nM).

2. Prepare solution of laminin with 10-fold higher concentration of the protein, i.e., 1.7 nM. Since molecular weight of laminin is 850,000 Da, the final laminin concentration will be 1.45 mg/mL.

3. Mix equal volumes of antibody and laminin solution. Incubate for 30 minutes at 37°C.

4. Centrifuge for 5 minutes at 10,000 g. Collect the supernatant; this is the solution of the ligand-blocked antibody to be used in your staining.

As a final piece of practical advice: keep your eyes wide open. The famous remark of Yogi Berra, "You can observe a lot just by watching," [6] is particularly true in this area of experimentation.

References

1 Davies DR, Cohen GH. Interactions of protein antigens with antibodies. *Proc Natl Acad Sci USA* 1996; **93**: 7–12.

2 Shi SR, Key ME, Kalra KL. Antigen retrieval in formalin-fixed, paraffin-embedded tissues: an enhancement method for immunohistochemical staining based on microwave oven heating of tissue sections. *J Histochem Cytochem* 1991; **39**: 741–748.

3 Cattoretti G, Pileri S, Parravicini C, Becker MH, Poggi S, Bifulco C, *et al.* Antigen unmasking on formalin-fixed, paraffin-embedded tissue sections. *J Pathol* 1993; **171**: 83–98.

4 Anversa P, Leri A, Rota M, Hosoda T, Bearzi C, Urbanek K, *et al.* Stem cells, myocardial regeneration, and methodological artifacts. *Stem Cells* 2007; **25**: 589–601.

5 Leri A, Kajstura J, Anversa P. Role of cardiac stem cells in cardiac pathophysiology: a paradigm shift in human myocardial biology. *Circ Res* 2011; **109**: 941–961.

6 Berra Y. *The Yogi Book*. New York: Workman Publishing, 1998, p. 95.

A murine model of cardiac arrest by exsanguination

Guangming Cheng,[1] Yiru Guo,[2] Harold K. Elias,[1] Carrie M. Quinn,[1] Arash Davani,[1] Yanjuan Yang,[1] Magdy Girgis,[1] Roberto Bolli,[2] and Buddhadeb Dawn[1]

[1] University of Kansas Medical Center, Kansas City, KS, USA

[2] University of Louisville, Louisville, KY, USA

Introduction

Cardiac arrest, a potentially terminal event, manifests as ventricular tachycardia/ fibrillation, asystole, or pulseless electrical activity in patients. The prolonged hypoperfusion of vital organs during arrest and resuscitation results in death or considerable morbidity even after a successfully resuscitated arrest. Notably, only approximately 11.4% of an estimated 382,000 patients experiencing out-of-hospital cardiac arrest, and 23% of an estimated 209,000 patients experiencing in-hospital cardiac arrest survive to discharge [1]. These facts underscore the acute need for increased awareness regarding the perils of cardiac arrest and for greater emphasis on resuscitative research.

However, an important problem with cardiac arrest research relates to the paucity of suitable animal models that mimic cardiac arrest in patients. The models of cardiac arrest in pigs, dogs, rats, and mice have thus far utilized asphyxia [2–6], ventricular fibrillation (VF) [7–13], or administration of KCl [14–17]. However, all of these models have their specific advantages and disadvantages, often related to the mode of arrest induction, that limit the utility of observations made. Moreover, the large animal models are often unsuitable or prohibitively expensive for genetic manipulation and molecular investigation. Hence we aimed to establish a mouse model of cardiac arrest that mimicked a real-life cardiac arrest with similar outcomes and yet with minimal confounding variables. We chose the mouse primarily because of its suitability for genetic manipulations. We chose exsanguination because this circumvents the use of extraneous agents and manipulations that may potentially interfere with accurate assessment of outcomes after a successful resuscitation. In this chapter, we describe this novel mouse model of cardiac arrest.

Materials and methods

Materials

Mice:
- Strains: C57BL/6
- Age: 10–12 weeks

Reagents/ equipment:
- Isoflurane and delivery system
- Mouse ventilator
- 20-G × 1″ i.v. catheter for endotracheal intubation
- 27-G needle for blood withdrawal
- 30-G needle attached to a PE-10 tubing (jugular vein cannulation)
- Heating pad and heating lamp

Manual of Research Techniques in Cardiovascular Medicine, First Edition. Edited by Hossein Ardehali, Roberto Bolli, and Douglas W. Losordo.

• AD Instruments PowerLab Data Acquisition System.

Methods

The investigation conforms to the principles of laboratory animal care according to the Guide for the Care and Use of Laboratory Animals (Department of Health and Human Services, NIH Publication No. 86-23, revised 1996). The experimental procedure described herein was approved by the Institutional Animal Care and Use Committee at the University of Kansas Medical Center.

Animals

Male mice (C57BL/6J, age 10–12 weeks) are purchased from the Jackson Laboratory (Bar Harbor, ME) and maintained at the Laboratory Animal Resources Center at the University of Kansas Medical Center. Mice are kept on a standardized diet and allowed to acclimatize to their new environment over a period of 48–72 hours, prior to any procedure. During this time, their circadian rhythm is maintained on a 12:12 hours alternating dark:light cycle.

Animal preparation

Following the induction of anesthesia (3% isoflurane), the anterior aspect of chest is shaved and the mouse placed in supine position with the limbs extended and restrained using adhesive tape. This is quickly followed by endotracheal intubation using a 20-G × 1″ i.v. catheter and mechanical ventilation using a mouse ventilator (Harvard MiniVent ventilator, Hugo Sachs Electronik, March-Hugstetten, Germany). The respiratory rate is maintained at 110 breathes/min and the tidal volume is adjusted according to the body weight to maintain arterial carbon dioxide tension within the physiological range (35–45 mmHg). Anesthesia is maintained with 1.5% isoflurane in 100% oxygen.

During the entire procedure, the core body temperature is monitored using a rectal probe and maintained very close to 37°C with the use of a heating pad and a heating lamp. A pressure–volume catheter (Mikro-Tip, 1F, Miller Instruments, Inc.) is then introduced into the right carotid artery connected to PowerLab16/30 Data Acquisition System (AD Instruments, Colorado Springs, CO) for arterial blood pressure monitoring.

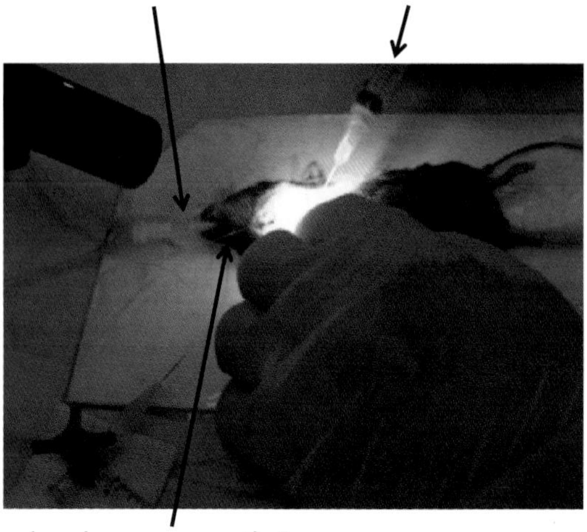

Endotracheal tube for mechanical ventilation   **Heparinized syringe with a 27-G needle for blood withdrawal**

Jugular venous catheter for blood reinfusion

Figure 29.1 Withdrawal of blood to induce cardiac arrest. A 27-G needle is introduced slowly and carefully through the left precordium to enter the left ventricular cavity. Blood is slowly withdrawn into the attached heparinized syringe by gentle suction. The direction of the needle is changed as necessary to facilitate blood withdrawal.

Electrocardiographic limb leads are used to monitor cardiac electrical activity and heart rate; and to document a state of electromechanical dissociation following exsanguination. For i.v. infusion of blood, fluid, and epinephrine, a 30-G needle connected to a PE-10 tubing is inserted into the right internal jugular vein. Both blood pressure and heart rate are recorded continuously starting at baseline (before cardiac arrest) until approximately 20 minutes after successful resuscitation.

Surgical procedure

Induction of cardiopulmonary arrest. Following instrumentation described previously, cardiac arrest is achieved by exsanguination. As shown in Figure 29.1, a 27-G needle is inserted percutaneously into the left ventricular cavity by penetrating the left precordium. The depth and direction of the needle are changed as necessary to achieve maximal blood withdrawal while avoiding traumatic injury to LV walls, lungs, and thoracic structures. With this

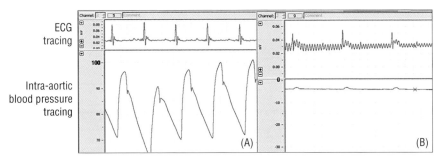

ECG
tracing

Intra-aortic
blood pressure
tracing

(A)   (B)

Figure 29.2 Heart rate and intra-arterial blood pressure before and during cardiac arrest. The heart rate and blood pressure tracings are recorded by LabChart (version 7) using PowerLab 16/30 Data Acquisition System. (A) Heart rate and blood pressure before the induction of cardiac arrest in a representative mouse. (B) Reduced heart rate (approximately 140 beats/min) and nearly undetectable blood pressure during cardiac arrest after blood withdrawal is complete. Together, these features constitute a pathological condition that mimics "pulseless electrical activity" in the clinical setting.

approach, blood is withdrawn directly from the LV cavity into a heparinized syringe by gentle suction. The target blood volume is estimated at 0.5 mL/10 g of body weight, which approximates to 1–1.5 mL of blood in mice weighing 25–30 g. The mechanical ventilation is stopped as soon as blood withdrawal is complete in order to establish a definitive and profound state of cardiorespiratory arrest. This state of circulatory collapse is maintained for 3.5 minutes. After blood withdrawal is complete, the syringe is kept at room temperature until reinfusion.

Resuscitation. After 3.5 minutes of cardiac arrest, heparinized autologous blood mixed with 5 μg of epinephrine is reinfused through the jugular vein. The ventilator is restarted at the beginning of blood infusion. In the event of a lack of sustained cardiac electrical activity on the monitor, a series of rapid yet gentle chest compressions are delivered using a fingertip until circulation is reestablished. Mice are extubated approximately 20 minutes after successful resuscitation and allowed to recover under close observation. During this period, the mouse is placed on a heating pad and kept in an incubator maintained at 37°C. The body temperature is monitored and the mouse is observed for continuation of spontaneous breathing and gradual recovery of ambulation and feeding behavior. If the mouse is noted to be lethargic and poorly responsive, the ECG leads are reattached to document any abnormal rhythm. In case of death during recovery, an autopsy is preformed to identify any traumatic injury to LV walls, large vessels, lungs,

and other mediastinal structures contributing to death. Following complete recovery, mice are returned to cages and subsequently to the animal facility.

Hemodynamic parameters. The heart rate and blood pressure before exsanguination in a mouse subjected to cardiac arrest are shown in Figure 29.2A. During blood withdrawal, intra-arterial blood pressure decreases progressively to approximately 0–5 mmHg at the completion of blood withdrawal (Figure 29.2B). During arrest, heart rate also decreases progressively to approximately 80–180 beats/min. Following infusion of blood and CPR, the heart rate and blood pressure increase gradually to reach near prearrest values. These changes in heart rate and blood pressure during the entire procedure are shown in Figure 29.3. These data indicate that exsanguination in this mouse model produces a hemodynamic state that faithfully mimics "pulseless electrical activity" in humans.

Assessment of outcomes. Since cardiac arrest inflicts systemic (whole-body) ischemia/reperfusion injury, dysfunction of brain, heart, and other organs is noted after this procedure. In order to detect such changes, we recommend that the following functional tests are performed along with this procedure:

1. Cardiac outcomes:
    a. complete echocardiographic evaluation of cardiac structure and function 4 days before

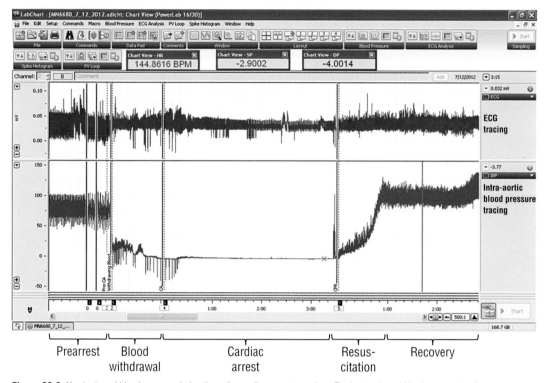

Figure 29.3 Heart rate and blood pressure during the entire cardiac arrest procedure. The heart rate and blood pressure tracings are recorded by LabChart (version 7) using PowerLab 16/30 Data Acquisition System. The hemodynamic tracings from a representative mouse show continuous recordings of heart rate and blood pressure before and during arrest and after successful resuscitation. The blood pressure drops conspicuously after blood withdrawal is complete, and remains at nearly undetectable levels through the entire 3.5 minutes of cardiac arrest. Following the infusion of normothermic blood, the blood pressure and heart rate recover progressively to near prearrest levels.

cardiac arrest, and at serial time points after resuscitation;

b. histological evaluation for myocyte apoptosis after sacrifice.

2. Neurological function and behavior:

a. memory and new learning, tested at serial time points using a modified Barnes maze;

b. neuromuscular coordination, tested at serial time points using the high-wire test;

c. behavior, movement and activity tested at serial time points by an automated device such as the Open Field system (AccuScan Instruments, Inc., Columbus, OH).

3. Renal and hepatic function to measure plasma levels of biochemical parameters.

In our experience, a 3.5-minute cardiac arrest in C57BL/6 mice is sufficient to cause apoptosis in various tissues and changes in cardiac and neurological function.

Discussion

Despite several changes in treatment algorithms, the outcomes of resuscitated cardiac arrest have not changed substantially [18]. Although more research efforts are clearly needed in this area, the lack of reliable and reproducible animal models of cardiac arrest, especially in small animals, has been a major barrier in this regard. Indeed, the current rodent models of cardiac arrest involve the induction of asphyxia in a rather unphysiological manner, or use KCl to produce cardiac standstill, resulting in changes in electrolyte levels, thereby introducing confounding variables. Notwithstanding these difficulties in producing a reliable model, the use of mice will greatly facilitate the investigation of molecular changes occurring during cardiac arrest and potential therapeutic interventions.

Although cardiac arrest in humans is frequently caused by ventricular arrhythmias, inducing arrhythmias in mice is difficult. Given the very high heart rate in mice, ventricular fibrillation (VF) in mice is quite challenging to induce as well as to maintain. We developed this mouse model of cardiac arrest with the perspectives discussed earlier. In this regard, this model of arrest by exsanguination offers several advantages: (i) the withdrawal of blood resulting in precipitous decrease in blood pressure and reduced heart rate creates a hemodynamic state that closely mimics pulseless electrical activity [19], a type of cardiac arrest frequently seen in patients; (ii) the induction of cardiac arrest with this method does not introduce extraneous electrolytes or chemicals into the circulation; (iii) it does not require the induction of arrhythmia, a highly unpredictable event in the mouse; (iv) the survival of approximately 40–50% mice allows meaningful studies; (v) the ease of genetic manipulations in the mouse makes it easier to test the functions of specific molecules in the setting of cardiac arrest in this model, and (vi) the mouse offers an inexpensive alternative for the initial hypothesis testing, before proceeding to costly preclinical experimentation in dogs or pigs. Moreover, the surgical technique for blood withdrawal is not overly difficult and the target blood volume can be withdrawn in the majority of mice. Indeed, necropsy studies revealed minimal damage to the myocardium in resuscitated mice. However, it should be noted that this mouse model is designed to recapitulate cardiac arrest as a result of "pulseless electrical activity" [19] and therefore the pathophysiology differs from that encountered during an arrhythmic cardiac arrest, in which the intravascular blood volume is preserved in the absence of effective circulation. In order to accurately reproduce an arrhythmic cardiac arrest, a large animal model (for example, a pig model [9,10]), may be used instead.

In summary, the mouse model of resuscitated cardiac arrest described herein produces pulseless electrical activity and may serve as a key platform for a broad range of investigations elucidating the physiological, biochemical, and molecular genetic changes associated with cardiac arrest. This model may therefore prove very useful for the identification of putative molecular targets for the management or prevention of cardiac arrest as well as for testing innovative therapies.

Acknowledgments

The authors gratefully acknowledge the expert secretarial assistance of Ms. Renee Falsken. This work was supported by NIH grant R01 HL-089939. The authors report no conflict of interest.

References

1 Roger VL, Go AS, Lloyd-Jones DM, Benjamin EJ, Berry JD, Borden WB, et al. Heart disease and stroke statistics – 2012 update: a report from the American Heart Association. *Circulation* 2012; **125**: e2–e220.

2 Katz L, Vaagenes P, Safar P, Diven W. Brain enzyme changes as markers of brain damage in rat cardiac arrest model. Effects of corticosteroid therapy. *Resuscitation* 1989; **17**: 39–53.

3 Hickey RW, Karasic RB, Bircher NG. ATP-MgCl2 pre-treatment in an animal model of asphyxial arrest. *Resuscitation* 1993; **25**: 109–118.

4 Liachenko S, Tang P, Hamilton RL, Xu Y. A reproducible model of circulatory arrest and remote resuscitation in rats for NMR investigation. *Stroke* 1998; **29**: 1229–1238; discussion 1238–1229.

5 McCaul CL, McNamara P, Engelberts D, Slorach C, Hornberger LK, Kavanagh BP, et al. The effect of global hypoxia on myocardial function after successful cardiopulmonary resuscitation in a laboratory model. *Resuscitation* 2006; **68**: 267–275.

6 Schreckinger M, Geocadin RG, Savonenko A, Yamashita S, Melnikova T, Thakor NV, et al. Long-lasting cognitive injury in rats with apparent full gross neurological recovery after short-term cardiac arrest. *Resuscitation* 2007; **75**: 105–113.

7 Bottiger BW, Schmitz B, Wiessner C, Vogel P, Hossmann KA. Neuronal stress response and neuronal cell damage after cardiocirculatory arrest in rats. *J Cereb Blood Flow Metab* 1998; **18**: 1077–1087.

8 Cerchiari EL, Safar P, Klein E, Cantadore R, Pinsky M. Cardiovascular function and neurologic outcome after cardiac arrest in dogs. The cardiovascular post-resuscitation syndrome. *Resuscitation* 1993; **25**: 9–33.

9 Tang W, Weil MH, Sun S, Gazmuri RJ, Bisera J. Progressive myocardial dysfunction after cardiac resuscitation. *Crit Care Med* 1993; **21**: 1046–1050.

10 Gazmuri RJ, Weil MH, Bisera J, Tang W, Fukui M, McKee D, et al. Myocardial dysfunction after successful resuscitation from cardiac arrest. *Crit Care Med* 1996; **24**: 992–1000.

11 Kern KB, Hilwig RW, Rhee KH, Berg RA. Myocardial dysfunction after resuscitation from cardiac arrest: an example of global myocardial stunning. *J Am Coll Cardiol* 1996; **28**: 232–240.

12 Song L, Weil MH, Tang W, Sun S, Pellis T. Cardiopulmonary resuscitation in the mouse. *J Appl Physiol* 2002; **93**: 1222–1226.

13 Fang X, Tang W, Sun S, Huang L, Chang YT, Huang Z, *et al*. Cardiopulmonary resuscitation in a rat model of chronic myocardial ischemia. *J Appl Physiol* 2006; **101**: 1091–1096.

14 Abella BS, Zhao D, Alvarado J, Hamann K, Vanden Hoek TL, Becker LB, *et al*. Intra-arrest cooling improves outcomes in a murine cardiac arrest model. *Circulation* 2004; **109**: 2786–2791.

15 Kofler J, Hattori K, Sawada M, DeVries AC, Martin LJ, Hurn PD, *et al*. Histopathological and behavioral characterization of a novel model of cardiac arrest and cardiopulmonary resuscitation in mice. *J Neurosci Methods* 2004; **136**: 33–44.

16 Neigh GN, Kofler J, Meyers JL, Bergdall V, La Perle KM, Traystman RJ, *et al*. Cardiac arrest/cardiopulmonary resuscitation increases anxiety-like behavior and decreases social interaction. *J Cereb Blood Flow Metab* 2004; **24**: 372–382.

17 Noppens RR, Kofler J, Hurn PD, Traystman RJ. Dose-dependent neuroprotection by 17beta-estradiol after cardiac arrest and cardiopulmonary resuscitation. *Crit Care Med* 2005; **33**: 1595–1602.

18 Nolan JP, Neumar RW, Adrie C, Aibiki M, Berg RA, Bottiger BW, *et al*. Post-cardiac arrest syndrome: epidemiology, pathophysiology, treatment, and prognostication. A Scientific Statement from the International Liaison Committee on Resuscitation; the American Heart Association Emergency Cardiovascular Care Committee; the Council on Cardiovascular Surgery and Anesthesia; the Council on Cardiopulmonary, Perioperative, and Critical Care; the Council on Clinical Cardiology; the Council on Stroke. *Resuscitation* 2008; **79**: 350–379.

19 Mehta C, Brady W. Pulseless electrical activity in cardiac arrest: electrocardiographic presentations and management considerations based on the electrocardiogram. *Am J Emerg Med* 2012; **30**: 236–239.

Part 4
Small Animal Imaging

30 Blood pressure, telemetry, and vascular measurements in the rodent model

Robert S. Danziger

University of Illinois at Chicago, Chicago, IL, USA

Introduction

Methods for recording cardiovascular physiology in rodents have advanced greatly in the last 10 years, prompted by the desire to phenotype a wide range of novel genetic mouse and rat strains. Measurements of peripheral arterial hemodynamics and vascular function are now possible using a variety of techniques.

Measurement of blood pressure

There are a variety of techniques available for measuring blood pressure (BP), and the one chosen should depend on the type of study, objectives, and resources available.

Noninvasive arterial BP monitoring (indirect methods)

Indirect methods for BP measurement are based for the most part on the application of various cuffs, which typically sense the point at which blood flow occurs during occlusion and release of blood flow through manipulation of the cuff pressure on an artery. These techniques utilize a variety of methods including photoelectric sensors, oscillometric sensors, Doppler sensors, chamber volume sensors, or acoustic sensors.

Indirect methods are recommended [1] for screening for frank systolic hypertension, large group differences in BP, substantial changes in systolic BP over time, and for screening BP in large numbers of rodents. Indirect methods are generally not recommended for quantifying relationships between BP and other variables, studying BP-independent effects of any intervention, analyzing intermittent or subtle forms of hypertension, measuring BP variability, determining diastolic BP or pulse pressure in conscious rodents, and making inferences about BP in a nonstressed, unrestrained animal.

The primary advantages of the noninvasive methods are that they do not require surgery, can be used in conscious animals, are less expensive than telemetry, can be used for repeated measurements, and are useful in screening a large number of animals [1]. Furthermore, they have been used for many of the rodent studies that have form the basis of clinical practices in humans.

The disadvantages are that: (1) they measure blood pressure over only a few cycles, making them not useful for measuring average BP over longer periods of time, for example day and night; (2) the restraint used provides stress and perturbs the cardiovascular system, thereby inducing increases in heart rate and blood pressure [2]; and (3) the accuracy of the indirect BP measurement systems has been questioned. Their ability to measure diastolic BP may also be inferior.

Manual of Research Techniques in Cardiovascular Medicine, First Edition. Edited by Hossein Ardehali, Roberto Bolli, and Douglas W. Losordo.
© 2014 John Wiley & Sons, Ltd. Published 2014 by John Wiley & Sons, Ltd.

Overview of the method. A cuff with a pneumatic pulse sensor is applied to the tail (i.e. "tail-cuff measurement"). Systolic and diastolic BP and HR are subsequently recorded, and three to ten measurements are usually made during a measurement session. Conventional noninvasive BP measurements in rodents are usually made after heating the animals; however, the need for this step has been questioned [3]. Animals are also usually "preconditioned" to reduce stress. This may include allowing the animals to habituate to the procedure for 5–10 days before data collection, placing the animals in the dark, using a single technician, or use of rewards [4].

There are a variety of currently available commercial systems, including ones made by IITC Life Science Inc. (Woodland Hills, CA); Columbus Instruments (Columbus, OH); and Kent Scientific Corporation (Torrington, Conn).

For a more extensive review of these technologies, see Kurtz *et al.* [1].

Invasive arterial BP monitoring (direct methods)

Direct, invasive BP monitoring involves placing a catheter or sensor directly into an artery. The primary advantages of direct BP measurement techniques are: the ability to quantify and identify relationships between BP and other variables; study BP-dependent and independent effects of interventions; analyze intermittent or subtle forms of hypertension; and study BP variability [1]. The ability to ascertain a large number of measurements over time allows for greater precision.

There are two general techniques for direct BP measurement, fluid-filled catheters and radiotelemetry.

Fluid-filled catheters

Catheter-based measurement of arterial BP is the oldest method for measuring BP. It is highly accurate because of ease of calibration and relatively inexpensive [5]. Fluid-filled catheters provide the additional advantage over other techniques of providing access to the vasculature for infusions of various experimental agents and solutions.

Catheter-based BP measurement shares many of the same advantages of the radiotelemetry method, and the two methods can be recommended for many of the same purposes. However, fluid-filled

catheters have the additional advantages of ease of recalibration and the ability to be used for infusions.

A disadvantage is that catheters are generally implanted for shorter periods of time compared to radiotelemetric devices, with maintenance of patent arterial catheters for a maximum of 4–5 weeks in mice. However, catheters can be used for long-term monitoring in larger animals (up to 1 year) with proper implantation [6].

Overview of technique. A catheter, generally filled with a heparinized fluid and connected to a calibrated pressure transducer, which is connected to an amplifier/ recording device, is inserted into a major artery, usually the aorta for rodents. These catheters can be used in both anesthetized animals and in conscious animals for long-term monitoring (up to a year in larger animals with proper implantation [6]). Complications include infection and thrombosis. However, if handled properly, a success rate of 90% can be attained. Several devices, such as "tether-swivel" devices, allow for relatively free movement by the animals during catheter-based BP measurements [7].

Systems are commercially available from ADInstruments (Bella Vista, NSW, Australia).

Radiotelemetry

Radiotelemetry, which has existed for 50 years, is the state-of-the-art method for measuring BP and other physiological parameters in freely moving, nonanesthetized rodents. This technique has been applied in numerous animal models, ranging from fish to monkeys. Implantable radiotelemetric monitoring is widely used and allows for high fidelity, continuous (24 hours per day), and effectively unlimited capacity, direct measurements of cardiovascular physiologic parameters [8]. Telemetry can be used to continuously monitor BP, sympathetic nerve activity (SNA), biopotentials (EMG, ECG, and EEG), oxygenation [9], and temperature using implantable sensors connected to external transducers. Using high-fidelity sensors, left ventricular, ocular, uterine, venous, and pleural pressures can be measured with great dynamic range. The technique has been used to establish the important effects of BP lability, beat-to-beat BP variation, "load," and diurnal BP variation in end-organ damage and outcomes.

The major disadvantage of radiotelemetry monitoring of BP is the expense and the need for greater surgical training/ skill. It is the most expensive of the commonly used BP measurement methods. This is both because of the initial investment and need for refurbishment of the catheters. However, the recent advent of reusable telemetry catheters and shorter implantation periods has reduced costs. In addition, newer sensors can be recharged *in vivo*.

Overview of technique. Radiotelemetry monitoring requires particular surgical training and careful attention to proper anesthetic techniques; however, the relative number of complications can be very low [10].

In rodents, a BP transducer is generally surgically inserted into either the abdominal aorta just caudal to the left renal artery or via the carotid artery under general anesthesia. The transducers come in a variety of sizes to accommodate different sized animals/ species. The transmitter is most commonly positioned in the peritoneal cavity. An alternative to this technique, in which thoracic aortic implantation of a pressure-sensing catheter is combined with subcutaneous placement of the transmitter along the flank, has been developed for studies in which peritoneal volume is critical (e.g. pregnancy). Experimental BP measurements are usually made 10–14 days after surgery. Radiotelemetry data is collected continuously, generally sampling at 5-minute intervals for 10 seconds and, depending on

data storage capabilities, may be recorded for days or weeks.

For additional details of the procedure and specific protocols, see Kurtz *et al.* [1].

Commercially available systems include ones from Data Sciences International (St. Paul, MN) and Biopac Systems, Inc. (Goleta, CA).

Vascular measurements

Doppler (*in vivo*)

Noninvasive Doppler velocity measurements [11] can be made in large and small arteries in anesthetized rodents, including mice. Using high ultrasonic frequencies with small transducers, measurement of a wide variety of parameters is possible (Figure 30.1). These include cardiac filling and ejection velocities, pulse wave velocity (through measurement of velocity pulse arrival times), peripheral blood velocity and vessel wall motion waveforms, jet velocity changes across stenoses for the calculation of pressure gradients, vascular resistance, and left main coronary artery velocity for estimation of coronary flow reserve. Doppler techniques have been employed to demonstrate changes in vascular stiffness in atherosclerosis, angiotensin II-induced injury, and effects of estrogen in rodents.

The major advantages of Doppler ultrasound imaging are that it is noninvasive, versatile, portable, safe, and economic. Commercially available units have spatial resolution similar to that of magnetic resonance microscopy. The limitations include that

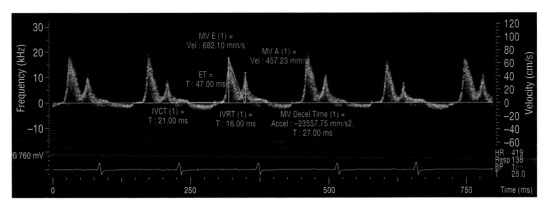

Figure 30.1 Left ventricular mitral flow in the normal mouse heart. Indexes of diastolic function are derived from this waveform and are critical to accurately assess diastolic dysfunction in the dilated and hypertrophic transgenic mouse model. Images were taken from the VisualSonics Vevo 770 Ultrasound Instrument.

it requires significant training and experience to generate reproducible and accurate measurements.

Overview of ultrasound technique. Ultrasound depends on the use of a probe that relies on acoustic differences or mismatch in tissue densities. Transducers are generally "hand held" but can also be placed on the tip of a catheter for intravessel (luminal) imaging. The higher the frequency, the better the spatial resolution. While transducers that image at frequencies of 9 MHz are often used for imaging rodent hearts, very high frequency and narrow beam width systems with 40- to 60-MHz transducers can have spatial resolutions of 50 μm. However, as frequency increases, sound wave penetration decreases and imaging may be possible of only 1 to 2 cm (versus 12 to 15 cm with lower frequencies). Temporal resolution is determined by the image frame acquisition rate, generally expressed in Hertz (Hz). With mice hearts beating in the range of 600 beats/min, a frame rate of 150 Hz or greater is desirable. A central processing unit (CPU) analyzes and constructs the images. The newest ultrasound devices have fully digital image processing capabilities. Both M-mode, which is generated from the transmission of one ultrasound beam over time, and two-dimensional (2-D) images are used. Spectral and color flow Doppler imaging determines blood velocity and direction of blood flow by utilizing Doppler shift. Ultrasound contrast agents, including microbubbles, can be used to improve visualization of vasculature and cardiac chambers. For a more detailed discussion of ultrasound techniques, see Coatney [12].

In vitro

The most common *in vitro* method for accessing vasculature in rodents is measuring tension in isolated aortic rings, which are fixed isometrically in perfused muscle chambers. Force of contraction is measured by a force-displacement transducer. An advantage of this methodology is that endothelium-dependent and independent responses can be easily discerned by denuding the endothelium in the rings.

Details of this procedure are provided in Van de Voorde and Leusen [13].

Developing technologies

At the time of the publication of this handbook, the feasibilities of a number of novel technologies are being tested to study cardiovascular physiology, including nuclear magnetic resonance (NMR) spectroscopy [14] and electron paramagnetic resonance [15].

Acknowledgements
Support is acknowledged from NIH-R21 and Veterans Administration Merit Award.

References

1 Kurtz TW, Griffin KA, Bidani AK, Davisson RL, Hall JE. Recommendations for blood pressure measurement in humans and experimental animals: Part 2: Blood pressure measurement in experimental animals: A statement for professionals from the subcommittee of professional and public education of the American Heart Association Council on High Blood Pressure Research. *Arterioscler Thromb Vasc Biol* 2005; **25**: e22–33.

2 Irvine RJ, White J, Chan R. The influence of restraint on blood pressure in the rat. *J Pharmacol Toxicol Methods* 1997; **38**: 157–162.

3 Kubota Y, Umegaki K, Kagota S, Tanaka N, Nakamura K, Kunitomo M, *et al.* Evaluation of blood pressure measured by tail-cuff methods (without heating) in spontaneously hypertensive rats. *Biol Pharm Bull* 2006; **29**: 1756–1758.

4 Bunag RD. Facts and fallacies about measuring blood pressure in rats. *Clin Exp Hypertens A* 1983; **5**: 1659–1681.

5 Kurtz TW, Griffin KA, Bidani AK, Davisson RL, Hall JE. Recommendations for blood pressure measurement in animals: Summary of an AHA scientific statement from the council on high blood pressure research, professional and public education subcommittee. *Arterioscler Thromb Vasc Biol* 2005; **25**: 478–479.

6 Palm U, Boemke W, Bayerl D, Schnoy N, Juhr NC, Reinhardt HW, *et al.* Prevention of catheter-related infections by a new, catheter-restricted antibiotic filling technique. *Lab Anim* 1991; **25**: 142–152.

7 Mattson DL. Long-term measurement of arterial blood pressure in conscious mice. *Am J Physiol* 1998; **274**: R564–570.

8 Kramer K, Kinter L, Brockway BP, Voss HP, Remie R, Van Zutphen BL, *et al.* The use of radiotelemetry in small laboratory animals: Recent advances. *Contemp Top Lab Anim Sci* 2001; **40**: 8–16.

9 Russell DM, Garry EM, Taberner AJ, Barrett CJ, Paton JF, Budgett DM, *et al.* A fully implantable telemetry system for the chronic monitoring of brain tissue oxygen in freely moving rats. *J Neurosci Methods* 2012; **204**: 242–248.

10 Schnell CR, Wood JM. Measurement of blood pressure and heart rate by telemetry in conscious unrestrained marmosets. *Lab Anim* 1995; **29**: 258–261.

11 Hartley CJ, Reddy AK, Madala S, Entman ML, Michael LH, Taffet GE, *et al.* Doppler velocity measurements from large and small arteries of mice. *Am J Physiol Heart Circ Physiol* 2011; **301**: H269 278.

12 Coatney RW. Ultrasound imaging: Principles and applications in rodent research. *ILAR J* 2001; **42**: 233–247.

13 Van de Voorde J, Leusen I. Endothelium-dependent and independent relaxation of aortic rings from hypertensive rats. *Am J Physiol* 1986; **250**: H711–717.

14 Chatham JC, Blackband SJ. Nuclear magnetic resonance spectroscopy and imaging in animal research. *ILAR J* 2001; **42**: 189–208.

15 Krishna MC, Devasahayam N, Cook JA, Subramanian S, Kuppusamy P, Mitchell JB, *et al.* Electron paramagnetic resonance for small animal imaging applications. *ILAR J* 2001; **42**: 209–218.

31 The setting: imaging conscious, sedated, or anesthetized rodents

Gene H. Kim and Roberto M. Lang
The University of Chicago Medical Center, Chicago, IL, USA

Preparation of rodent and equipment set-up

Ultrasonic assessment of murine hearts has been previously limited by: (1) low frame-rates relative to the rodent heart rates, and (2) inadequate transducer frequencies for near-field imaging. The recent development of high frequency probes (above 8 MHz), have allowed commercial echocardiographic equipment to have an axial resolution of approximately 0.2 mm with a lateral resolution of 0.3 mm when the image is zoomed and acquired at a depth of 1 cm. Most of the recently developed transducers are linear, which have the advantage of avoiding near field artifacts. High-frequency (30–50 MHz) mechanical probes have been recently developed, which are adequate for the murine chest and heart rate, allowing an axial resolution of approximately 50 µm at a depth of 5–12 mm. Most recently, these high-frequency mechanical probes have added color Doppler capabilities, enabling a complete evaluation of ventricular and valvular function. The following is a description of (1) the preparation of the rodent for imaging and (2) the confounding variables that may influence cardiac function.

Although the acquisition of echocardiograms in rodents is relatively simple, these studies are challenging because of the rodents response to stress. Cardiac ultrasound studies are further complicated by the small size, rapid contraction, and orientation of the rodent (especially mouse) heart. Following sedation, electrocardiographic electrodes (adhesive, needle, or metal conductors) should be placed on the animal paws (Figure 31.1A,B). To increase the transducer contact and reduce the presence of air bubbles, the area of the chest that is in direct contact with the transducer must be closely shaved and a depilatory agent used to remove all fur. The effects of anesthesia-induced changes in temperature on cardiac function and heart rate are well documented [1–6]; therefore, different methods to maintain thermoregulation should be used to avoid hypothermia. Ideally, the animal temperature should be maintained at approximately 37°C using a heated imaging platform, circulating warming pad, heating lamps, or autoregulated heating blankets. In addition, routine use of a warmed acoustic gel is recommended. Although the predominant concern regarding body temperature control is to avoid hypothermia, development of hyperthermia should be of equal concern. An unmonitored heating apparatus such as a simple heating pad or the presence of close proximity to halogen illumination can result in fast and dangerous elevation of body temperature. Since substantial body temperature fluctuations in either direction places the animal at risk, every attempt should be made to maintain normal body temperatures during and after surgery.

Also, the sonographer acquiring the images needs to avoid placing excessive pressure on the chest cavity with the transducer, since the weight of the transducer alone may result in bradycardia and hypotension. Accordingly, slight upward lifting of

Manual of Research Techniques in Cardiovascular Medicine, First Edition. Edited by Hossein Ardehali, Roberto Bolli, and Douglas W. Losordo.
© 2014 John Wiley & Sons, Ltd. Published 2014 by John Wiley & Sons, Ltd.

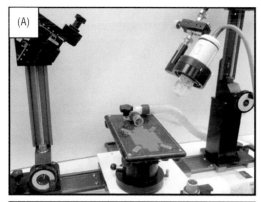

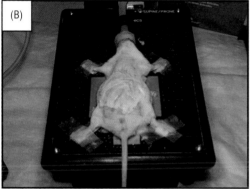

Figure 31.1 Equipment setup. Placement of imaging platform (A) and example of mouse prepped for imaging (B).

the transducer while maintaining contact with the murine chest wall is always recommended. The duration of image acquisition must also be kept to a minimum in order to reduce the physiologic and hemodynamic changes resulting from prolonged sedation.

The small size of the mouse heart beating with heart rates in excess of 500 beats/min, presents unique methodological challenges to cardiac ultrasound [7]. The mouse heart is more vertically oriented than the human heart. Parasternal long- and short-axis views despite the presence of narrow intercostal spaces are frequently easily obtained. However, the vertical heart's orientation and the small size of the rib cage may result in difficult and poorly reproducible apical views. The inability to consistently obtain apical views prevents the acquisition of mitral inflow Doppler required for the assessment of LV diastolic function. Furthermore, because of its small size and complex crescent shape,

as well as its anterior and shallow location, the right ventricle is not frequently well-visualized on transthoracic echocardiography. Chapters 32 and 33 will discuss optimal techniques for acquisition of echocardiographic data. In addition, adequate training and experience, both with anesthesia and image acquisition, are necessary in order to obtain high-quality, reproducible data.

Effects of anesthesia

Murine hemodynamics and ventricular function can be altered significantly by interventions such as anesthesia, ventilation, and surgical manipulations. Thus, the proper selection of anesthetic agents is crucial rodent studies. Studies on cardiac function acquired at suboptimal heart rates (averaging 300/minute) are not rare in the literature. Numerous aspects of cardiac physiology are greatly modified at slow heart rates and can confound the effects of the studied intervention on cardiac function.

Although anesthetic agents are frequently employed to immobilize and sedate rodents for better image acquisition during echocardiographic imaging, these drugs are known to have significant effects on cardiovascular function. Recently, increased attention has been placed on the variable effects of anesthetics on murine cardiac function during echocardiographic recordings. General anesthetics may directly affect organ function as well as blunt both respiratory drive and respiratory muscle function, potentially inducing cardiac dysfunction through hypoxia and acidosis. To minimize these confounding variables, investigators have routinely measured end-tidal carbon dioxide tension or mechanical ventilation parameters while simultaneously attempting to minimize the duration of anesthesia.

Heart rates in conscious normal mice have been reported to vary from 500 to 650 beats/min by telemetry methods [5,8,9]. The reduction in heart rate caused by anesthetics results in improved image quality due to better temporal resolution, but may simultaneously confound the physiological issue in question. Multiple general anesthesia regimens have been utilized in mice and rats, including intraperitoneal injections of ketamine: xylazine mixture, tribromoethanol, chloral hydrate, or barbiturates, as well as isoflurane or halothane

Table 31.1 Commonly used anesthetic regimens
for echocardiography

Compound	Delivery route	Usual dose
Ketamine : xylazine	i.p.	ketamine: 80–100 mg/kg xylazine: 10 mg/kg
Tribromoethanol	i.p.	0.02 mL/g
Pentobarbital	i.p.	30 mg/kg
Chloral hydrate	i.p.	0.5 mg/g
Isoflurane	Inhaled	Induction: 3–5% Maintenance: 1–2%
Halothane	Inhaled	Induction: 3–5% Maintenance: 1–2%

inhalation [1–6] (Table 31.1). When sedating mice, it is important to consider that most anesthetics, including barbiturates and inhalants, cause cardiovascular and respiratory depression. Although ketamine reportedly has less of a cardiodepressor effect, when administered with xylazine or diazepam, the combination results in hypothermia combined with negative inotropic and chronotropic effects. The intraperitoneal agents, tribromoethanol, ketamine–midazolam, or ketamine : xylazine, all cause early cardiodepression, resulting in decreased shortening fraction over the course of a 20-minute echocardiographic study, although tribromoethanol results in lesser hemodynamic compromise [4]. Comparatively, isoflurane anesthesia results in a relatively stable and reproducible end-diastolic dimension measurements and fractional shortening and during echocardiographic studies [6]. In addition, the use of isofluorane anesthesia enables dosing to be rapidly titrated to minimize cardiodepressive effects.

Anesthetic induction with injectable drugs can be challenging in rodents; their small body mass allows for only a narrow margin of safety when dispensing these type of agents. Likewise, maintenance of adequate anesthetic levels is difficult to administer in animals with high metabolic rates. Although not routinely used for surgery on mice, inhalation agents can significantly reduce the complications associated with general anesthesia. Isoflurane, for example, can

be delivered to the animal via a stream of oxygen with the use of a calibrated vaporizer resulting in rapid onset of action and adjustable anesthesia levels.

To avoid the confounding effects of anesthesia, echocardiographic recordings in conscious mice have been attempted. Ideally, echocardiograms should be performed on calm awake animals. This is truly feasible only after training the mice daily for several days prior to real data acquisition [9,10]. Training typically consists of simulating the echocardiogram procedure by holding the mice for 5 minutes at a time in the position required for echocardiographic image acquisition and touching the chest with the echocardiographic probe. Heated gel can also be used to simulate the echocardiographic procedure. Although avoiding anesthesia is appealing, echocardiographic acquisition in conscious mice requires additional training in animal handling while simultaneously increasing the operator's demand to focus on the animal and environmental conditions [11]. Conscious imaging is not possible in catheterized or instrumented animals. The consensus among investigators performing echocardiographic studies in murine models is that the choice of anesthetic, dosing regimen, and timing of data acquisition must be carefully adapted not only to the individual experiment, but also to the rodent strain, sex, age, and mutation [12].

General steps for preparing mice for imaging studies

1. Prior to the imaging study, anesthetize the mouse (2–3% isoflurane mixed with 0.5 L/min 100% O_2) in the induction chamber. Be sure to filter waste gas for the safety of the operator. Remove the animal from the induction chamber and use hair clippers to shave the fur from the neckline to mid chest level. Then remove the remaining body hair with hair removal cream.

2. Apply Duralube gel to both eyes to prevent drying of the sclera (avoid contacting the cornea with the gel applicator). Place the anesthetized mouse in a supine position atop a heating pad with embedded ECG leads in order to maintain body temperature.

3. Place the snout within a nose cone connected to the anesthesia system to maintain a steady-state

sedation level throughout the procedure (1.0–1.5% isoflurane mixed with 0.5 L/min 100% O_2). Perform a toe or tail pinch to confirm sedation. If necessary, the level of anesthesia can be adjusted to maintain a target heart rate of 450 ± 50 beats per minute (bpm).
4. Gently insert a rectal probe (after lubricating) to continuously monitor and adjust body temperature via the heating pad. It is important to maintain the body temperature within a narrow range ($37.0°C \pm 0.5°C$), as even moderate changes in temperature and heart rate affect cardiac function in mice.
5. Apply electrode gel to the four paws and tape them to the ECG electrodes.

References

1 Arras M, Autenried P, Rettich A, Spaeni D, Rulicke T. Optimization of intraperitoneal injection anesthesia in mice: drugs, dosages, adverse effects, and anesthesia depth. *Comp Med* 2001; **51**: 443–456.

2 Hart CY, Burnett JC Jr, Redfield MM. Effects of avertin versus xylazine-ketamine anesthesia on cardiac function in normal mice. *Am J Physiol Heart Circ Physiol* 2001; **281**: H1938–1945.

3 Kawahara Y, Tanonaka K, Daicho T, Nawa M, Oikawa R, Nasa Y, et al. Preferable anesthetic conditions for echocardiographic determination of murine cardiac function. *J Pharmacol Sci* 2005; **99**: 95–104.

4 Roth DM, Swaney JS, Dalton ND, Gilpin EA, Ross J, Jr. Impact of anesthesia on cardiac function during echocardiography in mice. *Am J Physiol Heart Circ Physiol* 2002; **282**: H2134–2140.

5 Takuma S, Suehiro K, Cardinale C, Hozumi T, Yano H, Shimizu J, et al. Anesthetic inhibition in ischemic and nonischemic murine heart: comparison with conscious echocardiographic approach. *Am J Physiol Heart Circ Physiol* 2001; **280**: H2364–2370.

6 Tarin D, Sturdee A. Surgical anaesthesia of mice: evaluation of tribromo-ethanol, ether, halothane and methoxyflurane and development of a reliable technique. *Lab Anim* 1972; **6**: 79–84.

7 Blizard DA, Welty R. Cardiac activity in the mouse: strain differences. *J Comp Physiol Psychol* 1971; **77**: 337–344.

8 Janssen B, Debets J, Leenders P, Smits J. Chronic measurement of cardiac output in conscious mice. *Am J Physiol Regul Integr Comp Physiol* 2002; **282**: R928–935.

9 Yang XP, Liu YH, Rhaleb NE, Kurihara N, Kim HE, Carretero OA, et al. Echocardiographic assessment of cardiac function in conscious and anesthetized mice. *Am J Physiol* 1999; **277**: H1967–1974

10 Rottman JN, Ni G, Brown M. Echocardiographic evaluation of ventricular function in mice. *Echocardiography* 2007; **24**: 83–89.

11 Gehrmann J, Hammer PE, Maguire CT, Wakimoto H, Triedman JK, Berul CI, et al. Phenotypic screening for heart rate variability in the mouse. *Am J Physiol Heart Circ Physiol* 2000; **279**: H733–740.

12 Hoit BD, Kiatchoosakun S, Restivo J, Kirkpatrick D, Olszens K, Shao H, et al. Naturally occurring variation in cardiovascular traits among inbred mouse strains. *Genomics* 2002; **79**: 679–685.

Echocardiography: standard techniques (M-mode, two-dimensional imaging, and Doppler)

Gene H. Kim,[1] Lauren Beussink-Nelson,[2] Sanjiv J. Shah,[2] and Roberto M. Lang[1]

[1] The University of Chicago Medical Center, Chicago, IL, USA
[2] Northwestern University Feinberg School of Medicine, Chicago, IL, USA

Introduction

Rodent models have been utilized extensively to investigate the mechanisms underlying normal cardiovascular development and function as well as the pathophysiologic origins of disease. *In vivo* techniques are necessary for the evaluation of the cardiac phenotype in these models; although *in vitro* assessments are also valuable, they are inherently limited given the functional complexity of the cardiovascular system. To fully characterize the rodent phenotype *in vivo*, it is necessary to employ an accurate, reliable, and reproducible noninvasive technique that allows for the serial evaluation of cardiac morphology [1]. With the appropriate noninvasive approach, longitudinal studies within the same animal are possible, permitting the continuous assessment of structure, hemodynamics, and response to interventions without significant impact on the animal or its physiology [2].

Echocardiography is the noninvasive method of choice in humans for defining cardiac parameters serially, assessing global and regional contractile function, and monitoring disease progression and treatment [3]. This technology has broad appeal because it is portable, relatively affordable, versatile, and safe [2,4]. Although technically challenging to perform in rodents due to their small size and rapid heart rate, significant technological advances in imaging capabilities have made echocardiography a powerful and sophisticated tool for the evaluation of cardiovascular function in the research setting. Echocardiography is now well established in rodent models, and has been validated against invasive measurements, magnetic resonance imaging (MRI), computed tomography (CT), and necropsy [5]. This extremely versatile tool has been extensively applied in the evaluation of cardiovascular function in mouse and rat models of disease to serially monitor cardiac performance, map the progression of dysfunction, and determine the effect of pharmacological, genetic, and surgical interventions. The goal of this chapter is to describe the basic protocol for the acquisition and analysis of echocardiographic images in the rodent and explain the derived parameters of systolic and diastolic function relevant to cardiovascular research.

Manual of Research Techniques in Cardiovascular Medicine, First Edition. Edited by Hossein Ardehali, Roberto Bolli, and Douglas W. Losordo.
© 2014 John Wiley & Sons, Ltd. Published 2014 by John Wiley & Sons, Ltd.

Materials

Ultrasound systems

Echocardiographic assessment in small animals has been limited in the past by the size of the rodent heart, low frame rate relative to high rodent heart rates, and transducer frequencies too low for near-field imaging [6]. These challenges have recently been overcome by the development of high-frequency transducers with a small imaging footprint, improved signal processing, and high frame rates, which can provide the superior spatial and temporal resolution necessary for visualizing anatomical structures and monitoring physiological activities on a small scale [7]. Both modified clinical systems and research-specific systems are used in the evaluation of the rodent heart.

Several modified commercial imaging systems have been adapted for use in rodent cardiovascular research. To visualize the small rodent heart, high-frequency linear transducers (10–15 MHz) are utilized, which are capable of generating high-quality images at very high heart rates. Many of these systems also come loaded with mouse- and rat-specific software to maximize imaging settings for these animals. In our labs we use the GE Vivid 7 system (GE Healthcare, Milwaukee, WI) with an i13L transducer (equipped with gray scale, color, and pulsed wave Doppler capabilities) as well as the VisualSonics Vevo Imaging Station platform (described in greater detail below); however, several other clinical echocardiographic platforms are also furnished with high-frequency transducers appropriate for rodent imaging.

Although commercial systems are capable of providing extensive physiologic information in these animals, they cannot always accurately assess detailed heart structures or small vessels, particularly in mice [8]. Dedicated research systems are ideal for visualizing the complete cardiovascular anatomy and physiology in the small animal with greater accuracy and reduced interobserver variability. The VisualSonics Vevo 2100 (VisualSonics, Toronto, Canada) comes with ultra-high-frequency linear array probes (up to 70 MHz), which are capable of achieving frame rates up to 1000 frames per second (fps), as well as animal handling platforms that allow for reproducible probe positioning, image optimization, and monitoring of body temperature and heart rate [2].

Additional equipment

- Anesthetic equipment
- Hair clipper with size 40 blade
- Chemical depilatory agent (such as Nair)
- ECG electrodes (needle, adhesive, or metal conductors)
- Heating pad
- Ultrasound gel and warmer
- Analysis software

Methods

Technical considerations

Rodent echocardiography is highly operator dependent and susceptible to significant variability. The reproducibility and accuracy of echocardiographic measurements relies on several factors, including the skill and experience of the sonographer and image analyzer, inherent animal characteristics, and the consistency of experimental conditions [9]. Therefore, although the protocol for performing and analyzing an echocardiogram may appear to be straightforward, caution must be applied to several aspects of this method in order to produce meaningful data [10].

Echocardiographic evaluation requires a well-trained and skilled sonographer to obtain accurate and reproducible high-quality images [11]. Considerable experience is necessary, and frequent sessions are required to maintain this skill. In addition to high-quality examination, careful data interpretation by an experienced operator is also essential to obtain reproducible and reliable data [2].

The hemodynamic state in rodents, and therefore the accuracy of the echocardiographic data, is dependent on the selection of an appropriate anesthetic and dosing regimen, as well as the timing of image acquisition relative to anesthesia induction. Considerations for appropriate anesthetic technique are described in detail in Chapter 31. Heart rate is closely related to cardiovascular function, and should be carefully monitored to maintain a similar level within each animal. Cardiac function is greatly modified at physiologically low heart rates, so every effort should be made to ensure that the heart rates are as high as possible under sedation, assuring stable contractility and echocardiographic measurements. The heart rate in conscious mice is generally 500–700 beats per minute (bpm), with a target heart rate under anesthesia of 450 ± 50 bpm; in rats, the conscious heart rate is 300–500 bpm, with a target heart rate under anesthesia of 300 ± 50 bpm [4,12]. The heart rate should be monitored throughout the exam, and across serial exams to decrease experimental variability [13].

Maintenance of normothermia is also a critical point of concern because cardiac function and heart rate are directly related to core temperature. Small animals are especially vulnerable to rapid hypothermia after the administration of anesthesia; long experimental protocols and shaving increase the risk [13]. The body temperature should be maintained near 37°C throughout the procedure with the aid of a heating pad or lamp; rectal thermometers may be used for monitoring if necessary [12].

Finally, it is important to avoid placing excess pressure on the chest wall with the transducer, since the weight of the transducer alone can cause bradycardia and hypotension [6,9]. Pressure on the chest may even result in deformation of the heart, particularly in mice [14,15]. To avoid these pitfalls, we typically use a large amount of acoustic gel and apply a slight upward lifting motion of the transducer while scanning.

Instrument settings

The following settings should be adjusted to optimize image quality in small animals:
• Simultaneous ECG recordings should be included with each image or clip.
• All two-dimensional (2D) images should be acquired as dynamic cine loops containing three to five cycles.
• Sweep speed should be maximized for M-mode measurements (200 mm/s) but shorter for storing images during the exam (50–100 mm/s).
• Gain and compression settings should be adjusted for visualization of endocardial and epicardial walls.
• Frame rate should be >100 fps.
  ◦ High frame rates can be obtained by narrowing the window of interest, decreasing the depth of imaging, reducing the frequency, and minimizing the number of focal points.
• Doppler settings

◦ All Doppler tracings should include five to ten cardiac cycles.
◦ The gain should be adjusted to just below the level where background noise appears to ensure a clear, well-defined Doppler waveform.
◦ Sweep speed should be maximized for measurements (200 mm/s) but shorter for storing images during the exam (50–100 mm/s).
◦ The smallest sample volume available should be used for recording all pulsed wave (PW) Doppler flow images.

Animal preparation and positioning

• After anesthesia, shave the animal from the left sternal border to the left axillary line, from the neckline down to the midchest level.
  ◦ This area should be further cleaned with a chemical depilatory lotion (Nair) to minimize ultrasound energy loss and reduce interference from remaining hair [7].
  ◦ The smallest possible area of hair should be removed to prevent excessive heat loss [12].
• Place the animal in a shallow left lateral decubitus or supine position on the warming pad.
  ◦ When imaging mice, secure the extremities to the examining surface with paper tape [16].
• Attach ECG electrodes to the animal's extremities.
• Apply a thin layer of pre-warmed gel to the chest wall.

Basic protocol

For a complete evaluation of cardiac morphology and physiology, three modes of imaging acquisition are broadly used: B-mode, M-mode, and Doppler. B-mode, or 2D imaging, is the most common format for general use, and produces a simple gray-scale image of cardiac structures [4]. M-mode images are obtained by displaying echoes from a single ultrasound beam over time [4]. Because this modality has very high temporal resolution (>1000 Hz), it has been widely used to phenotype the cardiovascular system in rodent models. Doppler imaging uses the Doppler shift principle reflected by a moving target (i.e. blood cells) to determine blood flow velocity and direction. An increase in the Doppler shift correlates with increasing blood flow velocity. The Doppler shift is affected by the alignment of the ultrasound beam and the flow of blood: the more parallel the beam, the less attenuation of the Doppler shift signal.

Two main Doppler applications are used in echocardiography: continuous wave (CW) and pulsed wave (PW). The major advantage of CW Doppler is that very high velocities can be measured accurately, although range resolution, or the determination of blood flow velocity from a precise location, is not possible; PW Doppler has accurate range resolution, but the maximum flow velocity that can be accurately determined is limited [17]. Transvalvular flow velocity waveforms obtained from Doppler echocardiography can be used to calculate peak velocity, ejection time (ET), and velocity time interval (VTI) [18,19].

Using these three techniques in combination, valves are evaluated for normal structure and function, cavity size and indexes of global and regional systolic function are calculated, and diastolic function is determined. Following the protocol described below, a complete study should take 20 minutes. To minimize variability, it is important to follow a standardized protocol and maintain the order and timing of the acquisitions between subjects, and for longitudinal measurements within a subject; in addition, all measurements should be averaged over three to five consecutive beats [9]. The protocol that follows is the standard in our laboratory; it may be altered as needed based on personal preferences and the priorities of the data acquired. Measurements may be performed during the study, but are more often performed offline on a workstation equipped with appropriate software. Normal values vary according to rodent strain, gender, and age; it is recommended that each laboratory establish a database of normal values in the commonly used strains of rats and mice [20]. In addition, measurements of individual parameters may vary in normal mice and rats up to 25% [23, 33], requiring a comparable control group to accurately estimate and assess minor changes.

Parasternal long axis (PLAX)

• Acquire the PLAX view by placing the transducer over the third or fourth intercostal space, along the axis of the left ventricle (LV), and orienting its notch toward the animal's right shoulder, at approximately 11 o'clock. (Figure 32.1B)

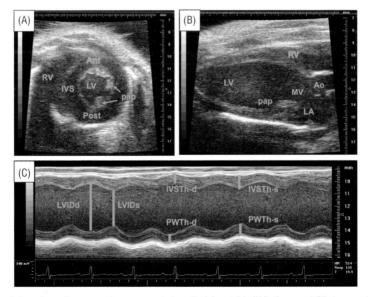

Figure 32.1 Representative echocardiograms and measurements from the left ventricle (LV) of a normal CD-1 mouse. The 2D parasternal short-axis image (A) and long-axis image (B) are shown at end diastole. The 2D guided M-mode image (C) was obtained at the level of the papillary muscles. Ant, anterior wall; Ao, aorta; d, diastole; IVS, interventricular septum; LA, left atrium; LV, left ventricle; LVID, LV internal diameter; PWTh, LV posterior wall thickness; MV, mitral valve; pap, papillary muscle; RV, right ventricle; s, systole.

∘ It is critical that this view includes the full length of the LV; foreshortening falsely minimizes the length of the LV and impairs the assessment of contractile function.

∘ Angulate or tilt the transducer to simultaneously visualize the left ventricular apex, mitral valve, aortic valve, and left atrium; take time to image through the entire heart to obtain a window in which all of these structures are present and the widest possible ventricular diastolic dimension is observed.

∘ A modified view may be necessary to view some structures optimally, such as the aortic root or ascending aorta.

∘ 2D measurements
- LV length
  - Measure the LV length from the apex to the middle of the mitral annulus at end diastole.
- Left ventricular outflow tract (LVOT) diameter
  - Measure the LVOT diameter at its maximum, during early systole.
  - Measure from the junction of the aortic leaflet with the septal endocardium to the junction of the leaflet with the mitral valve posteriorly, using the inner edge to inner edge method.

∘ In the PSAX papillary muscle view, trace the epicardium and endocardium during end diastole to obtain total and cavity areas.
- Images are considered adequate for measurement when >75% of the epicardial and endocardial contours can be adequately visualized [22].

∘ According to American Society of Echocardiography (ASE) recommendations, the endocardium is traced by covering the innermost border of the ventricle (extrapolating the border to avoid incorporating the papillary muscles), and the epicardium is traced by covering the first bright area immediately adjacent to the darker myocardium (excluding the strong epicardial echo) [16,23].

• Turn on 2D-guided M-mode and place the cursor just distal to the mitral leaflet tips, perpendicular to the long axis of the LV (while avoiding the papillary muscle); record an M-mode image.

• Pulmonary vein (PV) Doppler
∘ The mouse is distinctive in that it only has a single large pulmonary vein, which connects to the left atrium (LA) close to the atrioventricular groove; increased technical skill is required to locate this solitary vein [21].

∘ Rats have more than one pulmonary vein; Doppler tracings of the left lower pulmonary vein are obtained in a similar fashion to the mouse.

∘ From the PLAX window, the transducer is moved laterally and rotated 10–20° clockwise; the transducer is then tilted inferiorly and anteriorly until the aorta disappears and the pulmonary vein is visualized [21].

∘ The sample volume is placed 1 mm away from the LA–PV junction.

∘ In rodents, the flow pattern consists of a small S wave during systole, two forward D waves (D1 and D2) during diastole, and a small, reversed A wave during atrial contraction [21].

∘ The peak velocity of all four waves is measured, as well as the duration of the A wave and the deceleration time of the D2 wave (measured as the interval from the peak of the D2 velocity to its extrapolation to the baseline).

Parasternal short axis (PSAX)

• With the transducer in the PLAX position, rotate 90° clockwise so that the notch is directed at the animal's left shoulder, at approximately 3 o'clock, to obtain the PSAX view (Figure 32.1A).
∘ Rotate or tilt the probe as needed until a circular LV is obtained.

• Turn on 2D-guided M-mode and place the cursor at the mid-papillary level, perpendicular to the interventricular septum and posterior wall of the LV (Figure 32.1C).
∘ The papillary muscles should be clearly visualized, and the sampling line positioned through the center of the largest ventricular diameter (excluding the papillary muscles themselves).
∘ End-diastolic measurements
- Measurements are obtained at the point of maximal left ventricular diastolic dimension, peak of the R wave, or the frame after mitral valve closure.
- Interventricular septal thickness during diastole (IVSD), left ventricular end-diastolic dimension (LVEDD), and left ventricular posterior wall thickness during diastole (LVPWD) are measured.
- Most sources advise using the leading edge-to-leading edge method recommended by the ASE

[6,14,24,25], although some sources now report using the tissue–blood interface instead of the leading edge method due to improvements in resolution [9,26].

◦ End-systolic measurements

▪ Measurements are obtained at the time of the most anterior systolic excursion of the posterior wall associated with minimal chamber dimension, or the frame preceding mitral valve opening.

▪ Interventricular septal thickness during systole (IVSS), left ventricular end-systolic dimension (LVESD), and left ventricular posterior wall thickness during systole (LVPWS) are measured, using the methods described earlier.

◦ PLAX option

▪ Although cardiac dimensions can be measured from either the long or short axis M-mode tracings, most investigators rely on the PSAX view alone because it is rarely possible to align the M-mode cursor perpendicular to the long axis of the ventricle from the PLAX plane; however, either view can be used, depending on which one gives the best endocardial resolution.

• 2D PSAX images may also be obtained at the level of the apex and mitral valve, if desired.

• Pulmonary artery Doppler

◦ From the level of the papillary muscle, angle superiorly until the aorta, LA, right ventricular outflow tract (RVOT), and pulmonary artery are visualized.

◦ The PW sample volume is placed proximal to the pulmonary valve leaflets and aligned to maximize laminar flow; the following measurements are obtained from the RVOT, avoiding the opening and closing clicks of the pulmonary valve:

▪ Peak velocity

▪ VTI, obtained by tracing the outer edge of the Doppler profile.

▪ Pulmonary acceleration time (PAT), measured as the time from the onset of flow to peak velocity. This parameter should only be measured at sweep speeds below 200 mm/s; higher speeds may result in a less accurate assessment [27].

▪ ET, measured as the time interval between the onset and completion of systolic flow.

Apical four-chamber (A4C)

• Place the transducer at the cardiac apex, near the lower border of the ribs, and orient the notch toward the animal's left shoulder to obtain the A4C view.

◦ All four chambers should be visible, along with both atrioventricular valves and the interatrial and interventricular septum.

◦ Apical views are extremely difficult to obtain consistently in rodents, and do not exactly duplicate the corresponding views obtained in humans; the rodent heart is more vertically oriented, making acquisition of these views difficult [1].

◦ Positioning the animal in a steeper decubitus position and sharply angling the transducer anteriorly may be helpful.

• Mitral valve Doppler

◦ Turn on PW Doppler and place the sample volume between the tips of the mitral leaflets, with the beam parallel to mitral inflow and aligned to maximize laminar flow; angle correction may be used if necessary.

◦ Velocities are maximal at the leaflet tips; if the sample volume is placed closer to the annulus, the velocities will be lower due to the larger cross-sectional area for flow [9].

◦ Transmitral Doppler measurements may also be recorded from an angulated PLAX view (using angle correction no greater than 20°); this method is applied more often in mice due to the difficulty associated with obtaining apical views.

◦ Doppler measurements

▪ There are two waveforms associated with mitral inflow; the early (E) wave represents passive filling of the ventricle, and the later (A) wave represents active filling during atrial systole (i.e. atrial contraction) [28].

▪ The peak E and A wave velocities and the deceleration time of the E wave (from the peak E wave velocity to its extrapolation to the baseline) are measured.

▪ In reality, these parameters cannot always be measured because the high heart rate causes fusion of the two peaks [9]. The E and A waves fuse at heart rates of around 450–500 bpm in mice, and around 300 bpm in rats [3,4,29].

▪ However, the fused peak E velocity can still be used as a valuable measurement; even though the true peak velocity cannot be distinguished, many have found that this is still a useful index of function [9]. Using this method, the transmitral flow velocity at the start of atrial systole, known as the "E at A velocity" is measured [21].

Apical five-chamber (A5C)

• From the A4C window, tilt the transducer anteriorly, into a shallower angle relative to the chest wall, to simultaneously visualize the LVOT, aortic valve, and aortic root.
• Isovolumetric relaxation time (IVRT) Doppler
  ◦ Turn on PW Doppler and place the sample volume between the LVOT and the anterior mitral leaflet to simultaneously record mitral inflow and aortic outflow signals (both flow profiles should be distinct).
  ◦ IVRT is measured as the time between the closing of the aortic valve and the opening of the mitral valve.
• LVOT Doppler
  ◦ Move the sample volume to the level of the aortic annulus, proximal to the valve, and align the beam to maximize laminar flow; it is essential to angle the probe so that the Doppler beam is parallel to the flow, otherwise outflow measurements will be underestimated.
  ◦ When the sample volume is correctly positioned, the closing click of the aortic valve is noted.
  ◦ Measure the peak velocity, VTI, and ET.

Left ventricular structure and function

Chamber dimensions and wall thickness

Murine echocardiography has mostly been used in a variety of models and genetically modified mice for the assessment of LV size and function. B-mode images display 2D views of the heart (Figure 32.1) and other vasculature regions such as the aortic arch, pulmonary artery, and carotid artery. This mode allows a nonquantitative assessment of cardiac phenotype, chamber dimensions, and heart function as well as the visualization of fine cardiac structures such as mitral chordae, papillary muscles, and valvular leaflets. Short- and long-axis cine-loops may be traced in diastole and systole to assess cardiac function. Figure 32.1 illustrates B-mode images of a normal heart from a wild-type mouse showing

parasternal long-axis (Figure 32.1B) and short-axis views at the level of the papillary muscles (Figure 32.1A). In general, the right ventricle (RV) may not be clearly visualized in the short-axis views, in part because of the interference of the sternum, preventing a complete quantitative assessment of the RV. By allowing a regular distribution of lateral resolution over the entire field, B-mode can serve as a guidance platform for the operator to correct the positioning of structures that require further evaluation using other imaging formats such as M-mode and color Doppler imaging.

The modality most commonly used by investigators to perform LV measurements is M-mode, since its temporal resolution (>1000 Hz) is especially adapted to the fast mouse heart rate. M-mode echocardiography displays the position and motion of reflecting structures along one line (ice-pick view) as echo depth versus time, and thereby allows the high temporal resolution required for measurements of aortic diameter, LV chamber dimensions, and LV wall thickness. Measurements obtained with this modality are used in nearly all studies of murine cardiac physiology, thus proper data acquisition and adequate control settings are essential. Shown in Figure 32.1C is a typical M-mode obtained in a healthy adult mouse. Normal values for chamber dimensions and function have been reported [2,30–32]. However, it should be emphasized that cardiac dimensions vary according to mice strains, gender, and age, and rapidly change at different heart rates. It is important to verify that groups of mice are matched for these parameters. For these reasons, use of age, strain, and gender (ideally littermate) matched controls for each experiment should be used instead of reference values. In addition, measurements of individual parameters such as LVEDD and posterior wall thickness (PWTD) may vary in normal mice up to 25% [23,33], requiring a comparable control group to accurately estimate and assess minor dimensional changes. This variability may be explained not only by differences between strains but also due to differences in anesthetic regimens, heart rates, and loading conditions.

Left ventricular mass

LV mass is a commonly used descriptor of cardiac status. Longitudinal assessment of LV mass over

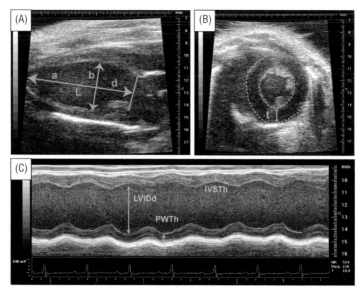

Figure 32.2 Representative echocardiograms and measurements for measurement of LV mass. The 2D parasternal long-axis image (A) and short-axis image (B) are shown at end diastole. The 2D-guided M-mode image (C) was obtained at the level of the papillary muscles. a, full major radius; b, minor axis radius; d, truncated major radius; IVSTh, interventricular septal thickness; L, LV length; LV internal diameter; LVID; PWTh, LV posterior wall thickness; t, myocardial wall thickness.

time is often required, thus limiting the use of necropsy specimens. Previous studies have examined the accuracy of M-mode and 2D LV mass measurement methods in small cohorts of predominantly normal mice [14,34]. The simplest method of LV mass calculation is the M-mode (cubed) method which is derived as follows:

LV mass

$$= 1.05[(IVSD + LVEDD + PWTD)^3 - (LVEDD)^3]$$

where IVS and LVPW are the interventricular septal and posterior wall thicknesses, respectively, and LVID is the LV internal diameter (Figure 32.2) [35].

Although M-mode echocardiography has yielded LV mass estimates with relatively good correlation with necropsy values in mice of uniform geometry [14,34], this method is limited in rodents with irregularly shaped hearts. With this method, images are obtained in a single plane and geometric assumptions are made. Accordingly, LV mass calculations derived from M-mode are subject to greater error than when formulas derived from multiplanar images are used.

In humans, 2D area–length-based estimates of LV mass have been shown to be more accurate than M-mode-based estimates [15,35,36]. With the 2D area–length method, LV mass is calculated as:

$$LV\ mass = [1.05(5/6\ A_1(L+t) - 5/6\ A_2 L]$$

where 1.05 is the specific gravity of muscle, A1 and A2 are the epicardial and endocardial parasternal short axis areas, respectively, L is the parasternal long-axis length, and t is the wall thickness calculated from A1 and A2 [36]. With the truncated ellipsoid method, LV mass is calculated as follows:

$$LV\ mass = \pi[(b+t)^2\{2/3(a+t)+d-d_3/[3(a+t)^2]\} \\ -b_2(2/3a+d-d_3/3a_2)]$$

where b is the minor axis radius of the LV measured at the level of the papillary muscle tip. Its placement determines the division of the measured LV length (L) into a full major radius (a) and a truncated major radius (d). The average wall thickness, t, is calculated from A1 and A2 (Figure 32.2) [23].

The Simpson rule can be applied for reconstructing infarct area size, LV mass, and derived LV ejection fraction. The Simpson rule is advantageous in experiments involving regional remodeling because in this method the LV cavity is represented as a stack of disks wherein the volumes of all disks are summed to obtain a close approximation of LV volume. LV mass is calculated by subtracting the volume of the LV cavity at end systole from the LV volume measured at end diastole and multiplying by the density of myocardium (1.055) [23,37].

Left ventricular systolic function

The most common measurement used to quantify LV systolic function is fractional shortening (FS) derived from M-mode (Figures 32.1 and 32.2). FS is calculated as follows:

$$\%FS = [(LVEDD - LVESD) / LVEDD] \times 100$$

Diastolic measurements are made at the time of maximal LV diastolic dimension, whereas LV end-systolic dimension are obtained at the time of the incisura of the aortic pressure tracing or at the time of minimal LV dimension. Intra- and interobserver variability between measurements of LVEDD, LVESD, FS, velocity of circumferential shortening (Vcf), and PWTD are approximately 10% either by 2D or M-mode method [33], which is acceptable for accurate measurements.

Ejection phase indices, including cardiac output, LV fractional area shortening, and ejection fraction, are other commonly used indices to measure LV systolic performance. In addition, traditional high-fidelity LV pressure tracings and their derived maximum rate of pressure generation (dP/dt_{max}) have also been commonly used. These indices are load dependent and as such are incapable of separating changes in ventricular contractility from those caused by altered loading conditions [19,38,39]. Cardiac output has been previously measured in mice with the use of radioactive soluble indicators and microspheres [40], while other investigators have employed implantable transit time flow probes or electromagnetic flow meters in the ascending aorta [41]. These methods are technically challenging and are not suitable for serial assessment.

To circumvent this limitation, investigators have estimated cardiac output as the difference between 2D-determined LV end-systolic and end diastolic volumes [41]. More recently, Doppler ultrasound techniques, which allow the noninvasive assessment of cardiac output multiple times per experiment and the ability to follow changes serially, have been used.

Stroke volume and ascending aortic blood velocity can be calculated from continuous wave aortic Doppler velocity recordings, acquired from the parasternal long-axis view using 12- to 15-MHz transducers and 2D-targeted M-mode echocardiographic measurements of the diameter of the proximal ascending aorta [42]. Other investigators have used different approaches, recording peak aortic velocities from the suprasternal approach or the apical window. More recently, with the advent of linear probes, high parasternal long-axis views have been used to record maximal aortic velocities [43–45]. Stroke volume (SV) can be calculated by multiplying the aortic VTI by the aortic cross-sectional area (CSA), which is calculated based on the diameter (D) of the aorta at the site of VTI measurement:

$$SV = VTI \times CSA, \text{ where } CSA = D^2 \times \pi / 4$$
$$= D^2 \times 0.785$$

Cardiac output can then be calculated as the product of SV and heart rate (Figure 32.3).

The major sources of error in estimating cardiac output using Doppler echocardiography in rodents include: (1) inadequate alignment between the sound beam and the aorta and (2) the inability to accurately measure the aortic diameter. With the development of new linear probes, flow alignment with the thoracic aorta can be optimized, resulting in less need for angle correction. Because of these constraints, as well as the limitation of frame rate, Doppler measurements of cardiac output are better suited for comparative, serial measurements rather than absolute determinations.

Load-independent assessment of myocardial contractility

The majority of studies assessing cardiac performance in mice using cardiac ultrasound have used ejection phase indices, such as ejection fraction, fractional shortening, and cardiac output, all of which are limited by their load dependence [19,38,39]. The ability to separate alterations in myocardial contractility from simultaneously occurring changes in loading conditions would enable a more physiological understanding of different cardiovascular phenotypes. Several relatively load-independent indices of LV performance, such as meridional

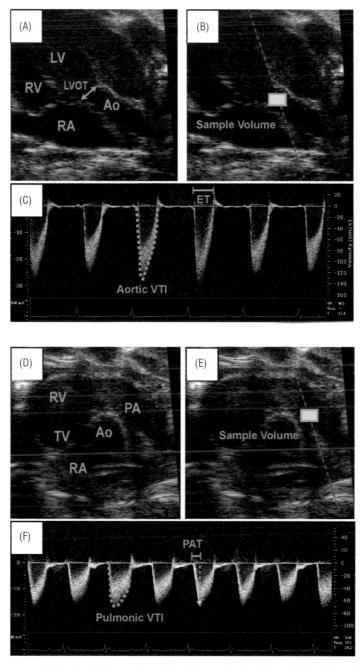

Figure 32.3 Doppler assessment of aortic and pulmonary flow. B-mode image of aortic outflow (A) obtained from apical approach. Schematic of pulsed-Doppler sample volume placement (B) with representative pulsed-Doppler tracing (C). B-mode image of pulmonic outflow (D) obtained from parasternal short-axis approach. Schematic of pulsed-Doppler sample volume placement (E) with representative pulsed-Doppler tracing (F). ET, ejection time; LVOT, left ventricular outflow tract; PA, pulmonary artery; PAT, pulmonary artery acceleration time; RA, right atrium; TV, tricuspid valve; VTI, velocity time interval.

end-systolic wall stress (σ_{es}) and rate-corrected velocity of fiber shortening (Vcf_c) relationship, have been used for the load-independent assessment of the contractile state in rodents [43]. The rate-corrected velocity of LV fiber shortening (Vcf_c) is calculated using the following formula:

$$Vcf_c = [(LVEDD - LVESD)/LVEDD]/ET_c$$

where ET_c is the rate-corrected LV ejection time divided by the square root of the preceding R–R interval. Compared with fractional shortening, Vcf_c has the advantage of being relatively preload and heart rate independent over the physiological range.

LV meridional systolic wall stress (σ), a measure of true LV afterload, can be calculated as a function of time using the following angiographically validated formula [46]:

$$\sigma(t) = [1.35][P(t)][D(t)]/[4][h(t)][1 + (h(t)/D(t))]$$

where σ is in g/cm^2, $[P]$ is aortic pressure, $[D]$ is LV internal dimension, $[h]$ is systolic LV wall thickness, and 1.35 is a unit conversion factor. LV pressures during LV ejection are assumed to be equal to systolic aortic pressures. It is possible that in the future, with the use of minimally invasive or accurate noninvasive (tail-cuff) determinations of aortic pressures, this index could be noninvasively determined.

Left ventricular diastolic function

Diastolic function has been studied in rodents using PW Doppler and color M-mode [47] Impaired LV relaxation has been associated with reduced early-to-late diastolic transmitral Doppler flow velocity ratios (i.e. decreased E/A ratio), prolonged isovolumic relaxation times (IVRT), and prolonged E wave deceleration times. However, multiple limitations have prevented widespread use of this methodology, including: (1) poor alignment of the Doppler beam with the transmitral flow, making it difficult to reproducibly compare tracings obtained in different animals; and (2) the high heart rate of rodents, which results in merging of the E and A waves and thus confounds mitral flow analysis. The main difficulty in studying mitral flow in rodent models is that in order to separate E and A waves, the heart rate may need to be slowed down

significantly. The physiological relevance of diastolic findings is unclear at abnormally slow heart rates.

The Tei index, also known as the myocardial performance index (MPI), is an echocardiographic Doppler index that combines systolic and diastolic function and has been utilized as a measure of myocardial function [49]. In humans, the Tei index is simple to calculate, reproducible, independent of heart rate and blood pressure, and characterized by a low interobserver and intraobserver variability. Its use has been applied to studies of rodents in the assessment of global LV function after myocardial infarction and the assessment of diastolic function [19,30,50,51]. The Tei index is calculated as follows:

$$\text{Tei index} = (IVRT + IVCT/ET) \text{ (Figure 32.4)}.$$

The velocity of flow propagation into the left ventricle, known as the propagation velocity (Vp), has been shown to provide an estimate of LV relaxation. Although traditional Dopplerindexes of diastolic function (such as IVRT and transmitral velocities) are load and rate dependent, color M-mode determined propagation velocity is a relatively load-independent index of LV filling [47]. Vp is obtained by placing the color Doppler sample box over the ventricle from valve to apex and adjusting the color scale to create aliasing, following which the M-mode sample volume is placed through the aliasing part of the inflow. Vp is measured by assessing the maximum slope of the first aliasing velocity as previously described [47]. Several studies have demonstrated that color M-mode flow propagation velocities and pulse wave Doppler echocardiography can be effectively used to noninvasively assess LV diastolic function in transgenic murine models [19,47,52,53]. The reliability of serial measurements of diastolic function remains to be determined.

Right ventricular assessment and pulmonary hypertension

To better understand the pathogenesis of pulmonary arterial hypertension (PAH), murine models have been developed using genetically modified mice [54,55]. In addition, surgical models using pulmonary artery banding or hypoxic exposure have been

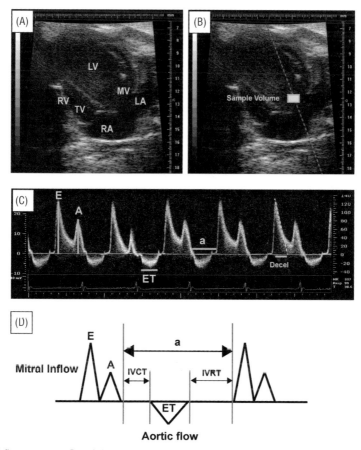

Figure 32.4 Mitral inflow assessment. B-mode image of apical four-chamber view (A) obtained from apical approach. Schematic of pulsed-Doppler sample volume placement (B) with representative pulsed-Doppler tracing (C). Schematic of mitral inflow Doppler pattern is seen in (D). Decel, deceleration time; ET, ejection time; IVCT, isovolumic contraction time; IVRT, isovolumic relaxation time; LA, left atrium; LV, left ventricle; MV, mitral valve; RA, right atrium; RV, right ventricle; TV, tricuspid valve.

utilized to study this condition. The spatial resolution of high-frequency probes (30–40 MHz) now allows for better visualization of the right ventricle. Nevertheless, 2D visualization of the right ventricle remains limited by the shape and position of the ventricle in rodents. Thus, hemodynamic assessment has become the tool more consistently used to assess the development of pulmonary hypertension.

In small animal models, right heart catheterization and measurement of right ventricular systolic pressure (RVSP), which is equal to pulmonary artery systolic pressure (PASP) in the absence of pulmonary stenosis, has been central in the detection and quantification of PAH. Right heart catheterization, however, is a terminal procedure in rodents that precludes longitudinal follow-up [56]. Indirect assessment of the severity of PAH by histological evaluation of postmortem heart and lung tissue also precludes serial assessment. Right ventricular systolic pressure can be estimated noninvasively in rodents using the peak tricuspid regurgitant flow velocity (where RVSP = $4V^2$). Echocardiography is able to detect acute and chronic changes in RVSP with high sensitivity and specificity and detect the effects of interventions on RVSP. However, the estimation of RVSP in rodents using echocardiography remains technically challenging. Apical and sub-costal views are not reliably obtained, preventing proper flow alignment and accurate measurement of tricuspid regurgitation by Doppler in these views. Furthermore,

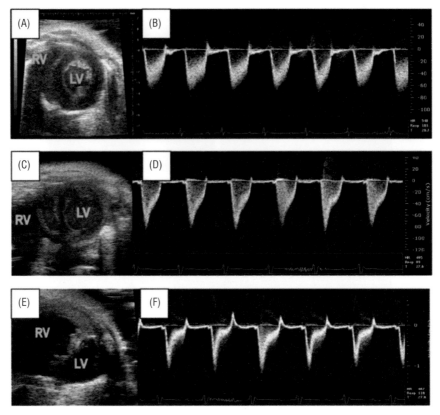

Figure 32.5 Pulmonary Doppler assessment of pulmonary hypertension. Representative B-mode short-axis images of the heart with mild (A), moderate (C), and severe (E) pulmonary hypertension. Note the degree of RV enlargement, RV wall thickness, and compression of LV cavity. Representative pulmonary artery Doppler tracings corresponding to the varying degrees of pulmonary hypertension in mild (B), moderate (D), and severe (F) elevations in pulmonary artery pressure. Note the changes in the Doppler waveform. LV, left ventricle; RV, right ventricle.

tricuspid regurgitation appears to be uncommon in rodents except at very high pulmonary pressures.

The pulmonary acceleration time (PAT, time from the onset of pulmonary flow to peak velocity by pulsed-wave Doppler recording) and the ratio of PAT to ET have been used as alternative indexes to estimate RVSP when tricuspid regurgitation is absent or of insufficient quality to reliably measure its peak velocity (Figure 32.5F). In response to an increase in pulmonary artery systolic pressure, the pulmonary valve tends to close prematurely, and peak flow velocity occurs earlier in systole. Therefore, pulmonary artery acceleration time decreases as pulmonary pressure increases [58,59]. Pulmonary acceleration time correlates inversely and linearly with mean pulmonary artery pressure in humans and with RVSP in rats and mice [27]. Figure 32.5

displays representative Doppler pulmonary artery tracings with increasing pulmonary hypertension and right ventricular dysfunction. In mice with high RVSP, the flow velocity accelerates rapidly to reach a peak early in systole, resulting in a shortened PAT [57].

Color Doppler

When using color Doppler imaging, a color-encoded map of flow velocity and direction is superimposed on the 2D image. Blood flowing toward the ultrasound transducer has an increase in echo frequency and is identified by the color red; flow away from the transducer has a decrease in echo frequency and is identified by the color blue. Each color has multiple shades, which become progressively lighter as velocity increases. Blood flowing horizontally is not detected; an alignment of the ultrasound beam as close as possible to the direction of the blood flow is, therefore, critical to enable detection directly toward or away from the transducer. Figure 32.6B illustrates color Doppler patterns through the aortic arch from a normal mouse. The colors red and blue show the direction of flow through the arch, and the various hues represent differing velocities. Doppler is particularly

useful to determine the severity of transverse aortic constriction (TAC) surgery to induce LV hypertrophy (Figure 32.6C,D). In the presence of turbulent flow, a mosaic of colors is present at the site of stenosis. Pressure/flow gradients attained through pulsed-wave Doppler allow for an assessment of the severity and reproducibility of the stenosis.

Both pulsed-wave Doppler and color Doppler imaging can be used to assess valvular disease. In different murine models, PW Doppler has

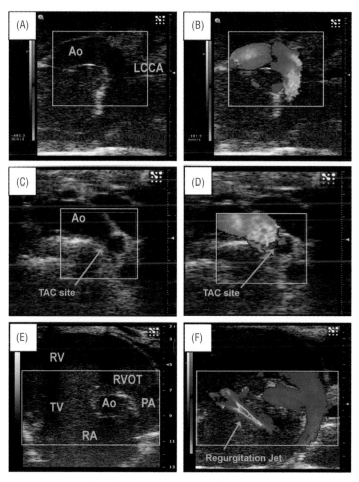

Figure 32.6 Example of color Doppler recordings. B-mode imaging of normal CD-1 mouse across the transverse aortic arch (A) with color Doppler imaging seen in (B), acquired from a high parasternal long-axis view, using a 56-MHz transducer. The probe was angled to align the maximal velocity flow across both the ascending and descending thoracic aorta. In (C), B-mode image of transaortic constriction site with corresponding color Doppler image see in (D). In (E), short axis image of an enlarged right atrial and ventricular chamber. Tricuspid regurgitation can be easily identified with color Doppler as seen in (F). Color flow Doppler images were obtained by centering the sampling area in a narrow region of interest. Note blue-colored velocity jet denotes flow away from the direction of the transducer, and red denotes flow toward the probe. Ao, aorta; LCCA, left common carotid artery; PA, pulmonary artery; RVOT, right ventricular outflow tract; TAC, transverse aortic constriction; TV, tricuspid valve.

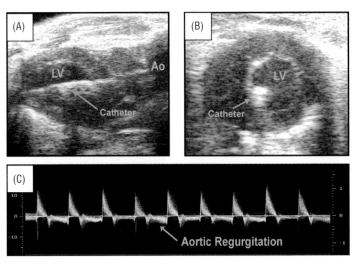

Figure 32.7 Echocardiographic evaluation of catheter placement. B-mode imaging of a catheter traversing the aortic valve in the left ventricular cavity. Images obtained in the long-axis (A) and short-axis (B) views. Note the highly echogenic catheter obscuring visualization of the aortic valve. Resultant aortic regurgitation seen in pulse-Doppler imaging is seen in (C). Ao, aorta; LV, left ventricle.

been used to verify the absence or presence of aortic insufficiency when a catheter is introduced retrogradely across the aortic valve [60] (Figure 32.7). Similarly, color Doppler can be used to identify valvular regurgitation (Figure 32.6F). Use of 2D superimposed color Doppler imaging allows for more rapid and consistent identification of regurgitant lesions. Pulse Doppler can be used for identification of regurgitation, however, this approach requires sampling of numerous regions without 2D guidance. Small or eccentric lesions may be overlooked and maximal velocity may not be measured. Color Doppler also allows the opportunity to evaluate for additional structural defects not easily seen by conventional B-mode imaging such as atrial and ventricular septal defects.

Assessment of embryonic and neonatal mice

Murine fetal echocardiography is a technically challenging technique. Until recently, imaging of embryonic mouse hearts frequently involved invasive methods. The embryo has to be sacrificed to perform magnetic resonance microscopy and electron microscopy or surgically delivered for transillumination microscopy. Mice measure between 15 and 20 mm at birth, which significantly

limits a variety of imaging modalities due to resolution constraints. In addition, the reported heart rate of embryos varies with the duration of gestation and is greatly influenced by technical issues such as temperature and anesthesia of the pregnant mouse. Fetal and perinatal death is a common feature when studying genetic alterations affecting cardiac development. In order to study the role of genes in the early development of cardiac function, ultrasound imaging of the live fetus has become an important tool for early recognition of abnormalities and longitudinal follow-up.

High-frequency ultrasound imaging of the fetus can provide detailed information on the early development of cardiac structures from E8.5 [64]. Conventional 2D and pulsed-wave Doppler imaging have been shown to provide measurements of cardiac contraction and heart rates at embryonic day E14.5 (Figure 32.8A–H) [61,62]. Fractional shortening measured in normal C57BL6 fetuses has been found to be approximately 50% at E16.5 and E18.5 [61]. Color Doppler has been particularly useful for *in utero* screening of valvular regurgitation and structural cardiovascular abnormalities in fetal mice [63]. High-frequency ultrasound imaging of the fetus has improved 2D resolution and can provide excellent information on the early development of cardiac structures from E8.5 [64].

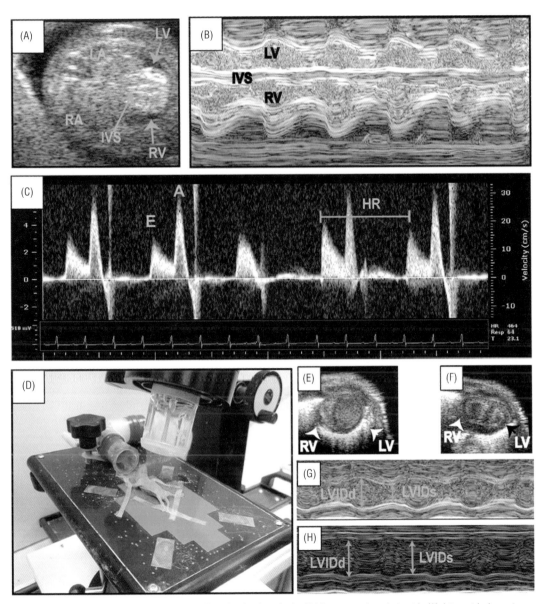

Figure 32.8 Fetal and neonatal echocardiography. B-mode of embryonic day E14.5 mouse embryonic heart in (A). Interventricular septum, right and left ventricular walls can be visualized in this image. M-mode image of E14.5 mouse is seen in (B). Mitral inflow Doppler pattern can be visualized as seen in (C), which will also allow for calculation of fetal heart rate. (D) Visualization of a newborn mouse undergoing a study. 2D short-axis view (E) and M-mode (G) of normal CD-1 neonatal mouse at the level of the papillary muscles. Right ventricular enlargement seen by b-mode in (F) due to a ventricular septal defect. Left ventricular dysfunction in a neonatal mouse detected by m-mode is seen in (H). IVS, interventricular septum; LVID, LV internal diameter.

This methodology can also be used as a guidance tool for interventional procedures such as injections and allows imaging of blood flow velocities for excellent hemodynamic assessment of the fetal circulatory system.

Overall, the heart rate in fetal mice appears to be slower than in adult mice (between 180 and 260 bpm after day E14.5). Optimal orientation of the fetus *in utero* may be difficult to achieve, precluding accurate M-mode measurements. To correct for inadequate orientation, investigators frequently exteriorize the uterus; however, the physiological repercussions of this procedure are unknown [65,66]. At very high frequencies, the blood appears echogenic due to the nucleation of fetal red blood cells. The echogenicity of the blood peaks at E13.5, making the differentiation of blood and myocardial walls difficult before E15.5 [67].

Until recently, neonatal mice have not been studied because of size and imaging constraints, as well as difficulty in delivering anesthesia. Recent advances in ultrasound technology have allowed the visualization of the cardiac anatomy of the newborn mouse and measurement of functional parameters. Before beginning the examination, the mouse should be placed in an inhalation chamber containing several gauze pads saturated with isoflurane for 30–60 seconds. When fully asleep, each animal is then placed supine on an internally heated platform, the temperature of which should be set and preheated to 40°C. The legs are then gently taped flat and Isoflurane at 0.5–1.0%, delivered via a conical tube fitted over the nose and mouth (Figure 32.8D). Anesthesia is deemed adequate when the animal lies quietly without struggling and when the heart rate and respiratory rates are stable.

Neonatal mice have slower heart rates and reduced contractile function when compared to adult mice. Although FS increases (from 34% to 45%) during the first week of life, neonatal heart rates (~300 bpm) remain slow [68]. Neonatal mice are extremely sensitive to hypothermia; when this occurs, heart rates will typically drop below 300 bpm with reduced fractional shortening, resulting in high mortality rate. Despite these limitations, neonatal pups can survive cardiac imaging and be taken back by their mother, which should facilitate the performance of serial studies on individual animals.

Assessment of aortic pathology

Numerous mouse models of atherosclerosis and aortic aneurysm are available today, illustrating various clinically-relevant phenotypes that can be evaluated using high-frequency echocardiography [69]. Measurement of atherosclerosis in the ascending aorta in mice has been shown to reflect total aortic plaque burden. Maximum plaque thickness and plaque area have been shown to

correlate highly with histology data [70]. The minor curvature of the aortic arch is subject to turbulent low shear flow, and is known to be an atherosclerosis-prone vascular site (Figure 32.9C). In mice, the common carotid artery is relatively free from atherosclerosis (Figure 32.9B), and plaque formations starts commonly at the aortic root and the ascending aorta. The innominate artery has also been proposed to be a representative site where atherosclerosis (Figure 32.9D), including spontaneous plaque rupture, can be assessed. The noninvasive nature of echocardiography makes this imaging modality particularly useful for serial assessment of plaque growth and response to interventions.

To image the aorta, a right parasternal long-axis view is used to visualize the ascending aorta, aortic arch, and the neck vessels in a single plane (Figure 32.9A). The vascular region proximal to the minor side of the aortic arch is known to be the initiation site of atherosclerotic lesions. This specific region is also recognized with the innominate artery branch as an anatomic landmark, which facilitates the exact localization of the measurement site during longitudinal studies. Subsequently, a parasternal short-axis view can be acquired to visualize the same arterial site in a cross-sectional view immediately proximal to the branch of the innominate artery.

Similar to atherosclerotic models, noninvasive measurement of aortic aneurysm development and progress using a high-frequency ultrasound imaging system has the advantages of low cost, rapid data acquisition, reproducibility, and high resolution (Figure 32.9E and F). Repeated monitoring of the progress of aneurysm development over time is feasible [71].

Conclusions

Rodent models represent a powerful tool for understanding the molecular mechanisms underlying both normal cardiovascular function and the pathophysiological basis of human cardiovascular disease. Recent advances in cardiac ultrasound have responded to the challenges imposed by small, fast-beating rodent hearts to make echocardiography a reliable means of quantifying the cardiac phenotype in mice and rats. Two dimensional/Doppler echocardiography currently provide a relatively inexpensive, accurate, and noninvasive method for

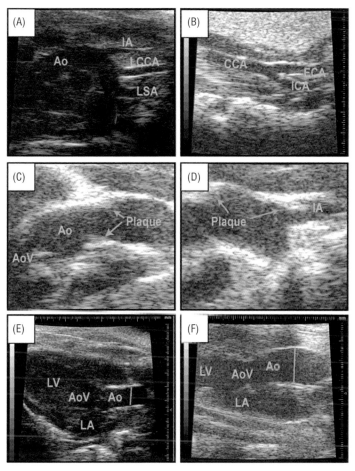

Figure 32.9 Assessment of aortic pathology. 2D image of the aortic arch obtained from a right parasternal long-axis view (A) allows for visualization of the three vessels branching from the aortic arch: innominate artery, IA; left common carotid artery; LCCA, and left subclavian artery, LSA. High-frequency ultrasound allows for visualization of the carotid artery (B). Visualization of aortic plaque in the proximal ascending aorta (C) and the ostia of the innominate artery (D). 2D image of normal aortic root and ascending aorta from a CD-1 mouse obtained from the parasternal long-axis view (E) compared to an aortic aneurysm seen in (F).

the serial assessment of cardiovascular structural and functional changes in a variety of rodent models.

References

1 Scherrer-Crosbie M, Thibault HB. Echocardiography in translational research: of mice and men. *J Am Soc Echocardiogr* 2008; **21**: 1083–1092.

2 Ram R, Mickelsen DM, Theodoropoulos C, Blaxall BC. New approaches in small animal echocardiography: imaging the sounds of silence. *Am J Physiol Heart Circ Physiol* 2011; **301**: H1765–1780.

3 Brown L, Fenning A, Chan V, Loch D, Wilson K, Anderson B, *et al.* Echocardiographic assessment of cardiac structure and function in rats. *Heart Lung Circ* 2002; **11**: 167–173.

4 Coatney RW. Ultrasound imaging: principles and applications in rodent research. *ILAR J* 2001; **42**: 233–247.

5 Stypmann J, Engelen MA, Epping C, van Rijen HV, Milberg P, Bruch C, *et al.* Age and gender related reference values for transthoracic Doppler-echocardiography in the anesthetized CD1 mouse. *Int J Cardiovas Imag* 2006; **22**: 353–362.

6 Collins KA, Korcarz CE, Lang RM. Use of echocardiography for the phenotypic assessment of genetically altered mice. *Physiol Genomics* 2003; **13**: 227–239.

7 Zhang L, Xu X, Hu C, Sun L, Yen JT, Cannata JM, *et al.* A high-frequency, high frame rate duplex ultrasound

linear array imaging system for small animal imaging. IEEE Trans Ultrason Ferroelectr Freq Control 2010; **57**: 1548–1557.

8 Okajima K, Abe Y, Fujimoto K, Fujikura K, Girard EE, Asai T, et al. Comparative study of high-resolution microimaging with 30-MHz scanner for evaluating cardiac function in mice. *J Am Soc Echocardiogr* 2007; **20**: 1203–1210.

9 Liu J, Rigel DF. Echocardiographic examination in rats and mice. *Methods Mol Biol* 2009; **573**: 139–155.

10 Scherrer-Crosbie M, Kurtz B. Ventricular remodeling and function: Insights using murine echocardiography. *J Mol Cell Cardiol* 2010; **48**: 512–517.

11 Balaban RS, Hampshire VA. Challenges in small animal noninvasive imaging. *ILAR J* 2001; **42**: 248–262.

12 Gao S, Ho D, Vatner DE, Vatner SF. Echocardiography in mice. *Curr Prot Mouse Biol* 2011; **1**: 71–83.

13 Rottman JN, Ni G, Brown M. Echocardiographic evaluation of ventricular function in mice. *Echocardiography* 2007; **24**: 83–89.

14 Gardin JM, Siri FM, Kitsis RN, Edwards JG, Leinwand LA. Echocardiographic assessment of left ventricular mass and systolic function in mice. *Circ Res* 1995; **76**: 907–914.

15 Kiatchoosakun S, Restivo J, Kirkpatrick D, Hoit BD. Assessment of left ventricular mass in mice: comparison between two-dimensional and m-mode echocardiography. *Echocardiography* 2002; **19**: 199–205.

16 Youn HJ, Rokosh G, Lester SJ, Simpson P, Schiller NB, Foster E, et al. Two-dimensional echocardiography with a 15-MHz transducer is a promising alternative for in vivo measurement of left ventricular mass in mice. *J Am Soc Echocardiogr* 1999; **12**: 70–75.

17 Otto CM. *Textbook of Clinical Echocardiography*, 4th edn. Philadelphia: Saunders/Elsevier, 2009.

18 Hartley CJ, Taffet GE, Reddy AK, Entman ML, Michael LH. Noninvasive cardiovascular phenotyping in mice. *ILAR J* 2002; **43**: 147–158.

19 Pollick C, Hale SL, Kloner RA. Echocardiographic and cardiac Doppler assessment of mice. *J Am Soc Echocardiogr* 1995; **8**: 602–610.

20 Syed F, Diwan A, Hahn HS. Murine echocardiography: a practical approach for phenotyping genetically manipulated and surgically modeled mice. *J Am Soc Echocardiogr* 2005; **18**: 982–990.

21 Yuan L, Wang T, Liu F, Cohen ED, Patel VV. An evaluation of transmitral and pulmonary venous Doppler indices for assessing murine left ventricular diastolic function. *J Am Soc Echocardiogr* 2010; **23**: 887–897.

22 Ghanem A, Roll W, Hashemi T, Dewald O, Djoufack PC, Fink KB, et al. Echocardiographic assessment of left ventricular mass in neonatal and adult mice: accuracy of different echocardiographic methods. *Echocardiography* 2006; **23**: 900–907.

23 Collins KA, Korcarz CE, Shroff SG, Bednarz JE, Fentzke RC, Lin H, et al. Accuracy of echocardiographic estimates of left ventricular mass in mice. *Am J Physiol Heart Circ Physiol* 2001; **280**: H1954–1962.

24 Reffelmann T, Kloner RA. Transthoracic echocardiography in rats. Evalution of commonly used indices of left ventricular dimensions, contractile performance, and hypertrophy in a genetic model of hypertrophic heart failure (SHHF-Mcc-facp-Rats) in comparison with Wistar rats during aging. *Basic Res Cardiol* 2003; **98**: 275–284.

25 Boluyt MO, Converso K, Hwang HS, Mikkor A, Russell MW. Echocardiographic assessment of age-associated changes in systolic and diastolic function of the female F344 rat heart. *J Appl Physiol* 2004; **96**: 822–828.

26 Lang RM, Bierig M, Devereux RB, Flachskampf FA, Foster E, Pellikka PA, et al. Recommendations for chamber quantification: a report from the American Society of Echocardiography's Guidelines and Standards Committee and the Chamber Quantification Writing Group, developed in conjunction with the European Association of Echocardiography, a branch of the European Society of Cardiology. *J Am Soc Echocardiogr* 2005; **18**: 1440–1463.

27 Jones JE, Mendes L, Rudd MA, Russo G, Loscalzo J, Zhang YY, et al. Serial noninvasive assessment of progressive pulmonary hypertension in a rat model. *Am J Physiol Heart Circ Physiol* 2002; **283**: H364–371.

28 Respress JL, Wehrens XH. Transthoracic echocardiography in mice. *J Vis Exp* 2010; (**39**). pii: 1738.

29 Watson LE, Sheth M, Denyer RF, Dostal DE. Baseline echocardiographic values for adult male rats. *J Am Soc Echocardiogr* 2004; **17**: 161–167.

30 Collins KA, Korcarz CE, Lang RM. Use of echocardiography for the phenotypic assessment of genetically altered mice. *Physiol Genomics* 2003; **13**: 227–239.

31 Hinton RB, Jr., Alfieri CM, Witt SA, Glascock BJ, Khoury PR, Benson DW, et al. Mouse heart valve structure and function: echocardiographic and morphometric analyses from the fetus through the aged adult. *Am J Physiol Heart Circ Physiol* 2008; **294**: H2480–2488.

32 Sebag IA, Handschumacher MD, Ichinose F, Morgan JG, Hataishi R, Rodrigues AC, et al. Quantitative assessment of regional myocardial function in mice by tissue Doppler imaging: comparison with hemodynamics and sonomicrometry. *Circulation* 2005; **111**: 2611–2616.

33 Hoit BD, Ball N, Walsh RA. Invasive hemodynamics and force-frequency relationships in open- versus closed-chest mice. *Am J Physiol* 1997; **273**: H2528–2533.

34 Manning WJ, Wei JY, Katz SE, Litwin SE, Douglas PS. In vivo assessment of LV mass in mice using high-frequency cardiac ultrasound: necropsy validation. *Am J Physiol* 1994; **266**: H1672–1675.

35 Devereux RB, Alonso DR, Lutas EM, Gottlieb GJ, Campo E, Sachs I, et al. Echocardiographic assessment of left ventricular hypertrophy: comparison to necropsy findings. *Am J Cardiol* 1986; **57**: 450–458.

36 Schiller NB, Shah PM, Crawford M, DeMaria A, Devereux R, Feigenbaum H, et al. Recommendations for quantitation of the left ventricle by two-dimensional echocardiography. American Society of Echocardiography Committee on Standards, Subcommittee on Quantitation of Two-Dimensional Echocardiograms. *J Am Soc Echocardiogr* 1989; **2**: 358–367.

37 Kanno S, Lerner DL, Schuessler RB, Betsuyaku T, Yamada KA, Saffitz JE, et al. Echocardiographic evaluation of ventricular remodeling in a mouse model of myocardial infarction. *J Am Soc Echocardiogr* 2002; **15**: 601–609.

38 Hoit BD, Khoury SF, Kranias EG, Ball N, Walsh RA. In vivo echocardiographic detection of enhanced left ventricular function in gene-targeted mice with phospholamban deficiency. *Circ Res* 1995; **77**: 632–637.

39 Milano CA, Allen LF, Rockman HA, Dolber PC, McMinn TR, Chien KR, et al. Enhanced myocardial function in transgenic mice overexpressing the beta 2-adrenergic receptor. *Science* 1994; **264**: 582–586.

40 Wang P, Ba ZF, Burkhardt J, Chaudry IH. Trauma-hemorrhage and resuscitation in the mouse: effects on cardiac output and organ blood flow. *Am J Physiol* 1993; **264**: H1166–1173.

41 Janssen B, Debets J, Leenders P, Smits J. Chronic measurement of cardiac output in conscious mice. *Am J Physiol Regul Integr Comp Physiol* 2002; **282**: R928–935.

42 Fentzke RC, Korcarz CE, Shroff SG, Lin H, Sandelski J, Leiden JM, et al. Evaluation of ventricular and arterial hemodynamics in anesthetized closed-chest mice. *J Am Soc Echocardiogr* 1997; **10**: 915–925.

43 Fentzke RC, Korcarz CE, Shroff SG, Lin H, Leiden JM, Lang RM, et al. The left ventricular stress-velocity relation in transgenic mice expressing a dominant negative CREB transgene in the heart. *J Am Soc Echocardiogr* 2001; **14**: 209–218.

44 Nemoto S, DeFreitas G, Mann DL, Carabello BA. Effects of changes in left ventricular contractility on indexes of contractility in mice. *Am J Physiol Heart Circ Physiol* 2002; **283**: H2504–2510.

45 Patten RD, Aronovitz MJ, Bridgman P, Pandian NG. Use of pulse wave and color flow Doppler echocardiography in mouse models of human disease. *J Am Soc Echocardiogr* 2002; **15**: 708–714.

46 Brodie BR, McLaurin LP, Grossman W. Combined hemodynamic-ultrasonic method for studying left ventricular wall stress: comparison with angiography. *Am J Cardiol* 1976; **37**: 864–870.

47 Schmidt AG, Gerst M, Zhai J, Carr AN, Pater L, Kranias EG, et al. Evaluation of left ventricular diastolic function from spectral and color M-mode Doppler in genetically altered mice. *J Am Soc Echocardiogr* 2002; **15**: 1065–1073.

48 Ichihara S, Senbonmatsu T, Price E, Jr., Ichiki T, Gaffney FA, Inagami T, et al. Angiotensin II type 2 receptor is essential for left ventricular hypertrophy and cardiac fibrosis in chronic angiotensin II-induced hypertension. *Circulation* 2001; **104**: 346–351.

49 Gabriel RS, Klein AL. Modern evaluation of left ventricular diastolic function using Doppler echocardiography. *Curr Cardiol Rep* 2009; **11**: 231–238.

50 Yuan LJ, Wang T, Kahn ML, Ferrari VA. High-resolution echocardiographic assessment of infarct size and cardiac function in mice with myocardial infarction. *J Am Soc Echocardiogr* 2011; **24**: 219–226.

51 Schaefer A, Meyer GP, Hilfiker-Kleiner D, Brand B, Drexler H, Klein G, et al. Evaluation of tissue Doppler Tei index for global left ventricular function in mice after myocardial infarction: comparison with pulsed Doppler Tei index. *Eur J Echocardiogr* 2005; **6**: 367–375.

52 Hoit BD. Spectral and color M-mode Doppler in genetically altered mice. Assessment of diastolic function. *Minerva Cardioangiol* 2003; **51**: 609–618.

53 Tsujita Y, Kato T, Sussman MA. Evaluation of left ventricular function in cardiomyopathic mice by tissue Doppler and color M-mode Doppler echocardiography. *Echocardiography* 2005; **22**: 245–353.

54 Steudel W, Ichinose F, Huang PL, Hurford WE, Jones RC, Bevan JA, et al. Pulmonary vasoconstriction and hypertension in mice with targeted disruption of the endothelial nitric oxide synthase (NOS 3) gene. *Circ Res* 1997; **81**: 34–41.

55 Beppu H, Ichinose F, Kawai N, Jones RC, Yu PB, Zapol WM, et al. BMPR-II heterozygous mice have mild pulmonary hypertension and an impaired pulmonary vascular remodeling response to prolonged hypoxia. *Am J Physiol Lung Cell Mol Physiol* 2004; **287**: L1241–1247.

56 Nemoto S, DeFreitas G, Carabello BA. Cardiac catheterization technique in a closed-chest murine model. *Contemp Top Lab Anim Sci* 2003; **42**: 34–38.

57 Thibault HB, Kurtz B, Raher MJ, Shaik RS, Waxman A, Derumeaux G, et al. Noninvasive assessment of murine pulmonary arterial pressure: validation and application to models of pulmonary hypertension. *Circ Cardiovasc Imaging* 2010; **3**: 157–163.

58 Litwin SE. Noninvasive assessment of pulmonary artery pressures: moving beyond tricuspid regurgitation velocities. *Circ Cardiovasc Imaging* 2010; **3**: 132–133.

59 Lavine SJ. Noninvasive estimation of right-sided pressures from spectral Doppler recordings of tricuspid and pulmonic regurgitant velocities. *Chest* 1999; **116**: 1–3.

60 Chiu HC, Kovacs A, Blanton RM, Han X, Courtois M, Weinheimer CJ, et al. Transgenic expression of fatty

acid transport protein 1 in the heart causes lipotoxic cardiomyopathy. *Circ Res* 2005; **96**: 225–233.

61 Spurney CF, Leatherbury L, Lo CW. High-frequency ultrasound database profiling growth, development, and cardiovascular function in C57BL/6J mouse fetuses. *J Am Soc Echocardiogr* 2004; **17**: 893–900.

62 Kim GH, Samant SA, Earley JU, Svensson EC. Translational control of FOG-2 expression in cardiomyocytes by microRNA-130a. *PLoS One* 2009; **4**: e6161.

63 Shen Y, Leatherbury L, Rosenthal J, Yu Q, Pappas MA, Wessels A, *et al.* Cardiovascular phenotyping of fetal mice by noninvasive high-frequency ultrasound facilitates recovery of ENU-induced mutations causing congenital cardiac and extracardiac defects. *Physiol Genomics* 2005; **24**: 23–36.

64 Srinivasan S, Baldwin HS, Aristizabal O, Kwee L, Labow M, Artman M, *et al.* Noninvasive, in utero imaging of mouse embryonic heart development with 40-MHz echocardiography. *Circulation* 1998; **98**: 912–918.

65 Ji RP, Phoon CK, Aristizabal O, McGrath KE, Palis J, Turnbull DH, *et al.* Onset of cardiac function during early mouse embryogenesis coincides with entry of primitive erythroblasts into the embryo proper. *Circ Res* 2003; **92**: 133–135.

66 Phoon CK, Ji RP, Aristizabal O, Worrad DM, Zhou B, Baldwin HS, *et al.* Embryonic heart failure in NFATc1/- mice: novel mechanistic insights from in utero ultrasound biomicroscopy. *Circ Res* 2004; **95**: 92–99.

67 Le Floc'h J, Cherin E, Zhang MY, Akirav C, Adamson SL, Vray D, *et al.* Developmental changes in integrated ultrasound backscatter from embryonic blood in vivo in mice at high US frequency. *Ultrasound Med Biol* 2004; **30**: 1307–1319.

68 Bose AK, Mathewson JW, Anderson BE, Andrews AM, Martin Gerdes A, Benjamin Perryman M, *et al.* Initial experience with high frequency ultrasound for the newborn C57BL mouse. *Echocardiography* 2007; **24**: 412–419.

69 Fuster JJ, Castillo AI, Zaragoza C, Ibanez B, Andres V. Animal models of atherosclerosis. *Prog Mol Biol Transl Sci* 2012; **105**: 1–23.

70 Gan LM, Gronros J, Hagg U, Wikström J, Theodoropoulos C, Friberg P, *et al.* Non-invasive real-time imaging of atherosclerosis in mice using ultrasound biomicroscopy. *Atherosclerosis* 2007; **190**: 313–320.

71 Hofmann Bowman M, Wilk J, Heydemann A, Kim G, Rehman J, Lodato JA, *et al.* S100A12 mediates aortic wall remodeling and aortic aneurysm. *Circ Res* 2010; **106**: 145–154.

Echocardiography: advanced techniques (tissue Doppler, speckle tracking, and three-dimensional imaging)

Lauren Beussink-Nelson,[1] Gene H. Kim,[2] Roberto M. Lang,[2] and Sanjiv J. Shah[1]

[1] Northwestern University Feinberg School of Medicine, Chicago, IL, USA

[2] The University of Chicago Medical Center, Chicago, IL, USA

Introduction

The widespread use of rodent models in the study of cardiovascular disease has increased the demand for advanced techniques to characterize the cardiac phenotype in these animals. Although standard echocardiographic methods are capable of providing extensive information about cardiac anatomy and physiology, there are several limiting factors associated with imaging the hearts of small animals that preclude a truly comprehensive evaluation of cardiovascular function. The echocardiographic indexes widely used to evaluate left ventricular (LV) systolic and diastolic function, such as M-mode derived fractional shortening (FS) and ejection fraction (EF) and pulsed wave (PW) Doppler interrogation of mitral inflow, can be greatly influenced by loading conditions, which limits their effectiveness in the assessment of myocardial contractility and relaxation [1]. In addition, the evaluation of regional function by two-dimensional (2D) echocardiography is typically performed visually, a subjective approach that frequently fails to detect alterations in ventricular function despite histologic evidence of injury [2,3]. Finally, standard echocardiographic techniques are also relatively insensitive to early or subtle alterations in cardiac performance, particularly in mice, due to limitations in spatial and temporal resolution [4].

Although these obstacles are significant, 2D echocardiography is still the primary tool for chamber quantification and evaluation of ventricular function in rodent models. However, new applications such as, tissue Doppler imaging (TDI), speckle tracking, and three-dimensional (3D) echocardiography have been introduced to improve the echocardiographic evaluation of cardiac function and overcome these limitations in both humans and rodent models [5]. These new techniques are capable of providing superior image resolution, greater precision and sensitivity, and a more refined evaluation of cardiac anatomy, function, and hemodynamic properties [6]. In addition, several of these new techniques are less load-dependent, giving investigators greater insight into ventricular mechanics and systolic function, and are able to quantify regional contractility with a degree of accuracy not attainable using standard methods [7].

The goal of this chapter is to describe the basic principles behind each of these new techniques and explain how they can be adapted to the evaluation of the cardiovascular phenotype in rodents.

Tissue Doppler imaging

Principles

In addition to spectral and color Doppler, a novel Doppler-based modality, TDI, can be used alternatively or in combination to assess global and regional cardiac function by evaluating the motion of the myocardial tissue with Doppler technology [8]. TDI-derived velocity estimation is based on the same principles as other Doppler modalities; however, while conventional Doppler flow measurements are based on the low-amplitude, high-velocity signals originating from moving blood cells, TDI measurements are based on the high-amplitude, low-velocity signals generated by the myocardium [9]. These signals are easily distinguished by adjusting the gain and velocity scales and using a low-pass filter to separate tissue-generated data from blood flow data [9,10]. The velocity of myocardial motion is measured directly using PW Doppler (with a sample volume placed at a specific site in the myocardium); alternatively, mean velocities for myocardial motion in the entire image plane can be displayed using color TDI [9].

TDI is readily available, sensitive, has excellent temporal resolution, and allows for quantitative evaluation of myocardial function; in addition, because this technique is largely automated, intraobserver and interobserver variability are reduced [10]. Both systolic and diastolic regional myocardial velocities and the timing of cardiac events may be quantified using TDI [2]. More recently, TDI technology has been used to evaluate strain rate (SR), which is a relatively load-independent index of regional function [11]. Although applying TDI to rodent hearts presents unique challenges, improved resolution has recently made it possible to record TDI in the rodent myocardium consistently and accurately [8,12,13].

Instrument settings

• Adjustments are made to display the velocity of the myocardium, rather than the blood flow velocity (as described previously); generally, the ultrasound system has a preset function to automatically optimize TDI signals.

• Scale:
  ◦ For PW TDI, a small velocity range is best (generally a scale of ±20 cm/s is applied); for color TDI, the velocity scale should be set to a range that just avoids aliasing in any region of the myocardium.

• Gain:
  ◦ PW TDI gain should be adjusted to eliminate background noise and ensure a clear signal; excessive gain should be avoided, as this causes spectral broadening and over-estimation of tissue velocity [10].
  ◦ Color TDI gain should be set just above the point at which random noise appears.

• Frame rate:
  ◦ A high frame rate is required to ensure accurate TDI-derived measurements; the same techniques employed to maximize frame rates using other modalities should be used to achieve a high TDI sampling rate.
  ◦ TDI frame rates over 200 frames/second (fps) are generally reported in rats (with even higher frame rates required in mice due to their higher heart rates) [11].

• Sample volume:
  ◦ PW TDI acquisition requires adjustment of the sample volume size and position so that it remains within the region of interest inside the myocardium throughout the cardiac cycle; generally, the smallest sample volume should be used [10].
  ◦ As with other Doppler modalities, both PW and color TDI are angle dependent, so the sample volume should be aligned with the direction of the motion to be interrogated.

Basic protocol

PW TDI velocities are recorded at a specific site in the myocardium; therefore, motion is measured only in the direction toward and away from the transducer, representing the component of regional velocity along the scan line [9]. PW TDI is generally used to measure longitudinal motion from the mitral annulus or regional radial motion from the myocardium of the inferolateral (posterior) wall; however, assessment from other segments is possible, as long as parallel alignment can be achieved. Color

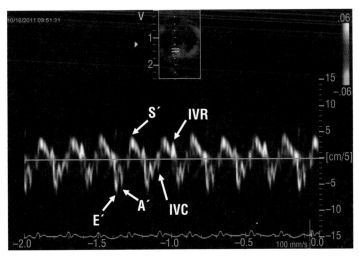

Figure 33.1 Tissue Doppler imaging of the septal mitral annulus. Tissue Doppler tracings recorded in a spontaneously hypertensive rat. A′, late (atrial) longitudinal tissue velocity; E′, early diastolic longitudinal tissue velocity; IVC, isovolumic contraction wave; IVR, isovolumic relaxation wave; S′, peak systolic longitudinal tissue velocity.

TDI velocities are used to qualitatively assess the velocity of myocardial motion toward and away from the transducer; in addition, a variety of functional parameters can be derived from the color TDI data set during offline analysis [10].

The apical window offers the best views for measuring tissue velocity in most segments because the motion of the ventricular walls is parallel to the ultrasound beam from this location. Although these views are difficult to obtain in rodents, an attempt should be made to record the TDI velocity on the septal portion of the mitral annulus by placing the sample volume near the junction of the anterior mitral leaflet and ventricular septum; a color TDI image may also be taken at this level. Due to the limitations associated with acquiring apical views in rodents, many researchers use the parasternal short axis (PSAX) window for TDI evaluation; however, from this view TDI assessment is not possible in most segments because parallel alignment with the direction of wall motion is difficult to achieve [10,14]. The most reproducible location for measuring TDI from the PSAX window is the inferolateral wall; anterior wall motion can also be aligned with the beam, but signals from this wall are more vulnerable to artifacts and variability due to close proximity to the chest wall and transducer [15]. To record the TDI velocity, place the sample volume within the inferolateral wall at the level of the papillary muscles; a color TDI image may also be taken at this level.

The PW TDI trace consists of three basic waveforms: systolic (S′), early diastolic (E′), and late diastolic/ atrial (A′) (Figure 33.1). The TDI curve is similar to the transmitral Doppler trace, but inverted and lower in velocity; importantly, the TDI values are also influenced by loading conditions, but to a lesser extent than conventional Doppler waves, especially in diastole [16]. The S′ wave begins after the initiation of the QRS complex and appears as a positive peak during systole, representing regional systolic contraction of the myocardium. The E′ and A′ waves measure the velocity of myocardial displacement as the ventricle expands during diastole, and correspond to passive and active LV filling, respectively; like the mitral inflow pattern, these waves are often fused at high heart rates, but the fused peak velocity may still be used for analysis [15].

In addition to measuring velocity waveforms, TDI is also well suited for determining the timing of myocardial events using the isovolumic contraction time (IVCT) and isovolumic relaxation time (IVRT) [5]. The IVCT is the first waveform that occurs during systole; its duration is measured as the time interval between the end of the A′ wave and the beginning of the S′ wave. The IVRT is the first waveform that occurs during early diastole; its duration is measured as the time interval between the end of the S′ wave and the beginning of the E′ wave. The IVCT and IVRT waveforms should not be confused with the tissue velocity waveforms; the isovolumic peaks are shorter and more variable in amplitude, while the true functional velocities (i.e. S′, E′, and A′) are longer and generally more consistent from cycle to cycle [2] (Figure 33.1).

Applications

Systolic function. TDI indexes have been validated as sensitive measures of systolic myocardial function in both large animals and rodents, and have been shown to detect subtle dysfunction earlier than conventional methods [3]. Systolic TDI measurements represent the regional function of the myocardium, which can be assessed in various segments by placing the sample volume in the area of interest; abnormalities of global dysfunction can also be identified if tissue damage occurs in a homogeneous manner [15]. The peak S′ velocity, as well at the time to peak and duration of the S′ wave, correlate well with ventricular systolic function. Reduced S′ velocities, as well as a shortened time to peak and S′ duration, indicate dysfunction [5,15].

Diastolic function. Diastolic function can be easily and reliably assessed by TDI, largely independent of loading conditions and heart rate [9,14]. Because most conventional diastolic function parameters have a bimodal distribution (e.g. E/A ratio is typically >1 in the setting of normal diastolic function but also in moderate and severe diastolic dysfunction) the presence and stage of diastolic dysfunction may be misinterpreted if transmitral flow alone is used for evaluation of diastolic function. Therefore, supplementing mitral inflow measurements with TDI is essential for the accurate assessment of diastolic function in small animals [2]. The peak E′ velocity is the best and most sensitive echocardiographic indicator of LV relaxation, and is reduced in the presence of diastolic dysfunction [5]. Changes in the E′/A′ ratio mirror the changes that occur in the transmitral E/A pattern during disease progression, with an increase in the A′ velocity early but a progressive decrease in A′ velocity as diastolic dysfunction worsens and atrial function decreases

[5,9]. In addition, the E/E′ ratio allows for the noninvasive estimation of LV end diastolic pressure (LVEDP) in rodents, even in the setting of fused inflow signals; the higher the E/E′ ratio, the higher the LVEDP [17].

Myocardial performance index (MPI). The MPI, also known as the Tei index, is a load-independent indicator of both systolic and diastolic cardiac function, and is described in detail in Chapter 32. Although typically calculated from PW Doppler signals, a major limitation of the PW Doppler Tei index is that, in most cases, all components of the MPI (i.e. ejection time, IVRT, and IVCT) cannot be measured within the same cardiac cycle. Therefore, changes in heart rate during inflow and outflow recordings may reduce the accuracy of this method, particularly in rodents under anesthesia, which often causes significant heart rate variation. TDI allows the measurement of both relaxation and contraction velocities simultaneously, independent of heart rate [18]. Figure 33.2 demonstrates the TDI-based calculation of the MPI. As with the PW Doppler MPI, a higher TDI-based MPI indicates worse overall cardiac function.

Limitations

As with all echocardiographic modalities applied to rodent research, TDI is challenging due to the small size and rapid heart rate of these animals, and like other Doppler modalities is inhibited by angle dependence. However, the main weakness of TDI is the effect of translational motion or myocardial tethering on the velocity waveform. TDI measurements are one dimensional, and only capable of detecting the component of motion parallel to the ultrasound beam; however, tethering, torsion, or translational motion may move the myocardium out of the sampling field, resulting in velocity measurements that do not reflect the true motion pattern of the region of interest [8].

Speckle tracking echocardiography

Principles

The recent development of advanced echocardiographic imaging techniques based on tissue deformation, including strain and strain rate, has enhanced our ability to accurately quantify the

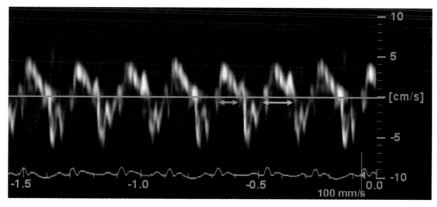

Figure 33.2 Calculation of the myocardial performance index using tissue Doppler imaging. The myocardial performance index is a marker of overall cardiac function. It is load-independent and accounts for both systolic and diastolic dysfunction. The MPI is calculated as the sum of isovolumic contraction time, ejection time, and isovolumic relaxation time (the end of the A′ wave to the beginning of the subsequent E′ wave; green arrow) divided by the ejection time (width to the S′ wave; orange arrow). A higher MPI indicates worse cardiac function.

complex events underlying myocardial contractility [8]. Strain is a measure of the deformation of a material, expressed as the fractional or percentage change from the object's original dimension; strain rate is the rate at which this deformation occurs [9]. When applied to the evaluation of cardiac function, strain is an index of the change in myocardial length during contraction and relaxation, and can have positive or negative values which reflect lengthening and shortening, respectively [5,10]. During each cardiac cycle, the ventricle undergoes a complex pattern of deformation in multiple planes in systole, followed by reverse changes during diastole [4]. Myocardial tissue deformation in these planes can be regionally and globally quantified using strain and strain rate.

Longitudinal strain represents deformation along the long axis of the ventricle and is typically measured from the apical four-chamber (A4C) view [8,9]. During systole, the myocardium contracts from the base to the apex of the heart, reflected as a shortening in the length of the wall; consequently, longitudinal strain decreases to a negative value during systole and moves back toward the positive direction during diastole [8]. Circumferential strain represents deformation along the curvature of the ventricle and can only be measured from the PSAX view [8,19]. During systole, the circumference of the ventricle decreases, reflected as a shortening of the wall; circumferential strain decreases to a negative

value during systole and moves back toward the positive direction with an increase in ventricular circumference during diastole [8]. Radial strain represents deformation towards the center of the ventricle and can be measured from multiple segments in both the PSAX and A4C views [8,19]. Unlike longitudinal and circumferential strain, which are represented by negative curves, radial strain is a positive curve reflecting increased myocardial thickness during systole and decreased thickness during diastole [8].

2D speckle tracking echocardiography (STE) is a non-Doppler based technique that enables the assessment of ventricular strain and SR by analyzing the movement of natural acoustic markers present in a standard 2D image [20]. STE, as the name implies, is based on tracking the motion of speckles, or small bright spots in the myocardium, as they move during the cardiac cycle [9]. These bright spots are the result of reflection, scattering, and interference patterns generated by small structures in the myocardium, which give rise to an irregular speckle pattern [5,19]. Tracking these unique speckle patterns provides local displacement information, from which strain and SR can be derived along the radial, circumferential, and longitudinal planes of the heart [10]. The STE image processing algorithm tracks user-defined regions of interest, which are comprised of stable blocks of speckle patterns. These blocks of speckles, or kernels, remain unchanged as they follow the myocardial wall, which allows them to be tracked from frame to frame [8,10]. The distance between the kernels in a defined myocardial segment is measured automatically and plotted over the cardiac cycle to generate strain and SR curves [21].

Instrument settings

• High frame rates result in high spatial and temporal resolution, which is necessary to generate high-quality tracking information.
  ◦ Frame rates should be >200 fps in mice, and have been reported as high as 375 fps; in rats, frame rates of 100–250 fps are acceptable [4,19,20,22].
• Gain and dynamic range should be adjusted to optimize contrast and endocardial definition and minimize artifacts; any artifact that resembles a speckle pattern will impact the quality of tracking, so care should be taken to avoid them [4,10].
• Apical foreshortening seriously affects the results of 2D STE; similarly, the PSAX images should be circular to ensure that deformation is assessed in the anatomically correct directions [10].

Basic protocol

Parasternal long axis views are preferred for performing longitudinal strain analysis in rodents because apical images are difficult to obtain in these animals. To analyze radial and circumferential strain, the PSAX view at the mid-papillary muscle level is used. STE analysis is performed offline using a speckle-tracking algorithm incorporated into a specialized workstation [7]. Two to three consecutive cardiac cycles are selected from the 2D loops based on frame rate, absence of artifacts, myocardial visualization, and contrast of endocardial and epicardial borders [4]. After selecting the appropriate cardiac cycles, the image is frozen at end-systole and the endocardium is traced, excluding areas of trabeculation and the papillary muscles [4]. After tracing of the endocardium is complete, the software automatically generates a corresponding epicardial tracing to define the region of interest. The width of this region may be adjusted manually to ensure that the entire myocardium is included and the outer tracing is just within the epicardial border (avoiding the pericardium) [22]. After the region of interest is defined, the software divides the wall into six

standard anatomic segments for regional speckle tracking analysis, automatically tracking and accepting segments of good quality and rejecting poorly tracked segments [22]. The quality of the speckle tracking should then be verified; if automated tracking does not fit with a visual inspection of wall motion, the region of interest should be manually adjusted until optimal tracking is achieved and at least five of the six segments track satisfactorily [20].

The speckle tracking algorithm then generates curvilinear strain graphs that provide a profile of strain with time (Figure 33.3). This quantitative data may also be presented as tables, segmental color wheels, or as a color display; however, the most effective way to quickly and accurately quantify strain and strain rate is by measurement of the computer-generated curves [8]. Peak strain and strain rate measurements are recorded from the six segments in each view, providing regional values; these values are then averaged across all six segments to generate global strain and SR measurements [4,10]. The total time for image acquisition and analysis should take less than 30 minutes for each animal.

Applications

Peak global and segmental systolic strain and SR values are commonly used to assess global myocardial contractility and regional function. The point at which peak strain and SR are measured is not constant across publications; the peak can be measured as the systolic maximum, the value at end-systole, or the peak overall value (regardless of timing) [10]. Any of these methods can be used to analyze strain and SR data, as long as the operator is consistent. Time to peak of the strain and SR curves is another tool used to evaluate myocardial contractility, as well as the synchrony of segmental contraction. During normal LV function, all segments contract at a similar velocity and peak at relatively similar times; in the setting of abnormal function, myocardial segments moving at different velocities are associated with a delayed time to peak [8].

STE-based calculations of strain and SR have proven to be highly reproducible and accurate quantitative parameters of global and regional contractile function that are more sensitive than

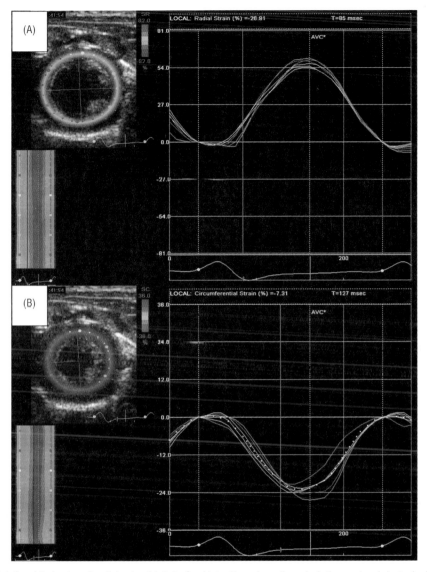

Figure 33.3 Left ventricular circumferential and radial strain. Speckle tracking echocardiography in the parasternal short axis view of a Wistar-Kyoto (WKY) rat demonstrating radial strain (A) and circumferential strain (B) curves.

conventional methods and less dependent on loading conditions [23]. An increase in stress on the heart wall, no matter the cause, results in a decrease in strain and SR; therefore, reductions in systolic strain and SR indicate the presence of myocardial dysfunction [7]. Strain and SR can be used to detect and evaluate a wide variety of myocardial disorders, including fibrosis, coronary artery disease, preclinical disease states, cardiomyopathies, myocardial toxicity, and transmurality, infarct size and tissue viability in ischemic models. Figure 33.4 displays a schematic of differences in regional strain curves as a result of an anterior myocardial infarction caused by ligation of the left anterior descending coronary artery. The use of STE in this setting has been shown to be an accurate marker of LV fibrosis [7]. Advancements in STE technology will likely broaden the availability and applicability of strain analysis in rodents to

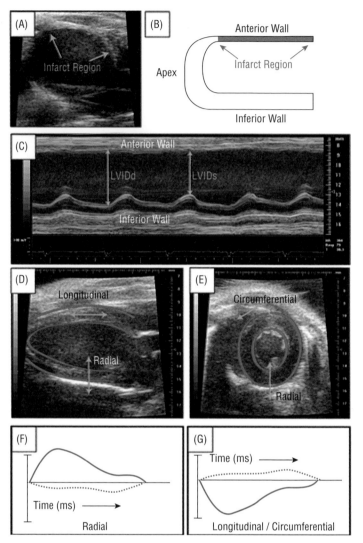

Figure 33.4 Schematic of left ventricular regional strain curves in the setting of an anterior myocardial infarction. In (A), left anterior descending coronary artery ligation results in anterior wall thinning, schematic seen in (B). Akinesis of the anterior wall visualized by M-mode imaging is seen in (C). Speckle tracking imaging schematic with parasternal long-axis (D) and short-axis (E) demonstrating strain in radial, longitudinal, and circumferential directions. Curvilinear strain data is depicted for radial (F) and longitudinal (G) planes (the solid red line corresponds to the inferior wall and the dotted red line corresponds to the infarcted anterior wall). Note the decreased absolute strain amplitude and dyskinetic motion of the anterior wall, as depicted by the strain curve. LVIDd, left ventricular internal dimension at end-diastole; LVIDs, left ventricular internal dimension at end-systole.

include other cardiac chambers and disease states in the future. For example, as reviewed in the previous chapter, echocardiographic imaging of the entire right ventricle (RV) is challenging in rodent models. However, it is relatively simple to identify the RV free wall on echocardiography even when the entire RV chamber is not well visualized. STE can be applied to the RV free wall (Figure 33.5) and can be a sensitive indicator of RV dysfunction.

Limitations

Although strain and strain rate technology are very appealing, they are still relatively new and evolving modalities and are associated with some important

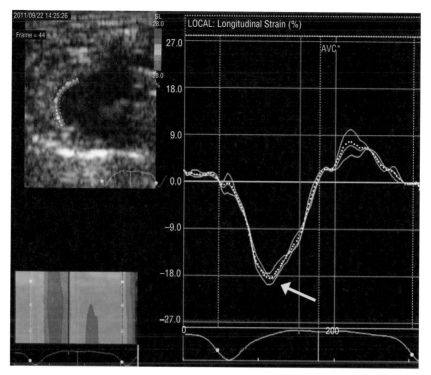

Figure 33.5 Right ventricular free wall strain. Speckle-tracking echocardiography analysis showing the longitudinal strain curves for three segments of the right ventricular free wall, along with average strain (dotted white line), in a control mouse. The arrow points to the peak longitudinal right ventricular free wall systolic strain.

limitations. The accuracy of strain and SR analysis is still dependent on image quality and frame rate; therefore, even though these techniques are semiautomated, they are still dependent on the skill of the operator to some degree [21]. Images must be of high resolution and high quality to result in optimal endocardial border tracking, which is significantly impaired by the presence of artifacts in the image [21]. This is particularly relevant to strain and SR analysis in rodents, whose thin ventricular walls and high heart rates often result in inaccurate tracking [16]. STE is also inhibited by the intrinsic nature of its 2D methodology. Foreshortened or misaligned views can limit the accuracy of STE; changes in the angle of incidence result in the capture of different fiber layers at different levels, leading to variability [4]. This problem is particularly significant in the PSAX views, where even small differences in angle can lead to highly variable strain measurements [4].

Three-dimensional imaging

Principles

3D echocardiographic technology complements and expands upon the diagnostic capabilities of 2D imaging. While M-mode and B-mode generate a grayscale display of anatomic data in one and two dimensions, respectively, 3D echocardiography facilitates the evaluation of the entire LV in three dimensions throughout the cardiac cycle, resulting in a more accurate and comprehensive appraisal of ventricular function and morphology [24]. 3D echo has evolved over the past two decades from an unwieldy technology with complicated acquisition and processing methods to a more streamlined clinical tool that can be used for rapid cardiovascular phenotyping [25,26]. As a result of these advancements in technology, 3D echo can now be used to assess ventricular anatomy and function in rodents, and has demonstrated excellent agreement with both MRI and histology for measurements of ventricular mass, volume, EF, and infarct size in normal and diseased rodent hearts [25].

Acquisition

A complete 3D study includes an assessment of ventricular function, valvular anatomy, and hemodynamic properties; alternatively, 3D echo can be performed on a more targeted basis to selectively complement 2D imaging, using a modified protocol [6]. There are two basic approaches for the acquisition and display of 3D datasets: reconstruction of a 3D image from 2D imaging in multiple planes, and real time volumetric imaging. No matter which approach is used, the technical factors associated with acquiring a high-quality 3D image are similar to those for 2D echocardiography; high temporal and spatial resolution, an experienced operator, and minimization of artifacts are the most important elements necessary for generating accurate and reproducible 3D images [24]. After the 3D dataset is acquired and volume rendered within the ultrasound system, a 3D volume is generated that can be rotated and viewed from any angle, permitting both external and internal views of the heart and providing optimal perspective for visualizing abnormalities [24]. This volume may then be sliced or cropped to assess the relationship, orientation, and motion pattern of anatomical structures and visualize blood flow from different perspectives [27].

3D reconstruction from 2D imaging

3D reconstruction of LV volumes and mass has been applied to quantify the cardiac phenotype in both normal and abnormal rodent models [25,28,29]. Through careful tracking of the transducer position, multiple 2D images can be recorded, aligned, and reconstructed offline into a 3D data set to accurately quantify ventricular mass and volume and visualize intracardiac structures from any point of view [6]. Serial images are acquired from multiple transducer positions combined with a locator system that records the position and orientation of each image; with the aid of ECG and respiratory gating, these images are then reconstructed offline into a 3D image that is near real-time and spatially precise [8]. Because other methods of 3D data acquisition

require specialized transducers that have not been miniaturized for use in rodents, this is the only method that has been broadly applied in rodent imaging.

Two main approaches have been reported in the literature using two different external locator systems for the reconstruction of 3D images in rodents. Using the method described by Scherrer-Crosbie *et al.*, preliminary 2D scanning is performed to locate the long axis of the LV, and a transparent ruler is taped to the rodent chest parallel to this axis [29]. Consecutive PSAX views are then obtained at 1-mm intervals, using the ruler for reference, and ventricular mass and volumes are reconstructed offline. The method used by Dawson *et al.* requires the construction of an adjustable platform with micrometer position capabilities and a holder device to secure the probe [25]. Consecutive PSAX views are obtained by moving the platform in 500-micrometer increments along the long axis of the heart, while the transducer remains stationary to reduce errors caused by angulation [30]. These clips are then reassembled offline into a 3D matrix, using the measured platform locations to position each image slice in the 3D dataset [25].

No matter which method of 3D reconstruction is applied, the quality of the dataset depends on several factors, including the quality and number of 2D images used for reconstruction, the ability to limit motion artifact, and adequate ECG and respiratory gating [6]. The greater the number of images obtained, the better the quality of the 3D reconstruction; however, this also lengthens scanning time and increases the risk of motion artifact [6]. The appropriate number of images for adequate reconstruction depends on the structure being examined; four to six is usually appropriate for the LV, with more images necessary to visualize complex structures such as valves [6]. Volume and mass quantifications from 3D reconstructions has proven to be more accurate and reproducible than those derived from 2D or M-mode images; data from multiple locations produces a more comprehensive dataset than from a single transducer location alone [9]. However, this method requires extensive offline data processing and is highly subject to artifacts [27]. To address these concerns, volumetric real-time data acquisition was developed.

Volumetric 3D imaging

In the early 1990s, specialized transducers capable of acquiring real-time volumetric datasets at high frame rates were developed [6]. These complex matrix array transducers typically contain thousands of elements, which can be steered in multiple directions to allow the acquisition and display of real-time 3D volume datasets from a fixed transducer position [24]. Rapid image processing then generates images that can be viewed in real time in any orientation on the screen [9]. Due to these advancements in transducer technology and improvements in analysis software, real-time 3D echo is now widely used in clinical practice; however, this technology has not yet been extended to small animals due to limitations in transducer footprint size, frame rate, and image resolution. The extremely rapid rodent heart rate makes it unlikely that real-time 3D echo will be applied to rodent studies in the near future [25].

Applications

As 3D technology has improved, its clinical applications have continually expanded; however, in rats and mice this technique is still largely limited to quantitative measurements of chamber mass and volume from reconstructed images. Regardless of which acquisition or analysis approach is used, 3D measurements of mass, volume, and EF are significantly more accurate and reproducible than 2D measurements [30]. To generate these measurements, the endocardial and epicardial borders are traced manually or using a semiautomated algorithm, and mass and volume are calculated using the summation of disks or other methods [30]. These volumes can also be segmented to analyze regional myocardial function [6]. The LV cavity is automatically divided into 16 segments, and the volume of each segment is calculated to generate a volume versus time curve of each segment throughout the cardiac cycle [27]. Because segmental volume changes are assumed to reflect segmental wall function, delayed or impaired changes in volume are recognized as indicators of abnormal function [27].

Limitations

The complex process behind acquiring and generating volumetric 3D datasets makes this technology vulnerable to several limiting factors. Regular heart rate and rhythm are required to ensure synchronization of the image clips across the entire 3D volume. In addition, the quality of 3D images is still inferior compared with 2D images due to reductions in resolution, and the process of offline data analysis is time-consuming [30]. Although 3D evaluation of the rodent heart is possible, these techniques are technically challenging in small animal models and are limited by relatively low frame rates [31]. At this time, none of the cutting-edge real-time 3D acquisition systems have the spatial or temporal resolution necessary to be adapted in rats and mice; only the more dated 2D reconstruction methods have been reported in the literature for application of 3D analysis in rodents.

References

1 Shimizu M, Konstantinov IE, Suess AM, Cheung M, McCrindle BW, Vogel M, et al. Noninvasive analysis of myocardial function using high-resolution Doppler tissue echocardiography in rats. *J Am Soc Echocardiogr* 2005; **18**: 461–467.

2 Sebag IA, Handschumacher MD, Ichinose F, Morgan JG, Hataishi R, Rodrigues AC, et al. Quantitative assessment of regional myocardial function in mice by tissue Doppler imaging: comparison with hemodynamics and sonomicrometry. *Circulation* 2005; **111**: 2611–2616.

3 Neilan TG, Jassal DS, Perez-Sanz TM, Raher MJ, Pradhan AD, Buys ES, et al. Tissue Doppler imaging predicts left ventricular dysfunction and mortality in a murine model of cardiac injury. *Eur Heart J* 2006; **27**: 1868–1875.

4 Bauer M, Cheng S, Jain M, Ngoy S, Theodoropoulos C, Trujillo A, et al. Echocardiographic speckle-tracking based strain imaging for rapid cardiovascular phenotyping in mice. *Circ Res* 2011; **108**: 908–916.

5 Oh JK, Seward JB, Tajik AJ. *The Echo Manual*, 3rd edn. Philadelphia: Lippincott Williams and Wilkins, 2007.

6 Hung J, Lang R, Flachskampf F, Shernan SK, McCulloch ML, Adams DB, et al. 3D echocardiography: a review of the current status and future directions. *J Am Soc Echocardiogr* 2007; **20**: 213–233.

7 Popovic ZB, Benejam C, Bian J, Mal N, Drinko J, Lee K, et al. Speckle-tracking echocardiography correctly identifies segmental left ventricular dysfunction induced by scarring in a rat model of myocardial infarction. *Am J Physiol Heart Circ Physiol* 2007; **292**: H2809–2816.

8 Ram R, Mickelsen DM, Theodoropoulos C, Blaxall BC. New approaches in small animal echocardiography: imaging the sounds of silence. *Am J Physiol Heart Circ Physiol* 2011; **301**: H1765–1780.

9 Otto CM. *Textbook of Clinical Echocardiography*, 4th edn. Philadelphia: Saunders/Elsevier, 2009.

10 Mor-Avi V, Lang RM, Badano LP, Belohlavek M, Cardim NM, Derumeaux G, *et al.* Current and evolving echocardiographic techniques for the quantitative evaluation of cardiac mechanics: ASE/EAE consensus statement on methodology and indications endorsed by the Japanese Society of Echocardiography. *J Am Soc Echocardiogr* 2011; **24**: 277–313.

11 Liu J, Rigel DF. Echocardiographic examination in rats and mice. *Methods Mol Biol* 2009; **573**: 139–155.

12 Weytjens C, Franken PR, D'Hooge J, Droogmans S, Cosyns B, Lahoutte T, *et al.* Doppler myocardial imaging in the diagnosis of early systolic left ventricular dysfunction in diabetic rats. *Eur J Echocardiogr* 2008; **9**: 326–333.

13 Syed F, Diwan A, Hahn HS. Murine echocardiography: a practical approach for phenotyping genetically manipulated and surgically modeled mice. *J Am Soc Echocardiogr* 2005; **18**: 982–990.

14 Schaefer A, Klein G, Brand B, Lippolt P, Drexler H, Meyer GP, *et al.* Evaluation of left ventricular diastolic function by pulsed Doppler tissue imaging in mice. *J Am Soc Echocardiogr* 2003; **16**: 1144–1149.

15 Matoba S, Hwang PM, Nguyen T, Shizukuda Y. Evaluation of pulsed Doppler tissue velocity imaging for assessing systolic function of murine global heart failure. *J Am Soc Echocardiogr* 2005; **18**: 148–154.

16 Gao S, Ho D, Vatner DE, Vatner SF. Echocardiography in mice. *Curr Protoc Mouse Biol* 2011; **1**: 71–83.

17 Slama M, Ahn J, Peltier M, Maizel J, Chemla D, Varagic J, *et al.* Validation of echocardiographic and Doppler indexes of left ventricular relaxation in adult hypertensive and normotensive rats. *Am J Physiol Heart Circ Physiol* 2005; **289**: H1131–1136.

18 Schaefer A, Meyer GP, Hilfiker-Kleiner D, Brand B, Drexler H, Klein G, *et al.* Evaluation of Tissue Doppler Tei index for global left ventricular function in mice after myocardial infarction: comparison with Pulsed Doppler Tei index. *Eur J Echocardiogr* 2005; **6**: 367–375.

19 Migrino RQ, Zhu X, Pajewski N, Brahmbhatt T, Hoffmann R, Zhao M, *et al.* Assessment of segmental myocardial viability using regional 2-dimensional strain echocardiography. *J Am Soc Echocardiogr* 2007; **20**: 342–351.

20 Peng Y, Popovic ZB, Sopko N, Drinko J, Zhang Z, Thomas JD, *et al.* Speckle tracking echocardiography in the assessment of mouse models of cardiac dysfunction. *Am J Physiol Heart Circ Physiol* 2009; **297**: H811–820.

21 Geyer H, Caracciolo G, Abe H, Wilansky S, Carerj S, Gentile F, *et al.* Assessment of myocardial mechanics using speckle tracking echocardiography: fundamentals and clinical applications. *J Am Soc Echocardiog* 2010; **23**: 351–369.

22 Treguer F, Donal E, Tamareille S, Ghaboura N, Derumeaux G, Furber A, *et al.* Speckle tracking imaging improves in vivo assessment of EPO-induced myocardial salvage early after ischemia-reperfusion in rats. *Am J Physiol Heart Circ Physiol* 2010; **298**: H1679–1686.

23 Scherrer-Crosbie M, Thibault HB. Echocardiography in translational research: of mice and men. *J Am Soc Echocardiogr* 2008; **21**: 1083–1092.

24 van der Heide JA, Kleijn SA, Aly MF, Slikkerveer J, Kamp O. Three-dimensional echocardiography for left ventricular quantification: fundamental validation and clinical applications. *Neth Heart J* 2011; **19**: 423–431.

25 Dawson D, Lygate CA, Saunders J, Schneider JE, Ye X, Hulbert K, *et al.* Quantitative 3-dimensional echocardiography for accurate and rapid cardiac phenotype characterization in mice. *Circulation* 2004; **110**: 1632–1637.

26 Abraham T. *Case Based Echocardiography Fundamentals And Clinical Practice*. London: Springer-Verlag, 2011.

27 Roelandt J. Three-dimensional echocardiography. In: Nihoyannopoulos P, Kisslo J, eds. *Echocardiography*. London: Springer, 2009, pp. 603–618.

28 Coatney RW. Ultrasound imaging: principles and applications in rodent research. *ILAR J* 2001; **42**: 233–247.

29 Scherrer-Crosbie M, Steudel W, Hunziker PR, Liel-Cohen N, Ullrich R, Zapol WM, *et al.* Three-dimensional echocardiographic assessment of left ventricular wall motion abnormalities in mouse myocardial infarction. *J Am Soc Echocardiogr* 1999; **12**: 834–840.

30 Lang RM, Bierig M, Devereux RB, Flachskampf FA, Foster E, Pellikka PA, *et al.* Recommendations for chamber quantification: a report from the American Society of Echocardiography's Guidelines and Standards Committee and the Chamber Quantification Writing Group, developed in conjunction with the European Association of Echocardiography, a branch of the European Society of Cardiology. *J Am Soc Echocardiogr* 2005; **18**: 1440–1463.

31 Collins KA, Korcarz CE, Lang RM. Use of echocardiography for the phenotypic assessment of genetically altered mice. *Physiol Genomics* 2003; **13**: 227–239.

In vivo tomographic cardiac imaging: positron emission tomography and magnetic resonance imaging

Bruno C. Huber, Patricia K. Nguyen, and Joseph C. Wu

Stanford University School of Medicine, Stanford, CA, USA

Introduction

Small animal models, especially genetically engineered mice, are increasingly recognized as useful tools in cardiovascular research. A major limitation is the need to sacrifice the animals to perform tissue or molecular analysis, which precludes *in vivo* observation of the processes (natural or perturbed) under study. *In vivo* visualization of biological processes is especially critical in the emerging field of stem cell therapy, where extensive discussions and controversies with regard to the basic mechanisms of cell therapy still predominate [1]. Functional, molecular, and morphologic quantitative imaging techniques are important tools for providing serial data about biochemical, genetic, and pharmacological processes *in vivo*. Platforms for small animal imaging include ultrasound, single-photon emission computed tomography (SPECT), positron emission tomography (PET), computed tomography (CT), magnetic resonance imaging (MRI), and optical techniques such as bioluminescence imaging (BLI) and catheter-based techniques [2,3].

MRI is generally accepted as the "gold standard" method for evaluating cardiac structure because it provides unrivalled images of heart anatomy *in vivo*, making it possible to conduct serial noninvasive assessments [4]. In addition to its classical functions such as assessing LV size, mass, and ejection fraction, MRI can accurately measure the myocardial infarct size by late gadolinium enhancement [5]. PET, on the other hand, has long been considered the "gold standard" for the assessment of myocardial viability and has emerged as a highly sensitive tool for investigating the *in vivo* biodistribution of transplanted cells for myocardial regeneration [6]. In this chapter, we will discuss the specific protocols for assessing myocardial structure/function and viability by MRI and PET, respectively, as well as tracking stem cell fate by other modalities.

Protocols

Here we describe standard protocols for using MRI to assess LV structure and function as well as protocols for using PET to image cardiac viability and track transplanted stem cells in mice.

Anesthesia of animals

(See Chapter 31 for additional information). We generally use the breathable halogenated ether

Manual of Research Techniques in Cardiovascular Medicine, First Edition. Edited by Hossein Ardehali, Roberto Bolli, and Douglas W. Losordo.

isoflurane (1.5–2%) with oxygen (2 mL/min) to anesthetize animals for MRI and PET experiments. Isoflurane is the most commonly used anesthetic because the anesthesia level is easily controlled and the depression of cardiac function is minimal. The quantity of isoflurane in the mixture is adjusted based on the vital signs of the animal during the scan. Anesthesia of animals can be achieved by other anesthetics such as ketamine and xylazine as well [7]; however, these agents cannot be as easily manipulated.

MRI

General

Our mouse cardiac imaging experiments are performed by a 7 Tesla animal scanner (Magnex/Varian, Palo Alto, CA; Figure 34.1A) using a 20-mm diameter coil for both transmitting and receiving the signal. MRI uses a very strong magnetic field that requires extreme caution. The high magnetic field is always on, even when the MR scanner is not being used. Any metallic object that comes into contact with such a high magnetic field will be strongly and rapidly attracted by the magnet. Therefore, researchers conducting MRI studies should be careful to remove any metallic objects from their clothing and the animals before entering the proximity of the instrument, and should ensure the surrounding environment is free from such objects.

Animal preparation

1. Place the mouse in the knock-down chamber and adjust the oxygen flow meter to 2 L/min. Then adjust the isoflurane vaporizer to 2.5% for about 2–3 minutes.

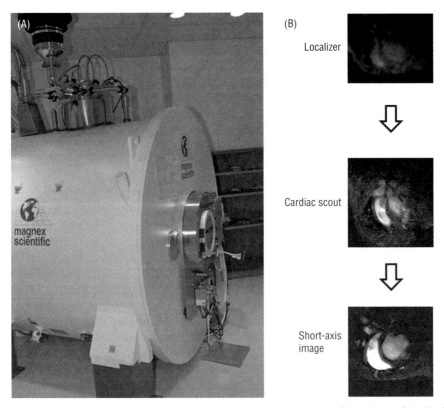

Figure 34.1 Evaluation of heart function by cardiac MRI. (A) 7 Tesla horizontal-bore animal scanner (Magnex/Varian, Palo Alto, CA) used for mouse cardiac imaging. (B) Protocol for obtaining short-axis cardiac images of mouse hearts. Initially, low-resolution localizer images are obtained to locate the heart. These images are used to get four-chamber and two-chamber images of the heart. Standard orientations consisting of two and four chamber long-axis and short-axis views are acquired.

2. After the animal is sedated, place it in an animal holder with its nose inserted into a nose cone to maintain sedation throughout the study. Animal holders are used to prevent potential motion. There are several types of commercial holders, but a custom-designed holder can be fabricated as well to accommodate any special requirements of an experimental setup. During the imaging period, reduce the isoflurane vaporizer to 1.2–1.5%. The expired gas coming from the mouse nose cone is collected by a pump and removed into an in-house vacuum.

3. A small animal monitoring system (Small Animals Instruments, Stony Brook, NY) is used to monitor the physiological parameters (heart rate, respiration, and body temperature) of the animal and to provide cardiac gating. The ECG leads are secured at the thorax of the animal. A pneumatic pillow is attached to the abdomen of the animal to monitor respiration. The core body temperature of the animal is monitored with a probe underneath the animal and maintained at $37 \pm 0.5°C$ using a warm air blower. To avoid motion due to the air flow, tape the wires of the ECG electrodes to the animal bed. Place the animal in the animal bed in the prone position and restrain it with medical tapes. Avoid binding too tightly as this can potentially restrict respiration.

4. Keep the eyes of the animal moist using a sterile eye lubricating ointment.

5. After securing on the bed, place the coil in the magnet to keep the heart of the animal at the isocenter of the magnet.

MRI experiment

1. Acquire scout images along three orthogonal orientations to create axial, coronal, and sagittal images, using standard nongated fast spin echo, gradient recalled echo (GRE) sequence. Suggested parameters for the GRE sequence include: TR (repetition time) = 2.6 ms, TE (echo time) = 2.9 ms, number of excitations (NEX) = 1, field of view (FOV) = 6 mm, matrix = 256 × 128, flip angle (FA) = 30°, slice thickness 2.0 mm, and spacing 1 mm.

2. Scout images allow identification of the heart for planning subsequent acquisitions (Figure 34.1B).

3. The next localization image acquired should depict the long axis of the heart, showing the mitral valve, tricuspid valve, and the apex to ensure the subsequent short-axis prescription will be acquired along the long axis of the heart. This is typically achieved by making a prescription on the axial scout images that bisects the mid right and left ventricles. Review of the accuracy of the prescription can be verified on the coronal and sagittal scout images. It may be necessary to make additional localization acquisitions to achieve the adequate four chambers based on the positioning of the mouse heart. These images are acquired using a cardiac gated, fast GRE sequence with the same parameters as for the scout images.

4. After acquiring an adequate four-chamber image, a stack of sequential short-axis slices spaced 1 mm apart are prescribed from the cardiac apex to the base using a cardiac gated fast spoiled GRE (FSPGR) sequence. For each sequence, 20 cine frames encompassing one cardiac cycle are obtained with the following sequence parameters: TR = 150 ms, TE = 1 ms, NEX = 2, FOV = 5.5 mm, matrix = 256 × 256, flip angle (FA) = 20°, slice thickness 1.0 mm, and spacing 0 mm.

5. After imaging, the animals will be taken out of the scanner and monitored to assure full recovery before they are returned to the cage. Animals should be monitored throughout the recovery process. Because anesthetized mice lose heat rapidly, we keep the animals warm by providing a heat source until they are recovered from anesthesia.

Image processing

• Transfer selected MR imaging data to a postprocessing computer. For data analysis, the MR images should be in a DICOM format for analysis with a contouring program, such as Osirix Version 3.81 or Mass software.

• The image analysis includes tracing the endocardial borders and identifying the frames depicting the end-diastolic and end-systolic phases. LV end-systolic volume (LVESV), LV end-diastolic volume (LVEDV), LV mass, and LV ejection fraction (LVEF) can be computed from the traced borders [8].

Additional MRI techniques

In addition to the described functional imaging of the mouse heart, various MRI methods originally developed for imaging in humans have been adapted for mice [9]. For studying myocardial scar, delayed contrast-enhanced MRI of the heart and T1 mapping techniques have been used to detect overt and patchy scar, respectively. For acquisition of delayed enhancement images, short-axis ECG gated inversion recovery gradient-echo MR images are acquired from base to apex 20 to 30 minutes after intraperitoneal injection of Gd-DTPA. Delayed enhancement images, however, have limited spatial resolution, decreasing its sensitivity to detect patchy fibrosis. T1 mapping techniques, in contrast, can detect subtle differences in regional tissue characteristics by calculating the relaxation time within an image pixel. High-resolution T1 mapping is performed before and 20 to 30 minutes after contrast administration. The Look-Locker and modified Look-Locker sequences (MOLLI) are used to measure left ventricular values for T1 mapping. The MOLLI sequence can determine the T1 at the same phase of the cardiac cycle, enabling more accurate T1 measurement with less heart rate dependence. These methods will be particularly suited for detection of changes in myocardial scar and fibrosis in preclinical trials evaluating potential new therapy [10].

PET

General

Radioisotopes should be used only by persons trained in radiation protection. Time, distance, appropriate shielding, and knowledge of the radioactive source are the four elements of practical radiation protection that always must be correctly observed in order to minimize the radiation dose received. Radioactive waste disposal must be handled in accordance with national regulations. Radio-isotopes must be handled in a designated area. We employ PET for assessing cardiac viability using F-18 fluorodeoxyglucose ([^{18}F]-FDG) radiotracer [11]. We also employ PET for tracking of stem cells transduced with the herpes simplex virus thymidine kinase (HSVtk) reporter gene using F-18 9-(4-fluoro-3-hydroxymethylbutyl) guanine ([^{18}F]-FHBG) reporter probe [12]. Our mouse PET imaging experiments are performed using a Siemens/Concorde Microsystems MicroPET rodent R4 scanner (Figure 34.2A).

Animal and tracer preparation

1. Prepare or order a sufficient amount of [^{18}F]-FDG or [^{18}F]-FHBG to meet imaging needs. If your institution does not have a cyclotron facility to produce [^{18}F]-FDG or [^{18}F]-FHBG, order this radiotracer from an established cyclotron facility.

2. Place a mouse in the knock down chamber and adjust the oxygen flow meter to 2 L/min. Then adjust the isoflurane vaporizer to 2.5% for about 2–3 minutes.

3. Draw approximately 100–150 mCi [^{18}F]-FDG or [^{18}F]-FHBG per animal into a 28.5-gauge insulin syringe. Record the exact activity within the syringe at the time of injection using a dose calibrator.

4. After knocking down the animal, administer the entire syringe contents of the tracer into the animal via tail vein injection and use the dose calibrator after administration to record the remaining activity within the syringe.

5. Bring the animal back to a heated chamber and allow time for it to recover. Wait 55–60 minutes for the PET tracer to biodistribute systemically before proceeding to imaging.

6. Prior to imaging, knock down the animal again using 2% isoflurane.

7. Place the animal on the bed of the PET scanner and secure the animal by taping.

Small animal PET experiment

• For our [^{18}F]-FDG myocardial viability imaging or [^{18}F]-FHBG reporter probe imaging, we generally use a 5 to 10-minutes static PET protocol to acquire images in the horizontal, coronal, and sagittal views.

• Figure 34.2 demonstrates the combination of [^{18}F]-FHBG reporter probe imaging (top row) and [^{18}F]-FDG myocardial viability imaging (middle row) in rats 2 weeks after transplantation of embryonic stem cells (ES) cells expressing the HSVtk reporter gene. The fusion of [^{18}F]-FHBG and [^{18}F]-FDG images (bottom row) shows the exact anatomic location of transplanted ES cells (arrow) at the anterolateral wall of the rat heart in horizontal, coronal, and sagittal views.

Image processing

• After data acquisition, we reconstruct the images using filtered back projection algorithms with a software program provided by the small animal PET manufacturer such as ASI PRO.

• A commercially available software package, such as ASI PRO or A Medical Imaging Data Examiner (AMIDE, SourceForge, Inc., Mountain

(A)

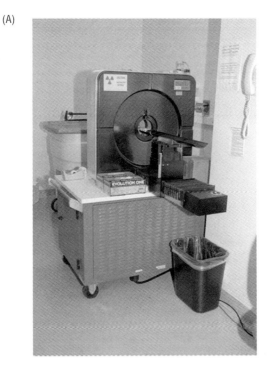

(B)

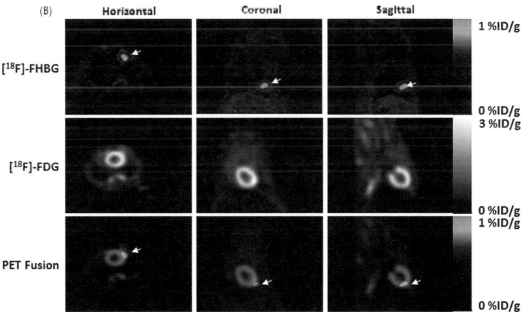

Figure 34.2 Small animal PET imaging for the assessment of viability and defining the tomographic location of transplanted ES cells in the myocardium. (A) The Siemens R4 microPET scanner is seen in the figure. (B) Combination of [^{18}F]-FHBG reporter probe imaging (top row) and [^{18}F]-FDG myocardial viability imaging (middle row) in a rat 2 weeks after cell transplantation defining the tomographic location of transplanted ES cells in the myocardium. The fusion of [^{18}F]-FHBG and [^{18}F]-FDG images (bottom row) shows the exact anatomic location of transplanted ES-TF cells (arrow) at the anterolateral wall in horizontal, coronal, and sagittal views. Notice that for the [^{18}F]-FHBG image, there is residual activity in the liver and bone due to hepatic clearance of tracer and free fluoride in systemic circulation. (Source: (B) Cao F 2006 [12]. Reproduced with permission from Wolters Kluwer Health).

View, California) [13], is used, to analyze the reconstructed images. Three-dimensional regions of interest (ROIs) encompassing the heart or the areas of uptake are drawn. For each ROI, counts/mL/min are then converted to counts/g/min and divided by the injected dose to obtain the image ROI derived [^{18}F]-FDG or [^{18}F]-FHBG percentage injected dose per gram of heart (% ID/g), as described previously [14].

Alternative approaches

Transthoracic echocardiography (Chapters 31–33) offers a low-cost method for the noninvasive evaluation of cardiac function in rodents and can be used to provide dimensional measurements of the mouse heart and to quantify cardiac systolic and diastolic performance [15]. Acquiring adequate echocardiographic planes, however, can be challenging due to the small size of the mouse heart. Echocardiography is also operator dependent and depends upon the quality of the acoustic window. Thus, investigators using echocardiography often estimate left ventricular function by calculating fractional shortening, which is based on a single short-axis view of the left ventricle. MRI, on the other hand, has superior image quality due to high spatial resolution and calculates ejection fraction based on a stack of short-axis views, which provides a more accurate evaluation of global LV systolic function.

Compared to physical labels used in MR, or to short-lived PET radionuclide tracers, biolumi-nescence imaging (BLI) is a highly sensitive method for tracking cell survival of transplanted stem cells [16]. In general, BLI requires incorporation of a reporter gene such as firefly luciferase (from *Photinuspyralis*), and photons are emitted when the optical probe, D-luciferin, administered intra-peritoneally or intravenously, is oxidized by the firefly luciferase enzyme, which is encoded by the *Fluc* gene [16]. The amount of background autofluorescence *in vivo* is low, so images are highly sensitive. Hence, BLI gives researchers an important tool to image transplanted cells *in vivo*, providing a greater understanding of their survival, migration, immunogenicity, and potential tumorigenicity in a living animal [12, 17]. Compared to other modalities such as PET-reporter gene imaging, BLI has limited

spatial resolution and reduced tissue penetration due to the relatively weak energy of emitted photons. For these reasons, it has not yet been applied in large animals and humans. However, bioluminescence has the advantages of being low-cost, high-throughput, and noninvasive, making it highly desirable for *in vivo* stem cell tracking in small animals [16].

Weaknesses and strength of the methods

Great advances in instrumentation and imaging technology have been made recently that are critical for the advancement and growth of cardiovascular imaging. Both PET and MRI can provide anatomic and functional assessment as well as visualization of biological processes at the cellular and molecular level. The relative strengths and weaknesses of PET, MRI, and BLI relative to their potential for cardiovascular and molecular imaging are summarized in Table 34.1. Selecting the most effective imaging technique requires a case-by-case determination of whether the imaging system can meet the specific requirements for spatial and temporal resolution, sensitivity, and penetration depth for visualization of the imaging target. In general, if assessment of myocardial structure and/or global systolic function is more important, the high spatial resolution of MRI may be preferred; however, viability and cell number can be more accurately tracked with direct radionuclide labeling using PET [1,3].

Conclusion

Recently, there have been rapid advances in small animal cardiovascular imaging. Both PET and MRI can provide anatomic and functional assessment as well as visualization of biological processes at the cellular and molecular level. In general, for assessment of myocardial function, the high spatial resolution of MRI is preferred, whereas PET may be superior in the evaluation of cardiac viability and cell tracking.

Acknowledgements

This work was supported by NIH R01EB009689, R01HL093172, CIRM DR2-05394 and TR3-05556 (JCW), ACCF/GE Healthcare Career Development Award in Cardiovascular Imaging (PKN), and

Table 34.1 Comparison of MRI, PET, and BLI: features, advantages and disadvantages of each modality

Imaging modality	Sensitivity, mol/L	Imaging time	Applications	Advantages	Disadvantages
MRI	10^3–10^5	Minutes to hours	Cardiac function, perfusion, infarct size, viability, *in vivo* cell tracking	Simultaneous molecular and anatomical data, high spatial resolution	Low sensitivity, low temporal resolution, inability to analyze diastolic function, long scaning or postprocessing time
PET	10^{11}–10^{12}	Minutes	Viability, *in vivo* cell tracking, detection of apoptosis, angiogenesis, remodeling, and regeneration, perfusion, infarct size	High sensitivity, quantitative	Radiation, relatively low spatial resolution, cyclotron or generator needed
BLI	10^{15}–10^{17}	Minutes	*In vivo* cell tracking	High sensitivity, high throughput, easy to operate, low cost	Low spatial resolution, not translational

German Research Foundation Grant DFG-Hu-1857/1-1 (BCH).

References

1 Nguyen PK, Lan F, Wang Y, Wu JC. Imaging: Guiding the clinical translation of cardiac stem cell therapy. *Circ Res* 2011; **109**: 962–979.

2 Buxton DB, Antman M, Danthi N, Dilsizian V, Fayad ZA, Garcia MJ, *et al.* Report of the national heart, lung, and blood institute working group on the translation of cardiovascular molecular imaging. *Circulation* 2011; **123**: 2157–2163.

3 Chen IY, Wu JC. Cardiovascular molecular imaging: Focus on clinical translation. *Circulation* 2011; **123**: 425–443.

4 Nahrendorf M, Hiller KH, Hu K, Ertl G, Haase A, Bauer WR, *et al.* Cardiac magnetic resonance imaging in small animal models of human heart failure. *Med Image Anal* 2003; **7**: 369–375.

5 Yang Z, Berr SS, Gilson WD, Toufektsian MC, French BA. Simultaneous evaluation of infarct size and cardiac function in intact mice by contrast-enhanced cardiac magnetic resonance imaging reveals contractile dysfunction in noninfarcted regions early after myocardial infarction. *Circulation* 2004; **109**: 1161–1167.

6 Beeres SL, Bengel FM, Bartunek J, Atsma DE, Hill JM, Vanderheyden M, *et al.* Role of imaging in cardiac stem cell therapy. *J Am Coll Cardiol* 2007; **49**: 1137–1148.

7 Hildebrandt IJ, Su H, Weber WA. Anesthesia and other considerations for in vivo imaging of small animals. *ILAR J* 2008; **49**: 17–26.

8 Huang M, Nguyen P, Jia F, Hu S, Gong Y, de Almeida PE, *et al.* Double knockdown of prolyl hydroxylase and factor-inhibiting hypoxia-inducible factor with nonviral minicircle gene therapy enhances stem cell mobilization and angiogenesis after myocardial infarction. *Circulation* 2011; **124**: S46–54.

9 Epstein FH. Mr in mouse models of cardiac disease. *NMR Biomed* 2007; **20**: 238–255.

10 Nacif MS, Turkbey EB, Gai N, Nazarian S, van der Geest RJ, Noureldin RA, *et al.* Myocardial t1 mapping with mri: Comparison of look-locker and molli sequences. *J Magn Reson Imaging* 2011; **34**: 1367–1373.

11 Li Z, Lee A, Huang M, Chun H, Chung J, Chu P, *et al.* Imaging survival and function of transplanted cardiac resident stem cells. *J Am Coll Cardiol* 2009; **53**: 1229–1240.

12 Cao F, Lin S, Xie X, Ray P, Patel M, Zhang X, *et al.* In vivo visualization of embryonic stem cell survival, proliferation, and migration after cardiac delivery. *Circulation* 2006; **113**: 1005–1014.

13 Loening AM, Gambhir SS. Amide: A free software tool for multimodality medical image analysis. *Mol Imaging* 2003; **2**: 131–137.

14 Toyama H, Ichise M, Liow JS, Vines DC, Seneca NM, Modell KJ, *et al.* Evaluation of anesthesia effects on [18F] FDG uptake in mouse brain and heart using small animal pet. *Nucl Med Biol* 2004; **31**: 251–256.

15 Scherrer-Crosbie M, Kurtz B. Ventricular remodeling and function: Insights using murine echocardiography. *J Mol Cell Cardiol* 2010; **48**: 512–517.

16 de Almeida PE, van Rappard JR, Wu JC. In vivo bioluminescence for tracking cell fate and function. *Am J Physiol Heart Circ Physiol* 2011; **301**: H663–671.

17 Sheikh AY, Huber BC, Narsinh KH, Spin JM, van der Bogt K, de Almeida PE, *et al.* In vivo functional and transcriptional profiling of bone marrow stem cells after transplantation into ischemic myocardium. *Arterioscler Thromb Vasc Biol* 2012; **32**: 92–102.

In vivo hemodynamics

Alexander R. Mackie[1], Kyle K. Henderson[2], Sol Misener[1] and Hossein Ardehali[1]

[1] Northwestern University Feinberg School of Medicine, Chicago, IL, USA
[2] Midwestern University, IL, USA

Introduction

The relationship between ventricular blood volume and the ventricular pressures that occurs over the cardiac cycle is conventionally known as the pressure–volume relationship. In-depth analysis of these parameters is frequently used in experimental settings to understand or investigate several fluctuating and instantaneous parameters of cardiac function. Naturally, understanding and evaluating the pressure–volume relationship requires the real-time, concurrent acquisition of both the pressure and volume variables in a live animal model. Additionally, the procedure requires the use of a specialized instrument known as a cardiac pressure–volume catheter along with a computer running dedicated software allowing for rapid data acquisition and analysis.

Other approaches, including the use of ultrasonic crystals, magnetic resonance imaging (MRI), and echocardiography, have been used to measure instantaneous volumes with varying degrees of success. These methods are often used to calculate load-dependent markers of systolic function such as ejection fraction, fractional shortening, and strain. While these can be valuable cardiac indices for measurement in laboratory animals, intrinsic contractility is a load-independent property of the ventricle. Pressure–volume analysis was developed as a method for measurement of cardiac chamber function in a load-independent fashion, and is currently the gold standard for the measurement of cardiac contractility. Pressure–volume catheter technology emerged several years ago [1,2] as a fairly reliable method to generate real-time ventricular PV loops in the intact heart. Additionally, recent advancements in the field, including the use of new "admittance" catheter technology in addition to the well-established "conductance" technology, provides several options for researchers who want to effectively evaluate the pressure–volume relationship in large mammals [3] and small rodents [4–9]. Considering the invasive nature of proper intracardiac catheter placement, the required occlusion of the carotid artery along with the potential damage to the aortic valve and the abdominal surgery required for reducing preload, catheter-based pressure–volume analysis in rodents is typically a terminal procedure.

Classically, instantaneous time-resolved pressure and volume data are plotted as continuous pressure–volume loops (PV-loops, Figure 35.1) with each individual PV-loop representing a single cardiac cycle. Analysis of PV-loops allows for the simultaneous assessment of several hemodynamic parameters of cardiac function, including stroke volume, stroke work, ejection fraction, cardiac output, compliance, chamber contractility, and muscle energetics, to name a few (Figure 35.2). Although the exact nature of the indices being evaluated will differ from study to study, the

Manual of Research Techniques in Cardiovascular Medicine, First Edition. Edited by Hossein Ardehali, Roberto Bolli, and Douglas W. Losordo.
© 2014 John Wiley & Sons, Ltd. Published 2014 by John Wiley & Sons, Ltd.

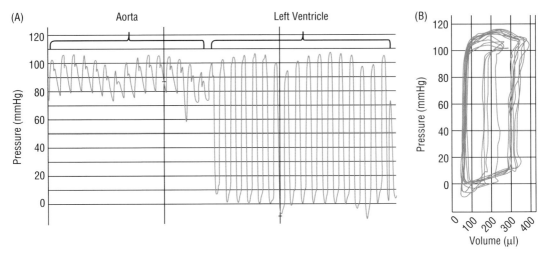

Figure 35.1 (A) A representative pressure recording depicting transition of the PV catheter from the aorta into the left ventricle. (B) A representative example of a PV-loop derived from pressure and volume recordings made in a rat.

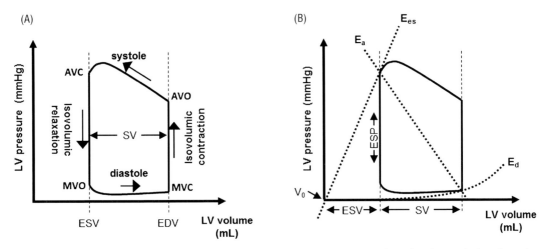

Figure 35.2 Shown in panel (A) is an example of a PV-loop including various parameters that can be evaluated over a single cardiac cycle. (B) Other examples of PV-loop parameters include end-systolic elastance (E_{es}), end-diastolic elastance (E_d), arterial elastance (E_a), ventricular–vascular coupling (E_a/E_{es}), and preload-recruitable stroke work (PRSW). AVC, aortic valve closes; AVO, aortic valve opens; EDV, end diastolic volume; ESV, end systolic volume; MVC, mitral valve closes; MVO, mitral valve opens; SV, stroke volume.

acquisition of the data needed to produce the PV-loop will allow for a significant number of off-line *post hoc* analyses.

There are several catheter manufacturers to choose from and this decision should be made carefully to ensure that the system requirements (i.e. the method used to estimate stroke volume, parallel conductance, etc.) and its capabilities (i.e. data output) fit the needs of the laboratory and the

experimental protocol(s). Regardless of the system selected, pressure–volume analysis can be applied to several experimental paradigms including: (1) animal models of cardiac dysfunction (i.e. acute myocardial infarction or models of cardiac hypertrophy); (2) assessment of novel and/or established pharmacological interventions (i.e. an on-table cardiac stress test with a dobutamine infusion), or (3) evaluation of knockout mice as a means to determine the function of specific genes as they pertain to cardiac function.

Lastly, although appreciating the complexity of the PV-loop and its associated analyses requires an in-depth understanding of cardiac physiology, this chapter will exclusively focus on the surgical procedures needed to achieve proper placement of the catheter in the left ventricle of a mouse or rat via the carotid artery. Several excellent resources are available to assist the reader with the associated PV-loop analysis as well as with the interpretation of any collected data [10,11].

Protocol

Please note that the following protocol details a nonsurvival, closed-chest left ventricular catheterization protocol for generating PV-loops. This procedure will describe the methodology using a rat as the research specimen and a video of the basic procedure can be accessed in the online materials supporting this text (see Video clip 35.1). Mice can also be used but will require adaptations to account for the smaller physiological size and anesthesia thresholds. Although the procedure below describes the use of isoflurane anesthesia, proper selection of general anesthesia procedures will be dictated by local institutional animal use committee guidelines. Selection of the anesthetic agent(s) also depends on the type of experimental model and requires knowledge of the effects of various anesthetics on hemodynamic variables to be measured during the study protocol. Several anesthesia comparison studies exist to help with this selection [10,12–15]. Lastly, laboratory personnel must follow the pre-experimental catheter preparation protocols, including any soaking of the catheter and/or required calibration as suggested by the specific manufacturer. All of the surgical tools and materials needed to complete these experiments can be found in Table 35.1.

1. Deeply anesthetize the rat with 3–5% isoflurane anesthesia in 100% O_2 via an induction chamber and then transfer the animal to a conical facial mask for the duration of the instrumentation and data collection. Once anesthetized, any required baseline blood samples should be collected under deep anesthesia (3–4% isoflurane). Ensure that any removed blood volume is replaced via injection

Table 35.1 Indwelling hemodynamic catheter equipment

FST S&T V vascular clamp size B-1, Cat. no. 00396-01
FST S&T JF-5TC forceps supergrip/ angled 45°, Cat. no. 00649-11
FST S&T JF-5 forceps standard/ angled 45°, Cat. no. 00109-11
FST Vannas spring scissors, Cat. no. 15002-08
FST extra fine Graefe forceps straight, Cat. no. 11150-10
FST extra fine Graefe forceps curved × 2, Cat. no. 11151-10
FST low cost cautery kit, Cat. no. 18010-00
FST fine iris scissors straight, Cat. no. 14090-09
3-0 and 6-0 black silk suture
2% Lidocaine HCl
Heating pad
1 cc TB syringe with 25-G needle
23-G needles for vascular picks
Cotton tipped applicators
2″ × 2″ gauze
Saline
Digital rectal probe and thermometer
Micro dissecting scope and/or magnifying glasses
Pressure volume catheter (ensure that the catheter is "primed" in physiologic saline for a minimum of 30 minutes prior to use)

(either i.v., i.p., or s.q.) of an equal volume of warmed sterile saline.

2. At this stage, mechanical ventilation can be achieved by intubating the animal. Several detailed techniques for intubation can be found in the literature [16,17]. A general guideline for ventilation settings for the rat are to use a tidal volume = $6.2 \times \text{mass}^{1.01}$ and respiration rate = $53.5 \times \text{mass}^{-0.026}$, with 1 cm H_2O positive end expiratory pressure to maintain airway patency [10].

3. Temporarily secure rat limbs to a heated table and anchor the intubation tubing to prevent accidental extubation. Importantly, minor changes in body temperature have significant effects on cardiovascular measures. As such, the body temperature of the rat should be maintained at 37.5° ± 0.5° with supplemental heat sources and monitored throughout the procedure with a rectal probe. Attach electrocardiographic (ECG) leads to monitor heart rate and electrical function if desired. Note: additional electrical signals or grounding in

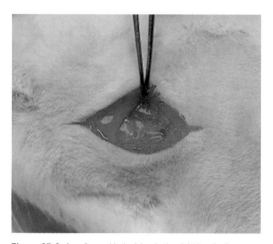

Figure 35.3 An ~2-cm skin incision in the right jugular furrow. (Note: The head of the rat is to the left in all images in this chapter.)

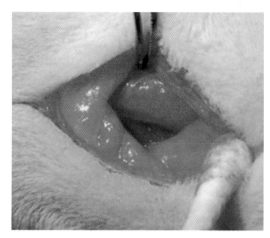

Figure 35.4 Depiction of the extent of blunt dissection required to visualize the sternohyoideus and sternomastoideus muscles overlying the carotid artery.

the vicinity of the PV catheter can create an electrical "sink" which can attenuate or impact accurate measurement of chamber volume.

4. Using fine hair clippers, shave the ventral aspect of the neck from the chin to the collar bone as well as the abdominal mid-line.

5. Ensure the depth of anesthesia is adequate for surgery by the absence of pedal, tail, and/or ocular reflexes. Make an ~2-cm incision along the medial aspect of the right jugular furrow (Figure 35.3). Muscle twitching in the neck is often involuntary and can be reduced through the modest application of 2% lidocaine solution, which is primarily used to keep the vessels moist.

6. The following steps describe how to use blunt dissection to isolate and separate the right carotid artery and the vagus nerve. Note: Given the important role of the vagus nerve on cardiovascular function, use extra precaution during the dissection to avoid damaging it.

7. Blunt dissection can be accomplished with blunt/round tipped scissors, forceps, or a small hemostat. Use of a dissecting microscope or magnifying glasses is highly advisable to avoid damaging surrounding tissues/ organs and blood vessels.

8. After making the incision, clear the connective tissue away using blunt dissection, taking care to avoid the jugular vein. Separate the overlying connective tissue and gently push the salivary glands

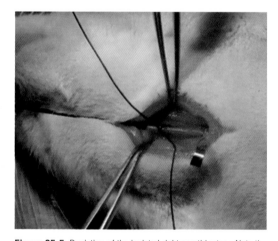

Figure 35.5 Depiction of the isolated right carotid artery. Note the presence of two ties, one rostral that is pulled immediately towards the head and a second caudal tie, that is loose and ready to be used to secure the catheter once in the artery. Also seen is the bulldog clamp, occluding blood flow at the caudal end of the isolated artery.

to the right. Continue until the sternohyoideus and sternomastoideus muscles are exposed (Figure 35.4).

9. At this muscular junction, go to the sternohyoideus and at approximately 30° to the right of the midline and along the same direction as the muscle fibers, use blunt dissection to a depth of ~1–3 mm (Figure 35.5) to expose the carotid artery and vagus nerve.

Continue dissection on both sides of the artery/ nerve to expose the greatest length possible. This is critical for simplifying the catheterization process.

10. If available, increase the microscope scope power or use magnifying glasses to better visualize the right carotid artery and nerve. Using 45° angled, fine-tipped forceps, gently scoop and separate the combined artery/ nerve from the surrounding fascia along the entire vessel length available. Then gently separate the nerve from the artery along the entire length (preferably ~13–15 mm in the rat).

11. Obtain a 40 cm length of 3-0 silk, moisten with saline, and fold in half. Lift the carotid artery slightly and gently pull the folded end of the silk underneath while constantly supporting the artery (dry silk can "saw" through the artery in a mouse). Cut the silk at the fold and position one piece at the upper most rostral end and the other piece at the caudal end of the artery. Using a surgeon's knot, place the rostral tie as high up (as close to the head of the animal as possible) to maximize the length of artery available for catheterization (Figure 35.5).

12. Place the vascular clamp (bulldog clamp) at the most caudal point of the carotid artery (a vascular clamp applicator is useful if the operator's hands are large). Place the caudal silk rostral to the clamp and use a single throw to create a loose pre-emptive tie (Figure 35.5). When the carotid artery is punctured, the vascular clamp will prevent bleeding and the loose caudal suture will be used to secure the catheter and prevent bleeding when the clamp is removed.

13. Several variations for catheterization are possible; two will be discussed here. Using the rostral suture, increase rostral tension on the carotid artery and anchor in place with tape. This greatly facilitates the catheterization process. Option 1: Using the very fine tips of Vannas Spring scissors, cut a small hole into the artery. A small flash of blood will occur as the artery empties its contained blood. Using fine-tipped forceps to hold the wall of the artery steady, advance the catheter into the lumen of the artery. Option 2: Obtain a 21-gauge needle, bevel side up. Using a hemostat, clamp ~5–10 mm down from the tip of the needle. Bend the hub of the needle away from the bevel to create a ~90° bend. This creates an inexpensive vascular pick that can be used to puncture the artery and facilitate insertion of the catheter. Additionally, instead of placing the bend in line with the bevel, a 45° offset will allow the shaft

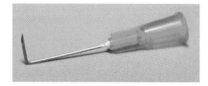

Figure 35.6 An example of the modified needle used to assist in the insertion of the PV catheter into the artery.

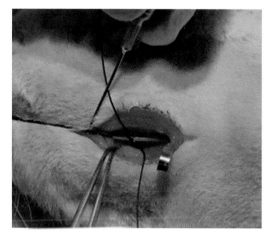

Figure 35.7 A depiction of the use of the modified needle to create a hole in the carotid facilitating entry of the PV catheter.

of the needle to be positioned to the side while keeping the needle's point/ bevel in line with the artery (Figure 35.6). Grasp the end of the PV catheter in one hand. Using the other hand, at the upper-most rostral region of the artery, puncture the artery with the 21-G needle (Figure 35.7). Importantly, keep the tip of the needle in the lumen of the vessel. Place the tip of the catheter below the needle and carefully advance the catheter into the lumen of the artery. Once the tip of the catheter is in the artery, carefully withdraw the needle to avoid damaging the PV catheter.

14. Advance the catheter until the tip reaches the vascular clamp. Ideally, the catheter's pressure and sensing electrodes will fit into the lumen of the vessel (Figure 35.8). If this is the case, secure the rostral suture with the two-throw tie using enough force to prevent bleeding while loose enough to advance the catheter. If the spacing prevents full insertion of the catheter's electrodes, apply additional rostral tension to the artery. The longitudinal tension increases radial traction of the vessel over the catheter and

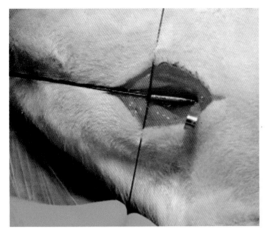

Figure 35.8 Tying the caudal tie to secure the PV catheter in the lumen of the carotid artery.

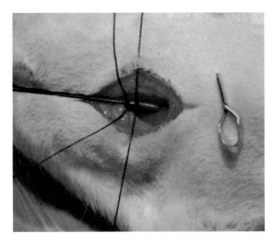

Figure 35.10 Loosening of the rostral tie as a means to facilitate easier advancement of the catheter towards the heart.

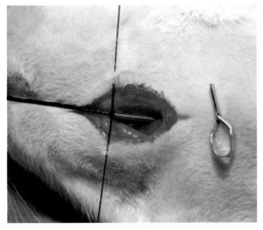

Figure 35.9 Removal of the bulldog clamp once the catheter has been inserted and advanced toward the heart.

minimizes blood loss when the vascular clamp is removed (Figure 35.9). Prepare the two-throw tie for quick occlusion and in successive actions remove the clamp, advance the catheter's electrodes past the rostral tie, and gently secure the tie to prevent blood loss. An additional tie can be used to secure the catheter and/or prevent blood loss (Figure 35.10).

15. At this stage the only visual guide for appropriate catheter placement will be the pressure readout signal indicative of appropriate carotid artery pressure waves.

16. For stability, ensure that the suture ends at the rostral end of the artery are still secured to the table

or fixed point, and advance the catheter gently. Resistance will typically be encountered once the catheter reaches the aortic valve. When the catheter passes the aortic valve, the pressure wave will change (Figure 35.1A) such that the diastolic pressure will now drop below 70–80 mmHg to approximately 5–8 mmHg in healthy animals. If the catheter stops at the aortic valve (forward resistance will be detected but no change in the pressure tracing will be observed) pull the catheter back slightly and attempt to advance again while rotating the catheter slightly. Be sure to avoid using any forceful movements and constantly monitor pressure tracings.

17. Movement of the catheter past the aortic valve requires practice. Over time, the catheter will assume the natural anatomical bends, thus facilitating future catheterizations. Frequently, extending the animals left foot will align the vasculature and promote entry. Gently shifting the chest to the left or right, and up or down can also facilitate entry of the catheter into the left ventricle.

18. When the catheter passes the aortic valve, the pressure sensor will record the left ventricular pressures (Figure 35.1A). Importantly, the distal electrodes will still be on the outside of the ventricle, typically resulting in the following PV trace (Figure 35.11). Please use Figure 35.11 as a guide for proper positioning of the catheter in the left ventricle. Proper positioning in the center of the ventricular chamber is critical for accurate, reliable generation of informative PV-loops.

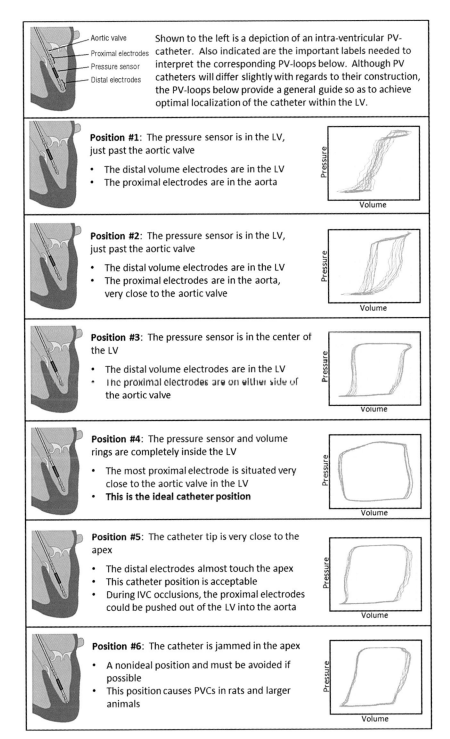

Figure 35.11 PV-catheter positioning guide.

19. Continue advancing the catheter, checking for optimal PV loops (isovolumic contraction and relaxations). Be mindful of the left ventricle's length during catheter advancement and use a delicate touch to sense resistance of the left ventricular apex. In mice and rats, it is relatively easy to puncture and damage the LV, respectively. Conductance catheters rely upon the investigator to obtain PV loops that are reflective of the specific research animals' ventricular volumes. Admittance catheters generate signals that reflect proximity to ventricular muscle, thus providing feedback to adjustments made to position the catheter in the center of the ventricle.

20. Once optimally located in the ventricular chamber, the experimental protocol can be started and data can be recorded. In order to acquire load-independent measures of left ventricular function, preload needs to be altered. To reduce preload, venous occlusion is sufficient. Briefly, increase the level of anesthesia and make a midline abdominal incision. Using blunt dissection, isolate the abdominal portion of the vena cava immediately superior to the renal vein. Following blunt dissection, place a 3-0 silk suture around (behind) the vena cava and carefully return the intestines to their normal position. Lower the isoflurane back to prior recording levels and wait until the blood pressure and PV-loops return to normal. Re-adjustment of the catheter may be necessary at this stage. Once steady state is re-established, lift up on the suture to occlude venous return. Occlusion of venous return will allow for determination of the end-systolic and end-diastolic pressure volume relationships (i.e. ESPVR and EDPVR), which are load-independent markers of contractility and diastolic compliance, respectively.

21. After collecting the data, slowly withdraw the catheter. As the electrical sensor becomes visible and before it touches the caudal suture, increase rostral tension on the rostral suture to minimize blood loss. Then loosen the caudal tie completely and carefully remove the catheter from the artery. The caudal tie can be retightened to prevent the animal from bleeding out and the heart can now be perfused and/or harvested for histology if needed.

Additional notes

• Each procedure should be performed as quickly as possible to minimize the influence of anesthesia,

body temperature loss, and fluid loss. If during the surgical preparation significant blood loss occurs, one should be cognizant of the impact that acute reductions in blood volume will have on the hemodynamic measurements being recorded.

• Isoflurane is ideal for survival surgery as well as approximating normal cardiovascular conditions (i.e. heart rate and blood pressure). Using a range of 1–5% isoflurane will accommodate deep anesthesia for blood draws and intubation while a predetermined level of light anesthesia should be used for recording functional data.

• If one wants to minimize respiratory artifacts during cardiac measures, a brief period of mechanical hyperventilation can be induced that will permit turning off the ventilator during a quick PV-loop recording. Bear in mind that repeated or prolonged hyperventilation will cause alkalosis that can independently influence cardiac function.

Alternative approaches

There are several other methodologies that assess ventricular volumes instantaneously including echocardiography or MRI. Importantly, standard echocardiography can only derive a 3D chamber volume measurement value by extrapolating from ventricular dimensions detected in 2D images. Therefore, this method can only provide an estimate for instantaneous blood volumes. However, the emergence of 3D echocardiography may diminish or eliminate the stated limitations of 2D echocardiography. Secondly, one can also determine the systemic, left ventricular and aortic pressures using far less sophisticated equipment than the PV catheter; however, catheter-based PV-loop acquisition is the only technique that simultaneously allows for the capture of a blood volume and pressure signal instantaneously making it the gold standard technique for evaluating cardiovascular function through pressure–volume analysis.

Strengths/ weaknesses of the method

The primary strengths of pressure–volume analysis are (1) the ability to provide load-independent measurements of cardiac chamber function such as contractility and diastolic compliance; and (2) the ability to measure several cardiac parameters simultaneously. A major weakness of the PV-loop acquisition technique is the fact that the procedure is almost always terminal. As opposed to other noninvasive methods that assess cardiac function such as echocardiography or MRI, acquisition of data at several time points in the same animal is virtually impossible. Therefore, for temporal analyses in experimental models, investigators must account for the added time and cost of making measurements in animals at various ages/ time points. Another minor weakness of the PV-loop technique is the inability to use the methodology presented here for the assessment of cardiac function in rodents that have undergone transverse aortic constriction/ banding. Due to the induced narrowing/ clamping of the aorta, one cannot advance the pressure–volume catheter to the heart thus precluding access to the aortic valve. An alternative method to circumvent this problem involves accessing the ventricle through an open-chest, apical puncture protocol which has been described elsewhere [10].

Conclusions

Pressure–volume analysis is the gold standard technique for the measurement of load-independent cardiac indices such as cardiac contractility and ventricular chamber compliance. Here we have described the basic surgical procedure for positioning a pressure–volume catheter into the left ventricle of a live, anesthetized rodent for the purposes of deriving the classical "pressure–volume loop" both at rest and with preload reduction maneuvers. Although many of the specific details of the procedure will be dictated by the specific catheter manufacturer, we have described the general techniques which can be useful for performing pressure–volume analysis. Pressure–volume analysis, once mastered, can be an indispensable technique for the measurement of valuable, load-independent cardiac function data in rodent models.

Acknowledgments

The authors would like to thank Anil Kottam, PhD at Science Systems Inc. for the images and graphics used in Figure 35.11.

References

1 Baan J, van der Velde ET, de Bruin HG, Smeenk GJ, Koops J, van Dijk AD, *et al*. Continuous measurement of left ventricular volume in animals and humans by conductance catheter. *Circulation* 1984; **70**: 812–823.

2 Sagawa K. *Cardiac Contraction and the Pressure-Volume Relationship*. New York: Oxford University Press, 1988.

3 Kass DA, Yamazaki T, Burkhoff D, Maughan WL, Sagawa K. Determination of left ventricular end-systolic pressure-volume relationships by the conductance (volume) catheter technique. *Circulation* 1986; **73**: 586–595.

4 Georgakopoulos D, Christe ME, Giewat M, Seidman CM, Seidman JG, Kass DA, *et al*. The pathogenesis of familial hypertrophic cardiomyopathy: early and evolving effects from an alpha-cardiac myosin heavy chain missense mutation. *Nat Med* 1999; **5**: 327–330.

5 Nagayama T, Takimoto E, Sadayappan S, Mudd JO, Seidman JG, Robbins J, *et al*. Control of in vivo left ventricular [correction] contraction/relaxation kinetics by myosin binding protein C: protein kinase A phosphorylation dependent and independent regulation. *Circulation* 2007; **116**: 2399–2408.

6 Takimoto E, Champion HC, Li M, Ren S, Rodriguez ER, Tavazzi B, *et al*. Oxidant stress from nitric oxide synthase-3 uncoupling stimulates cardiac pathologic remodeling from chronic pressure load. *J Clin Invest* 2005; **115**: 1221–1231.

7 Takimoto E, Champion HC, Li M, Belardi D, Ren S, Rodriguez ER, *et al*. Chronic inhibition of cyclic GMP phosphodiesterase 5A prevents and reverses cardiac hypertrophy. *Nat Med* 2005; **11**: 214–222.

8 Pacher P, Mabley JG, Liaudet L, Evgenov OV, Marton A, Hasko G, *et al*. Left ventricular pressure-volume relationship in a rat model of advanced aging-associated heart failure. *Am J Physiol Heart Circ Physiol* 2004; **287**: H2132–2137.

9 Pacher P, Vaslin A, Benko R, Mabley JG, Liaudet L, Hasko G, *et al*. A new, potent poly(ADP-ribose) polymerase inhibitor improves cardiac and vascular dysfunction associated with advanced aging. *J Pharmacol Exp Ther* 2004; **311**: 485–491.

10 Pacher P, Nagayama T, Mukhopadhyay P, Batkai S, Kass DA. Measurement of cardiac function using pressure-volume conductance catheter technique in mice and rats. *Nat Protoc* 2008; **3**: 1422–1434

11 Burkhoff D, Mirsky I, Suga H. Assessment of systolic and diastolic ventricular properties via pressure-volume analysis: a guide for clinical, translational, and basic researchers. *Am J Physiol Heart Circ Physiol* 2005; **289**: H501–512.

12 Jiang X, Gao L, Zhang Y, Wang G, Liu Y, Yan C, *et al*. A comparison of the effects of ketamine, chloral hydrate and pentobarbital sodium anesthesia on isolated rat hearts and cardiomyocytes. *J Cardiovasc Med* 2011; **12**: 732–735.

13 Zorniak M, Mitrega K, Bialka S, Porc M, Krzeminski TF. Comparison of thiopental, urethane, and pentobarbital in the study of experimental cardiology in rats in vivo. *J Cardiovasc Pharmacol* 2010; **56**: 38–44.

14 Matsuda Y, Ohsaka K, Yamamoto H, Natsume K, Hirabayashi S, Kounoike M, *et al*. Comparison of newly developed inhalation anesthesia system and intraperitoneal anesthesia on the hemodynamic state in mice. *Biol Pharm Bull* 2007; **30**: 1716–1720.

15 Saha DC, Saha AC, Malik G, Astiz ME, Rackow EC. Comparison of cardiovascular effects of tiletamine-zolazepam, pentobarbital, and ketamine-xylazine in male rats. *J Am Assoc Lab Anim Sci* 2007; **46**: 74–80.

16 Kastl S, Kotschenreuther U, Hille B, Schmidt J, Gepp H, Hohenberger W, *et al*. Simplification of rat intubation on inclined metal plate. *Adv Physiol Educ* 2004; **28**: 29–32.

17 Weksler B, Ng B, Lenert J, Burt M. A simplified method for endotracheal intubation in the rat. *J Appl Physiol* 1994; **76**: 1823–1825.

Part 5
Metabolism, Mitochondria, and Cell Death

36 Fractionation of cardiomyocytes and isolation of mitochondria

Christopher P. Baines

University of Missouri, Columbia, MO, USA

Introduction

The mitochondrion is critical for normal homeostasis of the cardiac myocyte. It is responsible for providing the vast amounts of ATP required for contraction, which it does through oxidative phosphorylation driven by the generation of NADH and FADH by the TCA cycle and β-oxidation. Mitochondria also help maintain ion homeostasis, especially with regard to Ca^{2+}, K^+, and Fe^+, and they are the initial site for the synthesis of many key substances, such as steroids and porphyrins [1–5]. However, under conditions of stress and disease, cardiac mitochondria also produce toxic amounts of free radicals and induce death-signaling programs through opening of the mitochondrial permeability transition pore and the release of apoptogenic factors, such as cytochrome c [2,3]. Thus, it is now well recognized that mitochondrial dysfunction plays a role in many cardiac disease states, including ischemia–reperfusion injury, drug-induced cardiotoxicity, myocarditis, and the cardiac aspects of Friedreich's ataxia, muscular dystrophy, and diabetes [2–5].

Consequently, it is imperative that we are able to isolate these organelles from cardiac tissue and/or cells to better understand the molecular mechanisms by which mitochondria control cardiac myocyte survival and death. Although there are many variations, the vast majority of techniques for the isolation of mitochondria follow a general theme. There is an initial disruption step, designed to rupture the plasma membrane while leaving the internal organelles intact [6,7]. The mitochondria are then separated from the other organelles by differential centrifugation, on the basis of their relative size [6,7]. Importantly, all steps are carried out in isosmotic buffer to prevent swelling and rupture of the mitochondria during the isolation procedure.

The procedures outlined below follow an extremely well-established protocol for the isolation of mitochondria (and other subcellular fractions) from both whole hearts and primary culture neonatal myocytes. It is a straightforward, quick, and reproducible method for generating washed mitochondria and we have used this extensively in our studies [8–12]. The mitochondria can then be utilized for a variety of analyses. Published examples include, but are certainly not limited to, immunoblotting and immunoprecipitations/pulldowns [8,9], mitochondrial swelling [10], mitochondrial respiration [13], fatty acid metabolism [14], Ca^{2+} uptake and release [15], Fe uptake [16], protein import assays [17], reactive oxygen species production [18], and mitochondrial proteomics [19]. Of course there are advantages and disadvantages with any methodology and we will discuss these at the end of the chapter.

Manual of Research Techniques in Cardiovascular Medicine, First Edition. Edited by Hossein Ardehali, Roberto Bolli, and Douglas W. Losordo.
© 2014 John Wiley & Sons, Ltd. Published 2014 by John Wiley & Sons, Ltd.

Protocols

Isolation of mitochondria from whole hearts

We describe below a well-established, standard protocol for the isolation of mitochondria from intact hearts (Figure 36.1). In this particular case, we describe the procedure for mouse hearts, as this is the most common species used in our laboratory as well as others. However, this protocol can be easily scaled up for the isolation of mitochondria from larger animal hearts, as we have done for the pig (where we take ~1 cm³ of left ventricular tissue). In order to maintain mitochondrial integrity, it is best to minimize the time of euthanasia and to keep everything on ice during the isolation procedure.

Preparation

1. PBS kept on ice for rinsing hearts.
2. Homogenization buffer: 250 mM sucrose, 10 mM Tris pH 7.4, 1 mM EDTA. Protease and phosphatase inhibitors can be added if required. Keep on ice.

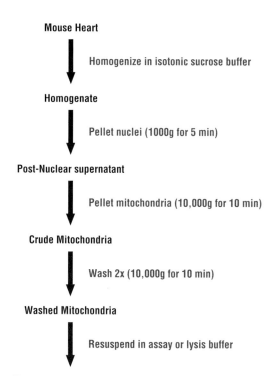

Mouse Heart

↓ Homogenize in isotonic sucrose buffer

Homogenate

↓ Pellet nuclei (1000g for 5 min)

Post-Nuclear supernatant

↓ Pellet mitochondria (10,000g for 10 min)

Crude Mitochondria

↓ Wash 2x (10,000g for 10 min)

Washed Mitochondria

↓ Resuspend in assay or lysis buffer

Experimental Mitochondria

Figure 36.1 Schematic depicting the basic procedure for isolating mitochondria from the mouse heart.

3. Dounce homogenizer with the tight-fitting "B" pestle (Kimble-Kontes 7 mL Cat. no. 885300-0007) prechilled on ice.
4. Prechill to 4°C a refrigerated centrifuge with a fixed rotor capable of holding 15-mL conical tubes, and capable of speeds up to 10,000 g (we use a Sorvall RT1⁺ centrifuge).

Harvest

1. Euthanize animals in necropsy, surgically remove hearts and immediately rinse in the ice-cold PBS.

Note. You can also remove the atria at this time if you wish to limit the preparation to ventricular tissue.

Fractionation

1. Place the whole mouse heart in the Dounce along with 1.5 mL of homogenization buffer.

Note. For larger animals such as pigs we typically use a 1-cm³ piece of left ventricular tissue that we mince up into smaller pieces with scissors prior to homogenization.

2. Homogenize the heart with "B" pestle – we usually find the 10–15 passes are sufficient. You will still have some fibrous tissue pieces in the mix but as long as the majority of the heart is broken up you should be fine.

Note. We often remove 200 µL of the homogenate at this point and add Triton X-100 (final concentration of 1%) to give a total lysate.

3. Place the homogenate in a 15-mL conical tube and centrifuge at 1000 g for 5 minutes to pellet the nuclei and unbroken cells/ debris.
4. Carefully, so as not to dislodge any of the fragile nuclear/ cell pellet, remove the supernatant with a serological pipette and decant into a clean 15-mL tube. Centrifuge this supernatant at 10,000 g for 10 minutes to pellet the mitochondria.
5. Remove the supernatant, add 5 mL of fresh homogenization buffer, and *gently* resuspend the mitochondrial pellet using a bulb pipette. Centrifuge again at 10,000 g for 10 minutes.

Note. The supernatant that is initially removed in this step can be further processed to generate light membrane and cytosolic fractions (see Step 8).

Note. If subsequent experiments involve calcium, the EDTA should be omitted from the homogenization buffer for these washing steps.

6. Repeat Step 5.

7. The washed mitochondrial pellet can now be *gently* resuspended in whichever solution is required for the experiment, i.e. lysis buffer for western blotting/ immunoprecipitation, respiration buffer for oxymetry, etc. For example, we typically resuspend the pellet in 200 μL of lysis buffer which yields ~1.5–3.0 μg/μL protein concentration depending in the size of the heart.

8. If light membrane and/or cytosolic fractions are also required, centrifuge the supernatant generated in Step 4 at 100,000 g for 60 minutes in a prechilled fixed rotor centrifuge (we use a Sorvall Mx120). The resultant pellet is the light membrane fraction (SR, Golgi, plasma membrane) and the supernatant is the cytosol.

The protocol mentioned earlier uses whole freshly isolated hearts. However, it is possible to generate sufficient mitochondria from small amounts of cardiac tissues, for example just with the left ventricle alone. Also we have successfully isolated mitochondria from previously frozen mouse hearts, although only for the purposes of western blotting [8]. Here, it is imperative that the heart is totally defrosted on ice before homogenization, otherwise the risk of fracturing mitochondria is greatly increased.

Although this process greatly concentrates the mitochondrial fraction, there are always going to be some issues with contamination from other subcellular compartments. Blotting for key proteins from these fractions can control for the amount of contamination. We typically blot for the ATP synthase (mitochondria), Na^{2+}/K$^+$ ATPase (sarcolemma), calnexin (ER/SR), and lactate dehydrogenase (cyotosol). Should extensive contamination occur, it maybe necessary to further purify the mitochondria by centrifugation through a Percoll (or equivalent) gradient [20]. However, while this will indeed further purify the mitochondria it will also further reduce the amount of final material and also runs the risk of stripping off key proteins associated with the mitochondrial outer membrane.

Isolation of mitochondria from cultured cardiomyocytes

The protocol we will describe for isolating mitochondria from cultured cardiomyocytes is essentially the same as detailed earlier in the chapter, but scaled down and with a couple of modifications. Here, we describe the procedure for isolating mitochondria from a 10-cm plate of ~3 × 10^6 neonatal rat ventricular myocytes, which we use routinely in our laboratory. This yields sufficient mitochondria for western blotting or some basic biochemical assays (~75–100 μg), but several plates will need to be pooled if the analyses are more extensive or require more starting matter.

Preparation

1. PBS at room temperature.

2. Homogenization buffer: 250 mM sucrose, 10 mM Tris pH 7.4, 1 mM EDTA. Protease and phosphatase inhibitors can be added if required. Keep on ice.

3. Dounce homogenizer with the tight-fitting "B" pestle (Kimble-Kontes 2 mL Cat. no. 885300-0002) prechilled on ice

4. Prechill to 4°C a refrigerated microcentrifuge with a fixed rotor capable of speeds up to 10,000 g (we use a Fisher Accuspin17RT microcentrifuge).

Harvest

1. Wash the cells once with PBS and scrape cells off using a cell scraper (we find Sarstedt's scrapers are by far the best). Pipette the cells into a 1.5-mL microcentrifuge tube and pellet by centrifuging at 15,000 g for 1 minute.

2. Remove the supernatant, resuspend the cell pellet in 200 μL of homogenization buffer, and incubate on ice for 10–15 minutes.

Note. We have found that allowing the cells to equilibrate with the sucrose buffer gives a better and cleaner yield than if you immediately homogenize them after resuspension.

Fractionation

1. Pipette the cell suspension into the Dounce.

2. Homogenize the cells with "B" pestle – we typically do 30 passes as we have found that it gives a better yield than the 10–15 passes used for the tissue (but without disrupting the mitochondria themselves).

3. Transfer the homogenate to a 1.5-mL micro-centrifuge tube and centrifuge at $800\,g$ for 10 minutes to pellet the nuclei and unbroken cells/ debris.

4. Carefully, so as not to dislodge the fragile nuclear/ cell pellet, remove the supernatant and transfer it to a clean 15-mL tube. Centrifuge this supernatant at $10,000\,g$ for 10 minutes to pellet the mitochondria.

5. Remove the supernatant (which can again be used to generate light membrane and cytosolic fractions), add 1 mL of fresh homogenization buffer, and *gently* resuspend the mitochondrial pellet. Centrifuge again at $10,000\,g$ for 10 minutes.

Note. Again, if subsequent experiments involve calcium, the EDTA should be omitted from the homogenization buffer for these washing steps.

6. Repeat Step 5.

7. The washed mitochondrial pellet can now be *gently* resuspended in whichever solution is required for the experiment.

8. If light membrane and/or cytosolic fractions are also required, centrifuge the supernatant generated in Step 4 at $100,000\,g$ for 60 minutes in a prechilled fixed rotor centrifuge. The resultant pellet is the light membrane fraction and the supernatant is the cytosol.

Alternative approaches

The vast majority of alternative methods focus on the technique by which the mitochondria are extracted from the cell. For example, if the cardiac tissue is particular fibrous, a prestep involving a tissue blender can be implemented [6], although of course this runs the risk of damaging mitochondria if care is not taken. With regards to cultured cells, one cycle of freeze–thawing may aid in the subsequent disruption of the cell membrane by the Dounce, thus increasing the number of mitochondria recovered. However, such freeze–thawing would render the mitochondria unsuitable for enzymatic/ metabolic assays. Alternatively, hypotonic swelling and rupture of the cells can be used [6,7]. Nitrogen cavitation, where nitrogen is forced into solution under high pressure, can also be used to disrupt cells [21]. When depressurized, the nitrogen is released as bubbles, which rupture the cells by shear stress. This procedure can be highly effective and has the advantage that the cells only go through one round

of disruption, as opposed to several with the Dounce approach. However, the nitrogen bomb instrument is relatively expensive compared to a Dounce (e.g. ~$2000 compared to ~$100).

There are several commercially available kits that can be used to isolate and purify mitochondria from both tissue and cultured cells. We have successfully used the Cell Fractionation Kit from Mitosciences (now Abcam) to generate relatively clean cytosolic and mitochondrial fractions for western blotting. However, this process relies on fractionation using detergents and so the final products are lysed. This in turn limits the use to immunoblotting, precipitation, and some enzyme activity assays. Mitosciences/ Abcam and Pierce also have mitochondrial fractionation kits that basically follow the same procedure detailed earlier. However, care must be taken as often the composition of the buffers in such kits is unknown due to proprietary reasons. This can be problem if EDTA is one of the constituents and you wish to do Ca^{2+}-dependent assays on the resultant mitochondrial preparation.

The use of mitochondria for functional/ metabolic assays requires the preservation of their $\Delta\Psi_m$ and function during the isolation procedure. In this regard, we have used mitochondria generated by these protocols for several functional assays, including swelling, mitochondrial respiration, and fatty acid oxidation, suggesting that mitochondrial functionality is indeed preserved. However, the isolation procedure can be modified to help ensure that this is the case. For example, resuspending the mitochondria in buffer containing ATP, Mg^{2+}, along with TCA cycle substrates, such as α-ketoglutarate and phosphoenol pyruvate plus pyruvate kinase, can help preserve function [16]. Additionally, the inclusion of BSA in the isolation and resuspension medium can bind free fatty acids and therefore help maintain mitochondrial membrane stability [22]. This appears to be especially beneficial for protein import assays [17].

Strengths and weaknesses of the method

There are several strengths to this method. It is relatively quick, with time from tissue or cell harvest to obtaining the washed mitochondrial pellet being less than 1 hour. It is straightforward, easy to learn, and does not require specialized chemicals or reagents. In particular, it does not involve gradients, which can be difficult to generate properly, are time consuming, and reduce the yield of mitochondria (although this may still be occasionally necessary). Moreover it is also comparatively inexpensive – assuming access to the necessary centrifuges, the biggest outlay is the homogenizer. Although the methods we have described here are for cardiac tissue and cells, this technique is transferable to other organ and cell culture systems (although the brain is a bit tricky), and can be scaled up or down depending on the amount of starting material.

A weakness is that the disruption process will inevitably rupture some mitochondria. This is especially true for cardiac tissue where the subsarcolemma mitochondria sit right under the plasma membrane that you are trying to disrupt. The extent of rupture can be visualized by western blotting for cytochrome c in the cytosolic fraction. Needless to say, too great a disruption of mitochondria will have a profound effect on functional assays. Consequently, in addition to determining cytochrome c in the cytosol, other assays can be employed to assess mitochondria integrity. These include measuring mitochondrial $\Delta\Psi_m$ by loading the mitochondria with Rhodamine 123 or Mitotracker Red [16,23]. Unbroken mitochondria with an intact $\Delta\Psi_m$ will take up the dyes and fluoresce. Alternatively, measurement of the state-3 to state-4 ratio of mitochondrial respiration using NADH-linked substrates (the so-called respiratory control ratio, RCR) can be used as an index of integrity. Mitochondria exhibiting an RCR of 4–5 are considered tightly coupled [6,23]. A third method is to measure O_2 consumption before and after the addition of exogenous cytochrome c. A large increase in respiration would indicate a pronounced rupture of the mitochondria such that the endogenous cytochrome c has been lost [6]. Should pronounced mitochondrial disruption be suspected, the number of passes with the Dounce can be reduced. While this will decrease the yield, it should help preserve integrity.

Finally, when homogenizing a whole heart you will obviously be including nonmyocyte mitochondria in the final prep. However, given that myocytes represent ~90–95% of a mouse or rat heart's volume [24,25] and ~30% of a myocyte's own volume is mitochondria, nonmyocytic mitochondria will only represent an extremely small proportion of the final fraction.

Conclusions

In summary, these basic protocols offer a quick, efficient, reproducible, and cost-effective way of isolating cardiac mitochondria for subsequent analysis. While there can be some drawbacks, especially concerning contamination with other fractions, we have found this to be a very useful technique. It is certainly an excellent first pass method for examining any potential changes to mitochondrial function, protein expression, etc., and the process can then be further refined should any positive findings be obtained.

References

1 Porter GA Jr, Hom J, Hoffman D, Quintanilla R, de Mesy Bentley K, Sheu SS, et al. Bioenergetics, mitochondria, and cardiac myocyte differentiation. *Prog Pediatr Cardiol* 2011; **31**: 75–81.

2 Whelan RS, Kaplinskiy V, Kitsis RN. Cell death in the pathogenesis of heart disease: mechanisms and significance. *Annu Rev Physiol* 2010; **72**: 19–44.

3 Baines CP. The cardiac mitochondrion: nexus of stress. *Annu Rev Physiol* 2010; **72**: 61–80.

4 Rosca MG, Hoppel CL. Mitochondria in heart failure. *Cardiovasc Res* 2010; **88**: 40–50.

5 O'Rourke B, Cortassa S, Akar F, Aon M. Mitochondrial ion channels in cardiac function and dysfunction. *Novartis Found Symp* 2007; **287**: 140–151.

6 Pallotti F, Lenaz G. Isolation and subfractionation of mitochondria from animal cells and tissue culture lines. In: Pon LA, Schon EA, eds. *Mitochondria*. San Diego: Academic Press, 2001, pp. 1–35.

7 Chaiyarit S, Thongboonkerd V. Comparative analyses of cell disruption methods for mitochondrial isolation in high-throughput proteomics study. *Anal Biochem* 2009; **394**: 249–258.

8 Baines CP, Zhang J, Wang GW, Zheng YT, Xiu JX, Cardwell EM, et al. Mitochondrial PKCε and MAPK form signaling modules in the murine heart: enhanced mitochondrial PKCε-MAPK interactions and differential MAPK activation in PKCε-induced cardioprotection. *Circ Res* 2002; **90**: 390–397.

9 Baines CP, Song CX, Zheng YT, Wang GW, Zhang J, Wang OL, et al. Protein kinase Cε interacts with and inhibits the permeability transition pore in cardiac mitochondria. *Circ Res* 2003; **92**: 873–880.

10 Baines CP, Kaiser RA, Purcell NH, Blair NS, Osinska H, Hambleton MA, et al. Loss of cyclophilin D reveals a critical role for mitochondrial permeability transition in cell death. *Nature* 2005; **434**: 658–662.

11 McGee AM, Baines CP. Complement 1q binding protein inhibits the mitochondrial permeability transition pore and protects against oxidative stress-induced death. *Biochem J* 2010; **433**: 119–125.

12 Emter CA, Baines CP. Cardiovascular remodeling in aortic-banded miniature swine is altered by aerobic interval training. *Am J Physiol* 2010; **299**: H1348–H1356.

13 Vinnakota KC, Dash RK, Beard DA. Stimulatory effects of calcium on respiration and NAD(P)H synthesis in intact rat heart mitochondria utilizing physiological substrates cannot explain respiratory control in vivo. *J Biol Chem* 2011; **286**: 30816–30822.

14 Ellis JM, Mentock SM, Depetrillo MA, Koves TR, Sen S, Watkins SM, et al. Mouse cardiac acyl coenzyme a synthetase 1 deficiency impairs Fatty Acid oxidation and induces cardiac hypertrophy. *Mol Cell Biol* 2011; **31**: 1252–1262.

15 Argaud L, Gateau-Roesch O, Augeul L, Couture-Lepetit E, Loufouat J, Gomez L, et al. Increased mitochondrial calcium coexists with decreased reperfusion injury in postconditioned (but not preconditioned) hearts. *Am J Physiol* 2008; **294**: H386–H391.

16 Ichikawa Y, Bayeva M, Ghanefar M, Potini V, Sun L, Mutharasan RK, et al. Disruption of ATP-binding cassette B8 in mice leads to cardiomyopathy through a decrease in mitochondrial iron export. *Proc Natl Acad Sci USA* 2012; **109**: 4152–4157.

17 McKee EE, Grier BL, Thompson GS, McCourt JD. Isolation and incubation conditions to study heart mitochondrial protein synthesis. *Am J Physiol* 1990; **258**: E492–502.

18 Korge P, Ping P, Weiss JN. Reactive oxygen species production in energized cardiac mitochondria during hypoxia/ reoxygenation: modulation by nitric oxide. *Circ Res* 2008; **103**: 873–880.

19 Agnetti G, Kaludercic N, Kane LA, Elliott ST, Guo Y, Chakir K, et al. Modulation of mitochondrial proteome and improved mitochondrial function by biventricular pacing of dyssynchronous failing hearts. *Circ Cardiovasc Genet* 2010; **3**: 78–87.

20 Pertoft H. Fractionation of cells and subcellular particles with Percoll. *J Biochem Biophys Methods* 2000; **44**: 1–30.

21 Gottlieb RA, Adachi S. Nitrogen cavitation for cell disruption to obtain mitochondria from cultured cells. *Methods Enzymol* 2000; **322**: 213–221.

22 Korge P, Honda HM, Weiss JN. Effects of fatty acids in isolated mitochondria: implications for ischemic injury and cardioprotection. *Am J Physiol* 2003; **285**: H259–H269.

23 Rajapakse N, Shimizu K, Payne M, Busija D. Isolation and characterization of intact mitochondria from neonatal rat brain. *Brain Res Brain Res Protoc* 2001; **8**: 176–183.

24 Reiss K, Cheng W, Ferber A, Kajstura J, Li P, Li B, et al. Overexpression of insulin-like growth factor-1 in the heart is coupled with myocyte proliferation in transgenic mice. *Proc Natl Acad Sci USA* 1996; **93**: 8630–8635.

25 Brüel A, Christoffersen TE, Nyengaard JR. Growth hormone increases the proliferation of existing cardiac myocytes and the total number of cardiac myocytes in the rat heart. *Cardiovasc Res* 2007; **76**: 400–408.

Assessment of glucose and fatty acid metabolism *ex vivo*

Darrell D. Belke[1] and E. Dale Abel[2]

[1] University of Calgary, Calgary, Alberta, Canada
[2] Carver College of Medicine University of Iowa, Iowa City, IA, USA

Introduction

The isolated working heart preparation has had a long and distinguished history in elucidating many aspects of cardiac physiology. Pioneering work in rat hearts over 40 years by John Neely set the stage for many studies in rodent hearts that established paradigms of metabolic regulation in the heart that still hold true today [1]. With the advent of the molecular era and the generation of genetically modified murine models of cardiovascular disease, the need arose for scaling these classical techniques to the murine heart. This chapter describes the approaches that have now been adapted and used by many groups for measuring myocardial substrate metabolism in isolated perfused mouse hearts.

Principle

The method is based upon the use of ^3H or ^{14}C radiolabeled glucose and ^3H palmitate. Glycolysis is characterized by the conversion of the 6-carbon containing glucose to 3-carbon pyruvate. The conversion of glucose to pyruvate results in the generation of H_2O at conversion of 2-phosphoglycerate to phosphoenolpyruvic acid (PEP) at the penultimate step in glycolysis by the enzyme enolase. The hydrogen that forms water in glycolysis comes from the 5 position of glucose. Because glucose is labeled

with tritium in the 5 position, the rate of generation of tritiated water reflects the rate of this reaction from which an overall estimate of glycolytic flux can be calculated. Glucose oxidation rates are derived by using uniformly labeled ^{14}C-glucose. Following the completion of glycolysis, ^{14}C-labeled pyruvate enters the TCA cycle, which will enrich the carbons of TCA intermediates with ^{14}C. CO_2 is generated at two steps in the TCA cycle (isocitrate $\rightarrow$ ketoglutarate and ketoglutarate $\rightarrow$ succinate). Thus trapping $^{14}CO_2$ from the perfusate or by releasing $^{14}CO_2$ from $H_2{}^{14}CO_3$ derived from dissolved $^{14}CO_2$ represents the basis for calculating the rate of oxidation of glucose. Palmitate oxidation rates are based on the use of palmitate that is labeled with ^3H at carbon 9 and 10. Long-chain fatty acid CoAs, such as palmitate, undergo beta-oxidation, which is an iterative process that sequentially generates the 2-carbon acetyl CoA moieties. The process of beta-oxidation generates the reducing equivalents NADH and $FADH_2$ (harboring the ^3H derived from the radiolabeled palmitate). These reducing equivalents provide electrons to the electron transport chain while the radiolabeled protons are pumped into the mitochondrial intermembrane space. These protons re-enter the mitochondrial matrix via ATP synthase to interact with molecular oxygen, producing water. The rate of generation of this ^3H_2O is used to calculate the rate of oxidation of the fatty acid palmitate.

Manual of Research Techniques in Cardiovascular Medicine, First Edition. Edited by Hossein Ardehali, Roberto Bolli, and Douglas W. Losordo.
© 2014 John Wiley & Sons, Ltd. Published 2014 by John Wiley & Sons, Ltd.

Methods

Working heart apparatus

The isolated working heart apparatus consists of five basic components (Figure 37.1): (1) a buffer reservoir holding sufficient buffer to maintain a constant supply of oxygen and substrates to the heart; (2) an oxygenator with sufficient surface area to oxygenate the buffer and permit gas (CO_2) exchange, attached to the heart via a preload line; (3) a cannula for mounting the heart and a chamber to contain it; (4)

a compliance chamber to mimic the elasticity of the aorta; and (5) an afterload / return line to ensure adequate coronary perfusion and to set the workload of the heart. Components 1–4 as well as the left atrial preload line need to be water jacketed to maintain a temperature close to 37°C. A pressure transducer for measuring aortic pressure development should be placed in the afterload cannula at a point as close to the aorta as possible to obtain an estimate of peak systolic pressure generated by the heart. High-fidelity pressure transducers, such as the 2.5-Fr

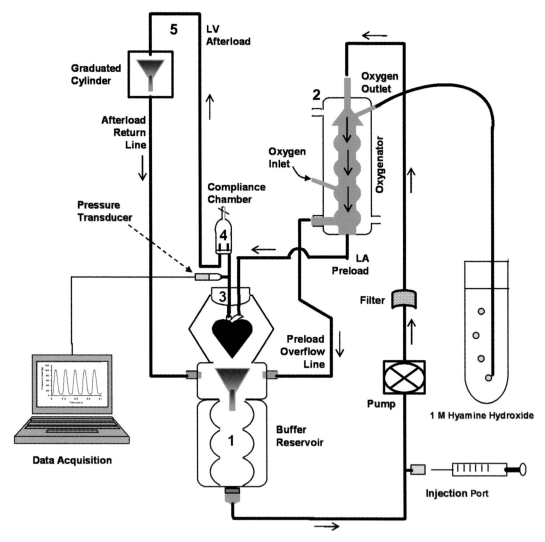

Figure 37.1 Schematic of isolated working heart perfusion rig. LA, left atrium; LV, left ventricle. 1, buffer reservoir; 2, injection port; 3, seal; 4, a compliance chamber; 5, height adjustment for determining afterload. See text for an explanation of the components. (Source: Modified from Belke DD 1999 [3]).

miniature pressure transducer produced by Millar Instruments (Houston, TX), can be integrated into small spaces [2]. Flow can be measured using in-line flow probes (Transonic Inc.) placed in the preload and afterload lines (coronary flow = preload − afterload flow rates); or graduated cylinders placed below the heart to obtain coronary flow, and in the return line to measure afterload flow rate. Flow meters for analysis of afterload and coronary flow rates must be integrated into the perfusion apparatus to obtain a gas-tight seal for metabolic measurements. Cardiac workload for the heart is determined as the product of total cardiac output (coronary and afterload flow) times peak systolic pressure.

Cannula geometry for the aorta and pulmonary vein is critical to ensure adequate perfusion of the heart and maintenance of a steady workload over sufficient time to perform a metabolic assessment. For mice, the aorta is cannulated with an 18-gauge plastic cannula (1.5 cm length, 0.95 mm ID, 1.30 mm OD), while the pulmonary vein is cannulated with a 16-gauge steel cannula (3 cm length, 1.14 mm ID, 1.52 mm OD) using 5-0 silk to secure the vessels to the cannula [2]. During the initial cannulation, the heart is perfused in Langendorff mode through the aortic cannula until the preload cannula is attached to the pulmonary vein. When switching from Langendorff perfusion to working heart mode, the left atrium is perfused by gravity from the oxygenator at a preload pressure of 15 mmHg; while the left ventricle contracts against a hydrostatic column on the aortic cannula set at a height equivalent to 50 mmHg of pressure. This is the minimum afterload recommended to maintain adequate coronary artery perfusion; however, afterload can be set at a higher pressure (greater height) if a greater level of work is required. Afterload should always be set to ensure continuous flow through the line as a result of cardiac output from the left ventricle, or coronary perfusion pressure will be altered during an experimental run.

Solutions

During the initial cannulation, the heart is Langendorff perfused with Krebs'–Henseleit bicarbonate (KHB) solution consisting of (in mM) 118.5 NaCl, 25 NaHCO$_3$, 4.7 KCl, 1.2 MgSO$_4$, 1.2 KH$_2$PO$_4$, 2.5 CaCl$_2$, 0.5 EDTA, and 11 glucose which is gassed with 95% O$_2$–5% CO$_2$ (pH 7.4) [3].

The working heart solution used for metabolic measurements is a modified KHB solution containing palmitate (generally 0.4 or 1.2 mM) bound to 3% BSA as a metabolic substrate in addition to 11 mM glucose [3]. To bind palmitate to BSA, palmitate is first dissolved in 25 mL of a water:ethanol mixture (60:40 vol/vol) containing 0.5–0.6 g Na$_2$CO$_3$/g palmitate and heated with constant stirring until the ethanol evaporates. The hot palmitate mixture is quickly added to the modified KHB solution containing BSA (without glucose) with rapid stirring to ensure adequate mixing and dissipation of heat to prevent the BSA from denaturing. This mixture is dialyzed overnight against 10 volumes of KHB solution (without glucose) using 8–12,000 mol. wt. cut-off SPECTRAPOR dialysis tubing (Spectrum Medical Industries, Los Angeles, CA). Dialysis is necessary to remove any remaining ethanol and Na$_2$CO$_3$, and to permit calcium binding to BSA to equilibrate free calcium at approximately 2 mM. Glucose (11 mM) is added to the modified KHB solution the next day, just prior to use. Hormones or drugs such as insulin, leptin, adiponectin, or catecholamines that may influence cardiac metabolism can then be added to the buffer at this point, prior to heart perfusions as described [4,5].

Radioactively labeled energy substrates

Anaerobic and oxidative metabolic flux is measured through the addition of radioactive-labeled energy substrates to the KHB solutions, which are subsequently metabolized by the different metabolic pathways (Figure 37.2). All isotopes are obtained from Perkin Elmer. Glycolytic flux is determined by measuring the amount of ^{3}H$_2$O released from the metabolism of 5-[^{3}H]glucose (specific activity = 400 Mbq/mol) by the triosephosphate isomerase and enolase steps of the glycolytic pathway. Glucose oxidation is determined by trapping and measuring ^{14}CO$_2$ released by the metabolism of [U-^{14}C]glucose (specific activity = 400 Mbq/mol). The ^{14}CO$_2$ released during glucose oxidation (pyruvate dehydrogenase and tricarboxylic acid cycle) is trapped using 1 M hyamine hydroxide (Figure 37.1) [6]. The total amount of ^{14}CO$_2$ released during glucose oxidation is the sum of that recovered from the exhausted gas passing through the oxygenator, and that liberated as bicarbonate from samples of the buffer solution.

Metabolic Pathways

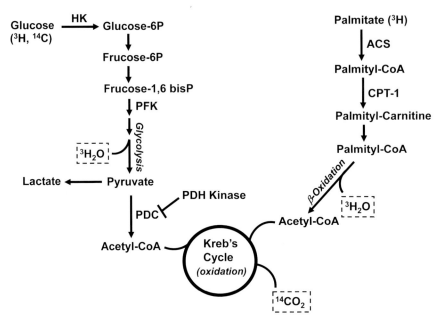

Figure 37.2 Metabolic pathway showing metabolism of radioactively labeled substrates into radioactive metabolites (dashed boxes). ACS, acyl-CoA synthetase; CPT-1, carnitine palmitoyl transferase isoform 1; HK, hexokinase; PDC, pyruvate dehydrogenase complex; PDH kinase, pyruvate dehydrogenate kinase; PFK, phosphofructokinase.

Palmitate oxidation is determined by measuring the amount of ^3H_2O released from 9,10-[^3H] palmitate (specific activity = 18.5 GBq/mol). While radioactively labeled glucose can be added to the KHB solution at any time, the radioactively labeled palmitate must be added during the initial step where palmitate is bound to BSA prior to dialysis. In general, either glucose metabolism (glycolysis and glucose oxidation) or oxidative metabolism (glucose and palmitate oxidation) can measured simultaneously in a single experimental run due to the different sources of metabolic signal (^3H_2O vs. $^{14}CO_2$), which can be physically separated from each other [7].

The ^3H_2O produced from glycolysis is separated from 5-[^3H]glucose and [U-^{14}C]glucose in the KHB solution samples through anion exchange resin (200–400 mesh Dowex 1-X4, obtained from Sigma) pretreated with 0.4 M potassium borate to activate the resin enabling it to bind glucose and allowing the ^3H_2O to flow through. Although the Dowex resin retains approx. 99% of glucose, a small amount

of 5-[^3H] glucose that passes through the resin contributes to the ^3H signal. To correct for this, the assay takes advantage of measuring the amount of [U-^{14}C] glucose that also passes through the resin as an internal standard to calculate the amount of contaminating 5-[^3H] glucose in the sample. As a result, the contribution of 5-[^3H] glucose to the ^3H_2O signal can be factored out.

The $^{14}CO_2$ released from glucose oxidation but retained in KHB solution as bicarbonate is released inside a sealed metabolic flask when combined with 9 N H_2SO_4 and trapped in a center well containing filter paper soaked in 300 μL of hyamine hydroxide. The ^3H_2O derived from the oxidation of palmitate can be separated from 9,10-[^3H]palmitate through a Bligh and Dyer extraction of polar and nonpolar substances [6]. If glucose oxidation is measured in the same preparation, the KHB solution sample must be passed through the anion exchange resin as outlined earlier, prior to the polar/ nonpolar extraction. After the extraction of metabolites from parent compounds, aliquots are counted using standard scintillation counting techniques, with ^3H_2O samples being counted using a water-soluble scintillation cocktail such as Ecolite (MP Biomedicals), and hyamine hydroxide samples using a scintillation cocktail such as CytoScint (MP Biochemicals). Calculations for converting counts per minute (CPM) or disintegrations per minute (DPM) values obtained from scintillation counting into metabolic rates have been published [8].

Experimental protocol

Once the heart is fully cannulated for the working heart mode, the Langendorff perfusion line is closed and the preload and aortic lines are opened. It may take the heart between 1 and 5 minutes to establish a stable heart rate and achieve constant flow through the afterload line. Once a steady heart rate and afterload flow is achieved, the heart is sealed within the perfusion apparatus to begin metabolic measurements. Any $^{14}CO_2$ evolving from the system as a result of gas exchange in the oxygenator is collected by bubbling the oxygen outflow through 15 mL of hyamine hydroxide (ICN, Irvine, CA). A total modified KHB solution of 35–50 mL is generally sufficient to permit analysis of metabolism in working mode for 60 minutes. At 20-minute intervals (starting at time = 0 min), a 2.5-mL sample of perfusate is withdrawn through an injection port mounted between the perfusate reservoir and the oxygenator (Figure 37.1). The perfusate samples are stored in scintillation vials under a 2-mL layer of paraffin oil to prevent the loss of $^{14}CO_2$. Up to 1 mL of the sample is injected into metabolic flasks containing an equal volume of 9 N H_2SO_4, while up to 0.5 mL of the remaining sample is used to measure glycolytic flux or fatty acid metabolism depending on experimental conditions. At the end of the experiment, the hearts are quickly frozen between metal blocks cooled in liquid N_2, weighed, and stored at −80°C. A sample of heart tissue (approx. 20 mg) is cut from the heart, weighed (wet wt), and then dried to remove all water (dry wt). The ratio of this sample (dry/wet wt) is used to calculate the total dry mass of the heart. Metabolic rates are calculated using the total dry mass of the heart to correct for variations in heart size. Alternately, metabolic rates can be normalized to cardiac power output (systolic pressure × cardiac output) to correct for variations in contractile performance [7].

Measuring myocardial oxygen consumption (MVO$_2$)

The development of flexible, fiber-optic oxygen (O_2) sensing probes has provided the ability to determine oxygen consumption rates in isolated working hearts and to use this data to determine cardiac efficiency. In perfused hearts, oxygenated buffer enters the coronary circulation at the coronary ostia in the aortic root. Oxygen is then extracted by the myocardium and the venous effluent enters the right atrium via the coronary sinus. Coronary sinus effluent can be collected in a sealed capillary tube [5] or can be cannulated directly with the fiber-optic O_2 sensing probe [9]. Prior to each experiment, the probe is calibrated in buffer preoxygenated with 100% O_2 (= 100), and with buffer containing a saturated solution of sodium hydrosulfite, which is an oxygen chelator (= 0).

The following formulae are used to determine myocardial oxygen consumption, cardiac hydraulic work, and cardiac efficiency:

$$MVO_2 \; (\mathbf{mL/min/g \; WHW}) = ((PaO_2 - PvO_2)/100)$$
$$\times (coronary \; flow/WHW) \times (725/760) \times (1000 \times C);$$

where C = Bunsen coefficient for plasma (i.e. 0.0212), PaO_2 = arterial partial pressure of oxygen and PvO_2 = venous partial pressure of oxygen (both in mmHg), 725 and 760 are atmospheric pressures at the University of Utah and at sea level, respectively (mmHg) and WHW is the wet heart weight in grams (g).

Cardiac hydraulic work (J/min/g WHW)
$$= CO \, (mL/min) \times DevP \, (mmHg)$$
$$\times 1.33 \times 10^{-4}/g \; WHW;$$

where CO = cardiac output and DevP = developed pressure.

Cardiac efficiency (%)
$$= hydraulic \; work/MVO_2 \times 100.$$

MVO$_2$ (mL/min) was converted to μmol/min by multiplying by the conversion factor 0.0393, and then to Joules (J/min) using the conversion of 1 μmol O_2 = 0.4478 J, as described by Suga [10].

Applications of this approach

Most groups have used this technique to measure glucose and fatty acid oxidation in aerobic perfused hearts. The set-up is not amenable to low-flow ischemia experiments. However, no-flow ischemia can be induced by discontinuing the pump for variable periods of time up to 20 minutes. Metabolic measurements are not possible during the ischemic period, but data measurements can resume upon re-perfusion. Other groups have used this technique to measure the relationship between cardiac work and metabolism. Metabolic work jumps are achieved by increasing the afterload, which is achieved by increasing the height of the afterload column; this can be combined by injecting an inotrope such as isoproterenol into the buffer reservoir. Finally, some groups have incorporated intraventricular catheters to obtain pressure–volume relationships at various workloads and to determine oxygen consumption in arrested hearts, which has provided insight into the oxygen cost for contraction and noncontractile functions in the heart.

Limitations and alternative approaches

A limitation of this approach is that it measures the rate of oxidation of exogenous substrates and does not allow for determination of oxidation rates of endogenous substrates such as glycogen or triglycerides. Furthermore, *in vivo* the majority of fatty acids that are oxidized by the heart are derived from lipolysis of triglyceride (TG) rich lipoprotein particles. Thus perfusing hearts with albumin-bound palmitate might not recapitulate the *in vivo* delivery of TG-derived lipids to the hearts, which are governed in part by the activity of lipoprotein lipase. Some groups have addressed this issue by perfusing hearts with radiolabeled chylomicrons. The second limitation is that the approach is limited by the fact that metabolism rates are limited in a given experiment to one ^{3}H and one ^{14}C-labeled substrate. Thus glycolysis and glucose oxidation or palmitate oxidation and glucose oxidation can be determined in a single heart but not all three pathways. Therefore it is often necessary to increase the number of hearts analyzed in groups by specific substrate pairs. Oxygen consumption cannot be measured when isotopes that are dependent on the release of $^{13}CO_2$ are being perfused, to minimize atmospheric loss. This means that in practice MVO_2 and cardiac efficiency is only measured during experiments in which palmitate oxidation rates are

being measured in hearts perfused with ^{3}H palmitate. Alternative approaches that enable the tracing of multiple metabolic pathways in the same heart, rates of metabolism of endogenous substrates, or flux rates of specific pathways such as anaplerosis can be achieved by perfusing hearts with deuterated substrates and analyzing their enrichment by NMR or mass spectrometry.

Conclusions

The isolated working mouse heart preparation is a technically challenging technique that has been used to shed important insights into the regulation of substrate metabolism in mouse hearts isolated from mice with a variety genetic mutations, cardiac hypertrophy, heart failure, metabolic disease such as diabetes and obesity, under conditions of normoxia or following ischemia and reperfusion. Despite the limitations of this approach, it provides a general measure of metabolic rates of major metabolic pathways that are utilized by the heart, and will provide an adequate index of substrate metabolism in the heart at a relatively low cost compared to approaches that rely on deuterated substrates. As our understanding of metabolic regulation in the heart becomes more sophisticated, it is anticipated that there will be an ongoing need for use of these protocols by many research groups to screen mutant mouse strains for metabolic phenotypes [9].

References

1 Neely JR, Morgan HE. Regulation of cardiac metabolism. A study of the isolated perfused rat heart as a model in the regulation of heart metabolism. *Penn Med* 1968; **75**: 57–61.

2 Larsen TS, Belke DD, Sas R, Giles WR, Severson DL, Lopaschuk GD, *et al.* The isolated working mouse heart: methodological considerations. *Pflugers Arch* 1999; **437**: 979–985.

3 Belke DD, Larsen TS, Lopaschuk GD, Severson DL. Glucose and fatty acid metabolism in the isolated working mouse heart. *Am J Physiol* 1999; **277**: R1210–1217.

4 Fang X, Palanivel R, Cresser J, Schram K, Ganguly R, Thong FS, *et al.* An APPL1-AMPK signaling axis mediates beneficial metabolic effects of adiponectin in the heart. *Am J Physiol Endocrinol Metab* 2010; **299**: E721–729.

5 Mazumder PK, O'Neill BT, Roberts MW, Buchanan J, Yun UJ, Cooksey RC, *et al.* Impaired cardiac efficiency

and increased fatty acid oxidation in insulin-resistant ob/ob mouse *Hearts Diabetes* 2004; **53**: 2366–2374.

6 Saddik M, Lopaschuk GD. Myocardial triglyceride turnover and contribution to energy substrate utilization in isolated working rat hearts. *J Biol Chem* 1991; **266**: 8162–8170.

7 Belke DD, Swanson E, Suarez J, Scott BT, Stenbit AE, Dillmann WH, *et al*. Increased expression of SERCA in the hearts of transgenic mice results in increased oxidation of glucose. *Am J Physiol Heart Circ Physiol* 2007; **292**: H1755–1763.

8 Barr RL, Lopaschuk GD. Direct measurement of energy metabolism in the isolated working rat heart. *J Pharmacol Toxicol Methods* 1997; **38**: 11–17.

9 How OJ, Aasum E, Larsen TS. Work-independent assessment of efficiency in ex vivo working rodent hearts within the PVA-MVO2 framework. *Acta Physiol* 2007; **190**: 171–175.

10 Suga H. Ventricular energetics. *Physiol Rev* 1990; **70**: 247–277.

Quantification and characterization of atherosclerotic lesions in mice

Abhinav Agarwal, Millicent G. Winner, Srinivas D. Sithu, and Sanjay Srivastava

University of Louisville, Louisville, KY, USA

Introduction

Cardiovascular disease is the leading cause of death worldwide. In 2010, one in four deaths was due to ischemic heart disease or stroke [1]. Atherosclerosis is the underlying cause of most of the ischemic diseases, including ischemic heart disease and stroke. It is a chronic inflammatory disease that develops slowly under the influence of genetic and environmental factors [2–4]. The most common risk factor for the development of atherosclerosis is hypercholesterolemia. Hypercholesterolemia results in excessive vascular accumulation of lipoproteins (Figure 38.1). Repeated failure of innate immune responses to clear subintimal low-density lipoprotein (LDL) results in the deposition of lipid-engorged macrophages, creating a nidus of expanding inflammation. Increased recruitment of smooth muscle cells into the lesions and deposition of fibrous tissues forms advanced plaques, which diminish luminal flow. Often, due to repeated erosion or acute fission, the plaque ruptures, leading to rapid intravascular thrombosis and a profound obstruction of blood flow.

Atherosclerosis is a highly complex and multi-factorial disease. Consequently, susceptibility to atherosclerosis in any given individual is determined by genetic risk factors, in concert with life style and diet [5]. In humans as well as in experimental animals, elevated plasma cholesterol is one of the most potent risk factors for atherosclerosis. In the apolipoprotein E (ApoE)-null mice, the lack of ApoE, which is a ligand for lipoprotein recognition and clearance by the lipoprotein receptor, results in delayed clearance of lipoproteins, and the mice develop a phenocopy of human type III hyperlipidemia with severe cholesterolemia on a normal chow diet due to the accumulation of chylomicrons and VLDL remnant lipoproteins [6,7]. Cholesterol levels in these mice are 400 to 600 mg/dL, as compared to <100 mg/dL in wild type mice. As they age, the ApoE-null mice develop atherosclerotic lesions spontaneously; the rate of atherogenesis is enhanced further by a western diet (42% fat, Harlan Laboratories diet TD88137), higher cholesterol (HF/HC) diet, which increases their cholesterol to ≥1000 mg/dL. The process of atherogenesis in these mice resembles the human disease in location, severity, and stage-specific progression. Similarly, pathological changes have been observed in the LDL receptor (LDLR)-null mice, which are a model of familial hyper-cholesterolemia [7]. On a normal chow diet, the LDLR-deficient mice develop moderate hyper-cholesterolemia with cholesterol levels around 250 mg/dL, due primarily to the accumulation of LDL cholesterol. The LDLR-null mice do not develop significant atherosclerotic lesions on normal chow diet. However, they are extremely sensitive to diet-induced hypercholesterolemia and in response

Manual of Research Techniques in Cardiovascular Medicine, First Edition. Edited by Hossein Ardehali, Roberto Bolli, and Douglas W. Losordo.
© 2014 John Wiley & Sons, Ltd. Published 2014 by John Wiley & Sons, Ltd.

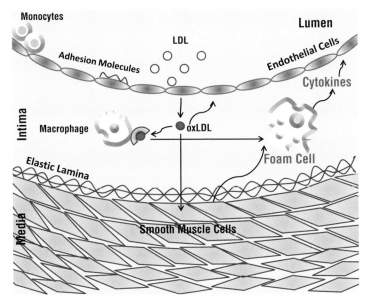

Figure 38.1 Fatty streak formation in the subendothelial space.

to western and HF/HC diet they display ≥1000 mg/dL serum cholesterol and robust atherosclerotic lesions throughout the aortic tree. Described below are the protocols to study atherogenesis in mice:

Protocols

Pathological screening of mice

To examine the contribution of genes of interest in atherogenesis, transgenic or knockout mice are generated on pro-atherogenic ApoE-null or LDLR-null background. Similarly, to examine the effect of a pharmaceutical agent or a toxicant, mice are exposed to that chemical for a prolonged period of time. Pathological screening of mice is performed as described [8–11]. Described below are the protocols for the factors that directly affect atherogenesis in mice.

Plasma lipoprotein analyses

Preparation of plasma.

1. At the completion of desired protocols, fast the mice for 16 hours.

2. Withdraw 1.0 mL blood by heart puncture using a tuberculin syringe with a 20-gauge needle containing 15 μL of 0.2 M EDTA (tetra sodium salt dihydrate).

3. Remove the needle and gently transfer the blood to a 2.0-mL plastic tube.

4. Centrifuge the blood at 500 g for 15 minutes at room temperature.

5. Aspirate the supernatant into a separate tube and centrifuge at 6000 g for 10 minutes at 4°C to obtain clear plasma.

Plasma cholesterol and triglycerides. Measure cholesterol and triglycerides level in the plasma on Cobas-Mira Plus automated chemistry analyzer, using commercial kits from Wako Chemicals Inc. (Ritchmond, VA) as per manufacturer's instructions [8–11].

Separation of lipoproteins. Cholesterol distribution in the lipoproteins is assessed by size-exclusion chromatography using a Superose 6B™ 100/300 GL column (Pharmacia LKB Biotechnology Inc.) attached to a Biorad Biologic Duo Flow FPLC (fast protein liquid chromatography) system.

1. Prepare the mobile phase (10 mM potassium phosphate, pH 7.4 containing 150 mM sodium chloride, 1 mM EDTA and 0.05% sodium azide).

2. Equilibrate the column overnight with the mobile phase at a flow rate of 0.5 mL/min.

3. Inject 100 μL plasma on to the column.

4. Elute the column with the mobile phase (isocratic) at a flow rate of 0.5 mL/min.

5. Collect fractions every minute for 30 minutes using a fraction collector.

6. Measure cholesterol and triglycerides in each fraction using the Wako kit.

NMR analysis of lipoproteins. Particle size and abundance of subclasses of lipoproteins are analyzed by NMR as described before [9,11].

Atherosclerotic lesion analyses

Mice on ApoE-null or LDLR-null background are weaned at 3 weeks of age and maintained on normal chow (NC). To measure baseline lipid profile, 50 μL blood is collected from the tail vein. At 10–12 weeks of age ApoE-null mice begin to display lipid deposition in the aortic valve and by 16–20 weeks of age visible lesions are observed in the aortic arch and the innominate artery (Figure 38.2). Subsequently, with time, lesions develop in the thoracic and

abdominal aorta. Described below are the protocols for the various processes involved in the etiology of atherogenesis and quantification and characterization of atherosclerotic lesions in mice.

Endothelial activation

The endothelium is a critical regulator of lesion formation and progression. The primary initiating event in lesion formation in the atherosclerotic mice is the accumulation of LDL in the subendothelial matrix in proportion to the circulating levels of LDL, which diffuse passively through the endothelial junctions and is retained in the vessel wall by the interactions between the apoB of the LDL particle and the matrix proteoglycans [12,13]. In the intima, LDL and related apoB containing proteins, such as lipoprotein(a), undergo a series of modifications including oxidation, lipolysis, proteolysis, and aggregation, of which lipid peroxidation is believed to be the key transformation that renders the intimal LDL atherogenic. Oxidized LDL (oxLDL)

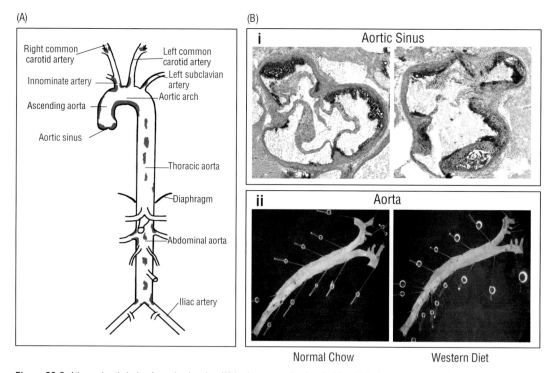

Figure 38.2 Atherosclerotic lesion formation in mice. (A) Lesion-prone sites (marked in red) in the mouse aorta. (B) Atherosclerotic lesion formation in the aortic sinus (i) and the aorta (ii) of apoE-null mice. Eight-week-old apoE-null mice were either maintained on normal chow, or fed western diet for 12 weeks. Mice were euthanized at 20 weeks of age and atherosclerotic lesion formation was examined. Lipids were stained with Oil Red O in the aortic sinus and Sudan IV in the aorta.

has proinflammatory properties. The proinflammatory properties of oxLDL, cause an increased generation of adhesion molecules and growth factors, such as macrophage colony-stimulating factor (M-CSF), in the overlying endothelium. Increased expression of adhesion molecules on endothelial cells facilitates adhesion of monocytes to the endothelium and their transmigration to the subendothelial space. In the subendothelial space the monocytes differentiate into macrophages, which express scavenger receptors for the uptake of oxLDL. This results in the formation of lipid-laden foam cells, which release proinflammatory cytokines, which in turn cause endothelial activation and smooth muscle cell proliferation (Figure 38.1). Described below are the protocols to examine endothelial activation.

Quantification of the expression of adhesion molecules

Aorta is pulverized and the powder is suspended in Lamelli buffer without glycerol. Expression of adhesion molecules is measured on western blots using anti-ICAM-1 [14] and anti-VCAM-1 [15] antibodies. The expression of ICAM-2, which does not change with atherosclerosis, diet, age, or cytokine stimulation [16], is used as a negative control. The steady-state levels of the mRNA for these adhesion molecules are measured by quantitative PCR. For the immunohistochemical analysis of adhesion molecules, sections of the innominate arteries and the aortic sinus are stained with appropriate antibodies (anti-ICAM-1, anti-VCAM-1, etc). Staining with anti-IgG1 or anti-IgG2 is used as a negative control. To minimize nonspecific staining, it is preferable to use fluorescence-tagged primary antibodies. A total of three or four serial sections from each animal are stained and analyzed by digital image analysis to quantify the extent of staining.

Complementary cellular studies are performed in cultured endothelial cells (mouse aortic endothelial cells, C57-6052, Cell Biologics, Inc. Chicago, IL; human aortic endothelial cells, CC-2535, Lonza, Walkersville, MD; and human umbilical vein endothelial cells (HUVEC), CC-2517, Lonza, Walkersville, MD) to obtain mechanistic insight about the reagents of interest on endothelial activation. Described below are the protocols for the measurement of markers of endothelial activation in HUVEC.

Surface expression of adhesion molecules

1. Incubate HUVEC in culture with reagents of interest (TNFα, LPS, oxLDL, etc.) for appropriate amount of time.

2. After washing cells with phosphate buffered saline (PBS), harvest cells in 5 mM EDTA and fix in 2% cold paraformaldehyde solution for 20 minutes.

3. Block cells with 1% bovine serum albumin-PBS for 30 minutes on ice.

4. Incubate cells with anti-ICAM-1 antibody (559047, clone LB-2 from BD Biosciences, San Jose, CA) for 1 hour on ice.

5. After incubation, pellet the cells by centrifugation and resuspend in PBS containing an Alexa488 conjugated anti-mouse IgG (A-11001 from Invitrogen, Grand Island, NY), and incubate for an additional 30 minutes.

6. After washing, analyze the fluorescence property of these cells using a flow cytometer (LSR II flow cytometer, BD Biosciences). Cells stained with an isotype control antibody are used to detect background staining, and the mean fluorescence intensity of these samples is subtracted from the mean fluorescence intensity of anti-ICAM-1-stained cells [17].

Monocyte adhesion assay

1. Culture HUVEC (5×10^4 cells) for 24 hours in 96-well plates and incubate with reagents of interest (TNFα, LPS, oxLDL, etc.) in endothelial cell culture medium for 18 hours.

2. Differentiate THP-1 cells (dTHP-1; human acute monocytic leukemia cell line, TIB-202; American Type Culture Collections, Manassas, VA) into macrophage-like cells by growing in 0.5 mM of dibutyryl cAMP (D0627; Sigma, St. Louis, MO) for 72 hours. Freshly isolated monocytes can also be used for monocyte adhesion assays. However, unlike THP-1 cells, primary cells do not have to be differentiated.

3. Label differentiated dTHP-1 cells with calcein acetoxymethyl ester (Invitrogen) (10 μM; 30 minutes at 37°C).

4. Allow dTHP-1 cells (5×10^4 cells/well; 1 hour at 37°C in HBSS with 0.1% glucose) to adhere to the endothelial monolayer in the presence Ca^{2+}/Mg^{2+}(1 mM).

5. Wash unadhered dTHP-1 cells thoroughly with PBS

6. Measure the adhesion of dTHP-1 cells to HUVEC using a florescent plate reader at 485 nm/530 nm [17]. Use wells with only endothelial cells to subtract background fluorescence.

Monocyte transmigration assay

Transmigration of differentiated monocytic THP-1 through the endothelial cells is measured as described before [17]. Similar method can be adapted for mouse cells.

1. Seed endothelial cells (4×10^4) on polycarbonate microporous membranes of 6.5 mm diameter and 5 μm pore size in Transwell chambers (Costar, Cambridge, MA) precoated with human fibronectin (10 μg/mL) at 37°C for 2 hours.

2. Allow the cells to grow in endothelial growth medium for 3–4 days.

3. Incubate with reagents of interest on endothelial monolayer on transwells.

4. Prior to monocyte transmigration assay, transfer transwells to a new 24-well plate with fresh growth media containing Ca^{2+}/Mg^{2+} (1 mM).

5. Differentiate THP-1 cells into macrophages as described earlier.

6. Add monocytic cells such as dTHP-1 cells (5×10^4 cells/transwell) in DMEM containing Ca^{2+}/Mg^{2+}(1 mM) and allow to transmigrate for 6 hours.

7. Collect the migrated monocytic cells. Detach monocytes attached to the bottom of the transwells with 5 mM EDTA in DMEM (15 minutes at 4°C), and then count under a light microscope.

Intravital microscopy

Intravital microscopy is used to study the leukocyte adhesion to the endothelium *ex vivo* [17].

1. For these assays, administer animals with reagent of interest or vehicle.

2. After appropriate time, anesthetize the animals with sodium pentobarbital.

3. Cannulate the trachea and the carotid artery to maintain airway patency and to directly monitor blood pressure, respectively.

4. Prepare the cremaster muscle for *in vivo* microcirculatory observation, positioned over an optic port in a specially designed plexiglass bath.

5. Fill the bath with modified Kreb's solution that is maintained at a temperature of 35 ± 0.5°C and a pH of 7.4 ± 0.5. The animal or the tissue bath is placed on the modified stage of a Nikon MM-11 microscope so that the microcirculation can be observed by transillumination of the cremaster muscle (a similar approach can be used for bigger vessels, like carotid artery).

6. Use closed-circuit television microscopy to observe and quantify the diameters of single, unbranched third-order venules that have basal diameters of 25–35 μm. Calibrate the video system with a stage micrometer, and measure the vessel diameters with a video caliper.

7. Measure the adhesion interactions between leukocytes and the vascular endothelium by quantifying the number of transiently (rolling) and firmly (sticking) adherent leukocytes.

8. Determine leukocyte rolling by counting the number of leukocytes passing an arbitrary reference point, and quantify leukocyte adhesion by counting, for each vessel, the number of adherent leukocytes in a 100-μm length.

Platelet activation and atherosclerosis

Blood platelets are the primary cells that initiate coagulation to prevent excessive blood loss due to vessel injury. We and others have shown that platelet activation could be involved in atherogenesis [9,18,19]. In humans, adherence of platelets to the damaged endothelium increases thrombus formation, accelerates atherogenesis, and increases the risk of ischemic heart disease. Studies in atherogenic mice suggest that deficiency of P-selectin, which enhances platelet–endothelial interaction, diminishes atherosclerotic lesion formation [18]. Massberg *et al.*, have shown that in apoE-null mice maintained on a western diet, platelet adhesion in the carotid artery precedes leukocyte adhesion, suggesting that platelets play a pivotal role in early atherosclerotic lesion formation [19]. Recently, we have shown Platelet factor 4 (PF-4) released from activated platelets causes endothelial activation and exacerbates atherosclerosis in ApoE-null mice [9,20].

Described below are the protocols for measuring platelet activation.

Isolation of platelets

1. Anesthetize the mice with sodium pentobarbital (0.1 mL; 50 mg/kg, i.p) and collect the blood from the heart using 1:9 (v/v) trisodium citrate (4%) as anti-coagulant.

2. Centrifuge the blood at 180 g for 20 minutes at 22°C. Aspirate the supernatant–platelet rich plasma (PRP) and centrifuge at 1000 g for 10 minutes at 4°C to sediment platelets.

3. Transfer the supernatant–platelet poor plasma (PPP) to a fresh tube.

4. Adjust the platelet count in the PRP to 3×10^8 cells/mL using PPP.

5. To obtain washed platelets (WP), wash the platelets three times with Tyrode buffer (137 mM NaCl; 20 mM HEPES, 1 mM $MgCl_2$, 2.7 mM KCl, 3.3 mM NaH_2PO_4, 5.6 mM glucose, 0.1% BSA, pH 7.4) and reconstitute in Tyrode buffer at a density of 3×10^8 cells/mL.

Platelet activation

Platelet aggregation. Platelet aggregation is a commonly used assay to assess platelet activation *in vitro* or *ex vivo* in response to agonists. Platelet aggregation is measured using a four-channel platelet aggregometer (Chrono-log Corp, Havertown, PA).

1. Incubate the PRP (adjusted to 3×10^8 cells/mL) for 2 minutes at 37°C with continuous stirring at 1000 rpm, and then stimulate with agonists such as adenosine 5′-diphosphate (ADP; 10 μM).

2. Measure the aggregation for 5 minutes by following change in light transmittance [20,21].

3. For measuring platelet aggregation in washed platelets, add $CaCl_2$ (2 mM) and fibrinogen (200 μg/mL) to the platelet suspension prior to the stimulation with ADP.

Platelet–leukocyte aggregates. Measurement of platelet–leukocyte aggregates *ex vivo* reflects platelet activation *in vivo* because activated platelets show enhanced propensity to bind blood cells or endothelial cells of the blood vessels. For these assays:

1. Collect the blood by heart puncture in Na_4·EDTA (0.2 M; 15 μL/mL blood).

2. Dilute aliquots of whole blood (100 μL) with 400 μL HEPES-Tyrode, pH 7.4, and fix the samples in 1% formaldehyde for 30 minutes at 4°C.

3. Lyze the red cells by dilution in water.

4. Collect the cells by centrifugation at 400 g for 8 minutes, wash with HEPES-Tyrode, pH 7.4, containing 1% BSA, and stain with FITC-labeled anti-CD41 and APC-labeled anti-CD11b or isotype matched controls for 30 minutes on ice [20].

5. Analyze the stained cells on a BD LSR II Flow Cytometer (BD Biosciences). For each sample, collect a minimum of 10,000 events. Platelet–leukocyte aggregates are defined as those events that are positive for both platelets and leukocytes and expressed as a percentage of total events.

Platelet–fibrinogen binding

Platelet–fibrinogen binding is another assay to assess platelet activation *in vivo*. While CD41 is the α subunit of the CD41/CD61 complex (GPIIb–IIIa; a noncovalently associated heterodimer), the activated CD41/CD61 complex is a receptor for soluble fibrinogen and plays a pivotal role in platelet aggregation and vascular hemostasis [20,22,23].

1. Incubate aliquots of blood (100 μL) with PE-labeled rat-anti-mouse CD41 antibody for 20 minutes at room temperature.

2. Dilute the samples with 4 volumes of HEPES-Tyrode solution and incubate with Alexa-flour488 fibrinogen (20 μg/mL) for 10 minutes at room temperature.

3. Fix the samples with paraformaldehyde (2%) for 20 minutes.

4. Lyze erythrocytes by adding 4.6 volumes of distilled water.

5. Centrifuge at 1000 g for 8 minutes, and wash the pellet with HEPES-Tyrode, pH 7.4 containing 0.1% D-glucose and 0.1% BSA (FACS buffer).

6. Resuspend the pellet in FACS buffer (1.0 mL) and analyze by flow cytometry [20].

Platelet factor 4 (PF-4) assay

Plasma PF-4 levels are assayed by a sandwich ELISA using DeoSet Mouse PF-4/CXCL4 ELISA kit (R&D Systems, Minneapolis, MN) according to the manufacturer's instructions.

1. Coat ELISA plates (96-wells) with a rat anti-mouse PF-4 capture antibody ($2\,\mu g/mL$ in PBS) for 16 hours at room temperature.
2. Wash the wells free of the unbound antibody and block with 1% BSA for 1 hour at room temperature.
3. Incubate the plasma samples or the PF-4 standards in the coated wells for 2 hours at room temperature.
4. Wash the wells three times and incubate with a biotinylated goat anti-mouse PF-4 antibody (100 ng/mL) for 2 hours at room temperature.
5. Wash the wells again and incubate with streptavidin conjugated to horseradish peroxidase for 20 minutes at room temperature. Repeat the washing step, add the substrate, tetramethylbenzidine (TMB) and incubate for 15 minutes.
6. Stop the reaction with $1\,N\,H_2SO_4$ and measure the developed color using a microplate reader at 450 nm.

Macrophages and atherosclerosis

Macrophages are key cellular elements in the pathogenesis of atherosclerotic plaques [24]. They play an essential role in all phases of atherogenesis. Fatty streaks, which are the earliest grossly visible vascular lesions, consist mainly of macrophages that have taken up massive amounts of cholesterol. Macrophages are also key determinants of plaque stability and rupture [25]. The importance of macrophages in atherogenesis is underscored by the observation that macrophage-deficient mice are resistant to atherosclerotic lesion formation [26]. Although the demonstrable ability of macrophages to accumulate cholesterol has attracted the most attention, macrophages could contribute to plaque pathogenesis by secreting inflammatory cytokines, which induce endothelial dysfunction and smooth muscle cell death, and matrix metalloproteases (MMPs), which could degrade extracellular matrix and cause plaque rupture. Described below are the protocols to elucidate the contribution of macrophage-derived foam cells in atherosclerosis.

Quantification of lipid laden lesions in the aorta

1. Remove the entire aorta from the heart, extending to the iliac arteries and including the subclavian right and left common carotid arteries and rinse with phosphate-buffer saline (PBS).
2. Remove periadventetial tissue under the dissecting microscope and cut the aortic arch and the distal aorta longitudinally to expose the intimal surface.

3. Pin the tissue *en face* on wax and stain the lipids with Sudan IV as described below:
   a. Incubate the enface aorta with 5 mg/mL Sudan IV (Sigma) in 15-cm dishes containing black wax in 70% isopropanol for 1 hour at room temperature.
   b. Remove excess dye by rinsing two times with 70% isopropanol.
   c. Rinse the aorta with PBS and acquire digital images.
4. Calculate percent lesion area by measuring the total surface area of the aorta and Sudan IV positive staining, using Metamorph 4.5 software [8–11].

Analysis of lesion formation in the aortic sinus

1. Freeze the upper half of the heart in OCT reagent.
2. Cut 8-μm thick cryosections from the origin of the aortic valve leaflets, throughout the aortic sinus as described by Paigen *et al.* [27].
3. Collect 9–12 serial sections from each mouse per slide.
4. Stain the slides with Oil Red O to detect the lipid deposition in these sections.

Protocol for oil red O staining

1. Bring the slides to room temperature and allow them to air dry for 15 minutes.
2. Place the slides in formalin for 10 minutes at room temperature. Remove excess formalin by rinsing in distilled water.
3. Place the slides in propylene glycol (Poly Scientific s264-32oz) for 2 minutes. Remove excess propylene glycol.
4. Incubate slides in filtered Oil Red O (0.5% in propylene glycol; Poly Scientific s-1848-32 oz) overnight at room temperature.
5. Pour off excess Oil Red O.
6. Place slides in propylene glycol (85% in distilled water) for 1 minute.
7. Thoroughly rinse excess propylene glycol with distilled water.
8. Stain the slides with filtered Mayer's modified hematoxylin (Poly Scientific s216-32 oz) for 30 seconds and rinse with running distilled water for 3 minutes.
9. Coverslip the slides with aqueous mounting medium (DAKO Faramount Aqueous Mounting Medium S3025).

10. Acquire digital images and calculate mean lesion area by quantifying total lesion area and Oil Red O positive area, using Metamorph 4.5 software.

Foam cell formation *in vitro* in macrophages

Complementary *in vitro* studies are performed to examine foam cell formation.

Oil Red O staining for foam cells:
1. Seed murine bone marrow-derived macrophages in four well chamber slides (150,000 cells per chamber) for 24 hours.
2. Incubate the cells with 0–50 μg/mL acetylated LDL (Ac LDL) or oxidized LDL (oxLDL) for 24–48 hours in lipoprotein-deficient RPMI 1640 medium.
3. Wash the cells with PBS and fix in formalin.
4. Stain the lipids with Oil Red O for 30 minutes followed by a wash with 60% isopropanol.
5. Counterstain the cells with hematoxylin. Acquire digital images and quantify Oil Red O staining by Metamorph.

Analysis of foam cell formation by fluorescence assisted cell sorting (FACS):
1. Seed bone marrow-derived macrophages in 12-well dish (1 × 10⁶ cells/well) in RPMI media supplemented with 1% penicillin/ streptomycin.
2. After 24 hours, add fresh media containing AcLDL or oxLDL (0–50 μg/mL) and incubate the cells for 24–48 hours.
3. Remove excess AcLDL/oxLDL and incubate the cells with Nile Red (100 ng/mL; Invitrogen, Carlsbad, CA) for 15 minutes.
4. Quantify lipid uptake by FACS [11]. A minimum of 10,000 events are measured.

Bone marrow transplantation studies to examine the contribution of macrophages in atherosclerosis

Bone marrow transplant studies are performed to specifically examine the contribution of macrophages or other hematopoietic cells, in mice of genotype of interest, to atherogenesis.

1. Subject 8-week-old male recipient LDLR-null mice to 950 cGy total body irradiation from a cesium source (Gamma-cell 40; Nordion, Ontario, Canada).
2. Twenty-four hours after irradiation, transplant mice with bone marrow cells (1 × 10⁷ cells/ mouse in 0.1 mL PBS) isolated from tibias and femurs of syngenic 8 to 12-week-old male experimental or corresponding wild type mice, through the retro-orbital plexus with 27-gauge needle.
3. After 4 weeks, confirm depletion of circulating cells and reconstitution of donor cells in all chimeric mice by PCR of blood genomic DNA. Collect blood through retro-orbital plexus with 27-gauge needle and extract DNA using QIAamp DNA Micro Kit (Qiagen). Perform PCR using PCR Master Mix (Promega Kit) and a set of three primers that amplify sequence either from the wild type or LDLR-knockout allele.
4. Characterize recipient mice for hematopoietic recovery by measuring cell surface markers of T cells (CD3), B cells (B220), granulocytes (Gr-1), and monocytes (CD11b), using FACS.

Mice with 85% or greater chimerism in the peripheral blood are used for further experiments. These mice are then placed on western diet for 8–12 weeks and atherosclerotic lesions are analyzed.

Characterization of lesion composition and nature

In atherosclerotic disease deposition of fat in the vessel wall narrows the lumen and eventually leads to the blockage of the blood flow. In humans the first stage of atherosclerosis comprises fatty-streak formation, which is characterized by lipid-laden macrophages in the subendothelial space. The second stage of lesions consists of fibrous plaques, comprising of smooth muscle cells and collagen. The third stage is thrombus formation with deposition of platelets, fibrin etc. A small unstable plaque rich in lipid-loaded macrophages and covered by a thin fibrous cap is more likely to rupture than a large stable plaque. The rupture of unstable plaques, especially coronary lesions, leads to morbidity and mortality. Atherosclerotic lesions in mice are similar to humans in many ways; however, lesions in mice usually do not rupture. Nonetheless, the composition and nature of the plaque are important determinant of plaque stability. Plaque composition, environment, and nature are usually examined in the aortic sinus or the innominate artery, as lesions is these sites are well defined and consistent. Composition of the lesion is examined by staining with Sirius Red to visualize collagen. Lesion cellularity is established by immunohistochemical staining for macrophages (MOMA-2), smooth muscle cells (α-smooth muscle actin), and T-lymphocytes (CD3) [10,11]. Appropriate nonimmune serum is used in place of the primary antibody as a negative control. The threshold is predetermined and remains the same for all the analyzed sections. The digital images are analyzed by a blinded observer [8–11]. The nature of the lesions is established by examining multiple parameters, including apoptosis, inflammation, etc. Described below are the protocols for establishing lesion cellularity and nature.

Sirius Red staining to visualize collagen
1. Fix air-dried slides containing frozen sections of aortic sinus in formalin for 10 minutes at room temperature. Remove excess formalin by rinsing with distilled water.
2. Place the slide in Picro-Sirius Red working solution (0.003%) (Sirius Red F3b, Raymond Lamb Inc.) for 1 hour at room temperature.
3. Dip the slide in 0.5% glacial acetic acid several times to achieve desired staining and remove acidified water from the slide by vigorously shaking.
4. Place slides in absolute ethanol for 30 seconds.
5. Repeat Step 4.
6. Place the slides in xylene for 30 seconds, with three changes and coverslip with Permount

Immunohistochemical staining for macrophages using anti-CD-68 antibody
1. Air dry slides of aortic sinus for 45 minutes at room temperature.
2. Place the slides in ice-cold acetone for 30 minutes for penetration of antibodies into the section.
3. Rinse the slides with Tris-buffered saline (TBS; 0.05 M Tris, pH 7.6 containing 1.5% NaCl) three times for 5 minutes each.
4. Incubate the slides in 10% fetal calf serum (FCS) in TBS for 30 minutes.
5. Drain the excess FCS and incubate the slides with 100 µL of the Alexa Fluor 647-conjugated anti CD-68 antibody (MCA 1957A647 from AbD Serotec, Raleigh, NC) at a 1:50 dilution in TBS containing 1% FCS overnight at 4°C.
6. Rinse the slides with TBS, three times of 5 minutes each.
7. Add DAPI (1 µg in 10 µL) to each slide and incubate for 15 minutes at room temperature.

8. Rinse sections with TBS three times for 5 minutes each.
9. Dip the slides in distilled water to remove the salts from buffer solution before mounting.
10. Drain the water from slides. Coverslip slides with a drop of mounting medium (e.g. Invitrogen's Slowfade Gold).
11. Cure the slides for 24 hours at room temperature. Acquire digital images.

Similar procedure is used for immune staining with anti-α-smooth muscle actin (Abcam), anti-CD3 (BD biosciences) antibodies or any other antibody of interest. Immunohistochemical approach is also used to examine lesion inflammation using antibodies raised against various cytokines and chemokines (IL6, MCP-1, etc). Quantitative PCR is used to measure the steady-state levels of the cytokines and chemokines in the aorta. Expression of MMP-3 and MMP-9 is measured in the frozen sections by zymography. Levels of MMP-3 and MMP-9 are also measured in the plasma by ELISA as indices of plaque stability.

Lesional apoptosis
In Situ Cell Death Detection Kit, Fluorescein (Roche Applied Science, Indianapolis, IN; Cat no. 11684795910) was used according to manufacturer's instructions to detect apoptosis in atherosclerotic lesions in frozen aortic sinus sections. It is based on the detection of single- and double-stranded DNA breaks that occur at the early stages of apoptosis. Apoptotic cells are fixed and permeabilized. Subsequently, the cells are incubated with the TUNEL reaction mixture that contains TdT and fluorescein-dUTP. During this incubation period, TdT catalyzes the addition of fluorescein-dUTP at free 3′-OH groups in single- and double-stranded DNA. After washing, the label incorporated at the damaged sites of the DNA is visualized by fluorescence microscopy.

1. Air dry the frozen tissue sections for 45 minutes.
2. Fix with 4% paraformaldehyde for 20 minutes at room temperature.
3. After washing with PBS (15 minutes, two times), incubate the slides with freshly prepared permeabilization solution (0.1% Triton-X in PBS) for 2 minutes on ice.
4. Wash the slides with PBS (15 minutes, two times).

5. Add TUNEL reaction mixture to the tissue sections and incubate in humidified atmosphere for 60 minutes at 37°C.

6. Wash the slides with PBS (15 minutes, two times).

7. Stain the nucleus with DAPI for 15 minutes.

8. Wash the slides (PBS, four times).

9. Cover slip the slides with a drop of Slow Fade Gold Reagent (Invitrogen) and observe under a fluorescent microscope using an appropriate filter. The apoptotic cells appear green.

Weaknesses and strength of the methods

Lesions in atherosclerotic mice

Mice are useful models to study chronic disease like atherosclerosis because their small size permits better quantification of atherosclerotic lesions, their use in sufficient numbers allows meaningful statistical comparison, and they are available with defined genetic backgrounds amenable to genetic changes. For the last two decades, LDLR-null and ApoE-null mice have been extensively used to study atherogenesis [6,28,29], because lesions in these mice resemble several features of atherosclerosis in humans. However, several drawbacks and limitations have also been noted with the murine models of atherosclerosis:

• Most of the atherosclerosis studies in ApoE-null mice are strain-dependant and ApoE-null mice on different backgrounds vary in plasma cholesterol levels as well as location and extent of lesion formation [30].

• Atherogenesis in humans is a slow chronic process and it takes several decades for the lesions to develop. However, in mice, atherosclerotic lesions develop at a significantly accelerated rate, and the process is further augmented by HF-diet. ApoE-null or LDL receptor-null mice maintained on western or HF/HC diet for 6–12 weeks develop profound lesions, especially in the aortic roots. Therefore, temporally, lesion formation in mice is distinctly different than humans.

• Since mice are small in size, it is very difficult to analyse lesion formation in them by ultrasound methods.

• Atherosclerosis in the coronary artery is the leading cause of morbidity and mortality in humans. However, atherogenic mice (LDLR-null and ApoE-null mice) have only sparse lesions (foam cells) in the coronary artery.

• In humans, atherosclerotic lesions erode and rupture. In contrast, murine lesions do not rupture.

Procedural problems

Measurement of cholesterol in the plaque. Staining with dyes like Oil Red O, Nile Red, or Sudan IV, while informative, is semiquantitative as measurements depend on a number of factors including the exposure time, washing, and quality of reagents.

Immunohistochemical analysis. Most of the lesion characterization is performed by immunohisto-chemical analysis. These assays are heavily dependent on the specificity of the antibody and even in the best case scenario, provide a semiquantitative analysis.

Contribution of a specific cell type to atherogenesis. It has been quite challenging to examine the contribution of various cell types present in the vessel wall or atherosclerotic plaque to the etiology of the disease. Cell-specific knockout mice have been made, however, often the promoter is leaky or is also expressed in other cells. For the contribution of macrophages to lesion formation, bone marrow transplant is extensively used. However, contribution of other hematopoietic cells in plaque formation in bone marrow-transplanted mice cannot be ruled out.

Alternative approaches

New models of atherosclerosis. Several investigators have developed other animal models of atherosclerosis which include, rats, rabbits, pigs, and nonhuman primates. However, similar to mice, lesions in these models are distinctly different than humans in location, extent, composition, and nature [31]. Therefore, new animal models of atherosclerosis resembling atherosclerosis in humans are urgently needed. Recently, we established a new LDLR-null rat model of atherosclerosis in which the LDLR is deleted by zinc finger nuclease technology. Plasma cholesterol level in these rats is threefold higher than the corresponding wild-type rats. Moreover, these rats are obese and insulin resistant. When maintained on HF diet (42% fat) for 34–52 weeks, these rats display atherosclerotic lesions throughout the aortic tree. Similarly, we observed that ApoE-null rats are hypercholesterolemic and when maintained on HF-diet for 28–42 weeks, they develop atherosclerotic lesions throughout the aorta. Composition and nature of atherosclerotic lesions in ApoE-null and LDL-null rats is being examined in our laboratory. Nonetheless, since these rats display multiple risk factors for atherosclerosis in humans, we expect them to be an improvement over the existing models of atherosclerosis in mice and other experimental animals. Moreover, since these rats are quite big (>1 kg) it is possible to perform ultrasound and angiographic studies to examine lesion size and location in live animals.

Measurement of cholesterol in the plaque. Mass spectrometry can also be used to measure cholesterol levels in the plaque. Mass spectroscopic methods are more quantitative than staining the plaques for neutral lipids. Moreover, it also provides information about the esterified and nonesterified cholesterol in the plaque.

Immunohistochemical analysis. Whenever possible, for example protein modifications in the lesions, mass spectrometry should be used as a complementary approach. For cells abundant in the plaques such as macrophages, it is recommended to digest the plaques to isolate macrophages and then perform appropriate measurement by FACS. Several laboratories have successfully adapted this approach to study the role of macrophages in atherogenesis.

Bone marrow transplant experiment. For bone marrow transplant experiments, a more useful approach will be to generate knockout mice, using for example the CD-68 promoter, and then perform the bone marrow transplant experiment. This will eliminate the contribution of CD-68 in nonhematopoietic cells on atherogenesis.

Conclusions

Atherogenic mice such as ApoE-null and LDLR-null mice are useful models to study certain features of atherosclerotic lesions in humans, or to examine the effect of pharmaceutical agents and toxicants on atherogenic processes. However, there remain a variety of limitations with these models. A number of procedural and technical complications also need

to be resolved. Emerging new experimental models in the field and technical advancement for the quantification and characterization of atherosclerotic disease in experimental animals are urgently needed.

References

1 Lozano R, Naghavi M, Foreman K, Lim S, Shibuya K, Aboyans V, *et al*. Global and regional mortality from 235 causes of death for 20 age groups in 1990 and 2010: A systematic analysis for the global burden of disease study 2010. *Lancet* 2012; **380**: 2095–2128.

2 Glass CK, Witztum JL. Atherosclerosis. The road ahead. *Cell* 2001; **104**: 503–516.

3 Libby P. Inflammation in atherosclerosis. *Arterioscler Thromb Vasc Biol* 2012; **32**: 2045–2051.

4 Rader DJ, Daugherty A. Translating molecular discoveries into new therapies for atherosclerosis. *Nature* 2008; **451**: 904–913.

5 Smithies O. Many little things: One geneticist's view of complex diseases. *Nat Rev Genet* 2005; **6**: 419–425.

6 Breslow JL. Mouse models of atherosclerosis. *Science* 1996; **272**: 685–688.

7 Fazio S, Linton MF. Mouse models of hyperlipidemia and atherosclerosis. *Front Biosci* 2001; **6**: D515–525.

8 Baba SP, Barski OA, Ahmed Y, O'Toole TE, Conklin DJ, Bhatnagar A, *et al*. Reductive metabolism of age precursors: A metabolic route for preventing age accumulation in cardiovascular tissue. *Diabetes* 2009; **58**: 2486–2497.

9 Srivastava S, Sithu SD, Vladykovskaya E, Haberzettl P, Hoetker DJ, Siddiqui MA, *et al*. Oral exposure to acrolein exacerbates atherosclerosis in apoe-null mice. *Atherosclerosis* 2011; **215**: 301–308.

10 Srivastava S, Vladykovskaya E, Barski OA, Spite M, Kaiserova K, Petrash JM, *et al*. Aldose reductase protects against early atherosclerotic lesion formation in apolipo-protein e-null mice. *Circ Res* 2009; **105**: 793–802.

11 Srivastava S, Vladykovskaya EN, Haberzettl P, Sithu SD, D'Souza SE, States JC, *et al*. Arsenic exacerbates atherosclerotic lesion formation and inflammation in apoe-/- mice. *Toxicol Appl Pharmacol* 2009; **241**: 90–100.

12 Lusis AJ. Atherosclerosis. *Nature* 2000; **407**: 233–241.

13 Ross R. The biology of atherosclerosis. In: Topol EJ, ed. *Comprehensive Cardiovascular Medicine*. Philadelphia: Lippincott-Raven, 1998, pp. 13–26.

14 Park JG, Yoo JY, Jeong SJ, Choi JH, Lee MR, Lee MN, *et al*. Peroxiredoxin 2 deficiency exacerbates atherosclerosis in apolipoprotein e-deficient mice. *Circ Res* 2011; **109**: 739–749.

15 Matsui R, Xu S, Maitland KA, Mastroianni R, Leopold JA, Handy DE, *et al*. Glucose-6-phosphate dehydrogenase

deficiency decreases vascular superoxide and atherosclerotic lesions in apolipoprotein e(-/-) mice. *Arterioscler Thromb Vasc Biol* 2006; **26**: 910–916.

16 Hajra L, Evans AI, Chen M, Hyduk SJ, Collins T, Cybulsky MI, *et al*. The nf-kappa b signal transduction pathway in aortic endothelial cells is primed for activation in regions predisposed to atherosclerotic lesion formation. *Proc Natl Acad Sci USA* 2000; **97**: 9052–9057.

17 Vladykovskaya E, Sithu SD, Haberzettl P, Wickramasinghe NS, Merchant ML, Hill BG, *et al*. Lipid peroxidation product 4-hydroxy-trans-2-nonenal causes endothelial activation by inducing endoplasmic reticulum stress. *J Biol Chem* 2012; **287**: 11398–11409.

18 Manka D, Collins RG, Ley K, Beaudet AL, Sarembock IJ. Absence of p-selectin, but not intercellular adhesion molecule-1, attenuates neointimal growth after arterial injury in apolipoprotein e-deficient mice. *Circulation* 2001; **103**: 1000–1005.

19 Massberg S, Brand K, Gruner S, Page S, Muller E, Muller I, *et al*. A critical role of platelet adhesion in the initiation of atherosclerotic lesion formation. *J Exp Med* 2002; **196**: 887–896.

20 Sithu SD, Srivastava S, Siddiqui MA, Vladykovskaya E, Riggs DW, Conklin DJ, *et al*. Exposure to acrolein by inhalation causes platelet activation. *Toxicol Appl Pharmacol* 2010; **248**: 100–110.

21 Srivastava S, Joshi CS, Sethi PP, Agrawal AK, Srivastava SK, Seth PK, *et al*. Altered platelet functions in non-insulin-dependent diabetes mellitus (niddm). *Thromb Res* 1994; **76**: 451–461.

22 D'Souza SE, Ginsberg MH, Burke TA, Plow EF. The ligand binding site of the platelet integrin receptor

gpiib-iiia is proximal to the second calcium binding domain of its alpha subunit. *J Biol Chem* 1990; **265**: 3440–3446.

23 D'Souza SE, Ginsberg MH, Matsueda GR, Plow EF. A discrete sequence in a platelet integrin is involved in ligand recognition. *Nature* 1991; **350**: 66–68.

24 Yan ZQ, Hansson GK. Innate immunity, macrophage activation, and atherosclerosis. *Immunol Rev* 2007; **219**: 187–203.

25 Li AC, Glass CK. The macrophage foam cell as a target for therapeutic intervention. *Nat Med* 2002; **8**: 1235–1242.

26 Smith JD, Trogan E, Ginsberg M, Grigaux C, Tian J, Miyata M, *et al*. Decreased atherosclerosis in mice deficient in both macrophage colony-stimulating factor (op) and apolipoprotein e. *Proc Natl Acad Sci USA* 1995; **92**: 8264–8268.

27 Paigen B, Morrow A, Holmes PA, Mitchell D, Williams RA. Quantitative assessment of atherosclerotic lesions in mice. *Atherosclerosis* 1987; **68**: 231–240.

28 Getz GS, Reardon CA. Diet and murine atherosclerosis. *Arterioscler Thromb Vasc Biol* 2006; **26**: 242–249.

29 Getz GS, Reardon CA. Animal models of atherosclerosis. *Arterioscler Thromb Vasc Biol* 2012; **32**: 1104–1115.

30 Maeda N, Johnson L, Kim S, Hagaman J, Friedman M, Reddick R, *et al*. Anatomical differences and atherosclerosis in apolipoprotein e-deficient mice with 129/svev and c57bl/6 genetic backgrounds. *Atherosclerosis* 2007; **195**: 75–82.

31 Xiangdong L, Yuanwu L, Hua Z, Liming R, Qiuyan L, Ning L, *et al*. Animal models for the atherosclerosis research: A review. *Protein Cell* 2011; **2**: 189–201.

Assessment of cell death in the heart

Russell S. Whelan, Klitos Konstantinidis, and Richard N. Kitsis

Albert Einstein College of Medicine, Bronx, NY, USA

Introduction

Apoptosis and necrosis are the principal means by which cardiomyocytes die in various heart diseases. Moreover, each of these forms of cell death has been shown to play critical roles in the pathogenesis of myocardial infarction and heart failure [1–3]. Apoptosis and necrosis differ in their morphological characteristics and are mediated by distinct, but intertwined, pathways. Although both processes ultimately result in cardiomyocyte death, they differ with respect to the collateral damage inflicted on the adjacent myocardium. Differences in signaling and effects on tissue architecture, and their implications for the development of potential anti-cell death therapies, provide a strong rationale for understanding apoptosis and necrosis both as individual processes and with respect to their combined effects on cardiomyocyte loss.

Death pathways

Apoptosis

Apoptosis is a highly regulated process that results in cell death and clearance without significant inflammation in the surrounding tissue. The primary effectors of this form of cell death are a class of proteases known as caspases [4]. Caspases are cysteine proteases that cleave specific proteins following aspartic acid residues. They exist as pro-enzymes (called procaspases) and become activated through a variety of mechanisms. Upstream pro-

caspases are activated primarily through induced proximity following their recruitment into multiprotein complexes (Figure 39.1). In contrast, downstream procaspases are activated by cleavage carried out by upstream caspases [5]. The downstream caspases go on to proteolyze a spectrum of cellular proteins – both structural and regulatory – to bring about the apoptotic death of the cell. At the morphological level, apoptosis is characterized by cellular shrinkage, fragmentation into apoptotic bodies, and phagocytosis of these corpses. These events take place with maintenance of plasma membrane/apoptotic body membrane integrity, thereby minimizing an inflammatory response and damage to adjacent tissue.

Activation of caspases during apoptosis occurs by two pathways: the extrinsic pathway, which is initiated by the binding of "death ligands" to cell surface "death receptors"; and the intrinsic pathway, which involves the mitochondria and endoplasmic reticulum. Both extrinsic and intrinsic apoptosis pathways have been shown to play important roles in cardiac disease[3].

The extrinsic pathway is activated by specialized ligands, some soluble and some present on the surface of other cells. The binding of ligand to receptor leads to formation of a multiprotein complex known as the DISC (death inducing signaling complex), within which procaspase-8, an upstream procaspase, is activated [6]. Caspase-8 then cleaves and activates downstream procaspases-3 and -7, which subsequently cut cellular proteins to bring about apoptotic cell death.

Manual of Research Techniques in Cardiovascular Medicine, First Edition. Edited by Hossein Ardehali, Roberto Bolli, and Douglas W. Losordo.

(A)

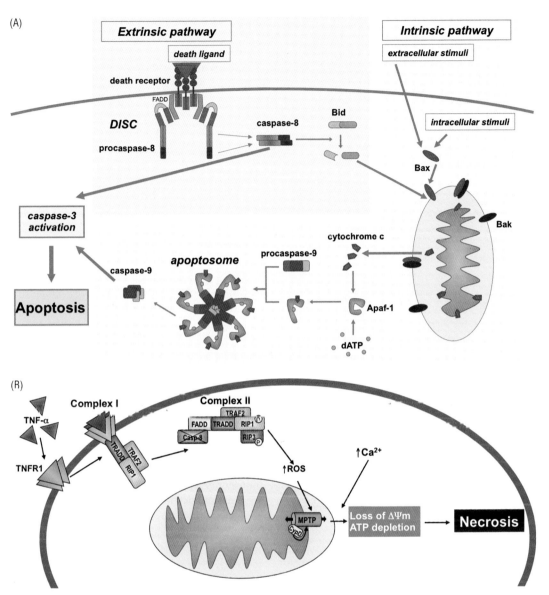

Figure 39.1 Apoptotic and necrotic pathways. (A) Apoptosis. Apoptosis is mediated by a proteolytic cascade involving caspases. The extrinsic apoptosis pathway is initiated by ligand binding to death receptors, which initiates the formation of a multiprotein complex called the death inducing signaling complex (DISC), in which procaspase-8 is activated. Caspase-8 then cleaves and activates procaspase-3, which itself proteolyzes cellular substrates to bring about apoptosis. The intrinsic apoptosis pathway integrates a wide variety of stimuli to induce Bax conformational activation and translocation to the mitochondria, resulting in permeabilization of the outer mitochondrial membrane (OMM) and cytochrome *c* release (see text). Cytochrome *c* in the cytosol triggers formation of the apoptosome, a multiprotein complex, in which procaspase-9 is activated. Caspase-9 subsequently cleaves and activates procaspase-3. Bid, a proteolytic substrate of caspase-8, connects the extrinsic and intrinsic apoptosis pathways. (B) Necrosis. The extrinsic necrosis pathway is illustrated by TNFα, which triggers formation of complex I. Complex I can promote survival through the activation of NF-κB (not shown). The conversion of complex I to cytosolic complex II (see text) signals cell death. Apoptosis results from the recruitment and activation of procaspase-8 in complex II. If caspase-8 is inhibited, necrosis results. Necrosis is dependent on phosphorylation events involving RIP1/3. The intrinsic necrosis pathway is mediated by opening of the mitochondrial permeability transition pore (MPTP) in the inner mitochondrial membrane (IMM). Opening of this pore precipitates immediate loss of the electrical potential across the IMM ($\Delta\Psi$m) (resulting in cessation of ATP synthesis) and influx of water into the mitochondrial matrix (resulting in mitochondrial swelling). The generation of ROS may connect extrinsic and intrinsic necrosis pathways.

In contrast, the intrinsic pathway is activated by a wider spectrum of death inducers. Extracellular stimuli include deficits in nutrients and survival factors, ischemia, and the presence of noxious stimuli such as reactive oxygen species (ROS) and UV radiation. Intracellular stimuli include ROS, proteotoxic stress, and DNA damage. These stimuli are relayed via a variety of pathways to Bax, a proapoptotic member of the Bcl-2 family. Once stimulated, Bax undergoes conformational activation, translocates from the cytosol to the mitochondria, and inserts into the outer mitochondrial membrane (OMM). Within this membrane, Bax, and the related protein Bak, undergo a complex series of homo- and hetero-oligomerization events that lead to permeabilization of the OMM, the defining event in apoptosis in the intrinsic pathway [7]. OMM permeabilization results in the release of several apoptogens, including cytochrome c. In the cytosol, cytochrome c triggers formation of the apoptosome, a multiprotein complex in which procaspase-9, another upstream procaspase, undergoes activation [8]. Caspase-9 then cleaves and activates downstream procaspases-3 and -7, resulting in apoptosis.

Programmed necrosis

In contrast to the morphological features of apoptosis, cells undergoing necrosis exhibit defects in plasma and organelle membrane integrity resulting in severe cellular and organelle swelling. A second feature of necrosis is marked deficits in ATP stores, resulting both from inadequate production and unrestrained consumption. Finally, necrosis is characterized by marked inflammation and damage to surrounding tissues. Because of these morphological and biochemical features, necrosis has traditionally been considered a passive process in which overwhelming environmental injury kills the cell. Work over the past 10–15 years, however, has shown that a significant proportion of necrotic deaths are, in fact, actively regulated (sometimes referred to as "programmed necrosis"). While the pathways that mediate necrosis are not as well fleshed out as those for apoptosis, it is clear that both death receptors and mitochondria are involved.

Necrosis mediated by death receptors (often called necroptosis) will be referred to herein as the extrinsic necrosis pathway [9,10]. This pathway is best illustrated by TNFα signaling. The binding of TNFα to TNF receptor 1 triggers the formation of complex I at the cell membrane, which includes the receptor and the serine/threonine kinase RIP1. Complex I can signal cell survival through a series of events that leads to NF-κB activation. However, the internalization of complex I combined with dissociation of the TNF receptor and deubiquitination of RIP1 results in formation of complex II in the cytosol, which signals cell death. The recruitment and activation of procaspase-8 in complex II results in the cleavage of downstream procaspases and apoptosis. Caspase-8 also precludes necrotic cell death by cutting RIP1 and RIP3 (another serine/threonine kinase), both of which are required for necrosis. When caspase-8 is inhibited, however, apoptosis does not take pace, RIP1 and RIP3 remain intact, and necrosis ensues. Necrosis in this setting involves a complex series of phosphorylation events involving RIP1 and RIP3. An understanding of the signaling events downstream of complex II remains murky, but some of these events (such as the production of ROS, as shown in Figure 39.1) likely connect the extrinsic necrosis pathway to the intrinsic necrosis pathway [11–13].

The intrinsic necrosis pathway involves the mitochondria [14]. The defining event is opening of an inner mitochondrial membrane (IMM) pore called the Mitochondrial Permeability Transition Pore (MPTP). Normally closed, this pore prevents the entry of ions (even protons), solutes, and water across the IMM into the mitochondrial matrix. This tight regulation is necessary to maintain $\Delta\Psi_m$, the electrical gradient across the IMM that drives ATP generation. In response to a necrotic stimulus, such as Ca^{2+}, the MPTP opens, an event that is sensitized by ROS. The consequences of MPTP opening include rapid dissipation of $\Delta\Psi_m$ (crippling ATP synthesis) and the influx of water into solute-rich mitochondrial matrix (resulting in mitochondrial swelling). While the core components of the MPTP are not known, positive regulators include cyclophilin D in the mitochondrial matrix and the adenine nucleotide translocase in the IMM.

Thus, the initial events in apoptosis and necrosis at the mitochondria appear to occur at two different membranes: opening on the MPTP in the IMM in necrosis and permeabilization of the OMM in apoptosis. The time scales for these events often differ as well. For example, Ca²⁺ elicits rapid opening of the MPTP in necrosis, while permeabilization of the OMM in apoptosis usually proceeds with slower kinetics. In contrast to the extrinsic pathway, the mechanisms that decide whether apoptosis or necrosis will take place at the mitochondria are not understood. It is clear, however, that necrosis and apoptosis signaling at this organelle are interconnected. For example, the early opening of the MPTP in necrosis that precipitates mitochondrial swelling sometimes leads to overt rupture of the OMM resulting in cytochrome *c* release and caspase activation. Conversely, activation of caspases in apoptosis may elicit necrosis by cleaving substrates in the IMM that trigger MPTP opening [15].

Caveats for the assessment of cell death in experimental models

Apoptosis and necrosis can be assessed using multiple assays that measure a wide range of parameters, including morphology, pathway activation, and terminal effects of these death processes (Table 39.1). These assays have varying sensitivities and specificities for the different forms

of cell death. Given that apoptotic and necrotic cells often co-exist in the same tissue, it is important to employ multiple modalities to be able to characterize the magnitude of each form of cell death with confidence.

Moreover, in light of numerous connections between apoptosis and necrosis signaling pathways, it is critical to assess a range of time points with each assay in order to delineate the initiating mode of cell death. Regarding this last point, special care must be taken when studying cell death *in vitro*, where there is no mechanism to clear apoptotic corpses. In contrast to *in vivo*, cells undergoing apoptosis in culture will eventually manifest plasma membrane breakdown and appear necrotic. Therefore, studies in cell culture must include early time points, and very late time points should be avoided, if possible. Model stimuli of the various death pathways provide useful positive controls (Table 39.2).

Another caveat pertaining to *in vitro* experiments is that cell death is usually accompanied by detachment from the plate. Discarding detached cells may result in underestimates of cell death and/or incorrect assessment of the modality of cell death.

Table 39.1 Important features of assays in apoptosis and necrosis

Assays	Apoptosis	Necrosis
Morphology (light/electron microscopy)	Cell shrinkage and fragmentation, chromatin condensation with margination, plasma membrane blebbing	Cell swelling, organelle swelling, loss of plasma membrane integrity
Caspase activation (e.g. western blots, immunostaining, substrate assays)	Present	Not classically present, but may occur following OMM rupture
TUNEL	Present (reflects downstream caspase activation)	Usually TUNEL negative, but can occur if caspases are activated by OMM rupture
Phosphatidylserine externalization (annexin V)	Annexin V-positive with intact plasma membrane integrity (PI negative)	Annexin V and PI positive
Propidium iodide staining (microscopy or flow cytometry)	PI excluded, (Late in cell culture PI may become positive)	PI staining occurs early
Extracellular release of cytosolicproteins (e.g. LDH, TnI)	Absent	Present
MPTP opening/loss of ΔΨₘ (e.g. TMRE)	Absent or occurs late *following* cytochrome *c* release	Occurs early

Table 39.2 Model stimuli for various death pathways

Apoptosis		Necrosis	
Intrinsic	Extrinsic	Intrinsic	Extrinsic
Staurosporine	Agonistic Fas Ab	Ionomycin	TNF-α + ZVAD with or without Smac mimetics
Etoposide	TNFα + cyclohexamide		

Accordingly, care should be taken to minimize disruption of cells during treatment and analysis. In addition, collection of both adherent and detached cells can be performed in some studies, and is described in further detail below.

Apoptosis

Caspase activation

Caspase activation can be assessed by procaspase cleavage. The rationale is that downstream caspases are activated by cleavage, and although cleavage is not the activating event for upstream caspases, it eventually occurs and provides a marker of activation.

Caspase cleavage is often assessed by immuno-blotting of cell/tissue lysates, although this can be challenging in mouse tissues because of the available antibodies. A variation of this approach is immunostaining of cells/tissues with antisera that recognize neoepitopes in active caspases that are revealed by the cleavage event.

Another approach to assess caspase activation is to measure the enzymatic activity of caspases in cell/tissue lysates using artificial tetrapeptide substrates that are relatively specific for that caspase. When artificial substrate assays are employed, an assessment of activation over time is preferable to measuring activity at a single time point. In addition, the use of artificial substrates to measure the activity of a given caspase may be more informative than the use of "specific" caspase inhibitors, which may not be specific at higher concentrations.

Another approach to measuring caspase activation is to assess cleavage of endogenous substrates. Thus, activation of procaspases-3/7 can be assessed by cleavage of PARP (poly (ADP-ribose) polymerase) [16](Figure 39.2). Activation of procaspase-8 can be assessed by cleavage of Bid (see Figure 39.1).

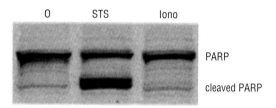

Figure 39.2 PARP cleavage. PARP is a known substrate of caspases-3/7. Induction of apoptosis with staurosporine (STS) results in the cleavage of PARP. In contrast, PARP cleavage is not observed when ionomycin is used to induce necrosis.

Using combinations of these approaches at early time points in apoptosis, one can determine whether the extrinsic pathway (cleavage of procaspase-8 and Bid) or the intrinsic pathway (cleavage of procaspase-9) is taking place. Activation of procaspases-3/7 is a measure of the final common pathway of caspase activation. A caveat is that late in the time course of apoptosis, connections between extrinsic and intrinsic pathways and feedback loops may obscure these readouts.

- Grow cells of interest in appropriate culture dish.
- Treat cells as desired.
- Following treatment with appropriate stimuli, wash cells once with PBS. Some death stimuli will promote detachment of cells from culture surface. Care should be taken minimize cell loss in this manner. If cell loss is a persistent issue, earlier time points or lower doses of the death stimulus can be employed.
- Administer sufficient lysis buffer (20 mM Tris-HCl, 150 mM NaCl, 2 mM EDTA, 1% Triton X-100, protease inhibitors) to cover the culture plate and incubate on ice for 5–10 minutes.
- Scrape plate gently with a cell scraper and collect in a 1.7-mL centrifuge tube.
- Sonicate these cells on ice for 2 × 5 second bursts at low intensity.

- Following sonication, spin the lysates down at 18,000 rcf for 10 minutes at 4°C.
- Collect the supernatant and measure the protein concentration by BCA or Lowry assay.
- Load equal amounts of protein (typically 15–30 μg is sufficient) onto a 10% acrylamide SDS-PAGE gel and run at 100 V for 1 hour to resolve bands in the 50–150 kDa range.
- Transfer to a nitrocellulose membrane using a wet apparatus for 60 minutes at 100 V–300 mA.
- Incubate in blocking buffer for 1 hour at room temperature.
- Incubate shaking overnight at 4°C with primary antibody (PARP [Cell Signaling]); in blocking buffer with 0.1% Tween-20.
- Wash and incubate with secondary antibody and visualize by enhanced chemiluminescence or fluorescence.

TUNEL

TUNEL is frequently used to assess apoptosis in cells/tissues. The cleavage of nuclear DNA during apoptosis is mediated by caspase-3-dependent events. TUNEL (terminal deoxynucleotidyl transferased UTP nick end labeling) is the principal technique to detect nuclear DNA degradation in cells/tissues. This assay reflects the abundance of free 3′hydroxyl groups made available by DNA cleavage during apoptosis [17]. TUNEL is more sensitive than analysis of DNA laddering by agarose gel electrophoresis. This protocol is based on that provided with the Roche TUNEL staining kit (*In Situ* Cell Death Detection Kit, TMR red), with alterations to improve staining in cardiac tissue samples.

- Fix hearts in 10% neutral buffered formalin for 24 hours at 25°C. Transfer hearts to 70% ethanol, paraffin embed for section preparation and slicing.
- Incubate paraffin-embedded slides at 65°C for 1 hour to remove excess paraffin and allow to cool at 25°C for 1 hour.
- Deparaffinize tissue section with serial washes: 3 × 5 minute xylene, 2 × 1 minute 100% EtOH, 2 × 1 minute 95% EtOH, 2 × 1 minute 70% EtOH, 2 × 1 minute PBS.
- Submerge slides in Antigen Retrieval Solution at 100°C for 30 minutes.
  - Antigen Retrieval Solution: 2.5 mL Antigen Unmasking Solution (Vector Laboratories-H-3300) in 250 mL dH$_2$O.

- Cool at 4°C for 10 minutes.
- Wash slides for 5 minutes in 1 × PBS.
- Wash slides for 5 minutes in 1 × PBS with 0.01% Triton (500 mL PBS + 50 μL triton).
- Incubate with Proteinase K at 20 μg/mL for 15 minutes at 25°C.
  - Proteinase K solution: 100 μL of Proteinase K (Millipore, 21627, 200 μg/mL) 900 μL of DNAse, RNAse free distilled water
- Wash 2 × 3 minutes in 1 × PBS. Perform the rest of the protocol in the dark.
- Mix the reaction mixtures as per Roche protocol, adding DNAse to the positive control.
- Cover each sample with 50–100 μL, enough to amply cover the tissue section, and incubate for 1 hour at 37°C in the dark.
- Wash slides 3 × 3 minutes in 1 × PBS.
- Block for 1 hour at 25°C with 10% goat serum in 1 × PBS/0.01% Triton.
- Keep incubation chamber well hydrated to prevent tissues from drying out.
- Counterstain for cardiomyocytes by incubating with primary antibody (Troponin I [Santa Cruz], 1:50 dilution in blocking solution) overnight at 4°C.
- Wash 2 × 3 minutes in 1 × PBS.
- Wash 1 × 5 minutes in PBS/0.01% Triton.
- Incubate with secondary antibody (1:1000) for 1 hour at 25°C.
- Wash 3 × 5 minutes in PBS/0.01% triton.
- Mount and coverslip slides using a medium containing DAPI (VECTASHIELD Vector Laboratories) and analyze slides by fluorescent microscopy.

Notes. TUNEL, which indicates activation of downstream procaspases-3/7, is taken as synonymous with apoptosis, and it is a good indicator of this process. However, if mitochondrial swelling during necrosis results in OMM rupture and cytochrome *c* is released, downstream procaspases may be activated, resulting in positive TUNEL staining.

Cytochrome *c* release

Cytochrome *c* release from the mitochondria to cytosol is a key event in the intrinsic apoptosis pathway. The method described below employs subcellular fractionation and subsequent immunoblot analysis (Figure 39.3).

(A)

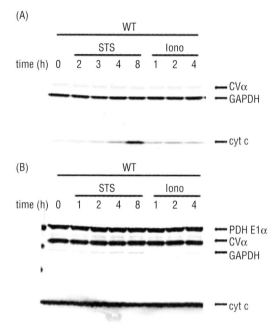

(B)

Figure 39.3 Cytochrome *c* release. (A) Cytosolic fraction. Cytochrome *c* is present in the cytoplasm of cells treated with the apoptosis inducer staurosporine (STS). In contrast, cytochrome *c* is not released into the cytoplasm after treatment of cells with ionomycin (Iono) to induce necrosis. Cytosolic fractions were blotted with both cytosolic (GAPDH) and mitochondrial (CVα) markers to determine fractional purity. (B) Mitochondrial fraction. The mitochondrial fraction should also be blotted for cytochrome *c* as well as both mitochondrial (PDH E1α and CVα) and cytosolic (GAPDH) markers. Reciprocal loss of cytochrome *c* may or may not be observed.

Digitonin lysis buffer. 10 mM KCl, 5 mM MgCl$_2$, 1 mM EDTA, 1 mM EGTA, 250 mM sucrose, 20 mM HEPES pH 7.2, 0.025% Digitonin (from 5% w/v stock solution), complete protease inhibitors. The lysis buffer can be made as a stock, but digitonin should be added immediately prior to mitochondrial isolation.
• Plate 5×10^5 cells in a 6-cm diameter dish for each sample the evening prior to experimentation. Use 2 mL of media for each 6-cm dish.
• When treating cells, pre-mix the desired stimulus with media warmed to 37°C. Gently replace the original media with the stimulus-containing media to minimize disruption to the cells. Do NOT add treatment directly to culture plates, as this does not provide a homogeneous treatment across the plate.
• For positive controls, treat with a necrotic (ionomycin, 10 μM) or apoptotic (staurosporine, 1 μM) stimulus.
• Harvest cells, including floating cells. Collect the media in a 15-mL tube. Wash the plate with PBS and collect the PBS in the same 15-mL tube. Add 0.5 mL trypsin for 5–10 minutes. Confirm cell detachment by microscopic examination. Add 1 mL of media to neutralize trypsin, and add the total volume (1.5 mL) to the 15-mL tube.
• Spin down at 500 rcf for 5 minutes at 4°C. Discard the supernatant. Wash cell pellet 1× with PBS. Spin down again at 500 rcf for 5 minutes at 4°C.
• Resuspend pellet in 100 μL Digitonin lysis buffer. Incubate for 5 minutes on ice.
• Immediately spin down lysate at 15,000 rcf for 10 minutes at 4°C.
• Transfer supernatant to a new tube. The supernatant is the cytosolic fraction.
• Lyse pellet in 100 μL PBS + 1% Triton X-100 + complete protease inhibitors, on ice for 1 hour.
• Spin down pellet at 15,000 rcf for 10 minutes at 4°. This supernatant is the mitochondrial fraction.
• Check the protein concentration of the cytosolic and mitochondrial fractions with BCA kit. Load equal amounts of protein (typically 15–30 μg is sufficient) onto a 12% acrylamide SDS-PAGE gel and run at 100 V for 1 hour to resolve bands in the 10–50 kDa range.
• Transfer to a nitrocellulose membrane using a wet apparatus for 60 minutes at 100 V–300 mA. Incubate in blocking buffer for 1 hour at room temperature.
• Incubate shaking overnight at 4°C with primary antibody (GAPDH (cytosolic), PDH-E1α (mitochondrial matrix), and Complex-Vα (inner mitochondrial membrane) [Mitosciences/Abcam]) in blocking buffer with 0.1% Tween-20.
• Wash and incubate with secondary antibody and visualize as desired.

Notes. Cytochrome *c* is a sensitive indicator of activation of the intrinsic apoptosis pathway. However, as described previously, mitochondrial swelling during necrosis may sometimes be of sufficient severity to result in OMM rupture and cytochrome *c* release.

Complementary approaches

Apoptosis is formally defined by morphology, and this can be evaluated by electron microscopy (EM). Cell shrinkage and fragmentation, chromatin condensation with margination, and plasma membrane blebbing are all findings indicative of apoptosis. In contrast, features of necrosis include mitochondrial swelling, poorly defined cristae, sarcomere disruption, and membrane abnormalities. Despite its strengths, however, EM also presents challenges. Preset criteria must be established to allow consistent analysis and quantification. An approach to random field selection is necessary to avoid operator bias. In addition, when comparing the magnitudes of apoptotic with necrotic cell death using EM, large necrotic cells may be easily identified than small apoptotic cells that may be fleetingly present. Therefore, rates of apoptosis relative to necrosis may be underestimated using EM.

Annexin V, which binds to phosphatidylserine, provides another assay for the detection of apoptosis. This approach is based on the movement of phosphatidylserine from the cytosolic to the extracellular face of the plasma membrane during apoptosis. Administration of fluorescently conjugated Annexin V will effectively label exposed phosphatidylserine, allowing for rapid analysis of apoptosis by fluorescence microscopy or flow cytometry, the latter sometimes challenging with cardiomyocytes but a less biased approach. There are several commercially available kits that allow for simultaneous assessment of Annexin V staining along with propidium iodide (PI) staining, which detects loss of plasma membrane integrity (see below). Healthy cells lack Annexin V and PI staining because phosphatidylserine is on the cytosolic face of the intact plasma membrane. Annexin V staining in the absence of PI staining is the most specific indicator of apoptosis. Double staining for Annexin V and PI is equivocal and may indicate necrosis or late stages of apoptosis with plasma membrane breakdown.

Necrosis

Entry of propidium iodide into the cell

Propidium iodide (PI) staining provides a direct assessment of plasma membrane integrity. In healthy cells, PI is excluded from the cell. In contrast, necrotic cells, which manifest defects in plasma membrane integrity, PI can enter the cell and intercalate with DNA resulting in intense nuclear staining that can be visualized by fluorescence microscopy or flow cytometry.

- Grow and treat cells as desired.
- Dilute propidium iodide to a final concentration of $1-5\,\mu g/mL$.
- Add propidium iodide to cells of interest and incubate for 5–10 minutes at 37°C.
- Counterstain cells with Hoechst 33452 for 5 minutes at 37°C.
- Analyze by fluorescent microscopy.

Notes. The ability of PI to gain entry into a cell provides a rapid assessment of necrosis. Hoechst, a nuclear stain that can cross membranes, allows evaluation of nuclear condensation/ fragmentation in apoptosis. The two stains can be combined to simultaneously assess necrosis and apoptosis in a given population of cells.

Release of intracellular proteins

Loss of membrane integrity allows for the release of intracellular contents into the extracellular milieu. Studies of necrosis have demonstrated release of LDH, HMGB1, and cyclophilin A, which can be assessed by immunoblotting or enzyme activity assays. Commercially available kits to measure LDH release by enzymatic activity employ LDH-mediated conversion of resazurin to fluorescent resorufin. This assay, which is performed in 96-well plates, is rapid, and requires limited processing and disruption of the cells being analyzed. Cardiomyocyte studies have also employed release of the cardiac-specific proteins such as troponin I in response to necrotic stimuli (Figure 39.4). These assays provide for rapid and specific analysis of plasma membrane dysfunction during necrosis.

- Plate and treat cells as desired.
- Collect $600\,\mu L$ of culture media, being careful not to disturb adherent cells.
- Spin collected media at 10,000 rpm for 10 minutes at 4°C.
- Remove $300\,\mu L$ of spun media and transfer to a fresh tube. Make sure not to disturb the pellet at the bottom.

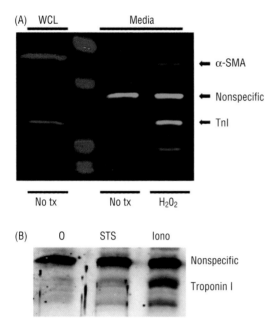

(A) WCL   Media

← α-SMA

← Nonspecific

← TnI

No tx   No tx   H₂O₂

(B)   0   STS   Iono

Nonspecific

Troponin I

Figure 39.4 Cardiac protein release. (A) Immunoblot of whole cell lysate (WCL) and cell culture media demonstrates the release of troponin I (TnI) and alpha-sarcomeric actin (α-SMA) from cultured neonatal rat cardiomyocytes treated with hydrogen peroxide. These proteins are not present in the media of untreated cells. (B) Immunoblot of cell culture media showing release of TnI in response to the necrosis inducer ionomycin, but not the apoptosis inducer staurosporine (STS).

• Take 15–30 µL of spun media, mix with equivalent volume of 2× Loading Buffer, and load onto a polyacrylamide gel and separate by size.
• Transfer to nitrocellulose membrane. Prior to blocking and blotting, a strip of the nitrocellulose membrane can be cut off and stained with Ponceau Red to be used as a loading control.
• Block for 1 hour with appropriate blocking antibody.
• Incubate shaking overnight at 4°C with primary antibody (Troponin I [Santa Cruz], α-sarcomeric actin [Abcam]) in blocking buffer with 0.1% Tween-20.
• Wash and incubate with secondary antibody and visualize as desired.

Notes. If bands cannot be detected in any samples (including a positive control), cells can be cultured in a smaller volume of media. Alternatively, media may be concentrated with the use of Amicon

concentration columns. Since secondary necrosis can occur in cultured cells after prolonged incubation times, prompt and careful assessment of cardiac protein release is essential. Simultaneous assessment of cell lysate to exclude apoptotic pathways (described in the apoptosis section) is recommended. Unused samples should be stored at −80°C. There is significant degradation that occurs following freezing, and more than one freeze–thaw cycle is not recommended.

Loss of inner mitochondrial membrane potential ($\Delta\Psi_m$)

Oxidative phosphorylation is the principal means of energy production in nearly every cell. This process requires the maintenance of an electrochemical gradient across the inner mitochondrial membrane known as $\Delta\Psi_m$, which drives the synthesis of ATP. Opening of the MPTP during necrosis results in a loss of $\Delta\Psi_m$, effectively disrupting ATP generation and causing mitochondrial swelling. Therefore, loss of $\Delta\Psi_m$ can be used to assess MPTP opening and necrotic injury in cultured cells. To determine $\Delta\Psi_m$, the voltage-dependent cationic lipophilic dye tetramethylrhodamine ethyl ester (TMRE) is employed. TMRE is capable of crossing membranes and accumulates in the mitochondrial matrix due to the negative charge present in this compartment. Once localized in the matrix, the ester is cleaved off trapping the TMRE in the matrix as long as the MPTP remains closed. Thus, TMRE accumulation in the matrix is a measure of $\Delta\Psi_m$. When the MPTP opens in response to a necrotic stimulus, such as Ca²⁺, the TMRE signal in the mitochondrial matrix rapidly dissipates as the dye redistributes throughout and exits the cell. These events can be monitored using microscopy or flow cytometry, the latter allowing for the rapid and unbiased assessment of a whole population of cells (Figure 39.5). In addition, flow cytometry allows for simultaneous processing of multiple samples.
• Plate 5×10^5 MEFs in a 6-cm diameter dish for each sample the evening prior to experimentation. Use 2 mL of media for each 6-cm dish.
• When treating cells, pre-mix the desired stimulus with media warmed to 37°C. Gently replace the original media with the stimulus-containing media to minimize disruption to the cells. Do NOT add treatment directly to culture plates, as this does

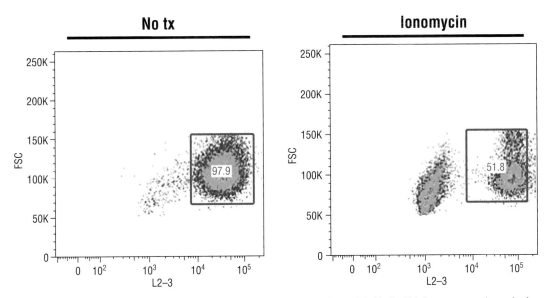

Figure 39.5 TMRE analysis using flow cytometry. Healthy cells maintain $\Delta\Psi_m$, as demonstrated by the high fluorescence on the x-axis of the cells enclosed in the box. Treatment with the Ca^{2+} ionophore ionomycin results in significant loss of TMRE staining indicative of loss of $\Delta\Psi$m (new population of cells shifted to the left).

not provide a homogeneous treatment across the plate.

• For positive controls, treat with a necrotic (ionomycin, 10 μM) or apoptotic (staurosporine, 1 μM) stimulus.

• Incubate for 30 minutes with 20 nM TMRE. Gently rock the plate in order to mix TMRE with media in the plate. Do NOT remove any media.

• Harvest cells (including floating cells). Collect the media in a 15-mL tube. Wash the plate with PBS and collect the PBS in the same 15-mL tube. Add 0.5 mL trypsin for 5–10 minutes. Confirm cell detachment by microscopic examination. Add 1 mL of media to neutralize trypsin, and add the total volume (1.5 mL) to the 15-mL tube.

• Spin down at 1200 rpm for 3 minutes at 4°C. Remove the supernatant and resuspend the cells in 500 mL of chilled 10% FBS (diluted in PBS) and keep at 4°C.

• Rapidly analyze the samples in a FACS machine. Healthy cells will demonstrate strong TMRE staining, and cells that have had necrotic MPTP opening will demonstrate a significant loss of TMRE staining and intensity.

Notes. Typically, rapid loss of TMRE occurs in response to necrotic stimuli. In situations where a prolonged incubation time is necessary, it is possible that secondary necrosis occurs following apoptosis. To determine whether TMRE loss is due to primary or secondary necrosis, it is advisable to assay for apoptosis as well. Cytochrome *c* release in parallel samples is recommended (described in the Apoptosis section). Absence of cytochrome *c* release in the presence of TMRE loss demonstrates that primary necrosis is occurring.

Assessing necrosis *in vivo*

While assessment of necrosis *in vivo* is challenging, several assays can be informative. Electron microscopy can be used to assess morphology, but has limitations – particularly with respect to comparing magnitudes of necrosis with those of apoptosis (discussed earlier). A time course of the release of intracellular proteins into the blood will provide an indirect measure of loss of plasma membrane integrity, and is used clinically to diagnose myocardial infarction. A more direct evaluation of plasma membrane integrity can be obtained by intraperitoneal injection of Evans blue dye, which gains entry into cells with damaged plasma membranes [18,19].

Conclusions

Apoptosis and necrosis are critical cell death processes in most cardiac disease. A thorough examination of the contributions of each form of cell death offers valuable insights into the underlying pathophysiology. The methods described in this chapter provide a strong framework for assessing cell death in culture and animal models. While each assay assesses an important aspect of cell death, use of multiple assays increases confidence in the results especially regarding the discrimination of apoptosis from necrosis. Moreover, given the interrelationships between apoptosis and necrosis signaling, the assessment of multiple time points is critical. Careful selection and application of the methods described in this chapter should be informative regarding the roles of cell death in cardiac disease and dysfunction.

Acknowledgements

This work was supported by NIH grants 5R01HL060665, 5U01HL099776, 1R03DA031671, The Harrington Project for Discovery and Development, and The Dr. Gerald and Myra Dorros Chair in Cardiovascular Disease of the Albert Einstein College of Medicine. We are grateful for the generosity and support of the Wilf Family.

References

1 Konstantinidis K, Whelan RS, Kitsis RN. Mechanisms of cell death in heart disease. *Arterioscler Thromb Vasc Biol* 2012; **32**: 1552–1562.

2 Kung G, Konstantinidis K, Kitsis RN. Programmed necrosis, not apoptosis, in the heart. *Circ Res* 2011; **108**: 1017–1036.

3 Whelan RS, Kaplinskiy V, Kitsis RN. Cell death in the pathogenesis of heart disease: mechanisms and significance. *Annu Rev Physiol* 2010; **72**: 19–44.

4 Pop C, Salvesen GS. Human caspases: activation, specificity, and regulation. *J Biol Chem* 2009; **284**: 21777–21781.

5 Boatright KM, Renatus M, Scott FL, Sperandio S, Shin H, Pedersen IM, *et al.* A unified model for apical caspase activation. *Mol Cell* 2003; **11**: 529–541.

6 Kischkel FC, Hellbardt S, Behrmann I, Germer M, Pawlita M, Krammer PH, *et al.* Cytotoxicity-dependent APO-1 (Fas/CD95)-associated proteins form a death-inducing signaling complex (DISC) with the receptor. *EMBO J* 1995; **14**: 5579–5588.

7 Chao DT, Korsmeyer SJ. BCL-2 family: regulators of cell death. *Annu Rev Immunol* 1998; **16**: 395–419.

8 Bao Q, Shi Y. Apoptosome: a platform for the activation of initiator caspases. *Cell Death Differ* 2007; **14**: 56–65.

9 Degterev A, Huang Z, Boyce M, Li Y, Jagtap P, Mizushima N, *et al.* Chemical inhibitor of nonapoptotic cell death with therapeutic potential for ischemic brain injury. *Nat Chem Biol* 2005; **1**: 112–119.

10 Holler, N., Zaru R, Micheau O, Thome M, Attinger A, Valitutti S, *et al.* Fas triggers an alternative, caspase-8-independent cell death pathway using the kinase RIP as effector molecule. *Nat Immunol* 2000; **1**: 489–495.

11 Cho YS, Challa S, Moquin D, Genga R, Ray TD, Guildford M, *et al.* Phosphorylation-driven assembly of the RIP1-RIP3 complex regulates programmed necrosis and virus-induced inflammation. *Cell* 2009; **137**: 1112–1123.

12 He S, Wang L, Miao L, Wang T, Du F, Zhao L, *et al.* Receptor interacting protein kinase-3 determines cellular necrotic response to TNF-alpha. *Cell* 2009; **137**: 1100–1111.

13 Wang Z, Jiang H, Chen S, Du F, Wang X. The mitochondrial phosphatase PGAM5 functions at the convergence point of multiple necrotic death pathways. *Cell* 2012; **148**: 228–243.

14 Halestrap AP. What is the mitochondrial permeability transition pore? *J Mol Cell Cardiol* 2009; **46**: 821–831.

15 Ricci JE, Muñoz-Pinedo C, Fitzgerald P, Bailly-Maitre B, Perkins GA, Yadava N, *et al.* Disruption of mitochondrial function during apoptosis is mediated by caspase cleavage of the p75 subunit of complex I of the electron transport chain. *Cell* 2004; **117**: 773–786.

16 Lazebnik YA, Kaufmann SH, Desnoyers S, Poirier GG, Earnshaw WC. Cleavage of poly(ADP-ribose) polymerase by a proteinase with properties like ICE. *Nature* 1994; **371**: 346–347.

17 Tanaka M, Ito H, Adachi S, Akimoto H, Nishikawa T, Kasajima T, Marumo F, *et al.* Hypoxia induces apoptosis with enhanced expression of Fas antigen messenger RNA in cultured neonatal rat cardiomyocytes. *Circ Res* 1994; **75**: 426–433.

18 Han R, Bansal D, Miyake K, Muniz VP, Weiss RM, McNeil PL, *et al.* Dysferlin-mediated membrane repair protects the heart from stress-induced left ventricular injury. *J Clin Invest* 2007; **117**: 1805–1813.

19 Miller DL, Li P, Dou C, Armstrong WF, Gordon D. Evans blue staining of cardiomyocytes induced by myocardial contrast echocardiography in rats: evidence for necrosis instead of apoptosis. *Ultrasound Med Biol* 2007; **33**: 1988–1996.

Assessment of mitochondrial function in isolated cells

Amy K. Rines and Hossein Ardehali

Northwestern University Feinberg School of Medicine, Chicago, IL, USA

Introduction

Mitochondria are the primary energy source in the cell, and their proper function is essential to maintaining cardiomyocyte and heart health. Oxidative phosphorylation occurs within the mitochondria, providing the majority supply of the high energy molecule adenosine triphosphate (ATP). As the heart requires high levels of ATP to maintain continuous contractions and proper ion homeostasis, disruptions in mitochondrial function and ATP production are particularly detrimental to heart function. Indeed, heart failure has been found to be accompanied by a gradual and steady decline in mitochondrial function [1], and chronic decreased mitochondrial function is also associated with ischemic heart disease, cardiac hypertrophy, and diabetic cardiomyopathy [2]. Thus, controlled regulation of mitochondrial function is essential to balancing the energetic needs of the heart.

Producing ATP from oxidative phosphorylation is a main function of mitochondria. The heart utilizes chiefly fatty acids (60–90% of total substrate) and less often glucose (10–40%) as substrate for producing acetyl-CoA [3]. Acetyl-CoA is processed through the tricarboxylic acid (TCA) cycle, making the reducing equivalents NADH and $FADH_2$ (Figure 40.1). NADH is also produced during glycolysis, pyruvate oxidation, and fatty acid β-oxidation. These reducing equivalents are then utilized by the electron transport chain to create an H^+ electrochemical gradient across the inner mitochondrial membrane that drives oxidative phosphorylation of ADP into ATP by ATP synthase. Measurements of several parameters of these processes can be used to provide information about overall mitochondrial function. In this chapter, we provide protocols for assaying mitochondrial respiration, cellular ATP, mitochondrial membrane potential, and mitochondrial mass and biogenesis.

Protocols

Respiration rates

Measuring respiration rates is the most direct assay of mitochondrial function, as oxygen is consumed during mitochondrial ATP synthesis. The Seahorse Bioscience XF extracellular flux analyzers currently provide the optimal setup for these measurements. These machines create a microchamber of media immediately above cells cultured in a 24-well or 96-well plate. Fluorescent biosensors can then detect extracellular acidification (an indicator of lactate levels and therefore glycolytic rate) and oxygen consumption rates directly in this microchamber of media with a high time resolution and after injection of compounds [4,5]. This setup provides significant advantages over traditional oxygen consumption analysis using a Clark electrode because it enables measurement of oxygen consumption without trypsinization or disruption to cells, requires a relatively small amount of cells, and has a higher

Manual of Research Techniques in Cardiovascular Medicine, First Edition. Edited by Hossein Ardehali, Roberto Bolli, and Douglas W. Losordo.

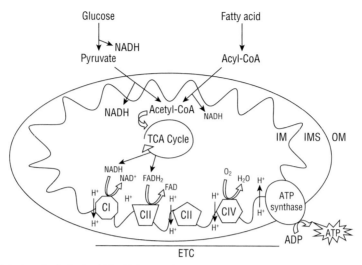

Figure 40.1 Simplified schematic of mitochondrial oxidative phosphorylation. CI–CIV, Complex I through IV; ETC, electron transport chain; IM, inner mitochondrial membrane; IMS, intermembrane space; OM, outer mitochondrial membrane.

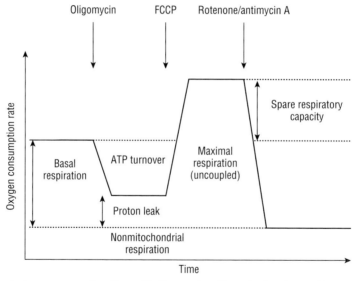

Figure 40.2 Components of oxygen consumption. (Source: http://www.seahorsebio.com/products/consumables/kits/cell-mito-stress.php).

throughput. However, a Clark electrode can also be used to make similar oxygen consumption measurements if necessary.

The Seahorse XF analyzer can measure basal respiration and respiration following injection of up to four compounds. With the appropriate pharmacological intervention, an investigator can determine basal respiration, ATP turnover and proton leak, maximal respiration capacity, and

nonmitochondrial respiration rates [6]. Basal respiration is composed of ATP turnover and proton leak (Figure 40.2). Treatment with oligomycin, which inhibits ATP synthase, will reveal the contributions of both processes. Oligomycin-sensitive respiration represents ATP turnover and coupling efficiency, and the remaining oligomycin-insensitive respiration represents proton leak. Maximum respiration capacity can then be determined by treatment with a mitochondrial uncoupler such as carbonylcyanide-*p*-trifluoromethoxyphenylhydrazone (FCCP), carbonyl cyanide *m*-chlorophenylhydrazone (CCCP), or 2,4-dinitrophenol (DNP). Spare respiratory capacity is measured by subtracting basal respiration from uncoupled respiration. Finally, nonmitochondrial respiration is measured after treatment with rotenone and antimycin A, which respectively inhibit complex I and complex III of the electron transport chain and block mitochondrial oxygen consumption. After measuring oxygen consumption rates in the machine, cells are trypsinized and counted with Trypan Blue or collected in lysis buffer and measured with a protein quantification assay for normalization of readings to viable cell count or protein content.

The manufacturer's protocol and advice for optimization for the particular machine model should be followed. Additionally, the protocol must be optimized in individual labs for each cell type and treatment. However, we have provided a general protocol for measuring oxygen consumption in cell culture with the Seahorse Bioscience XF analyzer:

1. Seed cells in a V7 cell plate with normal growth media and treat as needed. Leave four wells empty in different areas of the plate if including a background correction. Incubate in desired growth conditions, typically in a 5% CO_2 37°C incubator. The ideal number of cells must be calibrated, and should produce a baseline oxygen consumption rate (OCR) of 100–200. An initial calibration of 5000 to 50,000 cells per well is suggested.

2. On the day prior to the experiment, load 1 mL of Seahorse Bioscience calibration fluid into each well of the XF Assay cartridge plate. Incubate in a CO_2-free 37°C incubator to hydrate the sensors.

3. Prior to the day of the experiment, prepare unbuffered assay media and concentrated stock compounds of oligomycin (2 mg/mL in DMSO), FCCP (5 mM in DMSO), rotenone (20 mM in DMSO), and antimycin A (45.6 mM in 95–100% ethanol). Unbuffered assay media generally consists of DMEM with no phenol red containing 25 mM glucose, 2 mM glutamine, and 1 mM sodium pyruvate. Carefully adjust pH of all solutions to 7.2. Assay solution can be stored at 4°C, and stock compounds can be kept at −20°C for several months.

4. On the day of the assay, wash cells two times with 1 mL of unbuffered assay media warmed to 37°C. Add 500 μL of assay media and incubate cells in a CO_2-free 37°C incubator for 90 minutes.

5. Dilute stock compounds in assay media. Initial concentrations of oligomycin should be 10 μg/mL, FCCP should be 50 μM, rotenone and antimycin A should each be 100 μM. However, titration of these concentrations may be necessary. Load injection port A with 50 μL of oligomycin, port B with 55 μL of FCCP, and port C with 60 μL antimycin A/rotenone.

6. Calibrate assay cartridge and load plate when prompted. The program typically consists of an equilibration step and three to six baseline cycles of mix, measure, and wait steps, followed by injection of the ports each followed by three cycles of mix, measure, and wait steps. The time for each mix, wait, and measure step must be optimized and will depend on the OCR readings at baseline and after each injection (please consult the Seahorse Bioscience Training Course Workbook for additional information). Typical starting times are to mix 3 minutes, wait 2 minutes, and measure 3 minutes. Mix times need to be long enough to allow replenishment of oxygen within the well microchamber.

7. After the program has completed, collect the cells for normalization by cell number or protein content.

Problems typically associated with this procedure can often be avoided with careful calibration of the cell number, the concentration of the injected compounds, and the machine protocol. Additionally, maintaining the pH of every solution is very important and should not be overlooked. If problems persist, the polystyrene plate that is typically used may need to be exchanged for a polyethylene plate, which has decreased levels of gas diffusion and may increase sensor sensitivity.

The Seahorse Bioscience XF analyzer can also be used to measure function of isolated mitochondria. However, those protocols are beyond the scope of this chapter. Please consult Seahorse Bioscience for more information about how to measure function of isolated mitochondria.

Cellular ATP

Measurement of mitochondrial function can also be accomplished indirectly through assessment of cellular ATP. Maintenance of ATP levels can provide supportive data that mitochondria are capable of sustaining energy levels within the cell, with decreased ATP levels potentially indicative of mitochondrial dysfunction. However, this assay is an indirect measure of mitochondrial function, and should be used cautiously and only in combination with additional measures mentioned in this chapter, as cells can produce ATP through nonmitochondrial processes such as glycolysis. The most common method for measuring ATP uses the luciferin–luciferase system. Cell lysate is mixed with luciferin and luciferase, which hydrolyzes ATP from the lysate to generate luminescent light [7]. The more ATP is present in the lysate, the more luminescent signal is generated. As ATP is derived from several nonmitochondrial sources in the cell, it is essential to eliminate these sources of ATP and to measure only ATP derived from mitochondrial oxidative phosphorylation. Thus, ATP should be measured with and without oligomycin treatment in order to inhibit mitochondrial ATP synthesis and to determine the oligomycin-sensitive ATP that is made from oxidative phosphorylation.

There are several commercially available luminescence-based ATP assays, including the CellTiter-Glo Luminescent Cell Viability Assay from Promega, the ATP Bioluminescent Assay Kit from Sigma-Aldrich, and the ATP Determination Kit from Life Technologies. A standard curve of ATP should also be run simultaneously during these assays to ensure luminescent signals are within a linear detection range.

Although the protocol should be optimized and will depend on the exact kit that is used, we have provided a general protocol for measuring ATP using luminescence-based ATP assays.

1. Seed and treat cells as desired.
2. On day of assay, prepare ATP standard curve. Dilute ATP to $1\,\mu M$ in cell culture medium, make tenfold serial dilutions, and plate $100\,\mu L$ of each in an opaque 96-well plate.
3. Trypsinize cells, count, and dilute to optimized concentration in at least $700\,\mu L$ of media. The number of cells should be titrated to fall within the linear range of the ATP standard curve. An initial titration of 50 to 1000 cells in $100\,\mu L$ is recommended.

Remove $350\,\mu L$ of cells and add $1\,\mu g/mL$ final concentration of oligomycin. Add $100\,\mu L$ of untreated and oligomycin-treated cells in triplicate to the opaque 96-well plate. Also add $100\,\mu L$ media with no cells in triplicate for determination of background luminescence.
4. Equilibrate the plate for 30 minutes at room temperature.
5. Add $100\,\mu L$ of luminescence reagent and shake for 2 minutes to lyse cells.
6. Incubate the plate for 10 minutes at room temperature.
7. Read endpoint luminescence using an integration time of 0.25–1 second. Subtract background and oligomycin-treated readings from untreated readings to determine mitochondrial-specific ATP luminescence.

Mitochondrial membrane potential

Another measure of mitochondrial function is determination of the mitochondrial membrane potential ($\Delta\psi_m$). The mitochondrial membrane potential is the electrochemical gradient driven by accumulation of H^+ ions in the intermembrane space. This gradient is used by ATP synthase to fuel ATP synthesis, so maintenance of $\Delta\psi_m$ is indicative of the mitochondrial capacity to generate ATP [8]. Cellular stress can interfere with the mitochondria's ability to balance proton and ionic flux, leading to changes in $\Delta\psi_m$ and decreased efficiency in ATP production.

The mitochondrial membrane potential can be measured by several fluorescent dyes, including tetramethylrhodamine methyl (TMRM) and ethyl (TMRE) ester, JC-1, and rhodamine 23. These dyes are cationic and accumulate more in mitochondria with a more negatively charged matrix and more hyperpolarized $\Delta\psi_m$. Depolarization of $\Delta\psi_m$ leads to loss of dye accumulation. These dyes can be used in quenching or nonquenching modes. In quenching mode, a higher concentration of dye is used (typically $50\,nM–1\,\mu M$, with the optimal concentration determined empirically) so that accumulation of the dye in the mitochondria leads to signal quenching and reduced fluorescence. Depolarization of $\Delta\psi_m$ releases the dye from the mitochondria and unquenches the signal, leading to increased fluorescence. As quenching is a rapid and nonlinear event, this method is useful for studies involving an acute treatment that occurs after dye loading. For chronic treatments that must be performed before dye loading, the dyes should be used in nonquenched mode. Nonquenched dyes are used at lower concentrations (typically 0.5–30 nM) and have higher fluorescence when retained by a more hyperpolarized $\Delta\psi_m$, with fluorescent signal decreasing upon depolarization.

The choice of dye depends on the particular demands of the experiment [9]. TMRM and TMRE have the lowest mitochondrial binding and electron transport chain inhibition, which is generally more desirable, and have fast equilibration times across the plasma membrane which makes them more suitable for nonquenching studies. Rhod123 has a slower equilibration time, and is best used in quenching mode with rapid acute studies, as the dye will be retained in the cell longer after the unquenched burst. JC-1 has a dual color emission, creating a red signal when the dye aggregates in mitochondria with more hyperpolarized $\Delta\psi_m$, and green signal when the dye is released as monomers upon depolarization. This dual emission quality makes JC-1 generally suitable for detecting large changes in $\Delta\psi_m$, but not as precise in determining subtle changes in $\Delta\psi_m$. Additionally, the aggregate form of JC-1 has been reported to take around 90 minutes to equilibrate in cardiomyocytes [10], so this dye is not appropriate for studies conducted rapidly after loading. Moreover, JC-1 has been reported to aggregate irrespective of $\Delta\psi_m$ in certain cellular regions, so this dye must be used with caution. The signal readout for each dye can be determined by fluorescent or confocal microscopy, flow cytometry, or a fluorescent plate reader. Microscopy has the advantage of better resolving mitochondria-specific fluorescence and it is better suited for determining rapid changes in fluorescence, but flow cytometry and fluorescent plate readers are also valid for many studies. Regardless of the readout method, exposure to fluorescent light should be minimized to reduce photobleaching of the dyes. Additionally, oligomycin treatment can be used as a positive control for $\Delta\psi_m$ hyperpolarization, and CCCP or FCCP can be used as a positive control for depolarization to ensure the dyes are behaving as expected.

Mitochondrial mass and biogenesis

Assays of mitochondrial mass and biogenesis can also be used to measure overall mitochondrial function. Maintenance of a sufficient number of mitochondria is necessary to support the ATP demand of the cell. Mitochondrial biogenesis has been found to be impaired in during heart failure [11,12], and mitochondrial proliferation is often insufficient during hypertrophy [13], suggesting that decreased mitochondrial content is associated with cardiac dysfunction. However, excessive mitochondrial biogenesis is also maladaptive in some cardiomyopathies [14] and increased mitochondrial biogenesis can lead to cardiomyopathy [15], emphasizing that a carefully regulated level of mitochondrial content and biogenesis is necessary to maintain cardiovascular health.

Mitochondrial content and biogenesis can be assessed in isolated cells using several assays. First, electron microscopy can be performed to observe mitochondrial size and density in isolated cells. The precise protocols for conducting electron microscopy are dependent on the microscope used, so the institutional microscope facility should be consulted for suggested protocols on how to proceed with these experiments. There are also references available that discuss various electron microscopy protocols for the study of mitochondria [16–18].

Next, because mitochondria contain their own genome, the ratio of mitochondrial to nuclear DNA can be used as a measure of mitochondrial content per cell. Mitochondrial DNA can be determined by quantifying DNA levels of a mitochondria-encoded gene using quantitative real time polymerase chain reaction (qRT-PCR) and comparing its levels to that of a nuclear-encoded gene. Cytochrome *c* oxidase subunit I (COI), a component of Complex IV in the ETC, is commonly used for the mitochondrial gene, and 18S rRNA, a component of the 40S ribosomal subunit, is commonly used for the nuclear gene [12]. Total DNA can be isolated from cells using a commercially available kit such as the DNeasy Blood and Tissue Kit from Qiagen. qRT-PCR can be conducted using SYBR Green dye, between 0.1 and 1 ng of isolated DNA, and the following primer sequences:

Nuclear DNA for human, mouse, and rat (18S gene)
Forward: GTAACCCGTTGAACCCCATT
Reverse: CCATCCAATCGGTAGTAGCG
Human mitochondrial DNA (COI gene)
Forward: ACCCTAGACCAAACCTACGCCAAA
Reverse: TAGGCCGAGAAAGTGTTGTGGGAA
Mouse mitochondrial DNA (COI gene)
Forward: AGTGCTAGCCGCAGGCATTACTAT
Reverse: CTGGGTGCCCAAAGAATCAGAACA
Rat mitochondrial DNA (COI gene)
Forward: TCCTCCATAGTAGAAGCTGGAGCT
Reverse: CTAAGATAGAAGACACCCCGGCTA

Another method of measuring mitochondrial mass is to quantify fluorescence of dyes that localize to mitochondria largely irrespective of $\Delta\psi_m$. Examples of such dyes include 10-N-nonyl-acridine orange (NAO) and Mitotracker Green FM [19]. Fluorescence quantification is typically performed using flow cytometry. Cells are treated with 100–150 nM NAO or MitoTracker Green FM, incubated for 30 minutes at 37°C, washed, trypsinized, and resuspended in phosphate-buffered saline (PBS) before flow cytometry analysis. Some reports have found that NAO and MitoTracker Green FM fluorescence can be dependent on $\Delta\psi_m$ [20,21]. To avoid this potential complication, cells can be fixed prior to staining to eliminate any influence of $\Delta\psi_m$ on dye fluorescence. Prior to NAO staining, cells can be trypsinized and fixed in cold 70% ethanol at −20°C for 2 hours to several days. Before MitoTracker Green FM staining, cells can be fixed in 2% glutaraldehyde and 2% formaldehyde in PBS.

Quantification of mitochondrial enzyme activities can also serve as a measure of mitochondrial mass. Citrate synthase is commonly used for this purpose, as it localizes to the mitochondrial matrix and catalyzes the first step of the TCA cycle. Citrate synthase activity is measured by the addition of thiol to 5,5′-dithio-bis-(2-nitrobenzoic acid) (DTNB). Citrate synthase hydrolyzes acetyl-CoA, the first substrate of the TCA cycle, forming citrate and thiolyated CoA (CoA-SH). The thiol group from CoA-SH then reacts with DTNB to form TNB, causing an increase in absorbance at 412 nm [22] during the following reactions:

$$Acetyl\ CoA + Oxaloacetate$$
$$\rightarrow Citrate + CoA\text{-}SH + H^+ + H_2O$$

$$CoA\text{-}SH + DTNB \rightarrow TNB + CoA\text{-}S\text{-}S\text{-}TNB$$

This reaction can be assayed by commercially available kits (Citrate Synthase Assay Kit from Sigma Aldrich) or with the following protocol.

1. Lyse cells in 50 mM Tris-HCl, pH 7.5 with 0.3% Triton X-100 on ice.
2. Centrifuge lysates for 15 minutes at 13,000 rpm at 4°C and collect supernatant on ice.
3. Measure protein concentration by Bradford method or BCA assay.
4. Add 100 μg of protein to 1 mL reaction buffer containing 20 mM HEPES, 1 mM EGTA, 220 mM sucrose, 40 mM KCl, 0.1 mM DTNB, 0.1 mM acetyl-CoA, pH 7.4 at 25°C.
5. Measure absorbance in a cuvette at 412 nm in a spectrophotometer for 2 minutes to measure background absorbance.
6. Start reaction by adding 0.05 mM oxaloacetate, and monitor reaction at 412 nm for 3 minutes at 25°C.

Lastly, levels of genes involved in regulation of mitochondrial biogenesis can be used to assess the state of mitochondrial biogenesis in the cell. Peroxisome proliferator-activated receptor gamma coactivator 1-alpha (PGC-1alpha) is a transcriptional coactivator and master regulator of mitochondrial biogenesis through induction of nuclear respiratory factor 1 and 2 (NRF1 and 2) [23,24]. Levels of these genes can be assessed at the mRNA level by qRT-PCR and on the protein level by western blotting. Increased expression of these genes is often correlated with increased mitochondrial biogenesis and mass, but this must be confirmed with other functional assays discussed earlier.

Additional measures of mitochondrial function
There are several other parameters that can be used to assess mitochondrial health that will not be discussed here, but that are covered in more detail in other chapters of this book. Dysfunctional mitochondria with inefficient and leaky oxidative phosphorylation can lead to production of reactive oxygen species (ROS) [25]. Increasing levels of ROS can then overload antioxidant defenses, resulting in damage to DNA and other macromolecules within the mitochondria, and further functional damage. Thus, increased mitochondrial ROS can be indicative

of decreased mitochondrial function. Assays for measuring ROS are discussed in Chapter 42 *Measurement of reactive oxygen species in cardiovascular disease*. Mitochondria are also the initiating source of intrinsic proapoptotic cascade signaling, and decreased mitochondrial function can lead to mitochondrial damage and increased cytochrome *c* release and apoptosis [26]. Additionally, mitochondria have a primary role in handling calcium, which is essential for controlling oxidative phosphorylation, cell death, and calcium transients [27]. Thus, damage to mitochondrial function can also cause imbalances in calcium signaling. Methods of measuring apoptosis and calcium handling are detailed in Chapter 39 *Assessment of cell death in the heart* and Chapter 2 *Confocal imaging of intracellular calcium cycling in isolated cardiac myocytes*.

Alternative approaches

Alternative measures of respiratory function include assaying reduction of Alamar Blue (resazurin) or the tetrazolium salt MTT [3-(4,5-dimethylthiazol-2-yl)-2,5-diphenyl-2*H*-tetrazolium bromide] by metabolically active mitochondria. These methods are less precise and informative than measuring oxygen consumption, but can be used to crudely assess large changes in mitochondrial respiration. These assays are commercially available (CellTiter 96 AQ$_{ueous}$ Non-Radioactive Cell Proliferation Assay (MTS) from Promega, Alamar Blue from Life Technologies), and should also be normalized to viable cell number or protein content.

Weaknesses and strengths of the method

Although we have focused on measuring mitochondrial function in cell culture in this chapter, several of the methods mentioned here can be conducted either in intact cells or in isolated mitochondria. There are benefits to using either system depending on the needs of the experiment. Measuring function of isolated mitochondria gives the experimenter exclusive control over the substrates that are available to the mitochondria. Additionally, utilizing isolated mitochondria can allow the experimenter to selectively measure respiration driven by particular electron transport chain complexes. However, isolated mitochondria

also lack their cellular context, so experiments using mitochondria are generally less physiological. Furthermore, isolating mitochondria is a delicate procedure that often leads to mitochondrial damage and uncoupling. Thus, measuring mitochondrial function is often done in isolated cells unless precise measurements using particular substrates are needed, or if the procedures required to culture cells from primary tissue sources are particularly cumbersome. The researcher should make the final decision in determining whether isolated mitochondria or cells are most optimal for their experimental needs.

Conclusions

Healthy mitochondria are essential to maintaining the overall function of cardiomyocytes and heart tissue. Assaying mitochondrial function in isolated cells can be a crucial tool to determining mechanistic causes of altered mitochondrial function. Findings from mitochondrial function assays in isolated cells can be extrapolated to mechanistic insights in animal models or human disease, systems in which mechanistic studies of mitochondrial function can be difficult or impossible to perform directly. Together, the assays outlined in this chapter should help researchers study causes of altered mitochondrial function that may reveal important findings about overall cardiomyocyte and heart health.

Acknowledgements
Hossein Ardehali is supported by NIH grant K08 HL079387, R01 HL087149, and the American Heart Association.

References

1 Huss JM, Kelly DP. Mitochondrial energy metabolism in heart failure: a question of balance. *J Clin Invest* 2005; **115**: 547–555.

2 Lopaschuk GD, Kelly DP. Signalling in cardiac metabolism. *Cardiovasc Res* 2008; **79**: 205–207.

3 van der Vusse GJ, van Bilsen M, Glatz JF. Cardiac fatty acid uptake and transport in health and disease. *Cardiovasc Res* 2000; **45**: 279–293.

4 Wu M, Neilson A, Swift AL, Moran R, Tamagnine J, Parslow D, *et al.* Multiparameter metabolic analysis reveals a close link between attenuated mitochondrial bioenergetic function and enhanced glycolysis

dependency in human tumor cells. *Am J Physiol Cell Physiol* 2007; **292**: C125–136.

5 Ferrick DA, Neilson A, Beeson C. Advances in measuring cellular bioenergetics using extracellular flux. *Drug Discov Today* 2008; **13**: 268–274.

6 Brand MD, Nicholls DG. Assessing mitochondrial dysfunction in cells. *Biochem J* 2011; **435**: 297–2312.

7 Manfredi G, Yang L, Gajewski CD, Mattiazzi M. Measurements of ATP in mammalian cells. *Methods* 2002; **26**: 317–326.

8 Perry SW, Norman JP, Barbieri J, Brown EB, Gelbard HA. Mitochondrial membrane potential probes and the proton gradient: a practical usage guide. *Biotechniques* 2011; **50**: 98–115.

9 Scaduto RC, Grotyohann LW. Measurement of mitochondrial membrane potential using fluorescent rhodamine derivatives. *Biophys J* 1999; **76**: 469–477.

10 Mathur A, Hong Y, Kemp BK, Barrientos AA, Erusalimsky JD. Evaluation of fluorescent dyes for the detection of mitochondrial membrane potential changes in cultured cardiomyocytes. *Cardiovasc Res* 2000; **46**: 126–138.

11 Karamanlidis G, Nascimben L, Couper GS, Shekar PS, del Monte F, Tian R, *et al.* Defective DNA replication impairs mitochondrial biogenesis in human failing hearts. *Circ Res* 2010; **106**: 1541–1548.

12 Karamanlidis G, Bautista-Hernandez V, Fynn-Thompson F, Del Nido P, Tian R. Impaired mitochondrial biogenesis precedes heart failure in right ventricular hypertrophy in congenital heart disease. *Circ Heart Fail* 2011; **4**: 707–713.

13 Goffart S, von Kleist-Retzow JC, Wiesner RJ. Regulation of mitochondrial proliferation in the heart: power-plant failure contributes to cardiac failure in hypertrophy. *Cardiovasc Res* 2004; **64**: 198–207.

14 Sebastiani M, Giordano C, Nediani C, Travaglini C, Borchi E, Zani M, *et al.* Induction of mitochondrial biogenesis is a maladaptive mechanism in mitochondrial cardiomyopathies. *J Am Coll Cardiol* 2007; **50**: 1362–1369.

15 Russell LK, Mansfield CM, Lehman JJ, Kovacs A, Courtois M, Saffitz JE, *et al.* Cardiac-specific induction of the transcriptional coactivator peroxisome proliferator-activated receptor gamma coactivator-1alpha promotes mitochondrial biogenesis and reversible cardiomyopathy in a developmental stage-dependent manner. *Circ Res* 2004; **94**: 525–533.

16 Perkins EM, McCaffery JM. Conventional and immunoelectron microscopy of mitochondria. *Methods Mol Biol* 2007; **372**: 467–483.

17 Sasaki S. Determination of altered mitochondria ultrastructure by electron microscopy. *Methods Mol Biol* 2010; **648**: 279–290.

18 Bozzola JJ. Conventional specimen preparation techniques for transmission electron microscopy of cultured cells. *Methods Mol Biol* 2007; **369**: 1–18.

19 Maftah A, Petit JM, Ratinaud MH, Julien R. 10-N nonyl-acridine orange: a fluorescent probe which stains mitochondria independently of their energetic state. *Biochem Biophys Res Commun* 1989; **164**: 185–190.

20 Keij JF, Bell-Prince C, Steinkamp JA. Staining of mitochondrial membranes with 10-nonyl acridine orange, MitoFluor Green, and MitoTracker Green is affected by mitochondrial membrane potential altering drugs. *Cytometry* 2000; **39**: 203–210.

21 Jacobson J, Duchen MR, Heales SJ. Intracellular distribution of the fluorescent dye nonyl acridine orange responds to the mitochondrial membrane potential: implications for assays of cardiolipin and mitochondrial mass. *J Neurochem* 2002; **82**: 224–233.

22 Srere PA, Matsuoka Y. Inhibition of rat citrate synthase by acetoacetyl CoA and NADH. *Biochem Med* 1972; **6**: 262–226.

23 Wu Z, Puigserver P, Andersson U, Zhang C, Adelmant G, Mootha V, *et al.* Mechanisms controlling mitochondrial biogenesis and respiration through the thermogenic coactivator PGC-1. *Cell* 1999; **98**: 115–124.

24 Ventura-Clapier R, Garnier A, Veksler V. Transcriptional control of mitochondrial biogenesis: the central role of PGC-1alpha. *Cardiovasc Res* 2008; **79**: 208–217.

25 Turrens JF. Mitochondrial formation of reactive oxygen species. *J Physiol* 2003; **552**: 335–344.

26 Borutaite V, Brown GC. Mitochondria in apoptosis of ischemic heart. *FEBS Lett* 2003; **541**: 1–5.

27 Gunter TE, Yule DI, Gunter KK, Eliseev RA, Salter JD. Calcium and mitochondria. *FEBS Lett* 2004; **567**: 96–102.

Multinuclear NMR spectroscopy of myocardial energetics and substrate utilization in isolated perfused mouse hearts

Stephen C. Kolwicz, Jr. and Rong Tian

University of Washington School of Medicine, Seattle, WA, USA

Introduction

In experimental cardiovascular physiology, non-invasive and repeated measures of cardiac function, energetics, and metabolism provide a dynamic picture of myocardial performance during physiological or pathological perturbations. All of these parameters can be assessed in one sample by combining isolated perfused heart experiments with a multinuclear nuclear magnetic resonance (NMR) spectroscopic approach. This method is advantageous because simultaneous measurements of left ventricular (LV) function, myocardial energetics, and substrate utilization are made in a contracting heart.

NMR spectroscopy allows the user to measure metabolite content, as well as turnover rate, by assessing the content of a specific nucleus in biological samples [1,2]. For example, ^{31}P NMR spectroscopy can be used to quantify phosphorous-containing compounds in the sample. The most abundant phosphates in the cell are the high-energy phosphates phosphocreatine and ATP. Thus, ^{31}P NMR spectroscopy of the heart can assess myocardial energetics in various studies of bioengineered mouse models under pathological conditions [3–6]. With this method, dynamic changes in phosphocreatine and ATP can be assessed with repetitive measurements during physiological and/or pathological perturbations providing a detailed picture of energetic status.

Assessment of myocardial substrate utilization presents a unique challenge in that, although carbon-containing compounds are relatively abundant in the heart, the natural abundance of the NMR visible carbon isotope (^{13}C) is very low (~1–3%). Therefore, isotopic enrichment of substrates delivered to the isolated perfused heart is required. The specific ^{13}C-labeled substrates are chosen based on the ^{13}C-labeling pattern of the acetyl CoAs that are ultimately yielded. Since glutamate is easily detected by ^{13}C NMR spectroscopy and the enrichment pattern is similar to the TCA cycle intermediate, α-ketoglutarate under steady-state conditions, inferences of isotopic-enriched substrate entry into the tricarboxcylic acid (TCA) cycle can be made by examining the carbon labeling pattern of glutamate. As shown in Figure 41.1A, glucose with ^{13}C carbons in the 1st and 6th position (1,6-^{13}C glucose) will yield two acetyl CoA molecules with the ^{13}C carbon in the 2nd position (2-^{13}C acetyl CoA) once glycolysis and pyruvate decarboxylation are completed. Entry

Manual of Research Techniques in Cardiovascular Medicine, First Edition. Edited by Hossein Ardehali, Roberto Bolli, and Douglas W. Losordo.

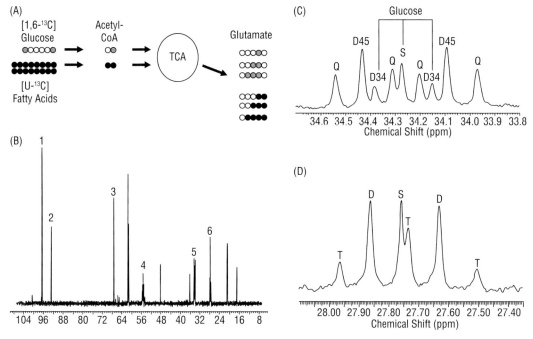

Figure 41.1 Representative data from ^{13}C NMR spectroscopy. (A) Diagram detailing the incorporation of ^{13}C labeled glucose and fatty acids into acetyl CoA and ultimately into glutamate. (B) Representative spectra from a mouse heart perfused with ^{13}C labeled substrates. 1, β-glucose; 2, α-glucose; 3, dioxane; 4, C2 of glutamate; 5, C4 of glutamate; 6, C3 of glutamate. (C) Representative multiplet of the C4 of glutamate. S, singlet; D34, doublet of C3 and C4; D45, doublet of C4 and C5; Q, quartet. (D) Representative multiplet of C3 of glutamate. S, singlet; D, doublet; T, triplet.

of the 2-^{13}C acetyl CoA into the TCA cycle will result in carbon labeling of glutamate. Likewise, fatty acids (FAs) that are uniformly ^{13}C-labeled (U-^{13}C) undergo beta-oxidation and create acetyl CoA molecules with both carbons labeled (1,2-^{13}C acetyl CoA). The 1,2-^{13}C acetyl CoA will create a distinct labeling pattern of glutamate. The presence of various ^{13}C labeled compounds or metabolic intermediates in an adequate enough concentration can be identified in the NMR spectra (Figure 41.1B). Visual inspection of the C4 glutamate spectra provide a hint towards the relative use of glucose versus FAs by comparing the peaks associated with the S and D34 (glucose) and the peaks associated with the Q and D45 (FAs), as illustrated in Figure 41.1C. Analysis of the individual peak areas of the C4 glutamate (Figure 41.1C) and C3 glutamate (Figure 41.1D) spectra and mathematical modeling can allow for the measurement of the relative use of one substrate versus another as well as relative flux through a particular pathway [7,8].

Protocol

For the NMR perfusion experiments, a typical protocol is divided into three stages: a preparatory day to create a fatty acid (FA) stock; single or multiple experimental days using isolated perfused hearts; and multiple days of tissue processing and data analysis (Figure 41.2).

Creation of fatty acid stock with ^{13}C stable isotopes

The lipophilic nature of long chain fatty acids (LCFAs) requires binding to bovine serum albumin (BSA) to increase solubility in the aqueous perfusate. A detailed protocol on the preparation and rationale of this has been previously published [9]. This protocol yields 4 liters of FA-based buffer at a final concentration of 0.4 mM and 1.2% BSA. Aliquots of the stock can be made and stored at −20°C. The most commonly used LCFAs in isolated heart perfusion experiments are palmitate and oleate. Alternatively,

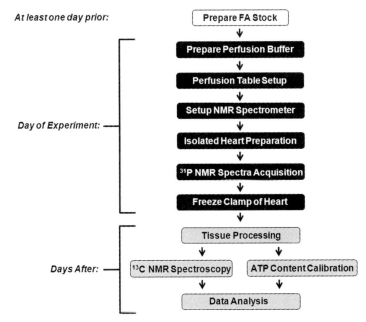

Figure 41.2 Experimental flow chart. The general steps of the entire experimental protocol are divided into three stages. At least one day before, the fatty acid (FA) stock solution is created. On the day of the heart perfusion experiment, several steps involving experimental setup and execution are required. In the days after the perfusion experiment, tissue processing and additional experiments are necessary to complete data analysis.

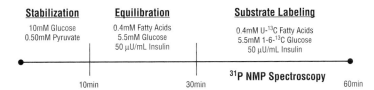

Figure 41.3 Overview of the isolated heart perfusion protocol. The perfusion protocol consists of three periods: stabilization, equilibration, and labeling. During the 10 minutes stabilization period, the heart is perfused with a modified Krebs Henseleit (KH) buffer supplemented with glucose and pyruvate. During equilibration, the perfusate is changed to a mixed, unlabeled substrate buffer with fatty acids, glucose, and insulin. During labeling, a mixed substrate buffer containing ^{13}C labeled fatty acids and glucose is used.

a mixture of saturated and unsaturated FAs (e.g. mixed fatty acids) can be used [5,6]. Depending on the experimental conditions, the stock can be modified to yield different concentrations of FA.

Langendorff heart perfusions combined with ^{31}P NMR spectroscopy

In Figure 41.3, the protocol scheme presented is designed to measure LV function, myocardial energetics, and substrate utilization under normal or baseline conditions. The heart is stabilized with a perfusate consisting of a modified Krebs Henseleit (KH) buffer (in mM: 0.5 EDTA, 5.3 KCl, 1.2 $MgSO_4$, 118 NaCl, 25 $NaHCO_3$, 2.0 $CaCl_2$, 10 glucose and 0.5 pyruvate). After stabilization, an unlabeled mixed substrate buffer with 5.5 mM glucose, 0.4 mM FAs, and 50 μU/mL of insulin is provided and the heart is allowed to equilibrate. After equilibration, the heart is perfused with a ^{13}C labeled mixed substrate buffer consisting of 5.5 mM 1,6-^{13}C glucose, 0.4 mM U-^{13}C FAs, and 50 μU/mL of insulin. During the labeling period, hearts are perfused for at least 30 minutes so that isotopic equilibrium of the TCA cycle can be achieved [10].

Since there are excellent references available regarding the Langendorff-isolated perfused heart protocol [11,12] details will not be discussed here. After preparation of the substrate buffers and Langendorff system, the NMR system is "calibrated" to facilitate acquisition of ^{31}P spectra. A standard containing 155 mM Na_2PO_4 and 25% deuterium oxide in a 10-mm NMR tube is placed into the bore of the magnet. "Calibration" refers to optimization of the spectrometer parameters in order to obtain the best possible phosphorous signal, accomplished by setting the radio pulse at the frequency at which the phosphorous signal resonates ("tuning") and making the field homogenous ("shimming").

Preparation of the isolated mouse heart in combination with ^{31}P NMR spectroscopy is as previously described with a few adaptations [5,6,11–13]. Initially, the heart is perfused at a constant flow of ~2 mL/min. The heart is carefully placed into a 10-mm NMR with a wide-bore "spinner" attached to help guide the sample into the NMR probe. Once the sample is safely in the probe, the perfusion pressure is set to a constant measure of 80 mmHg. Hearts are perfused at 37.0–37.5°C at a fixed end-diastolic (EDP) of ~8–10 mmHg. Multiple ^{31}P NMR spectra can be attained while simultaneously recording LV performance data (i.e. systolic pressure, EDP, heart rate, ±dP/dt, and coronary flow). At the completion of the experiment, the heart is removed from the NMR, freeze-clamped with Wollenberger tongs precooled in liquid nitrogen, and stored at −80°C until extraction.

Spectra are collected at a pulse angle of 60°, acquisition time of 0.4 seconds, and recycle time of 2.14 seconds. Spectra are obtained by averaging 120 free induction decays (FID) over a time period of 5 minutes. Frequency-domain NMR spectra are obtained by Fourier transformation of the FIDs [14]. Spectra are analyzed using 20 Hz exponential multiplication and zero and first order phase corrections.

Heart tissue processing and ^{13}C NMR spectroscopy of tissue extracts

For ^{13}C NMR spectroscopy, frozen heart tissues are powdered and homogenized in 1.2 M perchloric acid (PCA) in a 1:3 weight to volume ratio. The supernatant is neutralized with 5 M KOH to pH ~7.0. After centrifugation, the supernatant is filtered

through a resin column and rinsed with 3 mL of ultrapure water. The pH is then adjusted accurately to 7.0 with 1 M HCl. The sample is lyophilized and resuspended in 250 μL of deuterium oxide. As a reference standard, 1 μL of 25% 1,4-dioxane is added. The sample is filtered through a 0.2-μm syringe filter into a 3-mm NMR sample tube.

For ^{13}C NMR spectroscopy, the sample tube is placed in a 3-mm probe. Sample temperature is maintained at 21°C throughout the acquisition time. Proton-decoupled, ^{13}C NMR spectra are collected in a 600 MHz NMR spectrometer at a pulse angle of 60°, acquisition time of 1.5 seconds, and recycle delay of 2 seconds. Spectra are obtained by averaging ~4000–5000 FIDs over a time period of ~4–5 hours. Frequency-domain NMR spectra are obtained by Fourier transformation of the FIDs [14]. Spectra are analyzed using 1 Hz exponential multiplication and zero and first order phase corrections.

Analysis of NMR spectra

Converting NMR spectra into usable data requires multiple steps. First, each resonance peak of the ^{31}P spectra (Figure 41.4) is fitted to a Lorenztian function and the area determined. ATP is estimated by averaging the peak areas from γ-ATP and β-ATP. The α-ATP is not used because NAD^+ molecules contribute to an unknown portion of the signal. The ratio of phosphocreatine to ATP can be calculated (PCr:ATP) as an estimate of cardiac energetic status. Although ^{31}P NMR does not allow for direct quantification of PCr or ATP, the peak areas are proportional to the amount of phosphorous-containing compounds. Values for these signals are estimated by directly measuring ATP with a method such as high-performance liquid chromatography (HPLC). This value is used to calibrate the average ATP areas observed in the spectra.

The use of ^{31}P NMR spectroscopy in isolated perfused hearts also provides the most accurate measure of intracellular pH (pH_i) in a functioning organ. By analyzing the relative chemical shift of the inorganic phosphate (Pi) signal to the PCr signal, the researcher can monitor the "real-time" change of pH_i in the heart under different conditions (i.e. ischemia).

Several references are available regarding the analysis of ^{13}C NMR [7,8,15]. Spectra (Figure 41.1B)

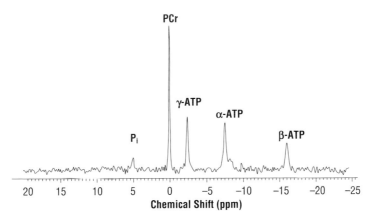

Figure 41.4 Representative ^{31}P NMR spectra of isolated mouse heart. Representative ^{31}P NMR spectra obtained by averaging 232 free induction decays (FIDs) over a 10-minute acquisition period. Notice the relatively small Pi peak. In an aerobically perfused heart supplied with pyruvate or fatty acids in addition to glucose, this peak should be minimal. During periods of ischemia, this peak increases while the PCr peak decreases. Notice the shoulder to the right of the α-ATP peak. This is the contribution of NAD$^+$ molecules. ATP, adenosine triphosphate; PCr, phosphocreatine; Pi, inorganic phosphate.

are referenced to the dioxane peak (~67.4 ppm). Of importance are the C4 and C3 carbons of glutamate that are centered at ~34.27 ppm and ~27.75 ppm, respectively (Figure 41.1B–D). The C4 glutamate has nine specific peak resonances while the C3 has six peak resonances in the respective multiplets [7,8,15]. Each of the resonance peaks is fitted to a Lorenztian function and the area determined. For the C4 multiplet (Figure 41.1C), the following ratios are determined: S/Total, D34/Total, D45/Total, and Q/Total [7,8,15]. Similar ratios are determined for the C3 multiplet (Figure 41.1D): S/Total, D/Total, and T/Total [7,8,15]. These ratios are subjected to isotopomer analysis using metabolic modeling, which estimates the contribution of the individual acetyl CoAs to the individual peaks in the multiplet [7]. The values calculated provide the relative contribution of FAs, glucose, and any unlabeled substrates (in this case, endogenous glycogen or triglycerides) utilized by the heart during the experiment.

Because the use of ^{13}C labeled substrates is based on the labeling position of the carbon from acetyl CoA that enters the TCA cycle, obtaining an all-inclusive substrate utilization profile requires additional experiments. Isolated hearts use both exogenous and endogenous substrates for energy production, which may change under certain conditions. Therefore, the use of different NMR

techniques [16], isotopic enrichment strategies [4–6], and data analysis may be required.

Variations of the protocol

The experiment described earlier can be adapted in various protocols to test additional hypotheses. For example, the perfusion protocol can be altered to include a period of ischemia/ reperfusion. Dynamic changes in high-energy phosphates can be plotted over a time course and compared in control and treatment groups [5]. Acute increases in energy demand utilizing high calcium or beta-adrenergic stimulation can also be examined [4,6]. In addition, different combinations of substrates in varying concentrations can be added to the perfusate [17]. Also, dynamic ^{13}C NMR spectroscopy can be performed in perfused hearts to provide more detailed information regarding metabolic flux [16]. Further examination of myocardial energetics can be made by measuring the creatine kinase reaction velocity or the ATP synthesis reaction velocity in the beating heart. This requires the use of ^{31}P magnetization transfer technique [4,18].

Alternative approaches

There are other strategies to assess cardiac function, energetics, and metabolism, either in concert or separately. The protocol presented herein is one way to accomplish this with perfused hearts of small animal models. However, *in vivo* analysis of cardiac function and energetics has been successfully completed in animal and human models with ^{31}P magnetic resonance spectroscopy (MRS) [19–22]. Furthermore, substrate metabolism can be assessed in an *in vivo* system using tracers or tracer analogs via magnetic resonance imaging (MRI) or positron emission tomography (PET) technology [23]. The utilization of these techniques is, however, limited by the availability of equipment and technical expertise.

More practical alternatives exist in the use of radioactive isotopes, such as radioactive carbon (^{14}C) or tritiated substrates (^{3}H), for the assessment of substrate metabolism in isolated perfused hearts [24–26] and cell culture systems [27]. Although this method is widely used, there are special requirements for the handling of radioactive materials as well as having the availability of a scintillation counter. Stable isotopes, such as deuterated compounds and ^{13}C substrates, can also be used in cell culture [28], perfused hearts [29], and *in vivo* models [30,31], and assessed using various mass spectrometry platforms. End-point measurements of ATP may be assessed using high-performance liquid chromatography (HPLC), which can provide an indication of energetic status in tissue extracts [32,33].

Strengths and weaknesses of method

The use of NMR spectroscopy in isolated perfused hearts is an experimental method with unique strengths in that simultaneous measurements of cardiac function, energetics, and substrate metabolism can be made. In addition, dynamic repeated measures can be made in a beating heart while direct functional and energetic responses are interrogated during physiological or pathological stress. However, despite the positives of this method, there are numerous limitations. The feasibility of performing such experiments requires the use of sophisticated and costly equipment. In addition, the use of ^{13}C-labeled compounds can be quite expensive for certain substrates. Moreover, since these are *ex vivo* experiments, generalizing findings to the *in vivo* condition must be done with caution since the interplay between systemic and cardiac metabolism could be important in modulating overall func-

tion and energetics. Lastly, the technically challenging nature of the experimental set-up and execution can limit the quality of the data. Therefore, it is imperative that the isolated perfused heart preparation be optimal so that cardiac function is stable for an extended time and PCr and ATP signals are adequate to obtain analyzable phosphorous spectra. Despite the limitations, the isolated perfused heart experiment, in conjunction, with multinuclear NMR spectroscopy remains a valuable research tool.

Conclusions

Assessment of cardiac function, myocardial energetics, and substrate utilization in isolated perfused mouse hearts in conjunction with multinuclear NMR spectroscopy is a technically challenging procedure requiring sophisticated equipment. However, the data it supplies to the researcher is invaluable in dissecting the effects of cardiac metabolism on function and energetics. The incorporation of bioengineered mouse models under physiological and/or pathological stressors in these experiments provides vital information in the understanding of the relationship between altered cardiac metabolism and myocardial performance.

References

1 Balaban R. NMR spectroscopy of the heart, part I. *Concepts Magn Reson* 1989; **1**: 15–26.

2 Fralix T, Balaban R. NMR spectroscopy of the heart: part II. *Concepts Magn Reson* 1989; **1**: 93–108.

3 Liao R, Jain M, Cui L, D'Agostino J, Aiello F, Luptak I, *et al*. Cardiac-specific overexpression of GLUT1 prevents the development of heart failure attributable to pressure overload in mice. *Circulation* 2002; **106**: 2125–2131.

4 Luptak I, Balschi JA, Xing Y, Leone TC, Kelly DP, Tian R, *et al*. Decreased contractile and metabolic reserve in peroxisome proliferator-activated receptor-alpha-null hearts can be rescued by increasing glucose transport and utilization. *Circulation* 2005; **112**: 2339–2346.

5 Luptak I, Yan J, Cui L, Jain M, Liao R, Tian R, *et al*. Long-term effects of increased glucose entry on mouse hearts during normal aging and ischemic stress. *Circulation* 2007; **116**: 901–909.

6 Yan J, Young ME, Cui L, Lopaschuk GD, Liao R, Tian R, *et al*. Increased glucose uptake and oxidation in mouse hearts prevent high fatty acid oxidation but cause cardiac

dysfunction in diet-induced obesity. *Circulation* 2009; **119**: 2818–2828.

7 Malloy CR, Sherry AD, Jeffrey FM. Evaluation of carbon flux and substrate selection through alternate pathways involving the citric acid cycle of the heart by 13C NMR spectroscopy. *J Biol Chem* 1988; **263**: 6964–6971.

8 Malloy CR, Sherry AD, Jeffrey FM. Analysis of tricarboxylic acid cycle of the heart using 13C isotope isomers. *Am J Physiol* 1990; **259**: H987–995.

9 Lopaschuk GD, Barr RL. Measurements of fatty acid and carbohydrate metabolism in the isolated working rat heart. *Mol Cell Biochem* 1997; **172**: 137–147.

10 Yu X, Alpert NM, Lewandowski ED. Modeling enrichment kinetics from dynamic 13C-NMR spectra: theoretical analysis and practical considerations. *Am J Physiol* 1997; **272**: C2037–2048.

11 Reichelt ME, Willems L, Hack BA, Peart JN, Headrick JP. Cardiac and coronary function in the Langendorff-perfused mouse heart model. *Exp Physiol* 2009; **94**: 54–70.

12 Sutherland FJ, Shattock MJ, Baker KE, Hearse DJ. Mouse isolated perfused heart: characteristics and cautions. *Clin Exp Pharmacol Physiol* 2003; **30**: 867–878.

13 Kolwicz SC, Jr., Tian R. Assessment of cardiac function and energetics in isolated mouse hearts using 31P NMR spectroscopy. *J Vis Exp* 2010; (42). pii: 2069.

14 Derome AE. *Modern NMR Techniques for Chemistry Research*. Oxford; New York: Pergamon Press, 1987.

15 Moreno KX, Sabelhaus SM, Merritt ME, Sherry AD, Malloy CR. Competition of pyruvate with physiological substrates for oxidation by the heart: implications for studies with hyperpolarized [1-13C] pyruvate. *Am J Physiol Heart Circ Physiol* 2010; **298**: H1556–1564.

16 O'Donnell JM, Zampino M, Alpert NM, Fasano MJ, Geenen DL, Lewandowski ED, *et al*. Accelerated triacylglycerol turnover kinetics in hearts of diabetic rats include evidence for compartment lipid storage. *Am J Physiol Endocrinol Metab* 2006; **290**: E448–455.

17 Jeffrey FM, Diczku V, Sherry AD, Malloy CR. Substrate selection in the isolated working rat heart: effects of reperfusion, afterload, and concentration. *Basic Res Cardiol* 1995; **90**: 388–396.

18 Spindler M, Saupe KW, Tian R, Ahmed S, Matlib MA, Ingwall JS, *et al*. Altered creatine kinase enzyme kinetics in diabetic cardiomyopathy. A(31)P NMR magnetization transfer study of the intact beating rat heart. *J Mol Cell Cardiol* 1999; **31**: 2175–2189.

19 Beer M, Sandstede J, Landschutz W, Viehrig M, Harre K, Horn M, *et al*. Altered energy metabolism after myocardial infarction assessed by 31P-MR-spectroscopy in humans. *Eur Radiol* 2000; **10**: 1323–1328.

20 de Roos A, Doornbos J, Luyten PR, Oosterwaal LJ, van der Wall EE, den Hollander JA, *et al*. Cardiac metabolism in patients with dilated and hypertrophic cardiomyopathy: assessment with proton-decoupled P-31 MR spectroscopy. *J Magn Reson Imaging* 1992; **2**: 711–719.

21 Gupta A, Akki A, Wang Y, Leppo MK, Chacko VP, Foster DB, *et al*. Creatine kinase-mediated improvement of function in failing mouse hearts provides causal evidence the failing heart is energy starved. *J Clin Invest* 2012; **122**: 291–302.

22 Gupta A, Chacko VP, Weiss RG. Abnormal energetics and ATP depletion in pressure-overload mouse hearts: in vivo high-energy phosphate concentration measures by noninvasive magnetic resonance. *Am J Physiol Heart Circ Physiol* 2009; **297**: H59–64.

23 van der Meer RW, Rijzewijk LJ, de Jong HW, Lamb HJ, Lubberink M, Romijn JA, *et al*. Pioglitazone improves cardiac function and alters myocardial substrate metabolism without affecting cardiac triglyceride accumulation and high-energy phosphate metabolism in patients with well-controlled type 2 diabetes mellitus. *Circulation* 2009; **119**: 2069–2077.

24 Buchanan J, Mazumder PK, Hu P, Chakrabarti G, Roberts MW, Yun UJ, *et al*. Reduced cardiac efficiency and altered substrate metabolism precedes the onset of hyperglycemia and contractile dysfunction in two mouse models of insulin resistance and obesity. *Endocrinology* 2005; **146**: 5341–5349.

25 Chambers KT, Leone TC, Sambandam N, Kovacs A, Wagg CS, Lopaschuk GD, *et al*. Chronic inhibition of pyruvate dehydrogenase in heart triggers an adaptive metabolic response. *J Biol Chem* 2011; **286**: 11155–11162.

26 Folmes CD, Sowah D, Clanachan AS, Lopaschuk GD. High rates of residual fatty acid oxidation during mild ischemia decrease cardiac work and efficiency. *J Mol Cell Cardiol* 2009; **47**: 142–148.

27 Spahr R, Jacobson SL, Siegmund B, Schwartz P, Piper HM. Substrate oxidation by adult cardiomyocytes in long-term primary culture. *J Mol Cell Cardiol* 1989; **21**: 175–185.

28 Metallo CM, Walther JL, Stephanopoulos G. Evaluation of 13C isotopic tracers for metabolic flux analysis in mammalian cells. *J Biotechnol* 2009; **144**: 167–174.

29 Bian F, Kasumov T, Jobbins KA, Minkler PE, Anderson VE, Kerner J, *et al*. Competition between acetate and oleate for the formation of malonyl-CoA and mitochondrial acetyl-CoA in the perfused rat heart. *J Mol Cell Cardiol* 2006; **41**: 868–875.

30 Castro-Perez J, Previs SF, McLaren DG, Shah V, Herath K, Bhat G, *et al*. In vivo D2O labeling to quantify static and dynamic changes in cholesterol and cholesterol esters by high resolution LC/MS. *J Lipid Res* 2011; **52**: 159–169.

31 Zhang XJ, Rodriguez NA, Wang L, Tuvdendorj D, Wu Z, Tan A, *et al.* Measurement of precursor enrichment for calculating intramuscular triglyceride fractional synthetic rate. *J Lipid Res* 2012; **53**: 119–125.

32 Neubauer S, Horn M, Naumann A, Tian R, Hu K, Laser M, *et al.* Impairment of energy metabolism in intact residual myocardium of rat hearts with chronic myocardial infarction. *J Clin Invest* 1995; **95**: 1092–1100.

33 Shen W, Asai K, Uechi M, Mathier MA, Shannon RP, Vatner SF, *et al.* Progressive loss of myocardial ATP due to a loss of total purines during the development of heart failure in dogs: a compensatory role for the parallel loss of creatine. *Circulation* 1999; **100**: 2113–2118.

Measurement of reactive oxygen species in cardiovascular disease

Mahmood Khan, Fatemat Hassan, Sashwati Roy, and Chandan K. Sen

Ohio State University, Columbus, OH, USA

Introduction

Recently, a lot of emphasis has been directed towards the pathological role of reactive oxygen species (ROS) and their contribution to cardiovascular disease. ROS have been implicated in the development and progression of heart failure, ventricular hypertrophy, ischemia–reperfusion injury, and even in atherosclerosis and hypertension [1–3]. In this chapter, we elaborate the different methods/techniques used for ROS measurements in the context of cardiovascular disease.

Oxygen possesses two unpaired electrons. Superoxide is a potent form of ROS that is formed when oxygen gains an extra electron. Superoxide can attract another electron, leading to the formation of another ROS molecule, hydrogen peroxide (H_2O_2). Molecular oxygen can be reduced to superoxide by several enzymatic electron transport systems; most prominent of which are mitochondrial electron transport complexes I and II, nonphagocytic NADPH oxidase (Nox), xanthine oxidase (XO), cyclooxygenase (COX), lipoxygenase (LOX), cytochrome P450 oxygenases, nitric oxide synthase (NOS) and also heme oxygenases [4]. Superoxide ($O_2^{\cdot-}$) and hydrogen peroxide (H_2O_2) act as progenitors for other ROS, including peroxynitrite ($ONOO^-$), hypochlorous acid, hydroxyl radical ($OH^\cdot$), lipid peroxides, lipid peroxy radicals, and lipid alkoxyl radicals [5]. $OH^\cdot$ is the most reactive and is released in negligible amounts.

The main source of ROS in the cardiovascular system is the mitochondrial electron transport chain and the nonphagocytic NADPH oxidase [6]. Under normal physiological conditions, the mitochondria release large amounts of free electrons in the process of producing energy. Normally, this process is tightly coupled to the production of ATP. Only 1–2% leak to form $O_2^{\cdot-}$ which is rapidly converted to H_2O_2 by superoxide dismutases (SODs), and any excess $O_2^{\cdot-}$ reacts with $NO^\cdot$ to form $ONOO^\cdot$. In physiological concentrations, almost all $O_2^{\cdot-}$ produced is scavenged by SODs, which include MnSOD (mitochondrial), Cu/Zn SOD (cytosolic), and ecSOD (in plasma membrane and extracellular spaces). During ischemia–reperfusion injury or with certain uncouplers like $NO^\cdot$, the electron transport chain is blocked and electrons are transferred directly to oxygen, forming large concentrations of superoxide free radicals, exceeding the capacity of MnSOD [5,7].

Small amounts of ROS are necessary for normal physiological function of cells [8], but acute or chronic release of large amounts of ROS has proven

Manual of Research Techniques in Cardiovascular Medicine, First Edition. Edited by Hossein Ardehali, Roberto Bolli, and Douglas W. Losordo.
© 2014 John Wiley & Sons, Ltd. Published 2014 by John Wiley & Sons, Ltd.

to be harmful. In the heart, acute release has been linked to cell death in myocardial infarction and ischemia–reperfusion injury [9], while chronic exposure has been implicated in the progression of end-stage heart failure [6]. Myocardial remodeling during progression of heart failure involves metalloproteinase activation, collagen deposition, and fibrosis, all of which are dependent on ROS [10,11].

There is an increasing body of evidence that ROS play an important role as physiological regulators in cardiovascular disease. Therefore, it has become crucial to develop and standardize accurate methods for the detection, quantification, timing, and localization of ROS both *in vitro* and *in vivo* systems. However, in the development and application of such techniques, many challenges are encountered. Antioxidant mechanisms are continuously scavenging different ROS, rapidly recycling these compounds, and rendering them intrinsically unstable. Subsequently, measurements at a particular time point might not reflect differences between treatment groups. Additionally, ROS production can be highly localized in certain cell compartments, limiting the accuracy of assays in an entire cell or tissue segments.

Measurement of the superoxide radical ($O_2^{\bullet-}$)

Electro paramagnetic resonance spectroscopy (EPR)

Principle. Specific forms of ROS can be measured directly at the site of production or as a footprint of their reaction with biological tissues. There is only one technique currently available for measuring ROS directly – electron spin resonance (ESR), also known as electron paramagnetic resonance (EPR) spectroscopy [12]. Using this approach, only the less-reactive and highly abundant radicals can be measured directly, such as the ascorbyl radical. EPR is too insensitive for measuring $O_2^{\bullet-}$ and •OH *in vivo*. Trapping mechanisms use spin traps to react with radicals generating stable adducts, which impart themselves to detection and quantification; this is very useful for *in vivo* studies

Although EPR can detect several specific forms of ROS, it is a relatively powerful tool to measure short-lived free radicals like $O_2^{\bullet-}$. EPR detects the paramagnetic properties of the unpaired electrons in free radicals. When a magnetic field is applied, these unpaired electrons arrange themselves either parallel or antiparallel to the imposed magnetic field. Application of electromagnetic radiation is absorbed by the unpaired electrons, which move to a higher energy level creating an absorption spectrum in the microwave region of the electromagnetic spectrum. A microwave generator, a resonator cavity, and a pair of electrical magnets on both sides of the resonator make up the EPR spectrometer. In brief, EPR measures the absorption of microwave radiation by an electromagnetic field in molecules with unpaired electrons like those present in free radicals. The absorbance spectrum is usually represented as its first derivative, which simply means that it is expressed as a rate of change of absorbance rather than absorbance itself. Most free radicals exist in low concentrations and are very short lived. Therefore, spin traps are used to produce long-lived adducts that can be measured by EPR spectrometers. Specific radical-trap adduct provides a signature EPR absorption spectra, where each radical has a specific *g* value (splitting factor), hyperfine structure, and line shape [13,14].

Commonly used spin traps include the nitrone compounds. Examples of traps often used to detect $O_2^{\bullet-}$ and •OH include PBN (α-phenyl-tert-butylnitrone), DMPO (5,5-dimethyl-1-pyrroline-*N*-oxide), and DEPMPO (5-[diethoxyphosphoryl]-5-methyl-1-pyrroline-*N*-oxide) [15]. Selection of spin trap is guided by several considerations. The trap should: (i) form a chemically stable adduct with the radical of interest; (ii) not be metabolized in biological systems; and (iii) react with the specific radical to generate a unique EPR spectrum. It is also important to identify the site where the probe will be localized in the living tissues. Spin traps can be used not only to identify, but also to quantify the specific radicals of interest.

Cyclic hydroxylamines are not spin traps *per se*, but are oxidized to form stable radicals that can be measured by EPR spectroscopy. They are relatively stable with half lives of several hours and undergo minimal bioreduction. Examples include CP-H (1-hydroxy-3-carboxy-2,2,5,-tetramethyl-pyrrolidine hydrochloride), CM-H (1-hydroxy-3-methoxycarbonyl-2,2,5,5-tetramethylpyrrolidine) and CAT1-H (1-hydroxy-2,2,6,6-tetramethylpiperidin-4-yl-

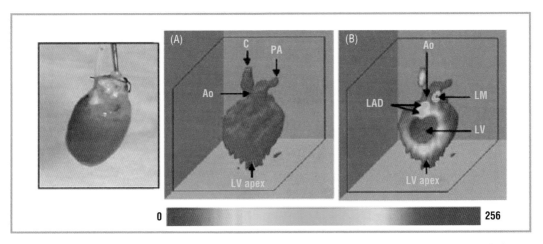

Figure 42.1 Three-dimensional image of rat heart infused with glucose char suspension: (A) full view of the heart; (B) a longitudinal cutout showing the internal structure of the heart; photograph of an isolated perfused rat heart is shown on the left. C, cannula; Ao, aortic root; PA, pulmonary artery; LM, left main coronary artery; LAD, left anterior descending artery; LV, left ventricular cavity. The void seen in the LV cavity is due to the inflated balloon. Image acquisition parameters: projections, 1024; magnetic field gradient, 50.0 G/cm; acquisition time, 78 min. (Source: Vikram, Rivera, Kuppusamy 2010. In Vivo imaging of Free Radicals and Oxygen. Methods in Molecular Biology, 2010, Volume 610, Part 1, 3–27. Reproduced with permission of Springer Science and Business Media).

trimethylammonium) [16]. These probes are more accurate than nitrone spin traps when used in cultured cells and intact tissues. CP-H and CM-H are cell-permeable probes and are well suited for measuring intracellular $O_2^{\cdot-}$. CP-H can also be oxidized by $ONOO^-$, so duplicate samples should be run with $ONOO^-$ scavenger to identify the specific ROS causing the reaction. CAT1-H is useful for measuring extracellular $O_2^{\cdot-}$ in intact tissue as it is resistant to auto-oxidation [16].

Materials and methods. To minimize auto-oxidation of hydroxylamines, stock solutions should be prepared in argon-bubbled ice-cold 0.9% NaCl with a chelating agent. Diethylenetriamine-penta-acetic acid or a combination of deferoxamine and diethyl-dithiocarbamate can be used as alternative chelating agents. Samples are incubated with Krebs/HEPES buffer containing the chelating agent along with the spin probe selected for 60 minutes at 37°C. Samples are then frozen in liquid nitrogen and EPR spectra are subsequently measured. If the spin probe selected is known to react with more than one free radical, duplicate samples can be preincubated in Krebs/HEPES buffer containing a scavenger that specifically extinguishes one of the reactive free radicals. For spin traps, the buffer is aspirated using capillary

tubing, snap frozen in liquid nitrogen and EPR spectra are recorded. Dikalov *et al.* described a detailed methodology [13].

Strengths. EPR directly measures short-lived free radicals, especially $O_2^{\cdot-}$. Nitrone spin traps are well suited for identifying free radicals when studying isolated enzymes. Cyclic hydroxylamines are useful to measure intracellular or extracellular $O_2^{\cdot-}$ when studying intact tissues and cells because they react with $O_2^{\cdot-}$ producing stable products that have long half-lives and are relatively resistant to bioreduction and auto-oxidation. EPR measurements can be restricted to a specific cellular compartment by proper selection of the spin probe [13]. Additionally, EPR enables imaging of tissue redox state *in vivo* and is useful for *in vivo* tissue oximetry (Figures 42.1 and 42.2) [17,18].

Limitations. The major limitation of EPR is the price and size of the spectrometers, which also require skilled staff and significant resources for maintenance. The bioreduction of highly unstable nitrone radical adducts into EPR-silent species limits their use in intact tissues and cells [19]. When DMPO and DEPMPO react with $O_2^{\cdot-}$ they form unique but short-lived adducts that can be identified

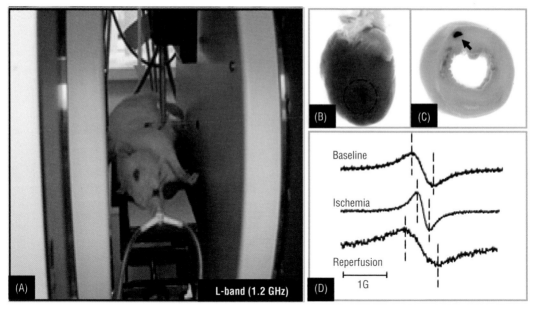

Figure 42.2 *In vivo* measurement of PO_2 in the rat heart using EPR oximetry. (A) Placement of a rat in the EPR spectrometer for monitoring of myocardial oxygenation. The animal, under isoflurane inhalation anesthesia, is placed in a right-lateral position with the chest open to the loop of a surface-coil resonator. (B,C) Implantation of oxygen-sensing microcrystals of LiNc-BuO in the left ventricular mid-myocardium. The probe particulates are seen as a black implant in the images of the whole heart and a formalin-fixed transverse slice through the left ventricle. The probe, which is nontoxic to tissue, responds to the partial pressure of oxygen (PO_2) at the site of placement. (D) Representative EPR signals obtained from a heart during preischemia (baseline), ischemia, and reperfusion. The peak-to-peak (indicated by dashed line) width of the signal is used to calculate PO_2 using a standard curve. Source: *Antioxid Redox Signal* 2009; **11**: 725–738. (Source: Khan M 2009 [18]. Reproduced with permission from Mary Ann Liebert, Inc).

through their hyperfine splits by EPR spectroscopy. Within seconds to minutes, they are rapidly converted to alcohols that produce EPR spectra identical to •OH adducts. Thus, the use of scavengers to discriminate between $O_2^{•-}$ and •OH is necessary. Caution should be exercised in selecting procedures for anesthesia and tissue processing; ketamine should be avoided as an anesthetic agent. Organic solvents should be used with caution because they can oxidize, trapping radicals and generating artifacts.

Chemiluminescence

Principle. At low basal levels, the source of ROS is hard to identify; however, under inducible conditions where copious amounts of ROS are produced, analytical systems can detect changes in ROS quantitatively. ROS signaling can be amplified by using sensitive $O_2^{•-}$-responsive chemiluminescent probes, most of which are cell permeable. The most commonly used probes are DCFH-DA (dichlorofluorescin diacetate), luminol, and lucigenin [20]. Luminol (5-amino-2,3-dihydro-1,4-phthalazinedione) is used to measure H_2O_2, HOCl, $OH^•$, and ONOOH [20]. Lucigenin (LC^{2+}) is more specific for $O_2^{•-}$ [21]. Lucigenin reacts with two $O_2^{•-}$ radicals, first forming a cation radical ($LC^{•+}$) which reacts with the second $O_2^{•-}$ forming the energy-rich dioxetane molecule (LCO_2), which subsequently emits a photon that can be detected by a luminometer [20,22]. $O_2^{•-}$ can also be measured by probes containing coelenterazine (2-methyl-6-phenyl-3,7-dihydroimidazol[1,2-a]pyrazin-3-1) [23]. Coelenterazine has been used to form CLA (cypridina luciferin analog) and MCLA (methylated-modified CLA) chemiluminescence probes.

Materials and methods. Krebs/HEPES buffer containing 5 μmol/L lucigenin is dark-adapted by incubating the buffer in a luminometer or

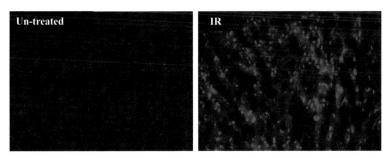

Figure 42.3 Measurement of superoxide in heart tissues subjected to ischemia–reperfusion injury (IR). Superoxide levels in the excised heart tissue were determined by histochemical staining and fluorescence microscopy at 10 minutes into reperfusion. (Source: Khan M 2010 [30]. Reproduced with permission from Aspect).

scintillation counter set to the out-of-coincidence mode until background counts stabilize. Samples are then added to the reaction vial and equilibrated for a few minutes. Five counts are then obtained every minute and averaged. While using luminol as a chemiluminescent probe, one should add specific scavengers to identify the specific ROS of interest. For example, catalase-sensitive signal may be interpreted as hydrogen peroxide specific. Similarly, urate may be used to detect peroxynitrite. Counts can be normalized to wet or dry weight used [21,24].

Strengths. The lucigenin-enhanced chemiluminescence approach is simple and widely used, as it is inexpensive and uses commonly available equipment [13]. Lucigenin is cell permeable, and thus can be used to measure intracellular $O_2^{\cdot-}$. Additionally, it is reasonably specific for $O_2^{\cdot-}$, and there is no need for a second measurement while using SOD. However, SOD must be modified in order to penetrate cells and dismutate $O_2^{\cdot-}$ at the site of lucigenin.

Limitations. Despite the broad usage of this technique, questions have been raised regarding its validity due to redox cycling through which lucigenin can produce $O_2^{\cdot-}$. Flavin-containing enzymes like XO and NOS can catalyze the reaction between lucigenin and oxygen, generating $O_2^{\cdot-}$. This redox cycling and artificial overestimation of $O_2^{\cdot-}$ is minimal when 5 μmol/L of lucigenin is used [21]. CLA and MCLA do not undergo such redox cycling. MCLA has also shown to have the highest signal : background ratio [25–27].

Fluorescence imaging

Principle. Dihydroethidium (DHE) exhibits a blue fluorescence in the cytosol, until it reacts with $O_2^{\cdot-}$ forming ethidium, which intercalates with nuclear DNA to produce a bright red fluorescence (Figure 42.3) [28]. DHE reacts with $O_2^{\cdot-}$ forming two main products: 2-hydroxyethidium, which is more specific for $O_2^{\cdot-}$, and ethidium, which reflects H_2O_2-dependent pathways involving metal proteins. Assessment of DHE fluorescence lacks specific quantification of each of its two main products, which are detected simultaneously. High-performance liquid chromatography (HPLC) separation and analysis of these two main products allows for more accurate quantitation of 2-hydroxyethidium [29]. DHE-based NADPH oxidase activity assays using HPLC or FACS analysis are commonly used. Such methods can enhance accuracy and allow better quantitation of vascular superoxide measurements [28].

Materials and methods. DHE is prepared in Krebs/HEPES buffer at 37°C at a concentration of 50 μmol/L. Tissues are incubated for 30 minutes. Sources of $O_2^{\cdot-}$ can be differentiated by preincubation with specific inhibitors such as oxypurinol as an XO inhibitor, apocynin as a NADPH oxidase inhibitor or N^G-nitro-L-arginine methyl ester as an inhibitor for the endothelial NO synthase. The tissue is then homogenized in 300 μL methanol and passed through a 0.22-μm syringe filter for subsequent HPLC analysis. A C-18 reverse column and a mobile phase at a flow rate of 0.5 mL/min containing 0.1% trifluoroacetic acid and an acetonitrile gradient are used to separate DHE, 2-hydroxyethidium and ethidium. Ethidium and 2-hydroxyethidium can be detected at an emission wavelength of 580 nm and an excitation wavelength of 480 nm [30]. DHE needs UV absorption at 355 nm [31].

DHE staining of tissues can instead be done by washing the OCT-embedded tissue sections with PBS for three times and subsequently incubating the tissue sections for 1 hour in 10 μM DHE at 37°C. In this case DHE should be prepared fresh in PBS and protected from direct light. Alternatively, when staining cells, DHE should be prepared in serum-free media rather than in PBS because cells should be alive in order to uptake the stain. DHE is available commercially from Molecular probes with an *excitation/emission wavelength* of 485 nm/590 nm. Because this approach lacks the power of HPLC separation, it is difficult to comment on the specific ROS being visualized unless additional measurements to address that concern are performed.

Strengths. Fluorescent DHE staining can indicate the exact location of $O_2^{\cdot-}$ production, thus solving the spatial challenge of ROS measurement. HPLC detection of 2-hydroxyethidium specifically quantifies $O_2^{\cdot-}$ in tissues.

Limitations. Experiments must be performed in a dark room due to the light sensitivity of DHE, which can react with oxygen in solution. DHE working solutions should be freshly prepared and stock solutions should be stored at −80°C in dark tubes using argon-purged buffers. HPLC also requires fairly expensive equipment and specific staining.

Measurement of superoxide radical in mitochondria

Superoxide can be measured using the previously discussed spectrophotometric methods [32]. CLA and MCLA provide highly sensitive chemiluminescent signals, but the main limitation in mitochondria is that CLA and its derivatives strongly inhibit complex I of the electron transport chain altering ROS production. DHE fluorescent staining of mitochondrial DNA is a reliable means for the estimation of ROS production [33]. This provides an advantage in isolated mitochondria over whole-cell measurements, where nuclear DNA can complicate the results.

Hydrogen peroxide (H₂O₂) assays

2′7′-dichlorofluorescein diacetate (DCFH-DA)

Principle. DCFH-DA is mainly used to measure H_2O_2, but can react with several other ROS, $ONOO^-$, lipid hydroperoxides, and minimally reacts with $O_2^{\cdot-}$. Nonfluorescent 2′,7′-dichlorodihydrofluorescein diacetate (DCFH-DA) is employed. DCFH-DA enters cells by passive diffusion. Inside the cytosol, esterases remove the acetate groups to form the nonfluorescent derivative 2′,7′-dichlorodihydrofluorescein (DCFH). Upon exposure to ROS as well as other oxidants such as reactive nitrogen species (RNS), DCFH undergoes two-electron oxidation, resulting in generation of the highly fluorescent DCF [34].

Materials and methods. DCFH-DA is available commercially from Molecular Probes (Eugene, OR). A stock solution can be prepared in DMSO and stored at −80°C. Cultured cells or frozen tissues preincubated with DCFH-DA prepared in serum-free media or PBS, respectively, at a final concentration of 10 μM for 1 hour. Precaution should be taken to address biological autofluorescence. DCFH-DA fluorescence can also be assessed in suspended cells using flow cytometry. One artifact of the method is the oxidation of dichlorodihydrofluorescein, which is released from tissues together with DCF during the extraction procedure. This problem may be resolved by decreasing pH during the extraction. The optimal conditions and the time for tissue incubation with DCFH-DA and for the extraction of DCF need to be determined on a case by case basis [35].

Strengths. DCFH-DA is able to measure intracellular ROS production, and to measure the spatial localization of ROS within tissues with single-cell sensitivity.

Limitations. Precautions should be taken while interpreting the results by this technique. Artificial amplification of DCFH-DA signal is a major concern. DCF is prone to photoreduction generating a semiquinone radical that can reduce oxygen to $O_2^{\cdot-}$. Peroxidases can also directly oxidize DCFH to DCF without interacting with superoxide. Moreover, DCF-free radical anion formed from redox reactions of DCF and DCFH can generate $O_2^{\cdot-}$ and react with antioxidants like ascorbate and thiols. Since DCFH-DA cannot measure $O_2^{\cdot-}$ directly, only the dismutated portion of $O_2^{\cdot-}$ to H_2O_2 will be measured, resulting in ROS signal amplification [36]. It is recommended to use the DCFH-DA for screening purposes, and that additional assays are used to quantify H_2O_2 [37].

HyPer: [H_2O_2]

Principle. HyPer is a genetically encoded fluorescent indicator used for measurement of intracellular H_2O_2 production by microscopic imaging [38,39]. HyPer consists of the fluorescent protein (cpYFP) and the H_2O_2-sensing regulatory domain of *Escherichia coli* (OxyR). OxyR consists of an H_2O_2-sensitive domain and a DNA binding domain. Upon oxidation by H_2O_2, OxyR undergoes a conformational change in order to expose the DNA binding domain, but at the same time exposing cpYFP and hence fluorescence [40].

Materials and methods. Cells are transfected with the HyPer-Cyto vector, preferably using the FuGENE 6 transfection reagent prepared in serum-free Opti-MEM. Cells are subsequently incubated for 16–24 hours in Opti-MEM supplemented with 2% FCS. Transfection can be confirmed using the GFP filter of the microscope. HyPer can be excited both at 420 and 500 nm with one emission peak at 516 nm.

Strengths. This method solves the problem of photoreduction encountered with DCF (dichlorofluorescein) derivatives, hence providing more accurate results. While DCF derivatives can be oxidized by several types of ROS and RNS, HyPer can only detect H_2O_2, making it more specific. The fact that HyPer is genetically encoded makes it suitable to be targeted to specific subcellular compartments. HyPer can be oxidized in physiological conditions at very low levels and also can detect relatively high pathological concentrations accurately. Taking real-time series images of HyPer can answer questions not only about the intensity of H_2O_2 generation, but also the temporal and spatial component of H_2O_2 production.

Limitations. At this time, HyPer represents one of the most acceptable approaches to study H_2O_2 in cellular compartments.

Measurement of hydrogen peroxide in mitochondria

To measure hydrogen peroxide in isolated mitochondria [41,42], scopoletin is still sometimes used, but DCFH-DA is used more commonly. DCFH-DA can be oxidized by other ROS molecules but predominantly H_2O_2. This method can be used in isolated mitochondrial preparations as well as in living cells. As long as additional approaches are employed to confirm the H_2O_2-sensitive component of DCFH-DA signal, the methodology is valuable.

Bio-markers

The following biomarker approaches rely on the indirect measurement of ROS by assessing the footprint of their reaction with biological tissues. ROS and RNS interact with DNA, proteins, and lipids in a characteristic way, producing specific biomarkers. Measurement of these products provides a quantitative means of measuring the impact of ROS, given that these products are unique to ROS biochemistry.

DNA damage

Principle. One of the most common targets of ROS is DNA, modifications of which have been associated with cellular transformation and genome instability [43–46]. There are a number of experimental strategies to assess oxidative modification of DNA bases, such as chromatography-based assays and indirect immunofluorescence. While the former provide quantitative assessment of oxidative modification, the latter is a much simpler assay for the qualitative determination of DNA base modification in very small sample sizes [47].

8-Oxo-2′-deoxyguanosine (8-oxo-dG) has emerged as a reliable marker for oxidative stress [48]. 8-oxo-dG is a mutagenic base modification product of ROS DNA damage that is excreted extracellularly into the plasma and urine [48]. Others have also used atomic force microscopy (AFM) to assess the distribution of double-strand breaks in DNA and hence assess and quantify the amount of oxidative damage to DNA [47].

Materials and methods. A detailed step-wise protocol for the method has been reported [49]. The HPLC system (Agilent 1100 Series, quaternary pump,

G1311A and microvacuum degasser, G1379A, Agilent Technologies Inc., Waldbronn, Germany), equipped with a nonthermostatted well-plate auto-sampler (G1313A),was linked to a 3200 QTRAPmass spectrometer from Applied Biosystems/MDS Sciex (MDS Inc., Concord, ON, Canada) for analysis. HPLC separation was achieved using a Chromolith Performance RP-18e column (4.6 mm ID × 100 mm L, particle size: 2 µm × 13 nm pore) (Merck KGaA, Darmstadt, Germany) secured by a guard cartridge (C18, 3 mm ID × 4 mm L) (Phenomenex, Torrance, CA). The isocratic mobile phase consisted of ammonium acetate (10 mmol/L adjusted to pH 4.3 with acetic acid) and acetonitrile (96.4 : 3.6 in volume). MS/MS analysis was performed in a positive-ion mode with a TurboIon Spray® source as described [49].

Strengths. Urine 8-oxodG represents a sensitive, stable and specific marker of oxidative stress in the whole body. The 8-oxodG molecules in urine are freely dispersed in the liquid matrix, and therefore it is not necessary to perform digestion or solid phase extraction before introducing the sample into HPLC. Because of the 100% recovery of 8-oxodG, an isotopic internal standard is not needed.

Limitations. A LC-MS/MS set-up and expertise is required for the assay.

Lipid peroxidation

Principle. Lipid peroxidation occurs during the reaction of lipid with molecular oxygen, and is associated with various pathological states [50]. A plethora of oxidation products are generated from lipid peroxidation reactions. One type of these oxidation products, the F2-isoprostanes, has reasonable stability in tissues and biological fluids and can act as a measure of oxidative stress status. Most of the oxidation products, however, have limited stability, and they either decompose or react with biomolecules, including proteins, lipids, and nucleic acids, to form adducts. Thus, the detection and quantification of these various oxidized lipids *in vivo* poses a significant challenge. Light emission during hydroperoxide-induced oxidation of luminol has been used as a chemiluminescence assay to assess lipid peroxidation [51]. This sensitive method combined with an HPLC separation has been used to analyze the levels of hydroperoxides from cholesterol esters and phospholipids in plasma samples. However, the thiobarbituric acid reactive substance (TBARS) and Fe(III)xylenol orange complex assays are the most frequently used methods to assess lipid peroxidation.

Materials and methods. The test is usually performed by heating a lipid peroxidation mixture and TBA in an acidic medium to form a red pigment, which has an absorption maximum at 532 nm and fluorescence emission at 553 nm [52]. To address the lack of specificity of conventional TBARS and diene methodologies, the Fe(III)xylenol orange complex assay was developed [53]. The ferric-xylenol orange (FOX) method for measurement of hydroperoxides is based on a technique that employs reduction of peroxides in an acidic condition by Fe^{2+} and formation of the colored ferric-xylenol orange (XO/Fe^{3+}) product with a peak at 560 nm. The 560 nm absorbance peak of XO/Fe^{3+} shifts to a 610 nm peak with high absorption intensity in the presence of phosphatidylcholine. This is useful for quantification of peroxides such as phospholipid hydroperoxides.

Strength. Both TBARS and FOX methods are simple assays that do not require specialized equipment.

Limitations. Both TBARS and the FOX assays are nonspecific methods, and caution is recommended when they are used for the analyses of oxidized biomolecules other than lipid hydroperoxides, such as endoperoxides [50].

Thiol-disulfide interchange

Principle. Thiol–disulfide interchange is a major component of most oxidative mechanisms carrying thiol to disulfide. Regulation of intracellular thiol–disulfide redox status is essential to cellular homeostasis and involves the regulation of both oxidative and reductive pathways, production of oxidant scavengers, and the ability of cells to respond to changes in the redox environment. In the cytosol, regulatory disulfide bonds can form in spite of the prevailing reducing conditions and may thereby function as redox switches. Such disulfide bonds are protected from enzymatic reduction by kinetic barriers and thus exist long enough to elicit the signal [54]. Thiol–disulfide redox switches regulate heme binding to proteins and modulate their activities. Methods to characterize heme-binding sites and to assess their physiological relevance represent powerful tools [55]. For thiol–disulfide interconversion to regulate activity of a system, the redox process must be reversible at the ambient redox potentials found within the cell. Thus, methods and their limitations need to be cautiously considered [55]. Several reversible oxidative post-translational modifications of protein cysteines also participate in cell signaling. Specific proteomic techniques are required to identify these modifications and to study their regulation in different cell processes that are collectively known as thiol redox proteomics.

Materials and methods. Fluorescence derivatization followed by two-dimensional electrophoresis is a relatively simple approach to "visualize" redox changes in a broad context. Such derivatization is now an established technique in general proteomics, mainly due to its use in two-dimensional fluorescence difference gel electrophoresis (DIGE) for quantitative proteomics. The protocol described below has been discussed in detail [56]. During extraction and sample preparation, it is critical to freeze thiols at their native redox state, which can be done by using TCA during the extraction to precipitate the protein samples. This method allows for a low pH during extraction that circumvents the formation of the thiolate form, which is more reactive in many oxidation and disulfide exchange reactions. After TCA precipitation, a washing step is performed to remove TCA. The samples can then be resuspended in a suitable buffer, preferably with a blocking agent such as N-ethylmaleimide (NEM) or 2-iodoacetamide (IAA). For sample labeling, infrared dyes DY-680 and DY-780 linked to maleimide have also been successfully used for redox proteomics. Once samples are labeled, standard protocol of DIGE is performed [57]. For two-dimensional electrophoresis (2-DE) image analysis, the labeled cysteine signals are analyzed with standard 2-DE software [56].

Strengths. This methodology is relatively accessible to many laboratories, unlike techniques that require extensive instrumentation such LC-MS. Multiple approaches and reagents are available for sample derivatization/ preparation. This method allows a relatively large number of samples and replicates to be compared at the same time.

Limitations. Specialized equipment is required for 2-DE and fluorescent imaging detection. Although the method is very sensitive for visualization of the variations in protein modification, it is difficult to identify the cysteines that are modified with the fluorophore from the digested spots.

Measurement of mitochondrial ROS in living cells

Cellular ROS measurement is often considered an indicator of mitochondrial function based on the assumption that mitochondria are the predominant generators of ROS [58]. That is not always accurate; for example in phagocytic cells the primary sources of ROS are NADPH oxidases. Even in nonphagocytic cells, novel sources of ROS are being reported constantly. When considering mitochondrial ROS, the major concern is that many probes inhibit complex 1 of the electron transport chain, altering the production of ROS and hence providing inaccurate results [32]. Reduced Mito Tracker Red CM-H_2Ros (Molecular Probes) is a mitochondria-specific probe for ROS measurements, both qualitatively and quantitatively. CM-H_2Ros is nonfluorescent, and fluoresces only when oxidized by intracellular hydrogen peroxide. CM-H_2Ros can only be oxidized, and hence can only fluoresce in actively respiring cells. Oxidation of CM-H_2Ros produces a positively charged fluorescent end product that covalently binds to mitochondrial proteins. Fluorescence can be detected at an emission wavelength of 590 nm. Precaution must be taken during incubation and permeation of the probe in live cells, because if the mitochondrial membrane potential collapses, the stain will diffuse to the nucleus and other cellular compartments [59]. The mitochondrial superoxide production can also be visualized by fluorescence microscopy using the MitoSOX™ Red reagent (Molecular Probes). MitoSOX™ Red reagent permeates in live cells where it selectively targets mitochondria and gets rapidly oxidized by superoxide, but not by other ROS and RNS [60]. The oxidized product is highly fluorescent upon binding to nucleic acid. Recently reported methods hold promise in delivering accurate quantitative and specific methodology for the measurement of mitochondrial ROS production; HyPer can be directed to mitochondria, where it is oxidized by hydrogen peroxide, exposing cpYFP (the circularly permuted yellow fluorescent protein) hence producing fluorescence (Section HyPer in this chapter). Wang *et al.* have recently used the circularly permuted yellow fluorescent (cpYFP) alone as a mitochondrial superoxide marker. The cpYFP fluorescence was achieved by dual excitation at 405 and 488 nm and an emission >505 nm [61]. These fluorescence-based techniques provide a reliable mitochondria-specific quantitative approach for measuring mitochondrial ROS production.

Conclusion

Prudent choice of appropriate analytical system(s) is undoubtedly the single most important consideration in the study of reactive oxygen species in biological systems. Cell biology studies must consider that the redox environment is not homogenous across the cell. The demonstrated presence of redox microenvironments within the cell requires that cell-compartment targeted probes (i.e. mitochondrial matrix, endoplasmic reticulum, etc.) be employed. Efforts to capture the kinetics of ROS production could be highly informative and should be seriously considered. While *in vitro* approaches are simpler, caution must be exercised when relating such findings to *in vivo* systems. EPR represents a direct *in vivo* approach to measure radical species, including molecular oxygen. Interpretation of EPR results must consider probe chemistry and how it interacts with the biological system in question. The study of tissue homogenates can be grossly misleading because homogenization under oxygen-rich ambience may cause several artifacts. Preanalysis storage of excised tissue is another critical factor. When possible, samples should be stored in liquid nitrogen to minimize *ex vivo* oxidation processes. In human studies, the opportunity to directly study reactive oxygen species is limited. In such scenarios, the study of biomarkers becomes valuable. As pointed out in this chapter, each and every assay system has its own advantages and limitations. The use of multiple assay systems, chosen with the biological system and specific hypothesis in mind, is recommended. Finally,

interpretation of data must exercise caution and account for the limitations of the assay systems used.

Acknowledgement

Relevant work in the authors' laboratory is supported by the following grants from the National Institutes of Health: HL073087 (CKS), GM069589 (CKS), GM077185 (CKS), NS42617 (CKS), NR013898 (CKS), and DK076566 (SR). MK was supported by AHA SDG 0930181N.

References

1 Manea A. NADPH oxidase-derived reactive oxygen species: involvement in vascular physiology and pathology. *Cell Tissue Res* 2010; **342**: 325–339.

2 Thirunavukkarasu M, Adluri RS, Juhasz B, Samuel SM, Zhan L, Kaur A, *et al.* Novel role of NADPH oxidase in ischemic myocardium: a study with Nox2 knockout mice. *Funct Integr Genomics* 2012; **12**: 501–514.

3 Elahi MM, Kong YX, Matata BM. Oxidative stress as a mediator of cardiovascular disease. *Oxid Med Cell Longev* 2009; **2**: 259–269.

4 Valko M, Leibfritz D, Moncol J, Cronin MT, Mazur M, Telser J, *et al.* Free radicals and antioxidants in normal physiological functions and human disease. *Int J Biochem Cell Biol* 2007; **39**: 44–84.

5 Sorescu D, Griendling KK. Reactive oxygen species, mitochondria, and NAD(P)H oxidases in the development and progression of heart failure. *Congest Heart Fail* 2002; **8**: 132–140.

6 Kuroda J, Sadoshima J. NADPH oxidase and cardiac failure. *J Cardiovasc Transl Res* 2010; **3**: 314–320.

7 Boveris A, Cadenas E, Stoppani AO. Role of ubiquinone in the mitochondrial generation of hydrogen peroxide. *Biochem J* 1976; **156**: 435–444.

8 Griendling KK, Sorescu D, Ushio-Fukai M. NAD(P)H oxidase: role in cardiovascular biology and disease. *Circ Res* 2000; **86**: 494–501.

9 Zweier JL, Kuppusamy P, Lutty GA. Measurement of endothelial cell free radical generation: evidence for a central mechanism of free radical injury in postischemic tissues. *Proc Natl Acad Sci U S A* 1988; **85**: 4046–4050.

10 Siwik DA, Pagano PJ, Colucci WS. Oxidative stress regulates collagen synthesis and matrix metalloproteinase activity in cardiac fibroblasts. *Am J Physiol Cell Physiol* 2001; **280**: C53–60.

11 Rajagopalan S, Meng XP, Ramasamy S, Harrison DG, Galis ZS. Reactive oxygen species produced by macrophage-derived foam cells regulate the activity of vascular matrix metalloproteinases in vitro. Implications for atherosclerotic plaque stability. *J Clin Invest* 1996; **98**: 2572–2579.

12 Halliwell B, Gutteridge JMC. *Free Radicals in Biology and Medicine*, 3rd edn. Oxford: Oxford University Press, 1999.

13 Dikalov S, Griendling KK, Harrison DG. Measurement of reactive oxygen species in cardiovascular studies. *Hypertension* 2007; **49**: 717–727.

14 Janzen EG. Spin trapping. *Methods Enzymol* 1984; **105**: 188–198.

15 Dikalov S, Jiang J, Mason RP. Characterization of the high-resolution ESR spectra of superoxide radical adducts of 5-(diethoxyphosphoryl)-5-methyl-1-pyrroline N-oxide (DEPMPO) and 5,5-dimethyl 1-pyrroline N-oxide (DMPO). Analysis of conformational exchange. *Free Radic Res* 2005; **39**: 825–836.

16 Dikalov SI, Kirilyuk IA, Voinov M, Grigor'ev IA. EPR detection of cellular and mitochondrial superoxide using cyclic hydroxylamines. *Free Radic Res* 2011; **45**: 417–430.

17 Kuppusamy P, Chzhan M, Wang P, Zweier JL. Three-dimensional gated EPR imaging of the beating heart: time-resolved measurements of free radical distribution during the cardiac contractile cycle. *Magn Reson Med* 1996; **35**: 323–328.

18 Khan M, Mohan IK, Kutala VK, Kotha SR, Parinandi NL, Hamlin RL, et al. Sulfaphenazole protects heart against ischemia-reperfusion injury and cardiac dysfunction by overexpression of iNOS, leading to enhancement of nitric oxide bioavailability and tissue oxygenation. *Antioxid Redox Signal* 2009; **11**: 725–738.

19 Bardelang D, Rockenbauer A, Karoui H, Finet JP, Biskupska I, Banaszak K, et al. Inclusion complexes of EMPO derivatives with 2,6-di-O-methyl-beta-cyclodextrin: synthesis, NMR and EPR investigations for enhanced superoxide detection. *Org Biomol Chem* 2006; **4**: 2874–2882.

20 Faulkner K, Fridovich I. Luminol and lucigenin as detectors for O2. *Free Radic Biol Med* 1993; **15**: 447–451.

21 Li Y, Zhu H, Kuppusamy P, Roubaud V, Zweier JL, Trush MA, et al. Validation of lucigenin (bis-N-methylacridinium) as a chemilumigenic probe for detecting superoxide anion radical production by enzymatic and cellular systems. *J Biol Chem* 1998; **273**: 2015–2023.

22 Maeda M. [Chemiluminescent assay for biological substances – chemiluminescent assay for alkaline phosphatase using lucigenin and its application to enzyme immunoassay]. *Rinsho Byori* 2004; **52**: 851–859.

23 Nakano M, Sugioka K, Ushijima Y, Goto T. Chemiluminescence probe with Cypridina luciferin analog, 2-methyl-6-phenyl 3,7 dihydroimidazo[1,2-a] pyrazin-3-one, for estimating the ability of human granulocytes to generate O2. *Anal Biochem* 1986; **159**: 363–369.

24 Li Y, Stansbury KH, Zhu H, Trush MA. Biochemical characterization of lucigenin (Bis-N-methylacridinium) as a chemiluminescent probe for detecting intramitochondrial superoxide anion radical production. *Biochem Biophys Res Commun* 1999; **262**: 80–87.

25 Bancirova M. Sodium azide as a specific quencher of singlet oxygen during chemiluminescent detection by luminol and Cypridina luciferin analogues. *Luminescence* 2011; **26**: 685–688.

26 Wang J, Xu M, Chen M, Jiang Z, Chen G. Study on sonodynamic activity of metallophthalocyanine sonosensitizers based on the sonochemiluminescence of MCLA. *Ultrason Sonochem* 2012; **19**: 237–242.

27 Hosaka S, Obuki M, Nakajima J, Suzuki M. Comparative study of antioxidants as quenchers or scavengers of reactive oxygen species based on quenching of MCLA-dependent chemiluminescence. *Luminescence* 2005; **20**: 419–427.

28 Laurindo FR, Fernandes DC, Santos CX. Assessment of superoxide production and NADPH oxidase activity by HPLC analysis of dihydroethidium oxidation products. *Methods Enzymol* 2008; **441**: 237–260.

29 Zhao H, Kalivendi S, Zhang H, Joseph J, Nithipatikom K, Vasquez-Vivar J, et al. Superoxide reacts with hydroethidine but forms a fluorescent product that is distinctly different from ethidium: potential implications in intracellular fluorescence detection of superoxide. *Free Radic Biol Med* 2003; **34**: 1359–1368.

30 Khan M, Meduru S, Mostafa M, Khan S, Hideg K, Kuppusamy P, et al. Trimetazidine, administered at the onset of reperfusion, ameliorates myocardial dysfunction and injury by activation of p38 mitogen-activated protein kinase and Akt signaling. *J Pharmacol Exp Ther* 2010; **333**: 421–429.

31 Fink B, Laude K, McCann L, Doughan A, Harrison DG, Dikalov S, et al. Detection of intracellular superoxide formation in endothelial cells and intact tissues using dihydroethidium and an HPLC-based assay. *Am J Physiol Cell Physiol* 2004; **287**: C895–902.

32 Degli Esposti M. Measuring mitochondrial reactive oxygen species. *Methods* 2002; **26**: 335–340.

33 Kruglov AG, Teplova VV, Saris NE. The effect of the lipophilic cation lucigenin on mitochondria depends on the site of its reduction. *Biochem Pharmacol* 2007; **74**: 545–556.

34 Reiniers MJ, van Golen RF, van Gulik TM, Heger M. 2′,7′-Dichlorofluorescein is not a probe for the detection of reactive oxygen and nitrogen species. *J Hepatol* 2012; **560**: 1214–1216.

35 Korystov YN, Emel'yanov MO, Korystova AF, Levitman MK, Shaposhnikova VV. Determination of reactive

oxygen and nitrogen species in rat aorta using the dichlorofluorescein assay. *Free Radic Res* 2009; **43**: 149–155.

36 Wrona M, Wardman P. Properties of the radical intermediate obtained on oxidation of 2′,7′-dichlorodihydrofluorescein, a probe for oxidative stress. *Free Radic Biol Med* 2006; **41**: 657–667.

37 Pase L, Nowell CJ, Lieschke GJ. In vivo real-time visualization of leukocytes and intracellular hydrogen peroxide levels during a zebrafish acute inflammation assay. *Methods Enzymol* 2012; **506**: 135–156.

38 Roma LP, Duprez J, Takahashi HK, Gilon P, Wiederkehr A, Jonas JC, et al. Dynamic measurements of mitochondrial hydrogen peroxide concentration and glutathione redox state in rat pancreatic beta-cells using ratiometric fluorescent proteins: confounding effects of pH with HyPer but not roGFP1. *Biochem J* 2012; **441**: 971–978.

39 Markvicheva KN, Bogdanova EA, Staroverov DB, Lukyanov S, Belousov VV. Imaging of intracellular hydrogen peroxide production with HyPer upon stimulation of HeLa cells with epidermal growth factor. *Methods Mol Biol* 2009; **476**: 76–83.

40 Belousova IE, Kazakov DV, Michal M, Suster S. Vulvar toker cells: the long-awaited missing link: a proposal for an origin-based histogenetic classification of extramammary paget disease. *Am J Dermatopathol* 2006; **28**: 84–86.

41 Loschen G, Azzi A. On the formation of hydrogen peroxide and oxygen radicals in heart mitochondria. *Recent Adv Stud Cardiac Struct Metab* 1975; **7**: 3–12.

42 Walker PD, Shah SV. Gentamicin enhanced production of hydrogen peroxide by renal cortical mitochondria. *Am J Physiol* 1987; **253**: C495–499.

43 Mao P, Reddy PH. Aging and amyloid beta-induced oxidative DNA damage and mitochondrial dysfunction in Alzheimer's disease: implications for early intervention and therapeutics. *Biochim Biophys Acta* 2011; **1812**: 1359–1370.

44 Lee SF, Pervaiz S. Assessment of oxidative stress-induced DNA damage by immunoflourescent analysis of 8-oxodG. *Methods Cell Biol* 2011; **103**: 99–113.

45 Pascucci B, D'Errico M, Parlanti E, Giovannini S, Dogliotti E. Role of nucleotide excision repair proteins in oxidative DNA damage repair: an updating. *Biochemistry (Mosc)* 2011; **76**: 4–15.

46 Kryston TB, Georgiev AB, Pissis P, Georgakilas AG. Role of oxidative stress and DNA damage in human carcinogenesis. *Mutat Res* 2011; **711**: 193–201.

47 Su M, Yang Y, Yang G. Quantitative measurement of hydroxyl radical induced DNA double-strand breaks and the effect of N-acetyl-L-cysteine. *FEBS Lett* 2006; **580**: 4136–4142.

48 Haghdoost S, Czene S, Naslund I, Skog S, Harms-Ringdahl M. Extracellular 8-oxo-dG as a sensitive parameter for oxidative stress in vivo and in vitro. *Free Radic Res* 2005; **39**: 153–162.

49 Lee KF, Chung WY, Benzie IF. Urine 8-oxo-7,8-dihydro-2′-deoxyguanosine (8-oxodG), a specific marker of oxidative stress, using direct, isocratic LC-MS/MS: Method evaluation and application in study of biological variation in healthy adults. *Clin Chim Acta* 2010; **411**: 416–422.

50 Yin H, Xu L, Porter NA. Free radical lipid peroxidation: mechanisms and analysis. *Chem Rev* 2011; **111**: 5944–5972.

51 Kawagoe M, Nakagawa K. Attenuation of luminol-amplified chemiluminescent intensity and lipid peroxidation in the livers of quercetin-fed mice. *Toxicol Lett* 2000; **114**: 189–196.

52 Meagher EA, FitzGerald GA. Indices of lipid peroxidation in vivo: strengths and limitations. *Free Radic Biol Med* 2000; **28**: 1745–1750.

53 Hermes-Lima M, Willmore WG, Storey KB. Quantification of lipid peroxidation in tissue extracts based on Fe(III) xylenol orange complex formation. *Free Radic Biol Med* 1995; **19**: 271–280.

54 Jensen KS, Hansen RE, Winther JR. Kinetic and thermodynamic aspects of cellular thiol-disulfide redox regulation. *Antioxid Redox Signal* 2009; **11**: 1047–1058.

55 Ragsdale SW, Yi L. Thiol/Disulfide redox switches in the regulation of heme binding to proteins. *Antioxid Redox Signal* 2011; **14**: 1039–1047.

56 Izquierdo-Alvarez A, Martinez-Ruiz A. Thiol redox proteomics seen with fluorescent eyes: the detection of cysteine oxidative modifications by fluorescence derivatization and 2-DE. *J Proteomics* 2011; **75**: 329–338.

57 Tewari AK, Roy S, Khanna S, Sen CK. Proteomic analysis of the mammalian cell nucleus. *Methods Enzymol* 2004; **381**: 192–201.

58 Orrenius S. Reactive oxygen species in mitochondria-mediated cell death. *Drug Metab Rev* 2007; **39**: 443–455.

59 Esposti MD, Hatzinisiriou I, McLennan H, Ralph S. Bcl-2 and mitochondrial oxygen radicals. New approaches with reactive oxygen species-sensitive probes. *J Biol Chem* 1999; **274**: 29831–29837.

60 Andre L, Gouzi F, Thireau J, Meyer G, Boissiere J, Delage M, et al. Carbon monoxide exposure enhances arrhythmia after cardiac stress: involvement of oxidative stress. *Basic Res Cardiol* 2011; **106**: 1235–1246.

61 Wang W, Fang H, Groom L, Cheng A, Zhang W, Liu J, et al. Superoxide flashes in single mitochondria. *Cell* 2008; **134**: 279–290.

Assessing autophagy

Roberta A. Gottlieb

San Diego State University, San Diego, CA, USA

Introduction

Macroautophagy involves protein nucleation and formation of a cup-shaped lipid double-membrane structure, which elongates to engulf the cargo (Figure 43.1). This requires the participation of enzymes homologous to E2 and E3 ubiquitin ligases, which transfer Atg12 onto an acceptor lysine of Atg5, and phosphatidylethanolamine onto LC3 after glycine is exposed at the C-terminus by Atg4. The lipidated form of LC3, referred to as LC3-II, has a faster mobility on SDS gels. LC3 lipidation attaches it to the autophagosomal membrane, thus the amount of LC3-II is generally proportional to autophagosomes abundance. LC3 has multiple homologs, which may be expressed in different tissues and may play nuanced roles in selective autophagy. A noncanonical form of macroautophagy – but also regulated by Ulk1 – involves membrane derived from the Golgi and participation of multiple Rab proteins (Figure 43.1). Little is known about noncanonical autophagy; however, in Atg5 or Atg7 knockout mice, noncanonical autophagy is unable to prevent the progressive development of heart failure. In either pathway of macroautophagy, the cup-shaped phagophore is recruited to the target cargo, such as a depolarized mitochondrion, where it encloses the target. Subsequently, it is transported via the microtubule network to fuse with a lysosome. Acidification of the vesicle is required for hydrolytic degradation of the contents. This dynamic process – from autophagosome formation to lysosomal fusion – is referred to as autophagic flux, and is a key consideration in evaluating autophagy. The number of autophagosomes at any moment reflects the balance of formation and lysosomal fusion.

Biological significance of autophagy in the heart

The role of autophagy in the heart has been the subject of numerous research articles and reviews in recent years, and is briefly summarized here. Autophagy plays a protective role as a part of the mechanism of ischemic and pharmacologic preconditioning, whereby mitochondria that may be more susceptible to ischemia–reperfusion injury are pre-emptively eliminated [1–5]. During ischemia, autophagy plays a beneficial role [6,7], likely by providing necessary nutrients and eliminating energy-consuming uncoupled mitochondria. However, Matsui et al. concluded that autophagy during reperfusion was detrimental [8]. This was based on observation of autophagosome abundance by microscopy and increased LC3-II and Beclin1 on western blots. However, they did not examine flux, although it had been shown that ischemia and reperfusion impaired flux in HL-1 cells, thus resulting in accumulation of autophagosomes and LC3-II [9]. To assess the functional significance of autophagy, they used Beclin1[+/−] mice, which exhibited reduced infarct size after ischemia and reperfusion, leading them to conclude that autophagy was deleterious in the setting of ischemia and reperfusion. However, more recent work with Beclin1[+/−] mice, in which flux was measured, led to the conclusion that Beclin1 interferes with flux, and

Manual of Research Techniques in Cardiovascular Medicine, First Edition. Edited by Hossein Ardehali, Roberto Bolli, and Douglas W. Losordo.

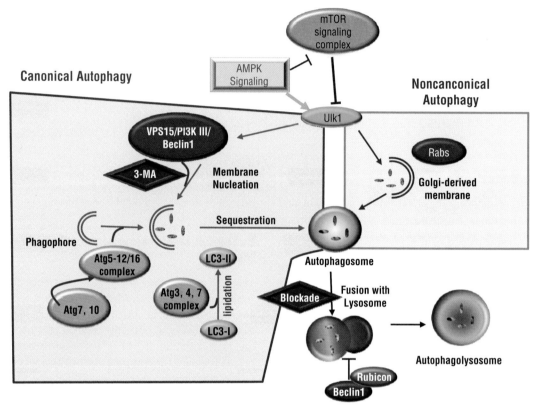

Figure 43.1 Simplified diagram of autophagy. Nutrient sensing is a key regulator of autophagy, mediated by the opposing input of mTOR to suppress autophagy and AMPK to activate it. Ulk1 is a central initiating kinase for both canonical and noncanonical autophagy. The VPS15/PI3K/Beclin1 complex mediates membrane nucleation, while two ubiquitin ligase-like systems mediate elongation of the phagophore and incorporation of LC3-II into the autophagosomal membrane. Various adaptor proteins mediate selective target engulfment (e.g. Parkin and p62/SQTM1 on depolarized mitochondria). Rab proteins, including Rab9, participate in noncanonical autophagy. The autophagosome traffics along microtubules and fuses with a lysosome, a process which requires acidification of the lumen, followed by degradation of the contents by hydrolytic enzymes including proteases, glycohydrolases, and lipases. Beclin1 in concert with Rubicon, interferes with autophagosome–lysosome fusion. Lysosomal dysfunction or blockade results in the accumulation of autophagosomes. (Source: Modified from http://www.cellsignal.com/reference/pathway/images/Autophagy.jpg).

that haploinsufficiency accelerates flux during ischemia–reperfusion [10]. Similar confusion arose from the study by Rothermel, which concluded from studies with Beclin1[+/−] mice that autophagy was maladaptive in load-induced heart disease [11]. There again, flux was not measured. More recent studies on ischemic injury, postinfarction remodeling, and aggregopathy-induced heart failure have led to the conclusion that autophagy plays a beneficial role [12–14]. This is not to suggest that autophagy is *always* a good thing. Excessive autophagy has been shown to be deleterious in

doxorubicin toxicity and ethanol-induced contractile dysfunction [15,16].

The isolated "snapshot" observation of increased autophagosomes and LC3-II after ischemia–reperfusion cannot reveal whether there is increased autophagy or impaired lysosomal clearance, just as a photo of cars on a freeway cannot reveal how fast they are moving (Figure 43.2). It can only be interpreted if flux is measured. In this chapter we will present methods to measure autophagic flux based on microscopy or western blot. Readers are referred to the definitive treatise on

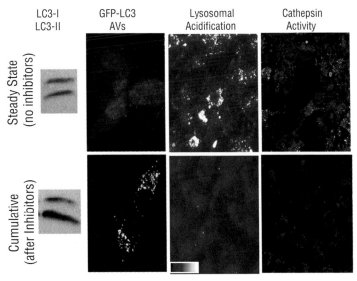

Figure 43.2 Autophagic flux. Autophagy can be assessed by western blotting of LC3. An increase in LC3-II *may* be consistent with increased autophagy, but may instead be a consequence of impaired lysosomal clearance. In the steady state, flux cannot be estimated. However, the rate of cargo transit can be determined by creating lysosomal blockade (a traffic jam) and monitoring the accumulation of cargo in a defined interval. The effect of lysosomal blockade is to prevent the clearance of autophagosomes (autophagic vacuoles, or AVs), which accumulate. The effect is seen on western blot as an increase of LC3-II, and by fluorescence microscopy (in cells expressing LC3-GFP) as an accumulation of puncta. Lysosomal blockade to prevent autophagosome–lysosome fusion is achieved by with neutralizing lysosomal pH with chloroquine or NH$_4$Cl; preventing lysosomal acidification with bafilomycin A1; inhibiting lysosomal proteases with pepstatin A; or blocking vesicle transport with colchicine or vinblastine. Here, lysosomal acidification is monitored with LysoTracker Red, with signal intensity plotted in false color (see inset); cathepsin D protease activity is monitored with Magic Red, again plotting signal intensity in false color. Lysosomal blockade with Bafilyomycin A1 and pepstatin A prevents LysoTracker Red accumulation and cathepsin-dependent generation of the fluorogenic product of Magic Red. Comparison of autophagy markers at steady-state and after blockade is used to determine autophagic flux (for interpretation, see Table 43.1). (Source: western blots: Allen Andres, Gottlieb lab, unpublished data; microscopy: Hamacher-Brady A, Brady NR, Gottlieb RA. *J Biol Chem 2006;* **281**: 29776–29787.)

measuring autophagy published by Klionsky *et al.* in 2008 [17].

Western blot analysis

Autophagic flux can be inferred from comparison of parallel samples with and without lysosomal blockade, either by western blotting or immuno-fluorescence. LC3-II abundance on western blot parallels autophagosome abundance detected by fluorescence microscopy. If autophagosomes (or LC3-II levels) increase after blockade, then autophagic flux is intact. If, however, autophagosome (or LC3-II) abundance increases minimally after blockade, then flux is impaired. This is the most broadly applicable method to determine flux *in vivo*.

1. Experimental design: For each data point, four or five animals are needed to have confidence in the results, as there is considerable biological variability. For flux determinations, another four or five animals will be required. Because of circadian effects on autophagy, all studies must be performed at a consistent time of day. There can be as much as a twofold variation in basal levels of autophagy over 4 hours; the magnitude of this change may be as large as the effect of an intervention. Factors including feeding, heat or cold stress, exercise, and anesthesia can affect autophagy. If a drug is to be administered, vehicle controls and nontreated controls must be assessed, as agents such as DMSO can induce autophagy. The interval between intervention and tissue harvest should be optimized for the system under study.

2. For the group of animals being used for flux comparison, administer chloroquine (10–50 mg/kg i.p.) [18] 2–4 hours before sacrifice. Alternative agents that can be used include bafilomycin (0.3 mg/kg i.p.) [12] or vinblastine (10 mg/kg i.p.) [19]. At the appropriate time point, the animal should be rapidly euthanized and the heart excised and snap-frozen in liquid nitrogen. As LC3 (particularly LC3-I) is labile, samples should be processed rapidly in protease inhibitors. To minimize degradation in SDS sample buffer, fresh samples should be boiled and assessed promptly and repeated freeze–thawing must be avoided. Homogenization of fresh or frozen tissue in RIPA buffer or solubilizing from nitrogen powder are two suitable methods for heart tissue samples.

3. SDS-PAGE gels should be optimized to allow separation of LC3-I and LC3-II, such as 4–20% or 10–20% Tris glycine gels (Invitrogen). Electrotransfer should use PVDF membranes rather than nitrocellulose to maximize binding of LC3-I. There are many homologs of LC3, including the GABARAP subset, but the LC3B isoform is abundantly expressed in heart and can be readily detected in rodent samples using the Cell Signaling antibody (Catalog no. 4108). An alternative antibody is from Novus (Catalog no. NB100-2220).

4. Measurement of p62/SQSTM1 can also be used to infer flux in conjunction with LC3-II. Soluble p62 is extracted in phosphate-buffered saline containing 1% Triton X-100 and protease inhibitors; the aggregate-associated p62 can then be detected by western blot after sonication of the Triton-insoluble fraction in 2% SDS in 50 mM Tris, pH 7.4. All buffers should contain protease inhibitors and samples must be kept on ice. Although soluble p62 is quickly upregulated in response to autophagic stimulation, the fraction of p62 that is associated with ubiquitinated protein aggregates is cleared when autophagic flux is intact. If flux is impaired, the amount of aggregate-associated p62 is unchanged.

5. Western blots of all samples to be compared should be processed concurrently and the images digitized for densitometric quantitation. In most cases, it is preferable to normalize to a housekeeping protein such as tubulin, actin, or GAPDH. For the particular system under study, it is important to confirm that the housekeeping protein doesn't change with the intervention (actin levels in the heart change considerably in response to mechanical unloading or hypertrophy; GAPDH changes in response to metabolic stress).

Microscopy

Transient transfection or adenoviral delivery of LC3-GFP is commonly used in cell culture to assess autophagy by fluorescence microscopy. Overexpression of LC3-GFP results in its diffuse distribution in the cytosol, but upon stimulation of autophagy, it is lipidated and incorporated into autophagosomal membranes. This allows visual scoring of the number of autophagosomes, although it is important to consider flux. After establishing a histogram profile of the number of autophagosomes per cell under basal and stimulated conditions for the cell type of interest, the cell population can subsequently be scored as the percentage of cells having "few" or "many" autophagosomes. For instance, in HL-1 cells under fed quiescent conditions, >80% of the cells have fewer than 20 puncta per cell, whereas under starved or autophagy-stimulated conditions, >80% of the cells will have more than 20 puncta per cell (often in excess of 60) [20,21]. This allows subsequent scoring to visually estimate each cell as few or many, and then to score the percentage of cells with many autophagosomes.

Another approach to monitoring autophagic flux with fluorescence microscopy employs tandem LC3-GFP-RFP [22]. Because GFP is more rapidly degraded in the lysosome than mRFP or mCherry, autophagosomes (before lysosomal fusion) exhibit fluorescence in both green and red channels, while autophagolysosomes only have red fluorescence. Impaired autophagic flux is characterized by an abundance of green-and-red puncta and few or no red-only puncta. LC3-fluorescent protein constructs: Many constructs are now available from AddGene. org. Transfect cells, or in the case of primary cells, infect with adenovirus carrying LC3-GFP, LC3-mCherry, or tandem LC3-EGFP-mCherry. The fluorescent protein moiety should be at the N-terminus, as the C-terminus is proteolytically processed to expose a glycine residue for subsequent lipidation. As transfection reagents can themselves stimulate autophagy, it is important to perform

Table 43.1 Guidelines to interpret autophagy assays

Microscopy (autophagic puncta)			Western Blot of LC3-II (flux assay)		Western Blot of LC3-II and p62 (inferred flux)		Interpretation
Free	Blocked	Tandem	Free	Blocked	LC3-II	p62	
Few	Many	Many puncta, many red only	+	+++	+ to +++	+	Active flux
Few	Few	Few puncta	+	+	+	+++	Initiation impaired
Some	Many	Some puncta, some red only	++	+++	+++	+ to ++	Active flux (or slightly impaired)
Some	Some	Many puncta, few red only	++	++	+++	+++	Flux impaired

appropriate controls and to allow a certain time for cell recovery.

1. Under parallel conditions, compare puncta formation in unstimulated and treated cells. It is important to conduct a time course when designing the study, as some agents induce autophagy within minutes, while others may require 12–24 hours.

2. For the tandem LC3-EGFP-mCherry construct, microscopy imaging in both red and green channels is performed; the fraction of puncta that are only seen in the red channel represent autophagolysosomes and can be used as an index of flux (perhaps represented as a % of total puncta), coupled with an estimate of the abundance of puncta (normalized to cell number, or the few/many estimate). The signal is unchanged with fixation.

3. In cells expressing a single fluor, flux analysis is accomplished by scoring autophagosome abundance without and with a lysosomal inhibitor such as chloroquine (3 μM) or bafilomycin (50–100 nM). Fluorescence microscopy is used to score the % cells with many puncta under steady state (Free) and lysosomal blockade (Blocked) conditions.

4. Transgenic mice expressing LC3-GFP, LC3-GFP/LC3-mCherry double transgenics, and mice expressing tandem LC3-GFP-mRFP/mCherry are available and permit similar analyses *in vivo* [23].

Interpretation

Interpretation of the results is not completely straightforward and requires an understanding of the dynamic nature of the process of autophagy and the specific nuances of the system under study. However, Table 43.1 can serve as a general guideline.

Strengths and weaknesses

Analysis of autophagic flux by comparing autophagic markers in the presence and absence of lysosomal blockade requires a considerable number of animals and is not feasible in settings where administration of a lysosomal inhibitor is impractical (e.g. large animal studies or human samples). In that case (as in human samples), western blot of LC3-II and Triton X-100-insoluble P62/SQSTM1 is helpful for interpreting autophagic flux. Microscopy is a useful tool where fluorescent LC3 fusion proteins can be employed, but it should be noted that overexpression of LC3 can have a modest stimulatory effect on autophagy, and LC3-fusion proteins can form aggregates that are easily mistaken for autophagosomes. Use of interventions to manipulate autophagy can be helpful in interpretation (see alternative approaches).

Alternative approaches

Few tools are available to measure autophagy in nontransgenic animals, including humans. Western blot analysis of biopsy samples, measuring both LC3 and p62 is, at present, the best method to assess autophagy and infer flux. Monodansylcadaverine (MDC) accumulates in acidic compartments including autophagolysosomes, but also functions as a solvent polarity probe, thus yielding greater fluorescence in the hydrophobic environment of the autophagosome double membrane [24,25]. MDC has not gained wide acceptance owing to its weak fluorescence, which is further reduced upon fixation, the problematic diffuse cytosolic staining, and controversy as to whether it is merely a lysosomal marker. However, we have used it successfully in cardiac studies, in which a dose of 1.5 mg/kg i.p. is given 1 hour before sacrifice [18]. AlexaFluor488™–cadaverine has better quantum yield fluorescence and is fixable, but it is costly and definitive evidence that it selectively labels autophagosomes is lacking. However, these dyes hold promise for use in tissues, if given systemically before tissue harvest [26]. There is an unmet need to be able to monitor autophagy *in vivo*, through the use of fluorescent or bioluminescent dyes, and eventually, contrast agents suitable for medical imaging.

Upregulation of autophagy in response to a stressor may be adaptive or deleterious. To understand the role of autophagy, one can inhibit the process and assess biological outcome. In all cases, the implications of increased (or decreased) autophagy must be ascertained through experiments in which autophagy is specifically manipulated. Drugs to inhibit autophagy initiation include PI3-kinase inhibitors wortmannin and 3-methyladenine, both of which have off-target effects that can confound their interpretation. Inhibitors of AMPK such as compound C (EMD Biosciences) should be used with caution as they may paradoxically induce autophagy [27,28]. Drugs to inhibit lysosomal flux include chloroquine (neutralizes lysosomal pH), Bafilomycin A1 (potent inhibitor of vacuolar proton ATPase), pepstatin A (inhibits lysosomal proteases), and colchicine (prevents transport of vesicles to lysosomes). The recombinant cell-permeable protein Tat-Atg5(K130R) functions as a dominant negative and was used in isolated perfused hearts to demonstrate a role for autophagy in cardioprotection; it has not yet been employed *in vivo* [1,3]. Beclin1[+/−] mice may yield misleading results because of Beclin1's complex roles to initiate autophagy yet reduce autophagosome–lysosome fusion [10]. Pharmacologic upregulation of autophagy may also provide insight into its functional significance. Commonly used agents include rapamycin, and agents that activate AMPK, such as AICAR or phenformin, may also be considered [29]. The mechanism by which a given agent induces

autophagy should be assessed before adopting it as a tool, as some agents may trigger autophagy by causing cellular stress (e.g. mitochondrial depolarization or ER stress).

Conclusions

Age, activity, metabolic status, circadian rhythm, drug exposure, and disease processes can all influence autophagy in the heart. These variables must be taken into account in experimental design. Interpretation of findings *must* take flux into account. For a given condition, it is essential to determine whether autophagy is functional (intact flux) or impaired, and whether it is part of a protective response or a contributing factor to the disease process. Use of appropriate methods and animal models will expand our understanding of the role of autophagy in heart disease.

References

1 Huang C, Liu W, Perry CN, Yitzhaki S, Lee Y, Yuan H, et al. Autophagy and protein kinase c are required for cardioprotection by sulfaphenazole. *Am J Physiol Heart Circ Physiol* 2010; **298**: H570–579.

2 Yitzhaki S, Huang C, Liu W, Lee Y, Gustafsson AB, Mentzer RM, Jr., et al. Autophagy is required for preconditioning by the adenosine A1 receptor-selective agonist CCPA. *Basic Res Cardiol* 2009; **104**: 157–167.

3 Huang C, Yitzhaki S, Perry CN, Liu W, Giricz Z, Mentzer RM, Jr., et al. Autophagy induced by ischemic preconditioning is essential for cardioprotection. *J Cardiovasc Transl Res* 2010; **3**: 365–373.

4 Sala-Mercado JA, Wider J, Undyala VV, Jahania S, Yoo W, Mentzer RM, Jr., et al. Profound cardioprotection with chloramphenicol succinate in the swine model of ischemia-reperfusion injury. *Circulation* 2010; **122** (**Suppl**): S179–184.

5 Huang C, Andres AM, Ratliff EP, Hernandez G, Lee P, Gottlieb RA, et al. Preconditioning involves selective mitophagy mediated by Parkin and p62/SQSTM1. *PLoS One* 2011; **6**: e20975.

6 Yan L, Vatner DE, Kim SJ, Ge H, Masurekar M, Massover WH, et al. Autophagy in chronically ischemic myocardium. *Proc Natl Acad Sci U S A* 2005; **102**: 13807–13812.

7 Takagi H, Matsui Y, Hirotani S, Sakoda H, Asano T, Sadoshima J, et al. AMPK mediates autophagy during myocardial ischemia in vivo. *Autophagy* 2007; **3**: 405–407.

8 Matsui Y, Takagi H, Qu X, Abdellatif M, Sakoda H, Asano T, *et al.* Distinct roles of autophagy in the heart during ischemia and reperfusion: roles of AMP-activated protein kinase and Beclin 1 in mediating autophagy. *Circ Res* 2007; **100**: 914–922.

9 Hamacher-Brady A, Brady NR, Gottlieb RA. Enhancing macroautophagy protects against ischemia/reperfusion injury in cardiac myocytes. *J Biol Chem* 2006; **281**: 29776–29787.

10 Foyil SA, Ma X, Hill JA, Dorn GW, 2nd, Diwan A. BNIP3 induced autophagy contributes to adverse ventricular remodeling. *J Cardiac Failure* 2010; **16** (**Suppl.**): S35.

11 Rothermel BA, Hill JA. Autophagy in load-induced heart disease. *Circ Res* 2008; **103**: 1363–1369.

12 Kanamori H, Takemura G, Goto K, Maruyama R, Ono K, Nagao K, *et al.* Autophagy limits acute myocardial infarction induced by permanent coronary artery occlusion. *Am J Physiol Heart Circ Physiol*; **300**: H2261–2271.

13 Kanamori H, Takemura G, Goto K, Maruyama R, Tsujimoto A, Ogino A, *et al.* The role of autophagy emerging in postinfarction cardiac remodelling. *Cardiovasc Res*; **91**: 330–339.

14 Tannous P, Zhu H, Johnstone JL, Shelton JM, Rajasekaran NS, Benjamin IJ, *et al.* Autophagy is an adaptive response in desmin-related cardiomyopathy. *Proc Natl Acad Sci* 2008; **105**: 9745–9750.

15 Xu X, Chen K, Kobayashi S, Timm D, Liang Q. Resveratrol attenuates doxorubicin-induced cardiomyocyte death via inhibition of p70 S6 kinase 1-mediated autophagy. *J Pharmacol Exp Ther* 2012; **341**: 183–195.

16 Guo R, Ren J. Deficiency in AMPK attenuates ethanol-induced cardiac contractile dysfunction through inhibition of autophagosome formation. *Cardiovasc Res* 2012 ; **94**: 480–491.

17 Klionsky DJ, Abeliovich H, Agostinis P, Agrawal DK, Aliev G, Askew DS, *et al.* Guidelines for the use and interpretation of assays for monitoring autophagy in higher eukaryotes. *Autophagy* 2008; **4**: 151–175.

18 Iwai-Kanai E, Yuan H, Huang C, Sayen MR, Perry-Garza CN, Kim L, *et al.* A method to measure cardiac autophagic flux in vivo. *Autophagy* 2008; **4**: 322–329.

19 Rez G, Csak J, Fellinger E, Laszlo L, Kovacs AL, Oliva O, *et al.* Time course of vinblastine-induced autophagocytosis and changes in the endoplasmic reticulum in murine pancreatic acinar cells: a morphometric and biochemical study. *Eur J Cell Biol* 1996; **71**: 341–350.

20 Brady NR, Hamacher-Brady A, Yuan H, Gottlieb RA. The autophagic response to nutrient deprivation in the hl-1 cardiac myocyte is modulated by Bcl-2 and sarco/endoplasmic reticulum calcium stores. *FEBS J* 2007; **274**: 3184–3197.

21 Yuan H, Perry CN, Huang C, Iwai-Kanai E, Carreira RS, Glembotski CC, Gottlieb RA, *et al.* LPS-induced autophagy is mediated by oxidative signaling in cardiomyocytes and is associated with cytoprotection. *Am J Physiol Heart Circ Physiol* 2009; **296**: H470–479.

22 Kimura S, Noda T, Yoshimori T. Dissection of the autophagosome maturation process by a novel reporter protein, tandem fluorescent-tagged LC3. *Autophagy* 2007; **3**: 452–460.

23 Terada M, Nobori K, Munehisa Y, Kakizaki M, Ohba T, Takahashi Y, *et al.* Double transgenic mice crossed GFP-LC3 transgenic mice with alphaMyHC-mCherry-LC3 transgenic mice are a new and useful tool to examine the role of autophagy in the heart. *Circ J* 2010; **74**: 203–206.

24 Munafo DB, Colombo MI. A novel assay to study autophagy: regulation of autophagosome vacuole size by amino acid deprivation. *J Cell Sci* 2001; **114**: 3619–3629.

25 Niemann A, Takatsuki A, Elsasser HP. The lysosomotropic agent monodansylcadaverine also acts as a solvent polarity probe. *J Histochem Cytochem* 2000; **48**: 251–258.

26 Perry CN, Kyoi S, Hariharan N, Takagi H, Sadoshima J, Gottlieb RA, *et al.* Novel methods for measuring cardiac autophagy in vivo. *Methods Enzymol* 2009; **453**: 325–342.

27 Meley D, Bauvy C, Houben-Weerts JH, Dubbelhuis PF, Helmond MT, Codogno P, *et al.* AMP-activated protein kinase and the regulation of autophagic proteolysis. *J Biol Chem* 2006; **281**: 34870–34879.

28 Vucicevic L, Misirkic M, Janjetovic K, Vilimanovich U, Sudar E, Isenovic E, *et al.* Compound C induces protective autophagy in cancer cells through AMPK inhibition-independent blockade of Akt/mTOR pathway. *Autophagy* 2011; **7**: 40–50.

29 Micic D, Cvijovic G, Trajkovic V, Duntas LH, Polovina S. Metformin: its emerging role in oncology. *Hormones (Athens)* 2011; **10**: 5–15.

Assessment of cardiomyocyte size

A. Martin Gerdes[1] and Alessandro Pingitore[2]

[1] New York Institute of Technology College of Osteopathic Medicine, Old Westbury, NY, USA

[2] Clinical Physiology Institute, CNR, Pisa, Italy

Introduction

Development of cardiovascular drugs that beneficially alter ventricular remodeling as well as function (e.g. angiotensin converting enzyme inhibitors, β-adrenergic receptor blocking agents) have led to improved outcomes in heart failure. In fact, heart failure research is currently in the "age of remodeling." Cumulative research using reliable and reproducible techniques indicates that myocyte shape largely accounts for underlying changes in chamber geometry [1–3]. Consequently, data on myocyte shape are important in understanding the cellular basis for beneficial and detrimental changes in chamber geometry. Ideally, the employed technique should include comprehensive information about **myocyte volume (V), length (L),** and **cross-sectional area (CSA)**. Chamber dilatation in progression to heart failure is largely due to myocyte lengthening from series addition of new sarcomeres. The increase in cell length is typically associated with no change in wall thickness, which is reflected at the myocyte level by an absence of change in myocyte CSA. Changes in myocyte CSA are related to alterations in wall thickness. Consequently, increased chamber diameter/ wall thickness ratio is associated with increased myocyte L/width ratio. With reliable determination of myocyte volume, changes in myocyte number can also be calculated by dividing total volume of myocytes by mean myocyte volume. Determination of myocyte number is important in studies examining cell death mechanisms or possible myocyte regeneration.

Myocytes make up about 75% of ventricular mass but are outnumbered by nonmyocardial cells. There are approximately 25 million myocytes per gram of tissue in normal mammalian hearts. Myocytes vary considerably in shape but, overall, are elliptical cylinders with the major transverse diameter running circumferentially and the minor transverse diameter running transmurally (Figure 44.1). Capillaries may also invaginate myocytes forming "tunnel capillaries," thus affecting myocyte shape. Myocytes branch extensively, largely at intercellular connections (intercalated discs). For a comprehensive overview of changes/ differences in myocyte shape associated with gender, species, growth, maturation, aging, cardiac hypertrophy of various etiologies, and failure, readers are referred to the review article, Gerdes 2002 [1].

Normally, myocyte remodeling is strictly linked to cardiac loading changes. In fact, increased afterload leads to an increase in wall thickness and myocyte CSA with minimal change in chamber volume or myocyte L. Increased preload leads to ventricular dilatation and an increase in L. With physiological adaptation to volume loading, the increase in L is accompanied by proportional increase in myocyte width (note: this translates to increases of approximately one-third in L and approximately two-thirds in CSA). Progression to dilated heart failure of ischemic and nonischemic etiologies is characterized by chamber dilatation with no change in wall thickness. This is reflected at the cellular level by an increase in myocyte L only. The absence of CSA growth during this process implicates

Manual of Research Techniques in Cardiovascular Medicine, First Edition. Edited by Hossein Ardehali, Roberto Bolli, and Douglas W. Losordo.

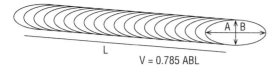

$$V = 0.785\ ABL$$

Figure 44.1 Cardiac myocyte shape is extremely variable but approximates that of an elliptical cylinder. A, major cross sectional diameter; B, minor cross sectional diameter; L, length; V, volume.

maladaptive remodeling of myocyte shape as a major contributor to elevated wall stress in progression to dilated heart failure.

Protocol

Collagenase isolation of myocytes

The collagenase method used for myocyte isolation from beating heart consists of the following steps:

1. Heart removal and cannulation
2. Heart perfusion
3. Heart digestion
4. Myocyte dissociation
5. Myocyte fixation

Heart removal and cannulation

When the animal is fully anesthetized, the heart is exposed by opening the thorax via the diaphragm, approaching from the peritoneal cavity. The heart is elevated and major vessels are quickly cut while being careful not to cut the aorta too close to the heart. It is important to retain enough of the ascending aorta to allow cannulation above the aortic valves. If the catheter pierces the aortic valves, coronary vascular perfusion pressure will be equal to intracavity pressure and impede proper vascular perfusion. Before cannulation, we recommend placing the beating heart into media containing heparin to inhibit clotting when trimming. Blot and weigh heart. Using fine-tip forceps, slide the aorta onto the cannula so that the tip of the cannula is just above the aortic valve. Slowly perfuse the heart by hand with a small syringe containing solution A (Table 44.1) with 0.4% heparin. It is good to minimize air bubbles by gently squeezing the heart to fill cannula with fluid when attaching to the syringe and when attaching to the perfusion apparatus.

Heart perfusion

Heart perfusion is provided in a retrograde manner on a Langerdorff apparatus with solution A. The

Table 44.1 Isolated myocyte protocol

	Volume (mL)		
	500	**1000**	**2000**
Primary solution			
Distilled H_2O (mL)	475	950	1900
Joklik's medium (g)	5.55	11.1	22.2
Na_2CO_3(g)	1.45	2.9	5.8
$MgSO_4$(g)	0.06	0.12	0.24
BDM (g)	1	2	4
pH value	7.2	7.2	7.2
Solution A:			
Primary solution (mL)	250	500	1000
EGTA (g)	0.022	0.083	0.088
Solution B:			
Primary solution	450 mL		
Collagenase	0.25 g (amount depends on activity, see text)		
BSA	0.45 g		

BDM, 2,3-butanedione monoxime; EGTA, ethylene glycol *bis*(B-amino-ethyl-ether)N,N'-tetra acetic; BSA, bovine serum albumin.

perfusion time is 5 minutes. It is important to maintain constant temperature of the perfusion system at 37°C with a flow rate of ~4 mL/min for a normal adult rat heart with some adjustments for smaller or larger hearts.

Heart digestion

After the initial "prewash" perfusion, the heart is perfused with Solution B containing collagenase while maintaining temperature and flow rate as before. The time of digestion is variable, usually around 25 minutes. During digestion the heart becomes swollen and turns slightly pale. Digestion can be considered finished when the heart feels spongy when gently pinched. *There may be variation in collagenase activity and efficacy between lots. So, the concentration may require adjustment.* The goal is a relatively slow, gentle digestion without "overcooking" as evidenced by damaged myocyte cell membranes. To optimize results, start with the above time and increase or decrease collagenase concentration based on quality of myocytes collected. It may be difficult to consistently obtain good myocytes from the right ventricle (RV) and left ventricle (LV) at the same time. Optimum digestion of LV myocytes often leads to slightly "over-cooking" the smaller RV myocytes. So, RV myocytes tend to have slightly lower quality when targeting optimum digestion for LV myocytes. Since the atria of rodents are often perfused by internal thoracic arteries rather than coronary arteries, this method may not yield good atrial myocytes.

Note. the isolated myocyte protocol provided here is *not* calcium tolerant but provides an unusually high percentage of well preserved, rod-shaped myocytes best suited for cell sizing and immunolabeling for epifluorescence or confocal microscopy. We routinely obtain preps with ~90% rod cells using this method.

Myocyte dissociation

Once enzyme digestion of the heart is complete, the heart is separated from the cannula, and atria are trimmed away. One can either mince whole ventricles or divide into RV-free wall and LV plus septum for chamber-specific determination of myocyte dimensions. In the past, we have also trimmed the outer and inner layer of the LV to obtain epi- and endomyocardial myocytes. The myocardial tissue is placed into a dish containing solution A. Tissue is cut into small pieces with fine scissors and, using a plastic transfer pipette, the heart tissue suspension is pippetted back and forth to disperse myocytes. The suspension is then filtered through nylon mesh (250 μm) into a 15-mL plastic test tube to collect myocytes. This can be repeated to increase yield. Cells can be fixed or frozen.

Myocyte fixation

We generally fill the 15-mL tube approximately half full with 1.5% glutaraldehyde in 80 mmol/L phosphate buffer or 2% paraformaldehyde in 80 mmol/L phosphate buffer if immunolabeling/confocal microscopy is desired. So, the cell suspension can be filtered directly into the fixative. The isolated cell suspension is then centrifuged for 5 minutes, the supernatant removed, and the tube topped off with the desired fixative. These isolated cells can be used for analysis or centrifuged through Ficoll if further removal of nonmyocytes is desired. Examples of mononucleate and binucleate isolated myocytes are shown in Figure 44.2. When stored in air-tight containers, glutaraldehyde-fixed cells can be maintained for many years with minimal change in volume.

Myocyte morphometry

Coulter Channelyzer determination of myocyte volume. Adult myocytes have large volumes but are

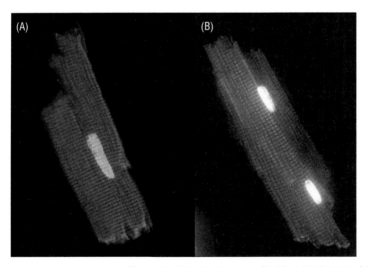

Figure 44.2 (A) Example of mononucleated myocyte; (B) example of binucleated myocyte. Nuclei are highlighted by DAPI labeling. Although in this example the mono- and binucleated myocytes have a similar size, binucleated myocytes are generally larger than mononucleated myocytes.

elliptical cylinders with relatively small diameters as they traverse the aperture in log-style fashion. So, their shape is quite different than that of spherical microspheres used to calibrate the instrument. The instrument has a built in shape factor of 1.5 based on a spherical particle. This shape factor is in the denominator of the equation used for calculation by the instrument. The correct shape factor for myocytes with an approximate length/width ratio of ~7–10 is ~1.05 [4]. Therefore, Coulter values for myocyte V should be multiplied by 1.43 (1.5/1.05 = 1.43) to correct for shape. Use of this shape factor was previously validated by our group. We use the median value for V determinations to minimize possible overestimation from cell clumps in the upper range of the histogram (although this is unlikely to be a problem because few counts accumulate at the high end of the histogram in a good cell preparation). The first narrow peak is comprised of nonmyocytes and cell debris and should be excluded by the lower threshold setting of the Coulter Channelyzer. One can confirm this by visually searching for the smallest viable myocytes on a microscope slide and estimating the volume based on dimensions.

When calibrating the Channelyzer, it is best to use microspheres as close to the target cell size range as possible. This allows improved precision by sampling from the full range of channels rather than having the histogram skewed to one side. With adult myocytes, however, smaller microspheres are necessary for proper calibration. To match the myocyte volume with a spherical particle of similar size for calibration, it would be necessary to use microspheres exceeding the instrumentation 20% upper limit for the ratio of particle diameter to aperture diameter. For adult myocytes, a 200-μm aperture works well. We use ~30-μm microspheres with an approximate V of 14,100 μm³ for calibration.

For myocyte sizing, place a pipette into the cell suspension and rapidly pipette the solution back and forth several times to mix the cells well. One can be fairly aggressive without damaging fixed cells. Place an aliquot of isolated myocytes into a Coulter cuvette containing Isoton for dilution. The goal is to measure between 3000 and 10,000 cells. If the Channelyzer model allows analysis of larger volumes, cells can be diluted more to build the histogram more slowly. An example of a typical myocyte histogram from an

adult female rat is shown in Figure 44.3. As indicated earlier, the median value of 19,640 would be multiplied by 1.43 to obtain the corrected value of 28,085 μm³ for this particular prep.

Microscopic measurements. Myocytes are approximately elliptical cylinders and settle on their flat side when placed on a microscope slide. Consequently, the **major diameter** (**A**) is viewed through the microscope. Using the following formula for an elliptical cylinder, the **minor diameter** (**B**) can be calculated if V, A, and L are known (Figure 44.1).

$$V = \pi/4 \cdot ABL$$

In general, the A diameter axis runs in a circumferential direction in the ventricular wall and may change during remodeling that affects chamber circumference. The A dimension is calculated from profile area/L. The B diameter axis runs in a transmural direction with changes related to alterations in wall thickness. So, these measurements can be helpful in understanding patterns of ventricular remodeling.

Cell length and sarcomere length can be measured by simply placing a drop of isolated myocytes on a slide and overlaying with a cover slip. It should be recognized, however, that evaporation along the edges causes compression of myocytes. While this does not affect myocyte length or sarcomere length, it will result in overestimation of A dimension as the cells flatten. Consequently, to determine A and B diameters, isolated myocytes should be placed in a welled slide or finger nail polish can be used to form a raised border for the cover slip to prevent flattening. Forty myocytes typically provides an adequate sample size. Only randomly sampled, rod-shaped cells with no visible membrane damage should be measured.

Sometimes it may be difficult to determine if one is visualizing an individual myocyte or a doublet, particularly in preps from individuals with severe cardiac hypertrophy where shape becomes more complex. We have adopted an approach that dramatically reduces the chance of inadvertently measuring a doublet. In rats, ~99% of myocytes are either binucleated or mononucleated. Cells with three or four nuclei comprise less than 1% of the population. So, we only sample from cells with one or two nuclei (Figure 44.2). Ignoring the other cells

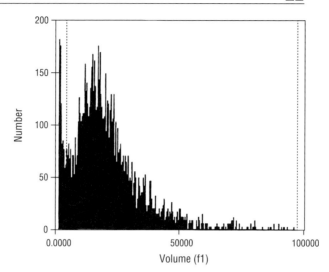

Cursor Statistics

Size at C1: 4577.00 fl
Size at C2: 97260.0 fl
Mean: 22920.0
Median: 19640.0
Mode: 17740.0
Standard Deviation:13750.0
Channelyzer Count: 8660

Statistical Results

Mean Cell Volume: 21290.0
Median: 18500.0
Mode: 2098.00
Std. Dev.: 14270.0

Figure 44.3 Typical Coulter Channelyzer histogram of isolated myocytes from a normal adult female rat. The first sharp peak represents debris/nonmyocytes and should be excluded by the lower threshold bar (C1). Myocytes represent a broad range of volumes as shown by the second peak. The median value for V should be corrected for shape as described in the text.

has minimal effect on mean L measurements and largely eliminates the possibility of inadvertently measuring a doublet or triplet. The location of myocyte nuclei is also helpful in the determination. Nuclei are centrally located in mononucleated cells and equally spaced from the cell center and ends in binucleated cells. To better visualize nuclei, myocytes are counterstained with the DNA marker 4′-6-diamidino-2phenylindole-HCL (DAPI) and visualized by UV light. Finally, the borders of myocytes are also helpful in making the determination. Myocyte borders rarely transition seamlessly to the next cell. Usually, there is an irregular junction since cells are generally offset from one another.

Finally, **sarcomere length (SL)** is measured at a higher magnification. For rats, resting, unloaded SL is ~1.90 μm. It is best to count 10 sarcomeres and divide by 10 to obtain the measurement. With the

protocol provided here, most well-preserved cells with no visible membrane damage will have mean SLs of ~1.90 μm due to arrest at resting, unloading conditions induced by BDM. Accurate cell lengths can be obtained from poorer preps, however, by normalizing cell length to this value by using the following formula:

Normalized L = measured L · 1.90/measured SL

When collecting profile area measurements to determine A and B dimensions, sampling should be only from cells with resting unloaded sarcomere length to minimize any contractile changes that could occur in transverse dimensions.

A summary of routinely collected parameters for myocyte sizing is:

1. *Myocyte L* (μm), defined as the longest length parallel to the longitudinal axis of the myocyte.

2. *SL* (μm) is calculated measuring 10 sarcomeres and dividing the obtained sum by 10.

3. *Normalized myocyte L* (μm) normalizes to resting, unloaded SL.

4. *Profile area* (μm^2) is obtained by tracing around boundaries of cells laying on their flat side.

5. *Myocyte V* (μm^3) obtained by Coulter Channelyzer using median V·1.43.

6. *Mean myocyte CSA* (μm^2) calculated as myocyte V/normalized myocyte L.

7. *Major transverse diameter* (A; μm) calculated as profile area/myocyte L.

8. *Minor transverse diameter* (B; μm) calculated using formula for elliptical cylinder.

Weaknesses and strength of the method

No other currently available method approaches the consistency, reliability, and comprehensive nature of this method. The accuracy and reproducibility of this technique can be gathered from data shown in Table 44.2, in which the parameters of cell morphometry collected from normal adult female rats of the Sprague–Dawley strain over a 10-year period are summarized. A weakness is that high-quality isolated myocytes are required for the measurements and this technique can be challenging

to establish. Additionally, digestion of tissue precludes the use of whole heart tissue for other purposes such as assessment of changes in the nonmyocyte compartment. Consequently, we often use matched sets of animals for isolations and whole tissue morphometry.

Alternative approaches

Many labs routinely measure myocyte CSA from histological preps. However, this approach has an overwhelming number of associated shortcomings that are rarely considered. For instance, values for CSA are typically overestimated due to difficulty in identification of good cross-sections and clear myocyte boundaries. Potential differences in contractile phase also affect measurements. Tissue shrinkage is often variable and significant. Many collect measurements at the nuclear level only, providing overestimation of mean myocyte CSA. Myocyte L or V can not be reliably determine with this approach. Consequently, measures are incomplete. Understandably, a quick survey of publications using this approach provides considerable confusion. For instance, many report dramatic increases in myocyte CSA despite no change in wall thickness after myocardial infarction

Table 44.2 Summary of isolated myocyte data from normal female rats obtained from the same source over a 10-year period

Body weight (g)	Myocyte volume (μm^3 × 10^3)	Myocyte length (μm)	Myocyte CSA (μm^2)	Reference
306 ± 13	26.6 ± 3.9	127 ± 5	210 ± 27	[2]
290 ± 18	25.6 ± 4.3	124 ± 6	206 ± 32	[7]
339 ± 27	29.0 ± 1.1	124 ± 6	234 ± 24	[8]
344 ± 21	28.3 ± 2.7	127 ± 7	222 ± 19	[9]
319 ± 20	28.0 ± 2.1	127 ± 5	230 ± 33	[10]
371 ± 31	29.1 ± 2.4	125 ± 7	233 ± 24	[11]
350 ± 26	25.7 ± 2.6	133 ± 3	193 ± 17	[11]
333 ± 17	29.2 ± 5	129 ± 5	225 ± 31	[12]
295 ± 25	29.1 ± 5.4	134 ± 8	217 ± 28	[13]
313 ± 5	25.1 ± 2.4	128 ± 7	195 ± 22	[14]
330 ± 12	26.0 ± 2.2	130 ± 6	199 ± 19	[14]
349 ± 34	29.5 ± 4	130 ± 6	224 ± 34	[15]

Each value is from a minimum of 6 animals. Animals were not obtained from one barrier exclusively, but nonetheless, data show minimal variability. Many different individuals were involved in data collection. Data are means ± S.D. Myocyte V was measured using a Coulter Channelyzer, Myocyte L was measured directly using a microscope, CSA was calculated from V/L.

(unlikely and quite different from the consistent result observed in our lab.). In our experience, this approach is not worth the effort and does not provide the level of precision or depth of information needed to understand changes in remodeling at the myocyte level.

In addition the collagenase isolated myocyte approach described here, we have also developed a method using KOH to isolate myocytes from whole fixed tissues for evaluation of myocyte length. This method has been described in detail elsewhere [5,6]. While the KOH method can provide reliable data for myocyte length and sarcomere length, extensive shrinkage in the B dimension precludes comprehensive assessment of other dimensions. The method is also rather challenging and difficult to establish.

Helpful advice

The method describe here is so reliable that one can easily identify relatively small differences between animals. On several occasions, we have discovered significant differences between normal rats of the same strain but obtained from different suppliers [7]. We have also observed significant differences between rats of the same gender, strain, and supplier but obtained from different barriers. These differences are, of course, within the range of normal but can adversely affect experimental outcomes if multiple shipments are used within a given study. Our advice is to obtain animals only from the same barrier. This should lead to optimum resolution of small differences related to an intervention. It should be pointed out that myocyte volume ranges from about 5000 to 150,000 μm^3 within a normal heart but the mean value for a large population of myocytes is very consistent (e.g. within a few percent for repeat Coulter Channelyzer runs).

The genetic variability between gender-matched siblings is greater than that of repeat measurements with the cell sizing approach outlined here. Consequently, there is no benefit from further refinement of the method. When the approach is implemented correctly and animal variability is minimized (e.g. consistent model, same animal source, minimal body mass differences), group-related cell remodeling changes can generally be

detected when heart mass changes exceed ~15% and sometimes less.

When a very effective lot of collagenase is identified, it is good to reserve or purchase a large supply if it will be used in a reasonable period of time. Collagenase solution A should be mixed in the morning and again in the afternoon during ongoing daily experiments since activity declines after several hours in solution. We generally have better luck with higher activity lots and this also provides cost savings since a lower concentration is needed.

Since many different individuals will likely be involved in data collection, good training is essential. Over the years, I have observed bias by some observers on cell length measurements. For instance, some may avoid large cells believing they could not possibly be a single cell. In some models with severe hypertrophy, such as Spontaneously Hypertensive Heart Failure rats, cells may reach 400 or 500 μm in length. So, this bias is not surprising. We recommend that a well-trained PI personally collect data from 5 or 10 isolated cell preps obtained from controls and several pathological models. These glutaraldehyde-fixed cells can be stored for many years and used to test and validate the reliability of new personnel.

Finally, we prefer using female rats in our experiments because they maintain body mass much better than males. Male rats tend to gain considerable body mass with age and many treatment interventions also affect body mass gain in males. Consequently, myocyte remodeling due to an intervention may often be masked in the background of body mass changes. If male rats are preferred for a given experiment, it may be worth considering minimal food restriction to ensure stable body mass during the study. While there is a high degree of gender bias among reviewers, we have often collected data from both genders in different pathological models and have never found a different myocyte remodeling response between the sexes independent of body mass changes.

Conclusion

A protocol to obtain precise, comprehensive measurements of cardiac myocyte dimensions has been outlined in detail. This approach provides significant insight into the underlying cellular basis of chamber remodeling. It also allows direct comparison of all published information using this method, regardless of species, gender, age, or underlying disease.

References

1 Gerdes AM. Cardiac myocyte remodeling in hypertrophy and progression to failure. *J Card Fail* 2002; **8** (Suppl): S264–268.

2 Gerdes AM, Moore JA, Hines JM, Kirkland PA, Bishop SP. Regional differences in myocyte size in normal rat heart. *Anat Rec* 1986; **215**: 420–426.

3 Gerdes AM, Kellerman SE, Malec KB, Schocken DD. Transverse shape characteristics of cardiac myocytes from rats and humans. *Cardioscience* 1994; **5**: 31–36.

4 Hurley J. Sizing particles with a Coulter counter. *Biophys J* 1970; **10**: 74–79.

5 Gerdes AM, Onodera T, Tamura T, Said S, Bohlmeyer TJ, Abraham WT, et al. New method to evaluate myocyte remodeling from formalin-fixed biopsy and autopsy material. *J Card Fail* 1998; **4**: 343–348.

6 Tamura T, Onodera T, Said S, Gerdes AM. Correlation of myocyte lengthening to chamber dilation in the spontaneously hypertensive heart failure (SHHF) rat. *J Mol Cell Cardiol* 1998; **30**: 2175–2181.

7 Campbell SE, Gerdes AM. Regional differences in cardiac myocyte dimensions and number in Sprague-Dawley rats from different suppliers. *Proc Soc Exp Biol Med* 1987; **186**: 211–217.

8 Campbell SE, Gerdes AM, Smith TD. Comparison of regional differences in cardiac myocyte dimensions in rats, hamsters, and guinea pigs. *Anat Rec* 1987; **219**: 53–59.

9 Gerdes AM, Moore JA, Hines JM. Regional changes in myocyte size and number in propranolol-treated hyperthyroid rats. *Lab Invest* 1987; **57**: 708–713.

10 Campbell SE, Gerdes AM. Regional changes in myocyte size during the reversal of thyroid-induced cardiac hypertrophy. *J Mol Cell Cardiol* 1988; **20**: 379–387.

11 Gerdes AM, Campbell SE, Hilbelink DR. Structural remodeling of cardiac myocytes in rats with arteriovenous fistulas. *Lab Invest* 1988; **59**: 857–861.

12 Liu Z, Gerdes AM. Influence of hypothyroidism and the reversal of hypothyroidism on hemodynamics and cell size in the adult rat heart. *J Mol Cell Cardiol* 1990; **22**: 1339–1348.

13 Bai SL, Campbell SE, Moore JA, Morales MC, Gerdes AM. Influence of age, growth, and sex on cardiac myocyte size and number in rats. *Anat Rec* 1990; **226**: 207–212.

14 Liu Z, Hilbelink DR, Crockett WB, Gerdes AM. Regional changes in hemodynamics and cardiac myocyte size in rats with aortocaval fistulas. 1. Developing and established hypertrophy. *Circ Res* 1991; **69**: 52–58.

15 Gerdes AM, Clark LC, Capasso JM. Regression of cardiac hypertrophy after closing an aortocaval fistula in rats. *Am J Physiol* 1995; **268**: H2345–2351.

Part 6

Manipulation of Gene Expression *in Vitro* and *in Vivo*

Generation of Cre-*loxP* mouse models for conditional knockout and overexpression of genes in various heart cells

Marisa Z. Jackson and Warren G. Tourtellotte

Northwestern University Feinberg School of Medicine, Chicago, IL, USA

Introduction

The study of human cardiovascular disease is often confounded by the multifactorial nature of the involved biological processes. In order to better understand the mechanisms underlying diseases such as hypertension, atherosclerosis, and heart failure, integrative physiology must be able to clearly distinguish cause from effect. While *in vitro* models continue to be useful to identify the most basic cellular processes involved in cardiomyocyte function, unraveling the connections between molecular pathways and their integrated physiological effects is best served by the experimental contexts that most closely emulate a particular disease. Conditional gene targeting in mice has emerged as a powerful technique for studying gene function *in vivo*, allowing experimental analysis to more clearly define the primary genetic/ molecular factors contributing to physiologic function and to correlate that with human disease.

Conventional gene knockout (KO) strategies create mutant mice carrying null alleles in the germ line, which, in the case of genes essential for development and survival, can lead to embryonic or perinatal lethality that preclude further analysis. In addition, many proteins have widespread tissue function, which makes it possible for some of them to functionally compensate during highly adaptable stages of development. Moreover, inactivating a gene in all tissues and at all stages of development often makes it difficult to study its cell autonomous function.

A further refinement to targeted mutagenesis utilizes the Cre-*loxP* system to conditionally ablate or overexpress genes. The bacteriophage P1-encoded Cre recombinase is a 38-kD protein that catalyzes DNA recombination between two 34-bp recognition sequences, known as *loxP* sites [1]. Targeting vectors introduce modified sequences containing these *loxP* sequences into the mouse genome, making it possible to induce recombination events in specific genomic DNA regions *in vivo*. With appropriate construct design, conditional gene inactivation (cKO) or overexpression (cKI) can be induced in mice carrying the *loxP*-flanked or "floxed" allele specifically in cells that express Cre recombinase (Figure 45.1).

The Cre-*loxP* system was developed over two decades ago and has since been enhanced to improve the temporal and spatial specificity of gene expression. Cre-recombinase expression can be regulated by tissue-specific gene promoters [2] as well as ligand-dependent Cre fusion proteins, wherein *loxP*-site recombination can be induced with the administration of ligands such as tamoxifen

Manual of Research Techniques in Cardiovascular Medicine, First Edition. Edited by Hossein Ardehali, Roberto Bolli, and Douglas W. Losordo.

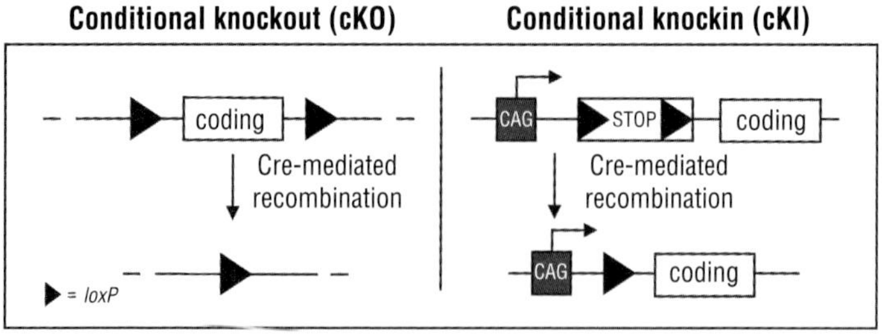

Conditional knockout (cKO)   **Conditional knockin (cKI)**

Figure 45.1 Strategies for conditional gain (cKI) and loss (cKO) of gene function in mice. For gene cKO, *loxP* sites are typically inserted into the genome flanking the desired segment of genomic DNA to be ablated *in vivo*. For gene cKI, a lox-STOP-lox (LSL) cassette is used to disrupt the regulatory control of the transgene by the desired promoter (in this case CAG). Removal of the LSL cassette by Cre-mediated excision enables irreversible expression of the transgene in Cre-recombinase expressing cells *in vivo*.

that localize the ligand-bound recombinase to the nucleus [3–6].

This chapter will present a generalized protocol for two of the most common vector designs: (1) the conditional knockout (cKO) for inactivation of gene function; and (2) the conditional knockin (cKI) for gene overexpression. Detailed discussions of the materials and general procedures outlined here can be found in previously published work [7–11].

Protocol

Conditional knockout (cKO) gene targeting
Identify bacterial artificial chromosome (BAC) mouse genomic DNA clone
The genomic structure of the gene to be targeted can be downloaded from an online database (e.g. UCSC Genome Browser, http://genome.ucsc.edu) and imported into analysis software (e.g. VectorNTI, Invitrogen, Carlsbad, USA) for visualization of exon and intron boundaries, alternatively-spliced transcripts, protein domains, etc.

The cKO gene targeting vector is based upon subcloned BAC genomic DNA isolated from an appropriate BAC that contains 100–200 kb of genomic DNA and the gene of interest. The UCSC Genome Browser is used to identify particular BAC clones that contain the gene of interest. The BAC clone can be obtained from clone repositories (e.g. CHORI, http://www.chori.org) and the appropriate clone is generally chosen so that the gene of interest is located approximately in the middle of the BAC DNA. This ensures the inclusion of sufficient flanking genomic DNA to accommodate the recombination arms for the construct and to obtain

the probes required for screening homologous recombinant ES cells by Southern blotting.

The targeting vector contains only a small portion of the gene to be targeted and recombination arms that flank any mutations that are to be introduced into the genome. Thus, a small amount of BAC genomic DNA must first be subcloned into a high copy plasmid (e.g. Bluescript, Agilent, Santa Clara, CA) using BAC DNA that has been amplified by traditional miniprep methods (e.g. QIAprep Spin Miniprep Kit, Qiagen, Valencia, USA) [10].

Materials and methods
Homologous recombination in *E. coli* (recombineering) is facilitated using *E. coli* strains that have been engineered to express the *Red* recombinase genes *exo*, *bet*, and *gam* under the control of a heat-inducible promoter [11]. Specific integration events can be engineered into a *target* DNA molecule using a *donor* fragment of DNA that has small homology domains with the target DNA and that flank a fragment of DNA to be inserted into the *target* molecule. Recombination between the two molecules within *E. coli* leads to a double cross-over event and strand exchange, leaving a precise insertion of the flanked DNA sequence and a selectable marker (e.g. *Neo*). For detailed discussion and method overview see [7,8].

Recombinogenic E. coli *strains.* This protocol is based upon recombinase-expressing *E. coli* strains that are substrains of the standard DH10B strain used to construct most BAC libraries. They contain a defective λ prophage expressing *exo, bet, and gam* recombinase proteins under the regulatory control of a temperature-sensitive promoter, rendering their expression inducible by heat shock. The *E. coli* strains and plasmid vectors used have been previously described in detail [8,11].

Recombinant E. coli:

DY380: Recombinase expression regulated by temperature-sensitive promoter.

EL250: Recombinase expression regulated by temperature-sensitive promoter and a second expression unit controlled by an arabinose-inducible promoter to express FLPe-recombinase.

EL350: Recombinase expression regulated by temperature-sensitive promoter and a second expression unit controlled by an arabinose-inducible promoter to express Cre-recombinase.

Vector DNA:

pBS-DT: a high-copy pBluescript KSII vector used for gap repair containing the negative ES cell selection cassette diphtheria toxin (DT-α) under the control of a Pol II promotor and cloned into the *Sma*I site of the vector polylinker. (Vector can be obtained from the Tourtellotte lab).

pL451 (also known as FNFL): contains *Neo* under the control of a eukaryotic and prokaryotic promotor (PGK) and flanked by two FRT sites and one 3′ *loxP* site in pBluescript KS.

pL452 (also known as LNL): contains *Neo* under the control of a eukaryotic and prokaryotic promotor (PGK) flanked by two *loxP* sites.

Transformation of BAC DNA into DY380 *E. coli*

In order to isolate a small fragment (8–14 kb) of mouse genomic DNA to be used to generate the targeting vector, the BAC must first be transformed into DY380 *E. coli*. A fresh DY380 *E. coli* colony is picked from selective LB plate (6.25 μg/mL tetracycline) and grown in selective LB overnight at 32°C. These strains must be kept at 32°C or lower for overnight incubations so that the recombinases are not induced until needed. DY380 cells are then made electrocompetent (glycerol washes) and the BAC is electroporated into them using standard protocols [10,11]. Chloramphenicol-resistant clones are selected and PCR using oligos that recognize a particular region of the gene of interest is used to confirm the presence of the appropriate BAC. A 10% frozen glycerol stock of the BAC in DY380

can be prepared and stored for at least 3 months at −20°C and much longer at −80°C.

Gap repair

Using the BAC plasmid as the template, homology domains (H1 and H2) are amplified by PCR (200–500 bp in length) to demarcate the ends of the DNA fragment to be subcloned. The primers contain restriction sites for enzymes permitting directional cloning into the pBS-DT polylinker with a unique restriction site between the two cloned homology domains to allow the retrieval plasmid to be linearized (Figure 45.2).

The DY380-BAC cells are treated by brief heat-shock (42°C for 15 minutes) and then made electrocompetent using glycerol washing on ice. The linearized gap repair retrieval vector (50–100 ng) is electroporated into the heat-induced DY380-BAC cells [10,11]. The electroporated *E. coli* are plated on ampicillin (Amp) plates and grown at 32°C to select Amp⁺ recombinants that are generated when successful gap repair of the high copy plasmid has occurred by homologous recombination. Control plates using uninduced electroporation-competent DY380-BAC cells should contain no Amp⁺ colonies. Colonies are screened (and sequenced) to ensure that the intended fragment of DNA has been retrieved from the BAC into the high-copy Gap repair retrieval vector (Figure 45.2). The resulting subclone (sub) is then shuttled to EL350 cells for subsequent recombineering procedures (EL350-sub).

Generating the conditional targeting construct

The overall strategy for generating a conditional knockout construct using recombineering has been previously described in detail [8]. In general, a region of genomic DNA to be conditionally ablated is flanked by similarly oriented *loxP* sites that are typically inserted into intron sequence to avoid altering gene expression from the *loxP* targeted allele. The targeting construct is generated using two rounds of homologous recombination that insert a 5′ *loxP* and a 3′ frt-flanked *Neo-loxP* cassette, both of which flank the DNA to be conditionally ablated. After embryonic stem (ES) cells have been targeted, the Neo-positive selection marker can either be removed by electroporation of a Flpe expression

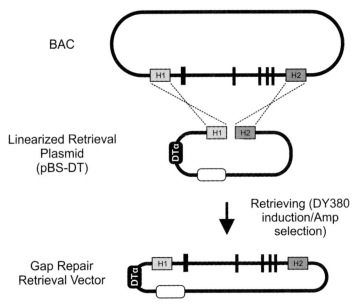

Figure 45.2 Strategy for subcloning a fragment of mouse genomic DNA for subsequent targeting vector construction. Gap repair and recombinase-expressing *E. coli* are used to retrieve the desired fragment of BAC genomic DNA into a high-copy plasmid vector.

plasmid into a targeted ES cell or by mating germline heterozygous animals to a mouse that expresses Flpe in the germline. Either method will remove the Neo selection cassette leaving a single closely juxtaposed Frt and *loxP* site in the genome. The *loxP*-site insertion positions can be precisely controlled because they depend upon homologous recombination events during construct design and not the presence of any particular restriction sites.

5′ loxP targeting. The 5′ *loxP* site is generated by cloning a targeting vector derived from the pL452 (LNL) plasmid. PCR primers with appropriate 5′ restriction sites are designed to amplify 100–200 bp homology domains that flank the desired insertion site. The homology domains (e.g. H3, H4; Figure 45.3) are cloned into the LNL vector, the plasmid is linearized and electroporated into heat-induced EL350-sub cells and grown on kanamycin plates to select clones with Neo inserts. Neo+ clones are screened for the appropriate recombination event and sequenced. A correctly targeted plasmid is electroporated into arabinose-induced EL350 cells that express Cre-recombinase to recombine the *loxP* sequences, thereby removing the Neo selection

marker and generating the 5′ *loxP* plasmid with a single precisely targeted *loxP* site (Figure 45.3A).

3′ loxP targeting. The 3′ *loxP* targeting vector is generated using primers designed to amplify 100–200 bp homology domains that flank the intended genomic DNA targeting region. The homology domains (e.g. H4, H5; Figure 45.3B), with appropriate restriction sites, are cloned into pL451 (FNFL). The targeting vector is linearized and electroporated into heat-induced EL350 cells containing the 5′ *loxP* plasmid (EL350-5′*loxP*) cells and the colonies are selected on kanamycin plates. Neo+ positive clones are screened and sequenced to identify the final conditional knockout targeting vector.

The final targeting vector can be tested *in vitro* to ensure that the Frt sites and *loxP* sites are performing nominally. Electroporation of the vector into either arabinose-induced EL350 (Cre) or EL250 (Flpe) cells will recombine the *loxP*/Frt sites so that the recombined plasmid can be sequence verified and the expected recombination events validated. Standard methods for culturing, selecting, and screening ES cells can then be used to identify

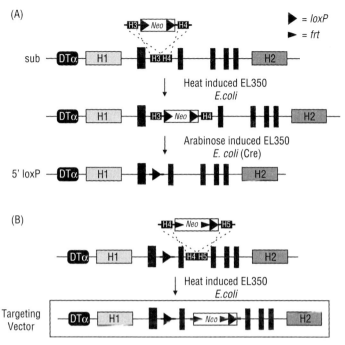

Figure 45.3 Strategy for designing a cKO construct using a two-step process to target 5′ *loxP* and 3′ *loxP* sites. (A) The 5′ *loxP* site is targeted by generating a targeting vector containing *loxP-Neo-loxP* (LNL) which is then recombined in *E. coli* to leave a single targeted *loxP* site. (B) The 3′ *loxP* site is targeted by generating a targeting vector that contains the *frt-Neo-frt-loxP* (FNFL) cassette to produce the final targeting construct (box).

targeted ES cells for generating chimeric mice after blastocyst injection.

Conditional knockin (cKI) gene targeting

The preferred method for conditionally overexpressing a protein of interest is to use gene targeting and homologous recombination to target the Rosa locus [12]. The Rosa locus is constitutively expressed and targeting efficiency in ES cells is very high. The method described is a slightly modified version of that previously described in detail by Srinivas *et al.* [9]. The method is based upon cloning the cDNA of interest into a standardized Rosa targeting vector that has been modified to use the strong chicken β-actin CMV (CAG) promoter to drive gene expression (pBIGT-CAG available from Tourtellotte lab). The cDNA to be overexpressed is placed downstream of a floxed PGK-*Neo* transcription stop cassette, which in turn is located downstream of the CAG promoter (Figure 45.4A).

Upon Cre-mediated recombination, the Neo-positive selection marker (which is used to select recombinant ES cells) and the strong polyA transcription termination sequence is excised, enabling strong CAG-mediated and conditional expression of the cloned cDNA [9].

The targeting vector is generated by cloning the cDNA into the multiple cloning site (MCS) of pBIGT-CAG. The pBIGT-CAG-cDNA cassette is then shuttled to the pRosa26-PA targeting vector using standard restriction site cloning. The pRosa26-PA vector contains a modified fragment of wild-type genomic Rosa locus DNA where the *Xba*I site (between the 5′ and 3′ recombination arms) has been replaced by rare eight-base *Pac*I and *Asc*I restriction sites. Standard cloning methods are used to shuttle the *Pac*I/*Asc*I fragment from pBIGT-CAG-cDNA to the *Pac*I/*Asc*I sites of pRosa26-PA to generate the final gene targeting vector (Figure 45.4B). This targeting construct is

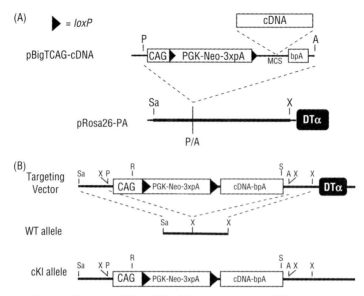

Figure 45.4 Strategy for designing a cKI construct. (A) The cDNA of interest is cloned into pBIGT-CAG and the cassette is shuttled to the targeting vector (Rosa26-PA). (B) The resulting targeting vector is recombined in ES cells using standard methods. A, *Asc*I; P, *Pac*I; Sa, *Sac*I; X, *Xba*I.

electroporated into ES cells, selected, and screened using the previously published methods without modification [9].

Strengths and weaknesses

Cre-*loxP* and *FlpE-frt* technologies provide powerful tools for manipulating the mammalian genome. Using a single mouse with a *loxP*- or *frt*-flanked gene, multiple recombinase-expressing transgenic lines can be used to either ablate or overexpress a gene of interest with precise spatial and temporal control. Moreover, tamoxifen-inducible Cre-recombinase driver mice provide an additional level of spatial and temporal control over gene expression [4]. In studies related to cardiovascular biology, the most commonly used Cre transgenic driver mouse uses the α-MHC promotor to express Cre-recombinase in cardiomyocytes and to recombine *loxP* sites in their genomic DNA [13]. However, it should be recognized that Cre-expression restricted to cardiomyocytes would not affect all cells in the heart, such as fibroblasts, endothelial cells, and vascular smooth muscle cells. Thus, a variety of other transgenic mice have been generated to express Cre-recombinase in different cardiac and vascular cells, some of which are indicated in Table 45.1.

Table 45.1 Selected Cre-driver mice for genetic studies in cardiovascular biology

Cre driver strain	Desired recombination	Original publication [Ref.]
Constitutive Cre		
αMHC-Cre	Myocardiocytes	[13]
Nppa-Cre3	Myocardiocytes (atrial)	[25]
ECsrp1[Cre]	Vascular smooth muscle cells	[26]
Tamoxifen-inducible Cre		
αMHC-CreER[T2]	Myocardiocytes (tamoxifen inducible)	[5]
HCN4-KiT	Pacemaker cells	[27]
Tie2-CreER[T2]	Endothelial cells	[28]
Tcf21-CreER[T2]	Epicardium, cardiac fibroblasts, valvular interstitial cells	[29]

There are several considerations when generating and using conditional gene targeted mice. For example, floxed alleles may be variably sensitive to Cre-recombinase expression depending on the location within the genome where the *loxP* sites are inserted and particular transgenic mice can express differing levels of Cre-recombinase. These issues can result in incomplete *loxP* recombination in a cell population, which can lead to incomplete loss- or gain-of-gene expression. Cre-recombinase-dependent reporter mice or PCR screens can be used to determine the efficiency of *loxP* recombination in the tissues of interest. Another major factor affecting the fidelity of conditional gene targeting is the temporal and spatial specificity of Cre-recombinase expression in a particular transgenic mouse. Often, particular promoters are assumed to have precise spatial and temporal expression but this is not often tested rigorously in many previously generated Cre-driver mice. Finally, there is also the possibility that high expression of Cre-recombinase can lead to cellular abnormalities. For example, high levels of Cre expression have been reported to arrest growth and lead to increased death in mammalian cells in some Cre-driver mice [14–16], although the majority of Cre-driver transgenic mice appear to develop normally.

Alternative approaches

The Flpe-*FRT* system can be used in a similar fashion to Cre-*loxP* and has been shown to mediate high-efficiency gene deletion [17]. More recently, an improved Flp deleter mouse has been developed expressing Flpo recombinase, a modified version of the site specific recombinase estimated to be five times more active than Flpe [18]. Additionally, the discovery of the Cre-like recombinase Dre, which acts on *rox* recognition sites, has been shown to mediate efficient recombination in transgenic lines and could serve as yet another tool in conditional gene targeting strategies [19,20].

Conclusion

Many studies have used site-specific Cre-*loxP* strategies to place Cre-recombinase under the control of cardiac-specific promoters to examine their role in cardiac function [21]. These approaches

have produced new insights into the mechanisms of myocardial hypertrophy [22], cardiomyocyte function and response to cardiac stress [23], and alterations in blood pressure [24], all within the context of cardiac-cell-specific gene mutations. The effort required to produce a conditional gain- or loss-of-function mouse model is only marginally increased above that associated with classical gene targeting strategies and thus, it is an attractive and preferred means of creating mutant mice to study gene expression in cardiac cell function *in vivo*.

References

1 Sauer B, Henderson N. Site-specific DNA recombination in mammalian cells by the Cre recombinase of bacteriophage P1. *Proc Natl Acad Sci U S A* 1988; **85**: 5166–5170.

2 Gu H, Marth JD, Orban PC, Mossmann H, Rajewsky K. Deletion of a DNA polymerase beta gene segment in T cells using cell type-specific gene targeting. *Science* 1994; **265**: 103–106.

3 Kuhn R, Schwenk F, Aguet M, Rajewsky K. Inducible gene targeting in mice. *Science* 1995; **269**: 1427–1429.

4 Feil R, Brocard J, Mascrez B, LeMeur M, Metzger D, Chambon P, *et al*. Ligand-activated site-specific recombination in mice. *Proc Natl Acad Sci U S A* 1996; **93**: 10887–10890.

5 Sohal DS, Nghiem M, Crackower MA, Witt SA, Kimball TR, Tymitz KM, *et al*. Temporally regulated and tissue-specific gene manipulations in the adult and embryonic heart using a tamoxifen-inducible Cre protein. *Circ Res* 2001; **89**: 20–25.

6 Metzger D, Clifford J, Chiba H, Chambon P. Conditional site-specific recombination in mammalian cells using a ligand-dependent chimeric Cre recombinase. *Proc Natl Acad Sci U S A* 1995; **92**: 6991–6995.

7 Lee EC, Yu D, Martinez de Velasco J, Tessarollo L, Swing DA, Court DL, *et al*. A highly efficient Escherichia coli-based chromosome engineering system adapted for recombinogenic targeting and subcloning of BAC DNA. *Genomics* 2001; **73**: 56–65.

8 Liu P, Jenkins NA, Copeland NG. A highly efficient recombineering-based method for generating conditional knockout mutations. *Genome Res* 2003; **13**: 476–484.

9 Srinivas S, Watanabe T, Lin CS, William CM, Tanabe Y, Jessell TM, *et al*. Cre reporter strains produced by targeted insertion of EYFP and ECFP into the ROSA26 locus. *BMC Dev Biol* 2001; **1**: 4.

10 Bouvier J, Cheng JG. Recombineering-based procedure for creating Cre/loxP conditional knockouts in the

mouse. *Curr Protoc Mol Biol* 2009; Chapter **23**: Unit 23.13.

11 Yu D, Ellis HM, Lee EC, Jenkins NA, Copeland NG, Court DL, *et al.* An efficient recombination system for chromosome engineering in Escherichia coli. *Proc Natl Acad Sci U S A* 2000; **97**: 5978–5983.

12 Soriano P. Generalized lacZ expression with the ROSA26 Cre reporter strain. *Nat Genet* 1999; **21**: 70–71.

13 Subramaniam A, Jones WK, Gulick J, Wert S, Neumann J, Robbins J, *et al.* Tissue-specific regulation of the alpha-myosin heavy chain gene promoter in transgenic mice. *J Biol Chem* 1991; **266**: 24613–24620.

14 Baba Y, Nakano M, Yamada Y, Saito I, Kanegae Y. Practical range of effective dose for Cre recombinase-expressing recombinant adenovirus without cell toxicity in mammalian cells. *Microbiol Immunol* 2005; **49**: 559–570.

15 Loonstra A, Vooijs M, Beverloo HB, Allak BA, van Drunen E, Kanaar R, *et al.* Growth inhibition and DNA damage induced by Cre recombinase in mammalian cells. *Proc Natl Acad Sci U S A* 2001; **98**: 9209–9214.

16 Schmidt EE, Taylor DS, Prigge JR, Barnett S, Capecchi MR. Illegitimate Cre-dependent chromosome rearrangements in transgenic mouse spermatids. *Proc Natl Acad Sci U S A* 2000; **97**: 13702–13707.

17 Dymecki SM. Flp recombinase promotes site-specific DNA recombination in embryonic stem cells and transgenic mice. *Proc Natl Acad Sci U S A* 1996; **93**: 6191–6196.

18 Kranz A, Fu J, Duerschke K, Weidlich S, Naumann R, Stewart AF, *et al.* An improved Flp deleter mouse in C57Bl/6 based on Flpo recombinase. *Genesis* 2010; **48**: 512–520.

19 Anastassiadis K, Fu J, Patsch C, Hu S, Weidlich S, Duerschke K, *et al.* Dre recombinase, like Cre, is a highly efficient site-specific recombinase in E. coli, mammalian cells and mice. *Dis Model Mech* 2009; **2**: 508–515.

20 Saxton TM, Henkemeyer M, Gasca S, Shen R, Rossi DJ, Shalaby F, *et al.* Abnormal mesoderm patterning in mouse embryos mutant for the SH2 tyrosine phosphatase Shp-2. *EMBO J* 1997; **16**: 2352–2364.

21 Ruiz-Lozano P, Chien KR. Cre-constructing the heart. *Nat Genet* 2003; **33**: 8–9.

22 Xiong D, Heyman NS, Airey J, Zhang M, Singer CA, Rawat S, *et al.* Cardiac-specific, inducible ClC-3 gene deletion eliminates native volume-sensitive chloride channels and produces myocardial hypertrophy in adult mice. *J Mol Cell Cardiol* 2010; **48**: 211–219.

23 Papanicolaou KN, Streicher JM, Ishikawa TO, Herschman H, Wang Y, Walsh K, *et al.* Preserved heart function and maintained response to cardiac stresses in a genetic model of cardiomyocyte-targeted deficiency of cyclooxygenase-2. *J Mol Cell Cardiol* 2010; **49**: 196–209.

24 Rindler TN, Lasko VM, Nieman ML, Okada M, Lorenz JN, Lingrel JB, *et al.* Knockout of the Na,K-ATPase alpha-isoform in the cardiovascular system does not alter basal blood pressure but prevents ACTH-induced hypertension. *Am J Physiol Heart Circ Physiol* 2011; **301**: H1396–1404.

25 de Lange FJ, Moorman AF, Christoffels VM. Atrial cardiomyocyte-specific expression of Cre recombinase driven by an Nppa gene fragment. *Genesis* 2003; **37**: 1–4.

26 Snider P, Fix JL, Rogers R, Peabody-Dowling G, Ingram D, Lilly B, *et al.* Generation and characterization of Csrp1 enhancer-driven tissue-restricted Cre-recombinase mice. *Genesis* 2008; **46**: 167–176.

27 Hoesl E, Stieber J, Herrmann S, Feil S, Tybl E, Hofmann F, *et al.* Tamoxifen-inducible gene deletion in the cardiac conduction system. *J Mol Cell Cardiol* 2008; **45**: 62–69.

28 Forde A, Constien R, Gröne HJ, Hämmerling G, Arnold B. Temporal Cre-mediated recombination exclusively in endothelial cells using Tie2 regulatory elements. *Genesis* 2002; **33**: 191–197.

29 Acharya A, Baek ST, Banfi S, Eskiocak B, Tallquist MD. Efficient inducible Cre-mediated recombination in Tcf21 cell lineages in the heart and kidney. *Genesis* 2011; **49**: 870–877.

46

Modulation of myocardial genes via use of adenoviral vectors and RNA interference approaches

Qianhong Li

University of Louisville, Louisville, KY, USA

Introduction

There have been dramatic advances in characterizing the phenomenon of RNA interference, which was first observed over a decade ago. In the elucidation of its mechanism, insights have been gained into cellular gene expression controls that have evolved into an invaluable tool for exploring pathognomonic roles of gene expression and translational products through knockdown. By harnessing cellular defense mechanisms and machinery believed to innately function in counteracting virally introduced double-stranded RNA, we are now able to design sequence-specific templates that serve to mimic microRNA translational control, thus targeting messenger RNA (mRNA), according to complementarity, and post-transcriptionally inhibiting phenotypic expression by directed mRNA degradation.

These relatively new tools have far reaching implications, both in basic science research and as potential novel therapeutic agents, as continued refinement for improved efficacy of *in vitro/in vivo* transduction techniques and targeting sequences emerge. However, despite few limitations on mRNAs that can be targeted, the techniques of siRNA post-transcriptional gene silencing do carry constraints and caveats that must be accounted for within experimental design and specific investigational protocols based on the desired degree and duration of knockdown. With this in mind, the recombinant adenoviral vector, as a means of siRNA transfer and continued expression for stable, sequence-specific, prolonged target gene silencing, has emerged as a staple approach within this technology. Methods for synthesis of these vectors have been well characterized and are readily reproducible. In time, the application of RNA interference by use of these adenoviral vector-mediated siRNAs, within the realm of cardiovascular medicine, will enable insights to be gleaned into pathophysiologic processes of the premier assailants of health worldwide.

RNA interference (RNAi) is the process of introducing or eliciting the synthesis of double-stranded RNA (dsRNA) molecules to post-transcriptionally suppress a gene of interest in a specific, sequence-dependent manner via degradation of its corresponding mRNA transcript. These dsRNA sequences are either transduced, to be transcriptionally generated within cell(s), or exogenously transfected into the cell(s) of interest. Once present, dsRNA is rapidly processed by the cytoplasmic RNase III-type enzyme Dicer into shorter (19–23 base pairs) RNA duplexes with distinct two-nucleotide overhangs at their 3′ termini and a phosphate at the 5′ termini [1]. The obtained small dsRNA fragments are designated as small interfering RNAs (siRNAs) and, after processing, serve as the pivotal elements for successful RNA interference [2]. In the presence of ATP, another endogenous enzyme complex, known as the

Manual of Research Techniques in Cardiovascular Medicine, First Edition. Edited by Hossein Ardehali, Roberto Bolli, and Douglas W. Losordo.

RNA-induced silencing complex (RISC) [3], binds the siRNA. Subsequently, the RISC complex initiates an unwinding of the siRNA strands yielding the antisense strand of the siRNA that remains bound to the RISC and the sense strand that undergoes cellular degradation [4]. The bound antisense strand of the siRNA is a single-stranded RNA (ssRNA), termed the guide strand, as it directs the RISC intrinsic Argonaute protein with "slicer" ability to endonucleolytically cleave homologous mRNA, which becomes complementarily recognized and bound to the antisense siRNA. Over many rounds, the target mRNAs are cleaved and depleted [5]. The Argonaute protein has many defined domains, each with specific, respective functions. However, this depth of detail is beyond the scope of this chapter. Essential for the RNAi process, the guide strand of ssRNA (i.e. the antisense strand of siRNA) functions as a probe to determine the target sequence specificity of the RNA interference response, thus leading to suppression of the homologous gene by down regulation of its mRNA transcript and consequentially its protein product [2–4,6–8].

The discovery of the RNAi phenomenon has rapidly yielded not only promising techniques used for functional genetics but also possibilities for therapeutic applications. Use of RNAi in cultured cells with the effective siRNAs to a specific target of interest is easily accomplished by introduction of siRNA into cells by lipid-mediated transfer. Synthetic siRNAs are inherently small (19–21 base pairs) and only need to cross the cell membrane, not the nuclear membrane, to be effective [3]. Additionally, synthetic, commercially prevalidated siRNAs are becoming increasingly available. However, synthetic siRNAs are short-lived in the cell and their longevity is also restricted by the rate of cell division, which if high will result in serial dilution of intracellular siRNA concentrations. This can have the result of transient effects on gene and translational silencing. In light of this, plasmid vectors have been designed to drive active expression of siRNAs through the use of RNA polymerase III promoters and can overcome these drawbacks.

Progress in elucidation of the mechanisms and machinery of endogenous RNAi in terms of microRNAs (miRNAs) suggests that RNAi might be induced in mammalian cells by introduction of synthetic genes that express mimics of endogenous miRNAs in the form of short hairpin RNAs (shRNAs) through plasmids containing RNA polymerase III promoters. After transduction, a plasmid vector containing an expression cassette with an RNA polymerase promoter can produce shRNAs. These shRNAs are subsequently processed into active siRNAs [9,10]. The shRNA-expressing plasmid vectors can produce a longer-lasting RNAi effect [5] but it is still time limited. Moreover, transfection efficiency is often low when shRNA plasmid vectors are transduced into nondividing primary cells, which are the most often used cell types for disease-related functional studies. The success of RNAi-mediated gene silencing *in vivo* depends on efficient, targeted siRNA delivery and retention within the organ of interest. Furthermore, the siRNA must remain stable while in transit until the construct can reach its ultimate destination within the tissue [3,5].

To address these issues, viral-mediated delivery of shRNA vectors have been developed and now function as a powerful alternative to transfection for primary cells, as well as having *in vivo* applications [11,12]. A number of shRNA viral systems have been reported. These include adenoviral, retroviral, and lentiviral systems [13–16]. The genomes of retroviral and lentiviral shRNA vectors integrate into the host genome, leading to long-term expression. In contrast, the adenoviral genome remains epichromosomal, resulting in a relatively transient expression profile. However, this characteristically avoids insertional mutagenesis problems that are possible with host genome integration. Additionally, intracellular adenoviral copy numbers are significantly higher than other models and facilitate high levels of intracellular shRNA expression, thus making adenoviral RNAi vectors particularly useful for RNAi-mediated gene silencing by downstream expression of siRNAs and effects of target gene knockdown. Moreover, adenoviral shRNA vectors can be produced with much higher titers than retroviral or lentiviral vectors, resulting in high-level transient expression with efficient transduction of both dividing and nondividing cells [14–16].

Although still in its infancy, use of RNAi technologies *in vivo* has already shown promise, and significant advances have been made in accessible tissues. Examples include the reduction of hematologic cholesterol transport within the mouse model [17], prevention of vascular smooth muscle cell proliferation in the injured rat carotid artery [18], targeted inhibition of oxidant signaling to provide a novel treatment for ischemic cardiomyopathy induced heart failure in mice [6,19], and others in the eye [20,21] and lung [22]. Despite the considerable complexities and need for further optimization of RNAi technologies and techniques, the increasing evidence for its application within whole-animal models provides powerful demonstration that genetic approaches can lead not only to novel insights in mechanistic aspects of molecular biology but also to clinical advances in therapeutic strategies for the treatment of disease.

Protocols

Guidelines for siRNA design

1. Select several (four or more) target sites for a single gene as not all designed siRNAs have equal effects on suppression of the target cellular gene product.
2. The selected siRNA target sequence is usually 19–21 nucleotides (nt) in length.
3. The potential siRNA target sites are AA dinucleotide sequences following 19 nt sequences.
4. Choose siRNA sequences with GC content around 30–50%.
5. Avoid selecting siRNA target sequences from the regions within 50–100 bp of the start codon and the termination codon.
6. Do not select intron regions as siRNA sequences.
7. Do not choose regions containing four or more consecutive As or Ts.
8. Avoid single nucleotide polymorphism (SNP) sequences.
9. Perform a BLAST homology search at http://blast.ncbi.nlm.nih.gov/ to confirm the potential siRNA sites in the same species database and to avoid off-target effects on other genes or sequences.
10. It is necessary to design negative controls by scrambling targeted siRNA sequence. The negative controls should have the same length and nucleotide composition as the siRNA. Perform a BLAST homology search at http://blast.ncbi.nlm.nih.gov/ to confirm the scrambling targeted siRNA sequence will not create new homology to other genes.
11. Customized services for design and preparation of siRNA are commercially available, including

Invitrogen, Santa Cruz, Dharmacon in Thermo Scientific Life Science Research, and QIAGEN.

Guidelines of shRNA design

1. Following the Guidelines of siRNA design, a 19 nt DNA sequence is selected homologous to the gene of interest. A construct is created with this 19 nt sequence (sense) followed by a short spacer (4–7 nt) and the inverted antisense with a poly-T fragment. This construct is inserted into the multicloning site (MCS) within a plasmid vector.
2. The plasmid vector should contain an expression cassette with an RNA polymerase promoter. The choice of RNA polymerase promoter is critical to ensure the effective production of shRNA. Within current literature, RNA polymerase III promoters, including U6 and H1, are reported to be strong promoters for stable shRNA expression in cells [23].

Considerations for RNAi transfer

Silencing gene expression through RNAi can provide valuable insights into gene function, but essentially requires efficient cellular delivery of siRNA or shRNA. Interfering RNA transfer is most commonly achieved either transiently by transfection of siRNA oligonucleotides, or by using shRNA expressed from a DNA containing plasmid or adenoviral vector. Determination of the ideal approach depends on the cell type being studied and whether transient or stable continuous knockdown is desired.

The most popular technique for transient transfection of unmodified siRNA or plasmid-encoded shRNA is by facilitated cytosolic delivery using cationic lipid-based reagents. siRNA oligonucleotides or plasmid-encoded shRNA sequences can be packaged into miniaturized lipid-based particulates called cationic liposomes, which are similar to cellular membranes. These lipid-based interfering RNA conglomerates fuse with cellular membranes, delivering their siRNA or shRNA contents into the cell's cytoplasmic compartment. This approach provides superior transfection efficiency and a lower requirement for interfering RNA concentrations, leading to more effective gene knockdown with minimal nonspecific effects. It is a simple, rapid protocol for consistent and reproducible results, and is suitable for delivering molecules across a diverse range of commonly used cell lines. For cell types not amenable to lipid-mediated transfection, adenoviral vector-mediated shRNA transfer is highly recommended secondary to its broad host range and ability to infect proliferating and quiescent cells. Additionally, adenoviral genomes do not integrate into the host cell chromosomes, making them safe vectors in respect to the mutagenesis potential for mediating transient gene expression silencing.

Determination of siRNA knockdown effects on gene expression in cells

It is critical to select the most effective siRNAs to four or more respective complementary siRNA target sites, along with proper dose titration, for adequate gene silencing. To screen the effect of the chosen siRNAs and delivery or expression methods, it is recommended to choose a cell line derived from the same species as the selected siRNA sequence(s). When the same species cell line with high transduction efficiency is available, the lipid-mediated siRNA transfection should be conducted to determine which siRNA has the optimal knockdown effect on gene expression prior to initiating construction of shRNA-encoding plasmid and adenoviral vectors. Several lipid-based reagents are commercially available, including Lipofectamine 2000 from Invitrogen, RNAiFect and HiPerfect from QIAGEN, Dharma*FECT* from Dharmacon, siIMPORTER from Upstate, and siLentFect from Bio-Rad. The following procedure is for Lipofectamine 2000-mediated siRNA transfection into adherent mammalian cells.

1. Set up the cells being treated with increasing concentrations of each siRNA at 0, 25, 50, 100, or 200 nm in triplicate for 48–72 hours.
2. Prepare the synthetic siRNA oligonucleotides (sense and antisense) in the RNase-free annealing buffer to obtain 20 μM of the final concentration for each oligonucleotide.
3. Anneal the oligonucleotide solution at 95°C for 4 minutes, followed by room temperature for 20 minutes.
4. The annealed siRNA solution can be stored at −20°C for future use.
5. Plate cells with the growth medium without antibiotics in six-well plates for 24 hours before transfection. The cells should be 40–50% confluent at the time of transfection, which is lower than

standard transfection experiments where cells are plated at 50–70% confluence.
6. Replace the growth medium with serum-free and antibiotics-free medium immediately before the next step.
7. Prepare the following mixture:
In tube A: add 10 μL of siRNA oligonucleotide solution (20 μM stock) into 175 μL of serum-free and antibiotics-free medium, mix gently. If the siRNA oligonucleotide solution is less than 10 μL, adjust its final volume to 10 μL with the annealing buffer.
In tube B: add 4 μL of Lipofectamine 2000 into 11 μL of serum-free and antibiotics-free medium, mix gently.
8. Add the mixture of tube B dropwise into tube A, mix gently two or three times. Incubate for 20 minutes at room temperature (the solution may appear cloudy).
9. After 20 minutes of incubation at room temperature, add 600 μL of serum-free and antibiotics-free medium into the mixture, mix gently –two or three times.
10. Aspirate serum-free and antibiotics-free medium from the culture plates.
11. Add the mixture dropwise onto the cells (800 μL/well).
12. Incubate the cells for 4 hours at 37°C in a 5% CO_2 incubator, stir plates gently once per hour.
13. Add 1.6 mL of growth medium per well containing 1.5× the normal concentration of serum without removing the transfection mixture.
14. Isolate RNA at 48 hours after transfection to demonstrate reduction of gene expression at the RNA level by real-time RT-PCR.
15. Or isolate protein at 72 hours after transfection to determine the level of protein knockdown by quantitative western blotting.

Construction of plasmid vector-based siRNA

An intrinsic limitation of synthetic siRNAs for RNAi in mammalian cells is the transient nature of siRNA. To address this issue, the plasmid vector-based system has been developed to facilitate expression of shRNA in mammalian cells. This involves a small DNA insert (about 50–70 bp) encoding a short hairpin RNA targeting the gene of interest cloned into a plasmid vector. In this expression cassette, the U6 promoter, an RNA polymerase III-dependent promoter [23], facilitates high-level, constitutive expression of the shRNA of interest in mammalian cells along with a polymerase III (Pol III) terminator for efficient transcription termination of the shRNA molecule. The resulting plasmid construct can be introduced by lipofactamine into dividing mammalian cells for transient expression of the shRNA of interest and initial RNAi screening. Expression of this RNAi cassette forms a shRNA molecule within the cell that will be processed and act as short interfering RNA (siRNA), thus generating the RNA interference effect. Once initial screening of the effect is complete, this U6 expression cassette can be easily and efficiently transferred into a plasmid for construction of an adenoviral-based shRNA vector. The following procedure is for generation of the U6 entry clone.

1. Follow the guidelines to design and synthesize two complementary DNA oligonucleotides encoding the shRNA of interest.
2. Prepare both the DNA oligonucleotides in the DNase/RNase-free annealing buffer to obtain 50 μM of the final concentration for each oligonucleotide.
3. Anneal the oligonucleotide solution at 95°C for 4 minutes, followed by room temperature for 20 minutes to create a double-stranded DNA oligonucleotide.
4. Dilute the double-stranded DNA oligonucleotide mixture to obtain 5 nM of the final concentration.
5. Clone the double-stranded DNA oligonucleotide into the pENTR/U6 vector by T4 DNA ligase.
6. Transfer the resulting ligation reaction into the competent E. coli and select for kanamycin-resistant transformants.
7. Perform lipofectamine-mediated transfer with the resulting pENTR/U6-shRNA entry construct into mammalian cells for transient RNAi analysis.
8. After initial shRNA screening, use the pENTR/U6-shRNA entry construct and pAd/BLOCK-iT-DEST for recombination reaction to create an adenoviral expression DNA clone.

Alternatively, oligonucleotides encoding the shRNA of interest are annealed and ligated via BamHI/EcoRI into pSIREN vector using Knockout RNAi Systems technology (Clontech, Mountain View, CA). The recombinant pSIREN is then transformed into E. coli. The resulting pSIREN construct is transfected into the cell line by lipofectamine 2000 in order to identify suppressing effects. After screening in the cells, the promising pSIREN construct is cut out with PI-SceI/I-CeuI and inserted into Adeno-X Viral DNA via PI-SceI/I-CeuI using Adeno-X Expression System 1 (Clontech). The resulting adenoviral vector is transfected into HEK293 cells and propagated, thereby generating the Ad-shRNA vector.

Construction of adenoviral vector-based siRNA

Adenoviral vector-mediated RNAi transduction in cell lines, particularly within primary human and cancer cell lines, can lead to an efficient, sequence-specific, prolonged reduction of the corresponding target mRNA. The result is a reduction of the target encoded protein level up to 7–10 days after transduction [1,24,25]. To accurately determine the efficacy of knockdown mediated by an RNAi vector, it is critical to ensure adequate transfer of the RNAi vector to as many cells in culture or organs in vivo as possible; otherwise, when measuring knockdown by quantitative real-time PCR or western immunoblot, the background mRNA or protein in nontransfected cells will interfere with the appraisal of gene knockdown in virally transduced cells; thus, knockdown could appear less effective than it actually is. Among the RNAi viral vector systems, adenoviral shRNA vectors with the aforementioned higher titer abilities can facilitate this higher efficiency of shRNA transfection within the cell cultures or organ systems of interest [10].

Adenoviral vectors are capable of transfecting the majority of human and many animal cell types. They are not dependent on active host cell division. As adenoviral vectors possess two highly desired features, that is high efficiency of construct delivery and high level of gene expression, adenoviral vectors are considered to be an outstanding vector for overexpressing siRNAs in a broad range of mammalian cells. Of note, it is preferred for RNAi in difficult-to-transfect cells. The following itemizes the protocol necessary for production of an adenoviral expression DNA clone.

1. Digest the adenoviral expression DNA plasmid with PacI to expose its inverted terminal repeats (ITRs).

2. Use lipofactamine 2000 to transfer the resulting plasmid into HEK293 cells.

3. Harvest adenovirus-containing cells when approximately 80% of cytopathic effect is observed (typically 10–12 days post-transfection).

4. Use the crude viral stock to amplify adenoviral shRNA vectors in HEK293 cells, and then purify and titrate adenoviral shRNA vectors with the standard procedures.

5. Transduce adenoviral shRNA vectors into the selected mammalian cell line to express the shRNA of interest and perform RNAi analysis before initiating RNAi experiments in the heart *in vivo*.

To investigate the biological effects of adenoviral shRNA vectors *in vitro*, the primary neonatal cardiomyocyte culture is a well-proven model because of the known fragility and instability in adult cardiomyocyte culture. The primary neonatal cardiomyocytes can be prepared from ventricular tissue of 1- to 3-day-old rat or mouse pups. Adenoviral shRNA vectors will be diluted in serum-free culture media to the desired concentration. The cells are precultured in six-well Nunc culture plates and are expected to be 70–80% of confluence after 24 hours of incubation. Then, the cells are rinsed once with serum-free culture media and incubated with adenoviral shRNA vectors for 1 hour. The necessary volume of complete culture medium is then added and cells are incubated for the desired time periods for *in vitro* studies.

Prior to use or construction of adenoviral vector-based shRNA, it is strongly recommended that the user should become thoroughly familiar with the safety considerations concerning the production and handling of adenovirus. Although the recombinant adenovirus type 5 (Ad5) used for shRNA is replication-defective and therefore incapable of establishing a productive viral infection in any animal or human, it is classified as a Class 2 agent and therefore must be handled as such in compliance with NIH Guidelines for Research Involving Recombinant DNA Molecules, October 2011 (available at http://oba.od.nih.gov/rdna/nih_guidelines_oba.html). For a description of laboratory biosafety level criteria, consult the Centers for Disease Control and Prevention web site at http://www.cdc.gov/biosafety/publications/bmbl5/index.htm.

Transfer of adenoviral vector-based shRNA into the heart

Modulation of genes within the heart using the adenoviral-mediated RNAi approach can be conducted by direct intramyocardial injection of adenoviral-shRNA vectors, most notably into the ischemic risk region of the left ventricle (LV). The murine model of intramyocardial injection with adenoviral vectors has been described previously [26,27]. After the anesthetized mouse's chest is opened via central thoracotomy, the mouse receives intramyocardial injections in the anterior LV wall with adenoviral RNA control vector or adenoviral shRNA vector. The intramyocardial injection is 10–20 μL in volume and performed with a 50-μL syringe with a 30-gauge needle; each mouse heart receives two injections in the soon-to-be-ischemic region of the LV. Two days later, the mice undergo an infarct protocol with a 30-minute coronary occlusion followed by 24 hours reperfusion. The cardiac regions transfected with adenoviral shRNA vectors are harvested at the designated time points to isolate RNA or protein for further determination of RNAi effects.

In the permanent infarction model, myocardial infarction is induced by surgical ligation of the left anterior descending (LAD) coronary artery, as described [26,27]. Immediately after permanent ligation, the mouse heart receives intramyocardial injections with adenoviral RNA control vector or adenoviral shRNA vector. A total of four injections (10 μL each) are administrated in the peri-infarct region in a circular pattern, at the border between infarcted and noninfarcted myocardium. The dose of adenoviral shRNA vectors injected may be up to 1×10^{10} viral particles via this route; injection of a higher volume of adenoviral vectors would not be feasible in the small mouse heart [28,29].

In the rat model of heart failure induced by the transaortic banding procedure, the aortic root is exposed and then a tantalum clip with an internal diameter of 0.58 mm is placed on the ascending aorta. After aortic-banded, it is necessary to wait about 3–4 months for rats to develop LV dilatation and a decrease in ejection fraction by 25% before cardiac gene transfer. An intracoronary administration is conducted to deliver adenoviral vectors into the heart. Briefly, a 22-gauge catheter is advanced from LV apex to the aortic root. The aorta and main pulmonary artery are cross-clamped for 30 seconds, during which time the rat heart receives an intracoronary infusion of adenoviral vectors ($\sim 3 - 5 \times 10^{10}$ pfu/200 μL). After a clamp time of 30 seconds, aortic flow is restored. Effects of cardiac-targeted RNA interference for heart failure is evaluated 1 month after gene delivery [28,30,31].

Because the adenoviral vector is replication-incompetent and does not integrate into the host genome, the adenoviral-mediated shRNA of interest will be expressed only as long as the viral genome is present within transduced cells. In actively dividing cells, the adenoviral genome is gradually diluted as cell division occurs. This results in an overall decrease in shRNA expression over time as evidenced by the observation that the target protein level generally returns to background level within 14 days after transduction. In nondividing cells or animal tissues, adenoviral-mediated shRNA expression is generally more stable and can persist for longer periods of time following transfection. If this is the first time transfection and RNAi has been attempted with adenoviral shRNA construct into the heart *in vivo*, it is highly recommended to perform a time-course experiment to determine the conditions for optimal target gene knockdown.

Weaknesses and strengths of the method

The RNAi targeting system controlling gene silencing in all living cells has contributed to a major advance in methodology for functional genomics. The strengths of the RNAi approach include identifying novel molecular targets, conducting functional studies in a gene-specific manner, creating model systems in cells *in vitro* and in animals *in vivo*, and developing novel therapeutic strategies to intercede with multiple disease-related genes [29,32,33]. It is costly and time consuming to develop conventional knockout mice due to homologous recombination-based gene targeting (knockout), embryonic stem cell manipulation, and animal breeding. However, by using viral vectors as delivery tools for shRNA, it is possible to generate *knockdown* animals in a few weeks rather than a few years. When conventional knockout is difficult, time consuming, or practically impossible in larger animals, the RNAi approach may greatly facilitate the generation of some specific disease models [33]. Additionally, developmental

effects are very significant in some knockout mice, which can generate poor animal models not suitable for use in physiological studies. This limitation may be overcome by the RNAi approach as this enables knockdown of a specific protein in adult animals that have developed normally [33,34].

The challenges should be acknowledged in using the RNAi approach in animals *in vivo* – in particular, how to deliver siRNA into the target cells [35]. Furthermore, adverse immune responses [36] and fatality in mice due to oversaturation of the cellular RNAi pathways [37,38] have been reported, demonstrating the necessity for optimization of therapeutic gene-silencing technologies. The "off-targeting" of siRNA also has some undesired effects, which are becoming concerns [39]. Thus, appropriate controls are critical for siRNA studies.

Alternative approaches

The application of single RNAi molecule knockdown strategies has presented great potential for use as a research tool and as a therapeutic approach for treatment of various diseases, including cancer [40] and neurodegenerative disorders [41]. The fact that natural miRNA hairpins have been found in clusters of multiple identical or different copies implies that multiple genes may be regulated together by encoding multiple shRNAs in a single transcript [42]. Thus, the combinatorial RNAi (co-RNAi) process may serve as an alternative approach to offer considerable advantages over the use of RNAi monotherapies by targeting multiple genes and by enhancing the levels of gene knockdown [43–45].

An additional alternative is to combine both RNAi and U1 inhibition (U1i) [38]. U1i is a novel post-transcriptional gene-silencing technique which inhibits polyadenylation and maturation of pre-mRNAs. As the actions of RNAi and U1i have distinct mechanisms in different cellular compartments, the combination of RNAi and U1i allows usage of minimal doses, thereby avoiding RNAi toxicity and weakness due to oversaturation of the cellular RNAi pathways [46,47].

Although the application of RNAi *in vivo* has been successfully demonstrated and clinical trials using RNAi-based therapeutics have been initiated, safety and delivery of RNAi still remain critical issues [48]. Among all viral vectors, the recombinant adenoassociated viral vector (rAAV) system has been accepted as the most promising viral vector for clinical gene therapy because of its capacities to express functional genes steadily in a relatively longer period (such as 1 year) and to specifically integrate into chromosome 19 of its host cell without inducing pathogenic and immunogenic reactions in the host [49–53]. rAAV is considered a safe vector as its viral vector backbone is devoid of all viral genes except the ITR sequences [50]. Additionally, rAAV vectors have great versatility and tissue-specific delivery potential through the availability of multiple serotypes (from rAAV1 to rAAV9), which can be further expanded by pseudotyping and capsid modification as desired [54]. Thus, the rAAV system can be predicted as a most promising alternative for shRNA delivery *in vivo*. To date, several independent studies on the use of rAAV vectors for shRNA expression in cells and in animals have been reported [34,53,55–57], demonstrating that rAAV is an ideal vector system for RNAi-based mechanism studies and gene therapy.

Conclusions

The discovery of the RNA interference phenomenon in controlling gene expression has markedly aided and advanced our understanding of gene regulation and function in the past decade. The potent, specific gene silencing effect of short interfering RNA sequences promises enormous potential in future studies of gene function and may help to revolutionize the treatment of disease. Recent progress in adenoviral vector-based RNAi offers the advantage of a broad host range and high gene transfer efficiency. Various primary cell types, which are most relevant for disease-related assays, along with organs *in vivo*, are able to be transfected, with subsequent molecular, functional, and phenotypic investigation. To date, targeted delivery is the most significant obstacle for the therapeutic use of siRNAs. If overcome, the impact on our understanding, and eventually therapeutic use, of siRNAs within cardiovascular diseases would be revolutionary.

Acknowledgement
The author thanks Drs. Roberto Bolli and Hossein Ardehali for critical review and advice.

References

1 Uchida H, Tanaka T, Sasaki K, Kato K, Dehari H, Ito Y, *et al*. Adenovirus-mediated transfer of siRNA against survivin induced apoptosis and attenuated tumor cell growth *in vitro* and *in vivo*. *Mol Ther* 2004; **10**: 162–171.

2 Moazed D. Small RNAs in transcriptional gene silencing and genome defence. *Nature* 2009; **457**: 413–420.

3 Hannon GJ, Rossi JJ. Unlocking the potential of the human genome with RNA interference. *Nature* 2004; **431**: 371–378.

4 Siomi H, Siomi MC. On the road to reading the RNA-interference code. *Nature* 2009; **457**: 396–404.

5 Inoue A, Sawata SY, Taira K. Molecular design and delivery of siRNA. *J Drug Target* 2006; **14**: 448–455.

6 Poller W, Hajjar R, Schultheiss HP, Fechner H. Cardiac-targeted delivery of regulatory RNA molecules and genes for the treatment of heart failure. *Cardiovasc Res* 2010; **86**: 353–364.

7 Gurlevik E, Woller N, Schache P, Malek NP, Wirth TC, Zender L, *et al*. P53-dependent antiviral RNA-interference facilitates tumor-selective viral replication. *Nucleic Acids Res* 2009; **37**: e84.

8 Ruvkun G. The perfect storm of tiny RNAs. *Nat Med* 2008; **14**: 1041–1045.

9 Taxman DJ, Livingstone LR, Zhang J, Conti BJ, Iocca HA, Williams KL, *et al*. Criteria for effective design, construction, and gene knockdown by shRNA vectors. *BMC Biotechnol* 2006; **6**: 7.

10 Grimm D, Kay MA. RNAi and gene therapy: A mutual attraction. *Hematology Am Soc Hematol Educ Program* 2007; **473–481**.

11 Mizuguchi H, Funakoshi N, Hosono T, Sakurai F, Kawabata K, Yamaguchi T, *et al*. Rapid construction of small interfering RNA-expressing adenoviral vectors on the basis of direct cloning of short hairpin RNA-coding dnas. *Hum Gene Ther* 2007; **18**: 74–80.

12 Hosono T, Mizuguchi H, Katayama K, Koizumi N, Kawabata K, Yamaguchi T, *et al*. RNA interference of ppargamma using fiber-modified adenovirus vector efficiently suppresses preadipocyte-to-adipocyte differentiation in 3T3-L1 cells. *Gene* 2005; **348**: 157–165.

13 Barquinero J, Eixarch H, Perez-Melgosa M. Retroviral vectors: New applications for an old tool. *Gene Ther* 2004; **11** (**Suppl 1**): S3–9.

14 Wadhwa R, Kaul SC, Miyagishi M, Taira K. Vectors for RNA interference. *Curr Opin Mol Ther* 2004; **6**: 367–372.

15 Wadhwa R, Kaul SC, Miyagishi M, Taira K. Know-how of RNA interference and its applications in research and therapy. *Mutat Res* 2004; **567**: 71–84.

16 Castanotto D, Rossi JJ. The promises and pitfalls of RNA-interference-based therapeutics. *Nature* 2009; **457**: 426–433.

17 Soutschek J, Akinc A, Bramlage B, Charisse K, Constien R, Donoghue M, *et al.* Therapeutic silencing of an endogenous gene by systemic administration of modified siRNAs. *Nature* 2004; **432**: 173–178.

18 Aubart FC, Sassi Y, Coulombe A, Mougenot N, Vrignaud C, Leprince P, *et al.* RNA interference targeting STIM1 suppresses vascular smooth muscle cell proliferation and neointima formation in the rat. *Mol Ther* 2009; **17**: 455–462.

19 Infanger DW, Cao X, Butler SD, Burmeister MA, Zhou Y, Stupinski JA, *et al.* Silencing Nox4 in the paraventricular nucleus improves myocardial infarction-induced cardiac dysfunction by attenuating sympathoexcitation and periinfarct apoptosis. *Circ Res* 2010; **106**: 1763–1774.

20 Campochiaro PA. Potential applications for RNAi to probe pathogenesis and develop new treatments for ocular disorders. *Gene Ther* 2006; **13**: 559–562.

21 Shen J, Samul R, Silva RL, Akiyama H, Liu H, Saishin Y, *et al.* Suppression of ocular neovascularization with siRNA targeting VEGF receptor 1. *Gene Ther* 2006; **13**: 225–234.

22 Lee YJ, Imsumran A, Park MY, Kwon SY, Yoon HI, Lee JH, *et al.* Adenovirus expressing shRNA to IGF-1R enhances the chemosensitivity of lung cancer cell lines by blocking IGF-1 pathway. *Lung Cancer* 2007; **55**: 279–286.

23 Hosono T, Mizuguchi H, Katayama K, Xu ZL, Sakurai F, Ishii-Watabe A, *et al.* Adenovirus vector-mediated doxycycline-inducible RNA interference. *Hum Gene Ther* 2004; **15**: 813–819.

24 Bain JR, Schisler JC, Takeuchi K, Newgard CB, Becker TC. An adenovirus vector for efficient RNA interference-mediated suppression of target genes in insulinoma cells and pancreatic islets of Langerhans. *Diabetes* 2004; **53**: 2190–2194.

25 Marzban L, Tomas A, Becker TC, Rosenberg L, Oberholzer J, Fraser PE, *et al.* Small interfering RNA-mediated suppression of proislet amyloid polypeptide expression inhibits islet amyloid formation and enhances survival of human islets in culture. *Diabetes* 2008; **57**: 3045–3055.

26 Li Q, Guo Y, Tan W, Ou Q, Wu WJ, Sturza D, *et al.* Cardioprotection afforded by inducible nitric oxide synthase gene therapy is mediated by cyclooxygenase-2 via a nuclear factor-kappab dependent pathway. *Circulation* 2007; **116**: 1577–1584.

27 Li Q, Guo Y, Ou Q, Cui C, Wu WJ, Tan W, *et al.* Gene transfer of inducible nitric oxide synthase affords cardioprotection by upregulating heme oxygenase-1 via

a nuclear factor-κb dependent pathway. *Circulation* 2009; **120**: 1222–1230.

28 Li Q, Guo Y, Ou Q, Chen N, Wu WJ, Yuan F, *et al.* Intracoronary administration of cardiac stem cells in mice: A new, improved technique for cell therapy in murine models. *Basic Res Cardiol* 2011; **106**: 849–864.

29 Li L, Haider H, Wang L, Lu G, Ashraf M. Adenoviral short hairpin RNA therapy targeting phosphodiesterase 5a relieves cardiac remodeling and dysfunction following myocardial infarction. *Am J Physiol Heart Circ Physiol* 2012; **302**: H2112–2121.

30 Suckau L, Fechner H, Chemaly E, Krohn S, Hadri L, Kockskamper J, *et al.* Long-term cardiac-targeted RNA interference for the treatment of heart failure restores cardiac function and reduces pathological hypertrophy. *Circulation* 2009; **119**: 1241–1252.

31 Sakata S, Liang L, Sakata N, Sakata Y, Chemaly ER, Lebeche D, *et al.* Preservation of mechanical and energetic function after adenoviral gene transfer in normal rat hearts. *Clin Exp Pharmacol Physiol* 2007; **34**: 1300–1306.

32 Eekels JJ, Sagnier S, Geerts D, Jeeninga RE, Biard-Piechaczyk M, Berkhout B. Inhibition of HIV-1 replication with stable RNAi-mediated knockdown of autophagy factors. *Virol J* 2012; **9**: 69.

33 Soustek MS, Falk DJ, Mah CS, Toth MJ, Schlame M, Lewin AS, *et al.* Characterization of a transgenic short hairpin RNA-induced murine model of tafazzin deficiency. *Hum Gene Ther* 2011; **22**: 865–871.

34 Cunningham SC, Kok CY, Dane AP, Carpenter K, Kizana E, Kuchel PW, *et al.* Induction and prevention of severe hyperammonemia in the spfash mouse model of ornithine transcarbamylase deficiency using shRNA and rAAV-mediated gene delivery. *Mol Ther* 2011; **19**: 854–859.

35 Oliveira S, Storm G, Schiffelers RM. Targeted delivery of siRNA. *J Biomed Biotechnol* 2006; **2006**: 63675.

36 Judge A, MacLachlan I. Overcoming the innate immune response to small interfering RNA. *Hum Gene Ther* 2008; **19**: 111–124.

37 Grimm D, Streetz KL, Jopling CL, Storm TA, Pandey K, Davis CR, *et al.* Fatality in mice due to oversaturation of cellular microRNA/short hairpin RNA pathways. *Nature* 2006; **441**: 537–541.

38 Koornneef A, van Logtenstein R, Timmermans E, Pisas L, Blits B, Abad X, *et al.* AAV-mediated *in vivo* knockdown of luciferase using combinatorial RNAi and U1i. *Gene Ther* 2011; **18**: 929–935.

39 Fedorov Y, Anderson EM, Birmingham A, Reynolds A, Karpilow J, Robinson K, *et al.* Off-target effects by siRNA can induce toxic phenotype. *RNA* 2006; **12**: 1188–1196.

40 Davis ME, Zuckerman JE, Choi CH, Seligson D, Tolcher A, Alabi CA, *et al*. Evidence of RNAi in humans from systemically administered siRNA via targeted nanoparticles. *Nature* 2010; **464**: 1067–1070.

41 Prakash S, Malhotra M, Rengaswamy V. Nonviral siRNA delivery for gene silencing in neurodegenerative diseases. *Methods Mol Biol* 2010; **623**: 211–229.

42 Kesireddy V, van der Ven PF, Furst DO. Multipurpose modular lentiviral vectors for RNA interference and transgene expression. *Mol Biol Rep* 2010; **37**: 2863–2870.

43 Liu YP, von Eije KJ, Schopman NC, Westerink JT, ter Brake O, Haasnoot J, *et al*. Combinatorial RNAi against HIV-1 using extended short hairpin RNAs. *Mol Ther* 2009; **17**: 1712–1723.

44 Grimm D. All for one, one for all: New combinatorial RNAi therapies combat hepatitis c virus evolution. *Mol Ther* 2012; **20**: 1661–1663.

45 Jahan S, Khaliq S, Samreen B, Ijaz B, Khan M, Ahmad W, *et al*. Effect of combined siRNA of HCV e2 gene and HCV receptors against HCV. *Virol J* 2011; **8**: 295.

46 Abad X, Razquin N, Abad A, Fortes P. Combination of RNA interference and U1 inhibition leads to increased inhibition of gene expression. *Nucleic Acids Res* 2010; **38**: e136.

47 Grimm D. The dose can make the poison: Lessons learned from adverse *in vivo* toxicities caused by RNAi overexpression. *Silence* 2011; **2**: 8.

48 Tiemann K, Rossi JJ. RNAi-based therapeutics-current status, challenges and prospects. *EMBO Mol Med* 2009; **1**: 142–151.

49 Henckaerts E, Linden RM. Adeno-associated virus: A key to the human genome? *Future Virol* 2010; **5**: 555–574.

50 Daya S, Berns KI. Gene therapy using adeno-associated virus vectors. *Clin Microbiol Rev* 2008; **21**: 583–593.

51 Li Q, Guo Y, Wu WJ, Ou Q, Zhu X, Tan W, *et al*. Gene transfer as a strategy to achieve permanent cardioprotection i: rAAV-mediated gene therapy with inducible nitric oxide synthase limits infarct size 1 year later without adverse functional consequences. *Basic Res Cardiol* 2011; **106**: 1355–1366.

52 Li Q, Guo Y, Ou Q, Wu WJ, Chen N, Zhu X, *et al*. Gene transfer as a strategy to achieve permanent cardioprotection ii: rAAV-mediated gene therapy with heme oxygenase-1 limits infarct size 1 year later without adverse functional consequences. *Basic Res Cardiol* 2011; **106**: 1367–1377.

53 McCown TJ. Adeno-associated virus (AAV) vectors in the CNS. *Curr Gene Ther* 2011; **11**: 181–188.

54 Pulicherla N, Shen S, Yadav S, Debbink K, Govindasamy L, Agbandje-McKenna M, *et al*. Engineering liver-detargeted AAV9 vectors for cardiac and musculoskeletal gene transfer. *Mol Ther* 2011; **19**: 1070–1078.

55 Han Y, Khodr CE, Sapru MK, Pedapati J, Bohn MC. A microRNA embedded AAV alpha-synuclein gene silencing vector for dopaminergic neurons. *Brain Res* 2011; **1386**: 15–24.

56 Koornneef A, Maczuga P, van Logtenstein R, Borel F, Blits B, Ritsema T, *et al*. Apolipoprotein b knockdown by AAV-delivered shRNA lowers plasma cholesterol in mice. *Mol Ther* 2011; **19**: 731–740.

57 Mayra A, Tomimitsu H, Kubodera T, Kobayashi M, Piao W, Sunaga F, *et al*. Intraperitoneal AAV9-shRNA inhibits target expression in neonatal skeletal and cardiac muscles. *Biochem Biophys Res Commun* 2011; **405**: 204–209.

Overexpression and downregulation of proteins *in vitro*

Marina Bayeva and Hossein Ardehali

Northwestern University Feinberg School of Medicine, Chicago, IL, USA

Introduction

Studying cardiac function in an *in vitro* system offers several advantages over the use of animal models, including relatively quick generation of data and the ability to conduct mechanistic studies. Despite losing several aspects of normal heart physiology, established cardiac cell lines such as H9c2 or HL-1 are commonly used in cardiovascular research due to their ease of culturing and commercial availability. Primary cardiomyocytes from neonatal or adult hearts provide a highly physiological system for the *in vitro* study of molecular signaling, calcium handling, contractility, and cellular mechanics in the heart. However, due to their short lifespan in culture, primary cardiomyocytes need to be freshly isolated prior to the experiments. The ability to modulate protein expression *in vitro* is a powerful tool which, unfortunately, is limited by the primary cardiomyocyte's resistance to the delivery of genetic material, such as DNA-based plasmids and synthetic small interfering RNAs (siRNA) [1,2].

Generally, the delivery of genetic material for overexpression and downregulation of proteins is achieved by **transfection**, when "naked" DNA or RNA is introduced into the cell, or through a virally mediated **transduction** with or without incorporation into the host's genome [3]. Adenoviruses and lentiviruses have been long employed to overexpress and downregulate proteins in cardiomyocytes with high efficiencies of gene delivery and relatively low toxicity [4,5].

The established cardiac cell lines are also susceptible to transfection and the standard protocols supplied by manufacturers can often be used successfully with very little optimization. On the contrary, primary cardiomyocytes are traditionally considered poor candidates for nonviral nucleotide delivery due to low transfection efficiencies. However, newer liposome-based reagents and optimization of protocols for electroporation have made the transfection approach much more popular among researchers in the cardiovascular field [3,6], although at times a virally based method may still be preferred to achieve satisfactory degree of protein overexpression or downregulation. This chapter discusses several tested protocols for transfection and transduction of established and primary cardiac cell lines, with a particular focus on protocols tested and successfully utilized in the primary cardiomyocytes. The summary of the techniques used to modulate protein expression *in vitro* is given in Figure 47.1.

Transfection is a relatively easy, inexpensive, and nontoxic method of gene delivery to the cell which, unlike the viral transduction, is less likely to disrupt cellular physiology and/or illicit immune response. The downsides of this method include low efficiency in primary cardiomyocytes and transient expression of the plasmid or siRNA construct [2]. **Lipofection**, or liposomal reagent-based transfection, exploits the ability of positively charged lipids to bind to anionic DNA/RNA and fuse with cellular membranes for the delivery of genetic material into the cell [7]. A broad

Manual of Research Techniques in Cardiovascular Medicine, First Edition. Edited by Hossein Ardehali, Roberto Bolli, and Douglas W. Losordo.

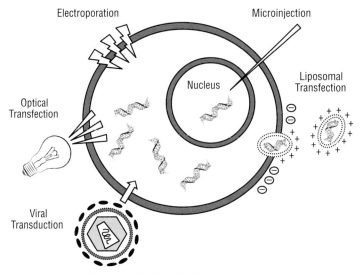

Figure 47.1 Methods for overexpression and downregulation of proteins *in vitro*.

range of liposomal reagents is commercially available; however, Lipofectamine 2000 (Invitrogen) remains the agent of choice for the transfection of cardiomyocytes and will be discussed in detail. Recently, chemically modified siRNA molecules, such as Dharmacon® Accell® siRNA (Thermo Scientific) have been shown to effectively reduce protein levels in cardiomyocytes without the use of transfection reagent [8]. Plasmid or siRNA delivery by **electroporation** is achieved through administration of brief electric impulses that permeabilize cellular membranes and allow for genetic material to pass through. A protocol combining electroporation and use of chemical solutions that stabilize cells in the electric field, termed **nucleofection**, was optimized for transfection of cardiomyocytes to increase nucleic acid delivery efficiency while minimizing cell death. Several companies have developed and tested nucleofection protocols for use with primary cardiomyocytes, with Amaxa® Rat Cardiomyocyte – Neonatal Nucleofector® Kit showing a promising 37% transfection efficiency with 60% cell viability [6]. The protocol for Amaxa nucleofection will be outlined. **Optical transfection** that uses focused laser light of a standard confocal microscope to create transient holes in membranes for DNA/RNA entry [9] allows for targeted transfection of cardiomyocytes in a heterogeneous culture [10]. Finally, microinjection technique can also be

used to deliver genetic material directly into the cell. However, low transfection efficiencies and technical challenges preclude the last two methods from being widely used and therefore they will not be discussed in detail. The reader is referred to the works by Nikolskaya *et al.* (2006) [10] for more information on optical transfection and to Bartoli *et al.* (1997) [11] for optimization of microinjection protocols.

The advantages of virally based transduction include fast, efficient, and stable transfer of genetic material without the need for cellular replication or high metabolic activity. Thus, viruses have traditionally been used for protein overexpression and downregulation in primary cardiac myocytes and other terminally differentiated, hard-to-transfect cells [12,13]. Some of the disadvantages include the lengthy and labor-intensive preparation of viral particles, and evidence of alteration of cellular physiology in response to viral infection [14]. Two classes of viruses are commonly used for targeted delivery of genetic material into cardiomyocytes. **Adenoviruses**, which can hold up to 35 kb of linear double-stranded DNA [15], are characterized by high infectivity with transduction efficiencies reaching 100% [13]. These viruses are particularly suitable for transient (up to 2 weeks) overexpression of proteins and therefore are ideal for many *in vitro* applications. It is important to note that adenoviruses are known to elicit immune response and therefore an empty vector must always be used for the control experiments. **Lentiviruses** are the RNA-based viruses that can infect nonreplicating cells and incorporate the transgene into the host genome [16], allowing for generation of stable cell lines. These viruses can accommodate up to 18 kb of genetic material [17], making them suitable for overexpression of certain proteins. Moreover, lentiviruses are extensively used for protein downregulation by delivering short hairpin RNAs and ensuring very high knockdown efficiency. Importantly, lentiviruses do not elicit inflammatory responses and are not associated with significant toxicity [15].

In summary, both transfection and transduction methods have been used in the established and primary cardiomyocyte cultures for modulation of protein expression. Several techniques validated for use in cardiomyocytes are summarized below, and a brief discussion of potential limitations and challenges is provided for each protocol.

Protocols

Lipofection

General considerations

A variety of liposome-based reagents have been developed and tested in cardiomyocytes, including FuGENE 6 (Roche, Germany), Lipofectamine PLUS (Invitrogen, USA), Lipofectamine 2000 (Invitrogen, USA), Metafectene (Biontex, Germany), GenePORTER (Gene Therapy Solutions, CA), and LipoGen (InvivoGen, CA). Most of the commercially available kits can be used with established cardiac cell lines and the manufacturers' protocols should be consulted to optimize the transfection efficiency. The two most suitable formulations for use in primary cardiomyocytes were shown to be FuGENE and Lipofectamine 2000 [2]. To date, Lipofectamine 2000 remains the reagent of choice for the transfection of cardiac cells, and is used extensively both for plasmid-based overexpression and siRNA-mediated knockdown of proteins. While protocols for the transfection of cardiomyocytes with Lipofectamine 2000 vary greatly between different studies, several factors were shown to be important for the successful delivery of nucleic acids. First, the optimal mass ratio of DNA to Lipofectamine 2000

was found to be around $1:2$ to $1:3$, but additional studies may be required to optimize this ratio for a given cell type and nucleic acid construct. The most suitable dilution of Lipofectamine 2000 is $1:25$ to $1:50$ and should be performed immediately before use. The optimal time for complex formation between Lipofectamine 2000 and nucleic acids is about 30 minutes of incubation, although the complexes were found to be stable for 2–6 hours after mixing. Finally, transfection of primary cardiomyocytes should be carried out 24–72 hours following isolation [18]. The viability of primary cardiac myocytes declines as a function of time, and significant toxicity can be observed in cells cultured for over 72 hours.

Protocol

Plasmid-based protein overexpression with Lipofectamine 2000 (24-well format)

1. Plate cardiomyocytes in complete growth medium 24–48 hours prior to transfection. One day before the transfection, remove medium and replace it with complete antibiotic-free medium to minimize toxicity of transfection.

2. Dilute 0.8 µg of DNA in 50 µL of Opti-MEM I (Invitrogen, USA) or another appropriate low or serum-free medium per well of a 24-well plate. Mix gently by pipetting up and down.

3. Dilute 2 µL of Lipofectamine 2000 in 50 µL of Opti-MEM I (or other low or serum-free medium). Mix by pipetting and incubate at room temperature for 5 minutes.

4. Mix diluted DNA with diluted Lipofectamine 2000 and incubate at room temperature for 20–30 minutes for the DNA-liposome complexes to form. The solution may appear cloudy, which will not affect the transfection efficiency.

5. Wash plated cells once with PBS and add 100 µL of the transfection mix to each well.

6. Incubate the cells at 37°C in 5% CO_2 for 4–6 hours for the gene transfer to occur, after which serum-containing, antibiotic-free medium may be added to each well. The removal of transfection complexes from cells is optional and will not affect the transfection efficiency.

7. Assess the expression of the gene of interest 24–48 hours later by quantitative RT-PCR, western blotting, or fluorescent microscopy if the protein is fluorescently tagged.

siRNA-based protein knockdown with Lipofectamine 2000 (24-well format)

1. Plate cardiomyocytes in complete growth medium 24–48 hours prior to transfection. One day before transfection, remove the medium and replace it with complete medium without antibiotic to minimize toxicity.

2. The amount of siRNA used for efficient knockdown varies, and the manufacturer's recommendations should be considered. Generally, 20 pmol of siRNA per 1 μL of Lipofectamine 2000 should be used. A single siRNA or a pool of several siRNAs can be used to knock down the gene of interest, while a scrambled siRNA should be used in control experiments. To minimize siRNA degradation, perform all experiments under RNAse-free conditions and use filtered pipette tips at all times.

3. Combine siRNA with 50 μL of Opti-MEM I and mix gently by pipetting.

4. Dilute 1–2 μL of Lipofectamine 2000 in 50 μL of Opti-MEM I and incubate at room temperature for 5 minutes.

5. Combine the diluted siRNA and Lipofectamine 2000 to a final volume of 100 μL per well, mix gently by pipetting, and incubate at room temperature for 20–30 minutes for the formation of complexes to occur. Make sure that all the tubes are tightly closed to avoid contamination with RNAses.

6. Wash cells once with PBS and add 100 μL of siRNA-Lipofectamine 2000 complexes to each well. Incubate at 37°C with 5% CO_2 for 4–6 hours and replace Opti-MEM I with antibiotic-free complete medium.

7. Assess the knockdown efficiency after 24–72 hours by western blotting or qRT-PCR.

Nucleofection

General considerations

Both small RNA molecules and large DNA plasmids can be introduced into a cell using nucleofection, thus this method is applicable for protein knockdown and overexpression [6,19]. Similar to liposome-based transfection, established cardiac cell lines are considered good candidates for nucleofection, while primary cells have been notoriously difficult to transfect using this method. However, new protocols are constantly being developed specifically for primary cardiomyocytes, leading to a more widespread use of this technology in the cardiovascular research.

About 37% transfection efficiency with 60% cell viability has been achieved for neonatal rat cardiomyocytes using Amaxa® Rat Cardiomyocyte – Neonatal Nucleofector® Kit [6]. However, transfection efficiencies remain low for adult cardiomyocytes, thus nucleofection is not suitable for this cell type. To minimize toxicity and optimize transfection efficiency, the following recommendations should be observed [20]. (1) Only freshly isolated neonatal primary cardiomyocytes are suitable for nucleofection. (2) All procedures should be carried out as quickly as possible, as viability of primary cardiomyocytes decreases with time. All reagents and materials must be ready prior to the isolation of the cells. (3) Larger pipette tips (1000 μL or more) should be used when transferring cells to avoid shearing. (4) It is essential to use DNA of high quality for nucleofection. Plasmids should be purified using QIAGEN EndoFree® Plasmid Kits or a similar product. The final DNA concentration should be between 1 and 5 μg/μL and A260:A280 ratio should be at least 1.8. (5) Optimal number of primary rat cardiomyocytes per sample is 2×10^6 and can range from 8×10^5 to 4×10^6. (6) Storage of cells in Nucleofector® solution will lead to increased mortality, so cells should be maintained in 37°C medium or PBS until ready for nucleofection. It is advisable to process one sample at a time. Do not store cells in Nucleofector solution for longer than 15 minutes. (7) The optimal voltage setting for electroporation will vary and manufacturer's guidelines should be consulted. The reported settings for neonatal cardiomyocytes on Amaxa nucleofector were: voltage = 360 V, resistance = 725 Ω, and capacitance = 50 μF.

Preparation

• Amaxa® Nucleofector I or Amaxa® Nucleofector II

• Amaxa® Rat Cardiomyocyte – Neonatal Nucleofector® Kit (Cat. no. VPE-1002) containing:
  ◦ Nucleofector solution and supplement
  ◦ Certified cuvettes
  ◦ Plastic pipettes
  ◦ pmaxGFP® positive control vector

• Coat 6-well plates with 1% gelatin solution sterilized by autoclaving.
• Prepare Nucleofector reaction solution by adding 18 μL of supplement to 82 μL of Nucleofector Solution to make 100 μL, keep at room temperature.
• Prepare culture medium for neonatal rat cardiomyocytes: DMEM/F12 medium supplemented with 5% horse serum, 0.2% bovine serum albumin, 2 mM L-glutamine, 3 mM sodium pyruvate, 0.1 mM sodium L-ascorbate, 1 μg/mL insulin, 1 μg/mL transferrin, 10 ng/mL sodium selenite, 0.02 mM cytosine-D-arabinofuranoside, 0.1 U/mL penicillin, 100 mg/mL streptomycin.
• Prewarm culture medium to 37°C (1.5 mL/ sample).
• Add 2 mL of supplemented culture medium to each well of the gelatin-coated 6-well plate, preincubate in a humidified incubator at 37°C with 5% CO_2.
• On the day of the assay, isolate and count primary neonatal rat cardiomyocytes. The cells should be kept in suspension at 37°C in culture medium until immediately prior to nucleofection.

Protocol

1. Collect 2×10^6 of freshly isolated neonatal rat cardiomyocytes per sample by centrifugation at 80 g for 1 minute at room temperature.
2. Carefully aspirate the medium and resuspend the cell pellet in 100 μL of Nucleofector reaction solution.
3. Add 1–5 μg of DNA or 30–300 nM of siRNA to each sample of cells suspended in the 100 μL of reaction solution.
4. Transfer 100 μL of nucleofection sample into the Amaxa-certified cuvette. Make sure that no air bubbles are present in the bottom of the cuvette. Close the cuvette with a cap.
5. Insert the cuvette into Nucleofector® and select Program G-009 for Nucleofector® II or G-09 for Nucleofector® I.
6. Once the program has finished, take out the cuvette, add 500 μL of the prewarmed medium and gently transfer cardiomyocytes using the provided pipettes into a well of a gelatin-coated 6-well plate with supplemented culture medium. Minimize handling of the sample and avoid repeated aspiration of the cells.

7. Following nucleofection, incubate cells for 24–72 hours at 37°C with 5% CO_2 and analyze transfection efficiency.

Adenoviral transduction
General considerations

Methods for preparation, propagation, purification, and viral titer determination of replication-deficient adenoviral vectors are beyond the scope of this chapter and for detailed protocols the reader is referred to [20]. Efficient overexpression of proteins in adult cardiomyocytes can be achieved with multiplicity of infection (MOI) of around 100, while lower virus titers of 5–20 MOI are suitable for the transduction of neonatal cardiac myocytes. A range of 5 MOI to 150 MOI has been reported for the established cardiac cell lines and can vary greatly depending on the protein of interest and duration of infection. A dose–response curve of increasing virus concentrations should be performed to determine the viral dose for optimal protein expression with minimal toxicity for each adenovirus tested. Importantly, the infectivity of recombinant viruses is greatly reduced by repeated freeze–thaw cycles. Thus, adenoviral vectors should be stored as a glycerol stock at −80°C and thawing should occur on ice. It is desirable to make small aliquots of the viral stock for use in the experiments.

Preparation

Before adenoviral stock can be used for protein overexpression, the most suitable MOI for the cells of interest must be determined. The MOI describes the number of particles needed to infect one cell. For example, an MOI of 100 means that 100 viral particles are required to effectively infect one cell. Since many recombinant viruses contain GFP or LacZ reporter genes, MOI can be determined with fluorescent or light microscopy. To determine the MOI of your viral stock, follow the steps below.

1. One or two days prior to transduction, plate 1×10^5 of cardiomyocytes per well of a 24-well plate.
2. Add sequential dilutions of the viral stock to each of the wells, leaving one well as a blank. The viral stock can first be diluted with 1 × PBS, combined with growth medium and added to cells.
3. After 48 hours of incubation at 37°C with 5% CO_2 image the cells by fluorescent microscopy. The

lowest MOI that renders the highest number of positive cells with minimal toxicity should be used for future experiments. In addition, the expression of a target protein should be quantified by western blotting at different MOIs and compared to GFP-only control adenoviral transduction and to noninfected cells.

Protocol

1. Plate primary rat cardiomyocytes 24–48 hours before the infection. Adult cardiomyocytes can be transduced as early as 2 hours following isolation. The established cell lines should be grown until 60–80% confluent.

2. Dilute the virus in serum-free medium to a concentration determined by dose–response titration and add to each well. Use the same MOI of a control virus encoding GFP or another inert protein to account for the effects of infection and protein overexpression on cellular physiology.

3. Incubate cells in a humidified incubator at 37°C with 5% CO_2. Depending on the vector and cell type, incubation times may vary widely, but many proteins are successfully overexpressed after 48–72 hours of incubation with adenovirus.

4. Following infection, virus-containing medium may be replaced with fresh serum-free medium. Alternatively, the expression of the protein of interest may be assessed immediately following infection.

Note on the transduction of adult murine cardiomyocytes. While the methods for transduction of neonatal and adult rat cardiomyocytes are well established, the adenovirus-mediated protein overexpression in adult murine cardiomyocytes remains challenging, primarily due to the significant degree of cell death. A study by Li *et al.* (2003) [21] found that medium formulation can dramatically affect viability and transduction efficiency of primary mouse cardiomyocytes, but not that of various other primary cells. Specifically, adenovirus-mediated transduction was shown to be virtually ineffective in myocytes cultured in M199 medium due to a failure of the virus to bind and get internalized. On the other hand, cells cultured in MEM supplemented with $NaHCO_3$ to 0.75 g/L retained viability for at least 48 hours after isolation procedure and were effectively transduced after 1

hour of incubation with 20 MOI of β-galactosidase adenovirus.

Lentiviral transduction
General considerations
Lentiviruses are capable of penetrating the intact nuclear envelope membrane and integrating its nucleic acid sequence into the host genome for long-lasting expression of the target gene. In addition to stable overexpression of proteins, lentiviruses are used extensively in protein knock down experiments by delivering plasmids that encode short hairpin RNAs (shRNA). The shRNA transcripts are rapidly processed into double-stranded siRNA molecules, resulting in a highly efficient inhibition of protein expression. The most commonly used lentiviral vectors are based on human immunodeficiency virus-type 1 (HIV-1) devoid of its accessory protein genes and therefore replication incompetent. The viral genome has been segregated into three plasmids: (1) vector plasmid carrying gene of interest and Rev expressor (pHR'CMV), (2) gag-pol packaging plasmid (pCMVΔR8.2), and (3) envelope construct (pCMV-VSV.G). Various constructs encoding lentiviral genome segments are commercially available. A replication-deficient virus is generated by co-transfection of the three plasmids into 293T cells, followed by the collection of viral particles and infection of cardiomyocytes or other target cells (Figure 47.2).

Protocol
1. Grow 293T cells in 10-cm dishes with 10 mL of DMEM supplemented with 10% FBS and penicillin/streptomycin until 50–60% confluent.

2. Co-transfect the subconfluent 293T cells with 15 μg of each of the three plasmids by calcium phosphate DNA precipitation method [20].

3. After 16 hours of incubation, replace the medium with DMEM plus 10% FBS supplemented with 10 mM of sodium butyrate and incubate cells for additional 8 hours. This step increases viral particle titers by more than 10-fold.

4. Gently wash 293T cells with PBS making sure that the cells do not detach from the plate. Incubate cells in fresh medium without sodium butyrate for additional 16 hours to allow for viral particle production.

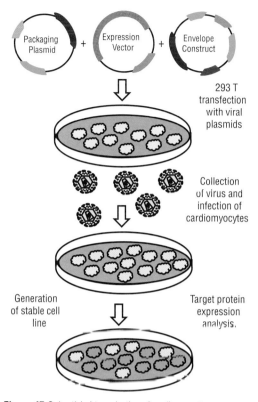

Figure 47.2 Lentiviral transduction of cardiomyocytes.

to some cells. Thus, the optimal concentration should be determined empirically.

8. For lentiviral transduction, plate the primary cells at 40 to 50% confluence and incubate them with the viral vector in polybrene-containing medium for at least 6 hours, but preferably overnight. Remove viral particles, add fresh medium without polybrene and incubate cells for additional 48 hours at 37°C with 5% CO_2, followed by the analysis of transgene expression or knockdown efficiency.

9. Many lentiviral vectors encode pyromycin, neomycin, or G418 selection markers, which can be used to establish stable transgenic cell lines. For this, cultured cells must be transduced for at least 24 hours in normal medium followed by application of selection medium containing the appropriate antibiotic. The selection medium should be changed every 3–4 days. Gently swirl the dish or flask to lift up dead cells before aspirating the old medium. Inspect the plate under the microscope to ensure that the majority of dead cells have been removed. Gently wash the cells with PBS, if needed. Replace the selection medium and repeat this processes two or more times, until significant degree of cell death is no longer observed. Passage cells as needed.

Weaknesses and strengths of the method

Modulation of protein expression is a widely used tool for the study of biochemistry, signaling, and cell physiology in the heart. It is a relatively fast and inexpensive way of investigating the function of a protein, compared to the generation of *in vivo* models. Moreover, certain mechanistic studies cannot be carried out in a mouse or rat model, and thus require a highly efficient and reliable *in vitro* setup. Despite significant improvements, the transfection efficiency of primary cardiac myoblasts by nonviral methods remains significantly lower than the viral delivery of genetic material [2]. Thus, liposome- or electroporation-based methods may not be suitable for experiments requiring high efficiency of protein overexpression or knockdown in primary cells, but remain extremely useful in the established cardiac cell lines. On the other hand, infection of cardiomyocytes by adenoviruses and lentiviruses may potentially alter cellular physiology and produce results that are inconsistent with *in vivo*

5. Harvest the viral particle-containing conditioned medium and filter it through 0.45-mm filters. This medium can be used to infect cardiomyocytes directly. Alternatively, a concentrated stock may be prepared.

6. To concentrate viral stocks, centrifuge the conditioned medium at 50,000 g at 4°C for 90 minutes. Discard supernatant and resuspend the pellet by incubating it overnight in Hanks' balanced salt solution at 4°C.

7. Prior to conducting experiments, determine the viral stock concentration by infecting cardiac myocytes with serial dilutions of viral stock in medium containing 2–10 μg/mL of polybrene (hexadimethrine bromide) and assess the expression of your gene of interest after 48 hours. Use the method for calculating MOI described for adenoviral transduction. Note that excessive exposure to polybrene, a cationic compound which facilitates viral interaction with cell membrane, may be toxic observations. Moreover, preparation of viral particles is a multistep process that requires cloning of nucleotide sequences into appropriate expression vectors, propagation, collection, and concentration of viral particles, and extensive testing to determine the effectiveness and infectivity of the virus for a particular cell type and protein of interest.

Modulation of protein levels *in vitro* has several potential limitations. A high degree of protein overexpression or modifications to its domains may result in misfolding and/or formation of protein aggregates. Moreover, plasmid-delivered genes may lack certain regulatory elements required for proper processing or targeting of the protein product. Changes in the levels of proteins that are a part of multimeric complexes may alter the stoichiometry of the complex components or disrupt certain interactions, resulting in difficult-to-interpret phenotypes or dominant-negative effects. siRNAs may have off-target effects, which can be minimized by using pools of three of four different siRNAs. However, this would be difficult to achieve in a lentiviral shRNA-based knockdown system. Moreover, many commercially available siRNA or shRNA particles have not been previously validated and therefore may not target the protein of interest for degradation even when successfully transfected or transduced into a cell. Certain proteins may be particularly resistant to overexpression or downregulation due to feedback inhibition or other regulatory mechanisms, and a thorough understanding of the signaling networks may be needed to overcome this limitation. Finally, the advancements gained through the *in vitro* study of protein function must be validated in an *in vivo* system, such as a knockout or transgenic mouse model, as even the primary cardiomyocytes are not 100% representative of the intact and working heart.

Conclusions

Established cardiac cell lines, such as H9c2 or HL-1, are good candidates for both transfection and transduction methods of delivering genetic material into a cell. Virus-based methods for modulation of proteins in primary cardiac myocytes often remain the technique of choice due to high efficiency of protein overexpression or knockdown. However,

many transfection-based nucleotide delivery protocols have been optimized for use in primary cardiomyocytes and are successfully employed by many investigators in the study of the heart.

References

1 Albert N, Tremblay JP. Evaluation of various gene transfection methods into human myoblast clones. *Transplant P* 1992; **24**: 2784–2786.
2 Djurovic S, Iversen N, Jeansson S, Hoover F, Christensen G. Comparison of nonviral transfection and adeno-associated viral transduction on cardiomyocytes. *Mol Biotechnol* 2004; **28**: 21–31.
3 Louch WE, Sheehan KA, Wolska BM. Methods in cardiomyocyte isolation, culture, and gene transfer. *J Mol Cell Cardiol* 2011; **51**: 288–298.
4 Mitcheson JS, Hancox JC, Levi AJ. Cultured adult cardiac myocytes: Future applications, culture methods, morphological and electrophysiological properties. *Cardiovasc Res* 1998; **39**: 280–300.
5 Zhou YY, Wang SQ, Zhu WZ, Chruscinski A, Kobilka BK, Ziman B, et al. Culture and adenoviral infection of adult mouse cardiac myocytes: methods for cellular genetic physiology. *Am J Physiol Heart Circ* 2000; **279**: H429–436.
6 Gresch O, Engel FB, Nesic D, Tran TT, England HM, Hickman ES, et al. New non-viral method for gene transfer into primary cells. *Methods* 2004; **33**: 151–163.
7 Felgner PL, Gadek TR, Holm M, Roman R, Chan HW, Wenz M, et al. Lipofection: a highly efficient, lipid-mediated DNA-transfection procedure. *Proc Natl Acad Sci U S A* 1987; **84**: 7413–7417.
8 Etzion S, Etzion Y, DeBosch B, Crawford PA, Muslin AJ. Akt2 deficiency promotes cardiac induction of Rab4a and myocardial beta-adrenergic hypersensitivity. *J Mol Cell Cardiol* 2010; **49**: 931–940.
9 Tsukakoshi M, Kurata S, Nomiya Y, Ikawa Y, Kasuya T. A novel method of DNA transfection by laser microbeam cell surgery. *Appl Phys B-Photo* 1984; **35**: 135–140.
10 Nikolskaya AV, Nikolski VP, Efimov IR. Gene printer: Laser-scanning targeted transfection of cultured cardiac neonatal rat cells. *Cell Commun Adhes* 2006; **13**: 217–222.
11 Bartoli M, Claycomb WC. Transfer of macromolecules into living adult cardiomyocytes by microinjection. *Mol Cell Biochem* 1997; **172**: 103–109.
12 Miyake K, Suzuki N, Matsuoka H, Tohyama T, Shimada T. Stable integration of human immunodeficiency virus-based retroviral vectors into the chromosomes of nondividing cells. *Hum Gene Ther* 1998; **9**: 467–475.
13 Kass-Eisler A, Falck-Pedersen E, Alvira M, Rivera J, Buttrick PM, Wittenberg BA, et al. Quantitative-

determination of adenovirus-mediated gene delivery to rat cardiac myocytes in vitro and in vivo. *Proc Natl Acad Sci USA* 1993; **90**: 11498–11502.

14 Schulick AH, Newman KD, Virmani R, Dichek DA. In-vivo gene-transfer into injured carotid arteries – optimization and evaluation of acute toxicity. *Circulation* 1995; **91**: 2407–2414.

15 de Muinck ED. Gene and cell therapy for heart failure. *Antioxid Redox Sign* 2009; **11**: 2025–2042.

16 Bonci D, Cittadini A, Latronico MV, Borello U, Aycock JK, Drusco A, *et al.* "Advanced" generation lentiviruses as efficient vectors for cardiomyocyte gene transduction in vitro and in vivo. *Gene Ther* 2003; **10**: 630–636.

17 Kumar M, Keller B, Makalou N, Sutton RE. Systematic determination of the packaging limit of lentiviral vectors. *Hum Gene Ther* 2001; **12**: 1893–1905.

18 Dalby B, Cates S, Harris A, Ohki EC, Tilkins ML, Price PJ, *et al.* Advanced transfection with Lipofectamine 2000 reagent: primary neurons, siRNA, and high-throughput applications. *Methods* 2004; **33**: 95–103.

19 Frias MA, Rebsamen MC, Gerber-Wicht C, Lang U. Prostaglandin E2 activates Stat3 in neonatal rat ventricular cardiomyocytes: A role in cardiac hypertrophy. *Cardiovasc Res* 2007; **73**: 57–65.

20 Metzger JM. *Cardiac Cell and Gene Transfer : Principles, Protocols, and Applications.* Totowa, NJ: Humana Press, 2003.

21 Li ZB, Sharma RV, Duan DS, Davisson RL. Adenovirus-mediated gene transfer to adult mouse cardiomyocytes is selectively influenced by culture medium. *J Gene Med* 2003; **5**: 765–772.

In vivo microRNA studies

Eva van Rooij

miRagen Therapeutics, Inc., Boulder, CO, USA

Introduction

MicroRNAs (miRNAs) are transcribed as precursor molecules called pri-miRNAs, derived either from annotated transcripts (as the introns of protein coding genes, the exons of noncoding genes, and the introns of noncoding genes) or from intergenic regions within the genome, and can encode a single or multiple miRNAs [1,2]. MiRNAs within known annotated transcripts can be under the direct transcriptional control of their host genes, while intergenic miRNAs are under their own control and in most cases are transcribed via the action of RNA polymerase II [2]. Pri-miRNAs fold into hairpin structures containing imperfectly base-paired stems and are processed by the endonuclease Drosha and its cofactor DiGeorge syndrome critical region 8 (DGCR8) into 60–100 nt hairpins known as pre-miRNAs [3–5]. The pre-miRNAs are exported from the nucleus to the cytoplasm by exportin5 [6], where they are cleaved by the endonuclease Dicer to yield imperfect miRNA–miRNA* duplexes [7]. The miRNA strand is selected to become a mature miRNA, while most often the miRNA* strand is degraded. The mature miRNA is incorporated into the RNA-induced silencing complex (RISC), which recognizes specific targets and induces post-transcriptional gene silencing [8]. The function of a miRNA is ultimately defined by the genes it targets and the effects it has on their expression. Two major silencing mechanisms have been identified for miRNAs: miRNAs can inhibit translational initiation, or can target mRNAs for degradation [9] (Figure 48.1). Under baseline conditions miRNAs appear to act as moderate regulators that function as a rheostat to maintain a certain cell fate, but appear to adopt a more pronounced function when a cell or tissue becomes stressed, like during disease.

The mature miRNA is responsible for the function of the miRNA, and can be detected by miRNA-specific detection through real-time PCR and northern blot analysis. While the expression level of miRNAs is cell type specific and is dynamically regulated during development and disease, the endogenous level of a miRNA can also be experimentally modulated by using oligonucleotide-based approaches.

Protocols

Protocol I: Northern blot analysis of miRNAs

Northern blotting is widely used to visualize specific miRNAs. Although it is fairly time consuming (at least 2 days) and requires large amounts of RNA (8 μg or more), it is the only approach that will visualize the expression of a miRNA, as well as the pre-miRNA.

1. MicroRNA northern blotting can be performed using a standard western blot electrophoresis/transfer system (Bio-Rad). Before use thoroughly clean all gel plates and gel apparatus.
2. Isolate total RNA from your tissue of interest using a regular TRIzol extraction and set the final concentration of your RNA sample at 1 μg/μL.
3. The small RNAs can be fractionated by electrophoresis on a 20% denaturing polyacrylamide gel. Make 20% acrylamide gels (per gel):

Manual of Research Techniques in Cardiovascular Medicine, First Edition. Edited by Hossein Ardehali, Roberto Bolli, and Douglas W. Losordo.
© 2014 John Wiley & Sons, Ltd. Published 2014 by John Wiley & Sons, Ltd.

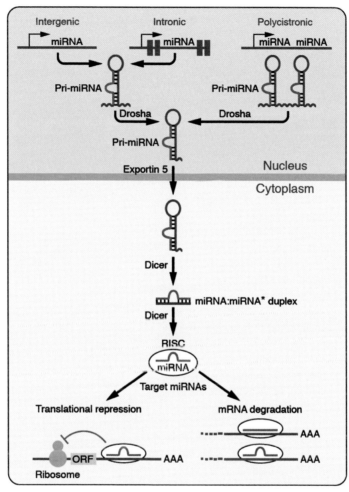

Figure 48.1 miRNA biogenesis. The primary transcripts of miRNAs, pri-miRNAs, are transcribed as individual genes, from introns of coding genes, or from polycistronic transcripts. The RNase Drosha further processes the pri-miRNA into 70–100 nucleotide, hairpin-shaped precursors, called pre-miRNA, which are exported from the nucleus by exportin 5. In the cytoplasm, the pre-miRNA is cleaved by Dicer into a miRNA duplex. Assembled into the RISC, the mature miRNA negatively regulate gene expression by either translational repression or mRNA degradation. ORF, open reading frame. (Source: Eva van Rooij 2011 [16]. Reproduced with permission from LWW).

7.5 g Urea

7.5 mL of 40% acrylamide Bis (29:1)

1.5 mL of 10× TBE

1.4 mL of dH$_2$O

100 µL of 10% APS

16 µL of TEMED

Spin solution (without APS and TEMED) for 30 minutes with stir bar and filter the solution through a 0.4-µm filter. Once filtered, add APS and TEMED and immediately pour your gel. Let your gel polymerize for ~1 hour, and clean out the wells with running buffer before loading each sample.

4. For detection of your miRNA use 10 µg of total RNA (load more if the miRNA is low expression) and add 12 µL loading buffer (90% formamide; 50 mM EDTA; 0.005% XCFF/BB). Prior to loading the sample, denature samples at 70°C for 5 minutes followed by incubating on ice for 5 minutes.

5. Run the gel for ~3 hours at 125 V in 1× TBE. The XCFF dye runs about small RNA size in 20% acrylamide gels.

6. Transfer your gel for ~1 hour at 80 V in cold room in 0.5× TBE onto a Bio-Rad Zeta-probe membrane (or something similar).

7. After transferring these small RNAs from the gel onto a membrane, the RNA can be fixed onto the membrane by UV crosslinking and/or baking the membrane. Cross-link the membrane in a UV Crosslinker (i.e. Stratagene's Stratalinker) and bake the membrane for 30 minutes at 80°C.

8. Prehybridize the membrane for 30 minutes in Rapid-Hyb buffer (Amersham) at 39°C.

9. Due to the small size and the low abundance of miRNA molecules, the use of an oligonucleotide probe with increased sensitivity is essential to detect the miRNA. The miRNA StarFire system from IDT provides an effective means of miRNA detection. In this system, the probe sequence is extended with a 3′ hexamer that binds to the 3′ end of the provided universal template oligonucleotide that consists of oligo-dT10 sequence at its 5′ end. Through a DNA polymerase extension reaction, radiolabelled α-^{32}P-dATP is added to the miRNA probe, resulting in a miRNA-specific probe containing a radioactive polyA. These probes enable efficient detection of miRNAs.

Label oligonucleotide probes using the StarFire kit protocol (IDT), *be sure the isotope is P^{32}-dATP*. Order StarFire custom oligo antisense to the mature miRNA of interest with standard desalting purification from IDT.

10. Label for 5–30 minutes at 37°C. Purify using microfuge columns.

11. Add probe and hybridize overnight at 39°C.

Protocol II: Real-time detection of miRNA levels

By far the most commonly used method to detect the expression level of an individual miRNA is miRNA-specific realtime PCR analysis.

A miRNA real-time reaction starts with reverse transcribing RNA into cDNA. The limited length of the mature miRNA (~22 nts), the lack of a common sequence feature like a poly(A) tail, and the fact that the mature miRNA sequence is also present in the pri- and pre-miRNA transcript poses several challenges for appropriate reverse transcription. One commercially available assay, developed by Life Technologies, utilizes stem loop reverse transcription primers that confer sequence specificity and binding stability. The stem–loop primers are designed to have a short single-stranded region that is complementary to the known sequence on the 3′ end of the miRNA, a double-stranded region (the

stem), and the loop that contains the universal primer-binding sequence. The resulting cDNA is then used as a template for qPCR with one miRNA-specific primer and a second universal primer (TaqMan® PCR, Applied Biosystems).

1. Prepare your total RNA by diluting samples to 12.5 ng/μL

2. Perform reverse transcription of your microRNA of interest and of the appropriate small RNA normalizer

Reaction mix for one sample:

12.5 ng/L total RNA	4 μL
10× RT buffer	1.5 μL
100 mM dNTPS	0.15 μL
target miR 5× RT primer	3 μL
small RNA control 5× RT primer	3 μL
MultiScribe™ RT (50 U/μL)	1 μL
ddH$_2$O	2.35 μL
final volume:	15 μL

Incubate:

30 minutes at 16°C

30 minutes at 42°C

5 minutes at 85°C

hold at 4°C.

3. In preparation for your microRNA PCR reaction, add 41.5 μL of ddH2O to the 15 μL RT reaction and mix well.

diluted RT reaction	5 μL
2× Gene Expression Master Mix	10 μL
target miR or small RNA control 20× microRNA assay probe	1 μL
ddH$_2$O	4 μL
final volume:	20 μL

4. Use a real-time thermal cycler to run your microRNA qPCR according to the following program:

10 minutes at 95°C

Cycle 40 times:

15 seconds at 95°C

60 seconds at 60°C (data collected at the end of this step)

Modulation of miRNA levels *in vitro*

In vitro miRNA manipulation can be achieved by straightforward transfection experiments and can serve to determine target regulation or to examine the physiological effect of the miRNA on processes such as the control of cell morphology, differentiation, proliferation, and survival. While miR mimics usually consist of double-stranded oligonucleotide chemistries, antimiRs are usually single-stranded molecules. The chemical design of these modulators determine the efficiency of miRNA regulation [10].

Transfection of a miRNA mimic or inhibitor can be achieved with commercially available reagents that serve to shield the negative charge of the oligonucleotide and facilitate cellular uptake. A variety of transfection reagents can be purchased from Thermo Fisher Scientific and Life Technologies. Specific cell types can respond differently to transfection, therefore it is best to optimize conditions by using a range of dose of transfection reagent, as well as a range of mimic or inhibitor. Titrating up and down in the low nanomolar range typically works well as a starting point.

In vitro UTR analysis

The most commonly used approach to verify a miRNA target site is by cloning the 3′ UTR of a predicted mRNA target into a luciferase reporter. By linking the target UTR to the luciferase reporter, a change in luciferase will indicate whether a miRNA can bind to the UTR and regulate the expression of the gene, either at the mRNA or protein level.

There are two approaches that can serve to determine whether a UTR is sensitive to binding of a specific miRNA. One approach is to transfect a cell line that expresses the miRNA of interest with a reporter containing either the wild-type UTR of a target gene or the UTR in which the miRNA binding site is mutated. If the construct containing the wild-type UTR shows a reduction in luciferase expression and this decrease is absent in the mutated version, this likely indicates that the endogenously expressed miRNA is capable of regulating that UTR. In this same set-up, one could employ a miRNA inhibitor to block miRNA function, which would then lead to an increase in luciferase.

Another option would be to transfect cells with both the luciferase reporter construct and increasing amounts of the miRNA of interest by either using an expression construct like pcDNA harboring the full length sequence of the pre-miRNA or by transfecting in chemically synthesized miRNA mimics. The advantage of introducing an miRNA is that if the miRNA actually targets the binding site in the UTR, a dose-dependent effect on luciferase read out can be determined, with this response being absent with the mutated construct.

To determine whether a UTR is susceptible to miRNA regulation, the complete sequence should be tested to assure that endogenous sequences that enhance or inhibit miRNA binding and gene regulation located distal to the miRNA binding site are also present in the reporter construct [11]. As in many aspects of miRNA biology, target regulation is under the influence of temporal and spatial specific mechanisms. The cell type, the differentiation state of the cell, and if a cell is under stress all appear to influence whether a miRNA regulates a target. Thus, to accurately assess whether miRNA/mRNA regulation actually occurs, transfection experiments should be performed in the cell type of interest, where all endogenously expressed cofactors are present [11].

Modulation of miRNA levels *in vivo*

AntimiRs are modified antisense oligonucleotides harboring the full or partial complementary reverse sequence of a mature miRNA, and can be used to specifically reduce the endogenous levels of a miRNA. Because miRNAs normally reduce the expression of target genes, antimiR treatment will result in an increase of expression by relieving this inhibitory effect on gene expression. There are several key requirements for an antimiR chemistry to achieve effective down regulation of a targeted miRNA *in vivo*. The chemistry needs to be cell permeable, cannot be rapidly excreted, needs to be stable *in vivo*, and should bind to the miRNA of interest with high specificity and affinity (reviewed in [12–14]). Several modifications have been used *in vivo* so far. These chemical modifications include 2′-O-methyl-group (OMe)-modified oligonucleotides, and LNA-modified oligonucleotides, in which the 2′-O oxygen is bridged to the 4′ position via a methylene linker to form a rigid bicycle, locked into a C3′-endo (RNA) sugar conformation [15]. Another chemical modification applied to enhance oligonucleotide stability is the balance between phosphodiester and phosphorothioate linkages between the nucleotides, with phosphorothioate providing more stability to the oligonucleotide and making it more resistant to nucleases (Figure 48.2).

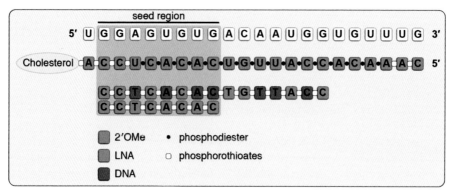

Figure 48.2 AntimiR chemistries. The most commonly used antimiRs are antagomirs or locked nucleic acid (LNA)-modified antimiRs. Antagomirs are oligonucleotides that harbor various modifications for RNase protection and to enhance pharmacological properties like cellular uptake and delivery. They differ from normal RNA by complete 2'-*O*-methylation (2'OMe) of the sugar, phosphorothioate backbone and a cholesterol moiety at the 3' end. Introducing LNA-modifications leads to a thermodynamically strong duplex formation with complementary RNA due to their high binding affinity. A fully phosphorothioated, 15 or 16-nucleotide LNA/DNA mixmer, or an 8-nucleotide fully modified LNA oligomer directed against the seed region of a miRNA is sufficient to establish *in vivo* miRNA inhibition. (Source: Eva van Rooij 2011 [16]. Reproduced with permission from LWW).

Antagomirs are complementary to the mature miRNA sequence and are conjugated to cholesterol to facilitate cellular uptake (Figure 48.2). The high binding affinity for LNA-containing antisense oligonucleotides allows inhibition with shorter LNA oligonucleotides (Figure 48.2). A fully phosphorothioated LNA/DNA oligo directed against the 5' portion of the mature miRNA, containing roughly 50% LNA bases or eight nucleotides fully modified LNA oligomer complementary to the seed region of the miRNA is sufficient to establish a functional effect *in vivo*. While both the antagomir and LNA-modified oligos can effective target a miRNA, the LNA-modified chemistries require lower doses based on their higher binding affinity.

Protocol III: Preparation of antimiRs for *in vivo* administration

AntimiRs can be dissolved in saline or PBS and injected into the animal intravenously or subcutaneously.

1. Dilute each antimiR to a predetermined theoretical concentration. Dissolve each oligonucleotide chemistry in sterile 0.9% aqueous solution of NaCl. For mouse studies, start with a theoretical concentration of ~12.5 mg/mL. For rat studies, start with a theoretical concentration of ~15.0 mg/mL.

2. Before injecting the animals, calculate the OD from the dissolved antimiR chemistry. To do so, take a small aliquot (~10 μL) from the resuspended oligo and dilute 1:10 or 1:100. Measure the absorbance at 260 nm in a cuvette with a 1-cm path length. Calculate the total OD using the following equation:

$$OD = A_{260} \times \text{original volume} \times \text{dilution factor}$$

As an example, if you diluted the oligo in 15 mL of 0.9% saline, diluted this 1:10 for absorbance measurements, and measured A_{260} of 50.00, total OD = 50.00 × 15 × 10 = 7500.

3. Next determine the total nmoles for each antimiR chemistry. The total nmoles can be calculated for each oligonucleotide based on the extinction coefficient at 260 nm and the total OD. To calculate nmoles, use the following equation:

$$\text{nmoles} = OD / \varepsilon_{260} \times 10^6$$

4. To continue from the example shown here, if the extinction coefficient = 192300.00, then nmoles = 7500/192300 × 10^6 = 39001 nmoles. A weblink to calculate the extinction coefficient of an oligonucleotide chemistry is http://www.idtdna.com/analyzer/applications/oligoanalyzer/ Determine the total number of milligrams (mg) for each oligo. The total number of mg can be calculated for each oligo based on the total nmoles and the MW of each oligo. Calculate the total number of mg using the following equation:

$$mg = nmoles/10^6 \times MW$$

To continue from the example shown here, if the MW = 5467.379, then mg = 39001/10^6 × 5467.379 = 213.233 mg. This is your true quantity of antimiR.

5. **Prepare a common stock.** For mouse studies, a stock solution of 10 mg/mL is sufficient to dilute down to most *in vivo* doses. In keeping with the example mentioned earlier, this would require 21.3233 mL of 0.9% NaCl to = 10 mg/mL. Since you already have 15 mL, you would only need to add 6.3233 mL of 0.9% NaCl.

Prepare solutions for *in vivo* administration. Once the stock solutions are prepared, it is easy to prepare working stocks based on the dose desired. We prefer to dose in a volume of 250 µL as this gives a large enough volume to minimize error while not overloading the animal with too much volume. The following equation can be used to calculate the desired concentration:

$$\text{Concentration (mg/mL)} = \text{mouse wt (g)} \\ \times \text{dose (µg/g)/volume of dose (µL)}$$

As an example, if you have a mouse that weighs 30 g and you would like to dose this mouse at a 25 mg/kg dose, in a 250 µL volume, it would be: Concentration = 30 × 25/250 = 3 mg/mL solution. So dilute your stock concentration down to 3 mg/mL, inject 250 µL and your mouse is dosed at 25 mg/kg.

Weaknesses and strengths of the methods

As with any research method, detecting miRNAs by northern blotting has some pros and cons. Currently, miRNA northern blotting is the only detection method that allows for visualization of both the mature miRNA and the pre-miRNA. However, a disadvantage, in addition to the requirement of relatively large amounts of RNA, is the inability of the northern blot probe to distinguish between related miRNAs. Often, related miRNAs differ by only one or two bases in their 3′ sequence, which makes it difficult to prevent the

probe from cross-reacting with the different miRNA family members.

Even though there are several very useful and effective methods to reverse transcribe a miRNA, the specificity and sensitivity of any real-time assay is dependent on the design of the miRNA-specific primer. Because the binding affinity of a primer is determined by the sequence, the GC content of a miRNA determines the T_m against the complementary sequence of the miRNA-specific primer. One should be cognizant of the fact that the binding affinity of a primer is miRNA specific and determines the efficiency of miRNA amplification, making it difficult to use qPCR to determine the relative abundance of different miRNAs. One way to circumvent this issue is to run a standard curve in parallel for samples containing known quantities of synthetic miRNA copies. At the same time, the assay is confounded by the existence of closely related miRNAs that often only differ by several bases in sequence. Although the primers are designed to be miRNA-specific, due to the high degree of homology between miRNAs, these assays are susceptible to cross-reactivity among different miRNA family members. If family member specificity is critical for the interpretation of the experiment, then it is recommended that the specificity of the real time assay be tested with synthetic templates for each family member.

In vitro or *in vivo* use of an antimiR to study the function of a miRNA is far less time consuming than generating a genetic deletion of your miRNA of interest. Like other oligonucleotide chemistries, antimiRs or mimics can be transfected into your cell type of interest while antimiRs for *in vivo* experiments can be dissolved in saline and injected into the animal intravenously or subcutaneously. While these antimiR approaches are very effective in inhibiting an miRNA *in vivo*, one should consider that systemic delivery might induce unknown off-target effects and that the effect observed might be due to effects outside of the target tissue.

An additional potential artifact can be introduced by the *in vivo* sequestering of the antimiRs into extracellular or intracellular compartments (e.g. endosomes). Although systemic delivery results in efficient uptake of antimiR in the cells, the antimiRs are taken up in endosomes which slowly release the antimiR; endogenously they only inhibit miRNAs when released from these compartments. However, tissue homogenization after systemic delivery can cause these captured antimiRs to be released and bind to the mature miRNA, causing an overestimation of binding efficiency of the antimiR *in vivo*. For this reason it is essential to look for biological target read-outs rather than simply measuring miRNA inhibition.

Conclusions

Even though we just started to scratch the surface of understanding miRNA biology, the techniques that are currently available for detection aid enormously in helping us move forward in our learning about the regulation of these small RNAs. The ability to regulate miRNA levels by antimiRs *in vivo*, not only provides a very useful experimental tool, but additionally represents a first step in the development of novel therapeutics. Although we need to remain focused on developing better assays and continue to expand our understanding about how miRNAs truly function, this chapter will hopefully provide a first step for researchers to start exploring the influence of miRNAs in their research area of interest.

References

1 Cai X, Hagedorn CH, Cullen BR. Human microRNAs are processed from capped, polyadenylated transcripts that can also function as mRNAs. *RNA* 2004; **10**: 1957–1966.

2 Lee Y, Kim M, Han J, Yeom KH, Lee S, Baek SH, *et al.* MicroRNA genes are transcribed by RNA polymerase ii. *EMBO J* 2004; **23**: 4051–4060.

3 Denli AM, Tops BB, Plasterk RH, Ketting RF, Hannon GJ. Processing of primary microRNAs by the microprocessor complex. *Nature* 2004; **432**: 231–235.

4 Gregory RI, Yan KP, Amuthan G, Chendrimada T, Doratotaj B, Cooch N, *et al.* The microprocessor complex mediates the genesis of microRNAs. *Nature* 2004; **432**: 235–240.

5 Lee Y, Ahn C, Han J, Choi H, Kim J, Yim J, *et al.* The nuclear RNAse iii drosha initiates microRNA processing. *Nature* 2003; **425**: 415–419.

6 Yi R, Qin Y, Macara IG, Cullen BR. Exportin-5 mediates the nuclear export of pre-microRNAs and short hairpin RNAs. *Genes Devel* 2003; **17**: 3011–3016.

7 Chendrimada TP, Gregory RI, Kumaraswamy E, Norman J, Cooch N, Nishikura K, *et al.* Trbp recruits the dicer complex to ago2 for microRNA processing and gene silencing. *Nature* 2005; **436**: 740–744.

8 Khvorova A, Reynolds A, Jayasena SD. Functional siRNAs and miRNAs exhibit strand bias. *Cell* 2003; **115**: 209–216.

9 Filipowicz W, Bhattacharyya SN, Sonenberg N. Mechanisms of post-transcriptional regulation by microRNAs: Are the answers in sight? *Nat Rev Genet* 2008; **9**: 102–114.

10 Lennox KA, Behlke MA. A direct comparison of anti-microRNA oligonucleotide potency. *Pharm Res* 2010; **27**: 1788–1799.

11 Bartel DP. MicroRNAs: Target recognition and regulatory functions. *Cell* 2009; **136**: 215–233.

12 Manoharan M. 2′-carbohydrate modifications in antisense oligonucleotide therapy: Importance of conformation, configuration and conjugation. *Biochim Biophys Acta* 1999; **1489**: 117–130.

13 Prakash TP, Bhat B. 2′-modified oligonucleotides for antisense therapeutics. *Curr Top Med Chem* 2007; **7**: 641–649.

14 Stenvang J, Kauppinen S. MicroRNAs as targets for antisense-based therapeutics. *Expert Opin Biol Ther* 2008; **8**: 59–81.

15 Weiler J, Hunziker J, Hall J. Anti-miRNA oligonucleotides (amos): Ammunition to target mirnas implicated in human disease? *Gene Ther* 2006; **13**: 496–502.

16 Eva van Rooij. The Art of MicroRNA Research. *Circulation Research* 2011; **108**: 219–234.

Part 7

Model Systems

Vascular and cardiac studies in zebrafish

Hans-Georg Simon, Molly Ahrens, and Brandon Holtrup

Northwestern University Feinberg School of Medicine, Chicago, IL, USA

Introduction

The zebrafish *Danio rerio* offers unique advantages for studying cell biological processes during vertebrate organogenesis, as zebrafish embryos develop externally and embryos and early larvae are practically transparent (Figure 49.1A). The optically clear zebrafish embryo, with its relatively small size and fast development (the heart starts beating at 18 hours post fertilization (hpf) followed with circulation initiated at 24 hpf), allow for direct noninvasive observation of developmental processes at high resolution. Importantly, zebrafish embryos can survive for an extended developmental time period with a seriously impaired or nonfunctional cardiovascular system, which is especially advantageous to analyze cardiac defects [1,2]. The simple architecture of the zebrafish heart, composed of an inflow region, two major chambers (an atrium and a ventricle), and an outflow tract, further aids in the analysis [3]. With a genome sequencing project completed, it is clear that the major genes and pathways underlying cardiovascular development are conserved between zebrafish and mammals, making the fish an ideal vertebrate research model to address unsolved questions concerning the morphogenesis of this vital organ *in vivo*, including the origins of defects in heart size, shape, and function.

The possibility to reduce or enhance gene function by microinjection of gene-specific morpholino (MO) antisense oligonucleotides and synthetic mRNA, respectively, make the zebrafish a fast functional read out system [4,5]. In addition, during the past decade, transgenesis became feasible and large-scale genetic screens have discovered a multitude of fish lines with cardiac mutations [6–9]. Zebrafish mutants recapitulating inherited human cardiac disorders, such as arrhythmias, aortic coarctation, cardiomyopathy, and Holt–Oram syndrome, have become important disease models [10–14].

The adult zebrafish is less accessible for direct visual cardiac analysis due to the opacity beyond its developmental stages. However, adult zebrafish models of heart disease and assessment of function are on the rise. For example, an ultrasound biomicroscopy (UBM) system has been developed to study cardiac function and physiology [15]. To facilitate microscopic observation into adulthood, a transgenic zebrafish reporter line that combines the lack of melanocyte and iridophore production with a red fluorescent heart has been generated [16], which allows for the quantification of the shortening fraction as well as heart rate *in vivo*, in both the embryo and adult zebrafish.

Most methodologies needed for zebrafish work are readily accessible and should facilitate characterization of cardiac and vascular phenotypes in a wide range of laboratories. Here we provide a brief introduction to the analysis of cardiovascular phenotypes in the zebrafish embryo, but for a more

Manual of Research Techniques in Cardiovascular Medicine, First Edition. Edited by Hossein Ardehali, Roberto Bolli, and Douglas W. Losordo.
© 2014 John Wiley & Sons, Ltd. Published 2014 by John Wiley & Sons, Ltd.

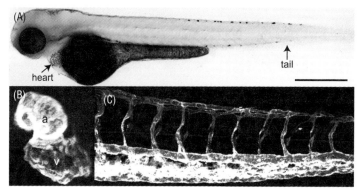

Figure 49.1 Zebrafish embryo with cardiovascular system. (A) Lateral view of zebrafish embryo at 72 hours post fertilization (hpf). (B) Ventral view of the heart at 72 hpf visualized by transgenic line *Tg(myl7: egfp)*. (C) Lateral view of vasculature in the tail at 72 hpf visualized by transgenic line *Tg(kdrl: mcherry)*. a, atrium; v, ventricle. Scale bar 400 μm.

in depth discussion of techniques we refer to *The Zebrafish Book: a Guide for the Laboratory Use of Zebrafish (Danio rerio)* [17], A guide to analysis of cardiac phenotypes in the zebrafish embryo [18], and Modeling cardiovascular disease in zebrafish [19].

Protocols

Morpholino (MO) or mRNA microinjection of zebrafish embryos

If mutant zebrafish lines are not available for phenotype analysis, the cellular level of the protein of interest can be manipulated in the zebrafish embryo via injection of MOs or mRNA. Beyond the brief summary protocol below, a more complete protocol can be found in the following references [4,17,20].

Prepare:

1. Set up breeding tanks the afternoon/ evening before the microinjection day.

2. Prepare 1% agarose (with egg water, 60 μg/mL of Instant Ocean®) dishes with furrows to hold embryos in place (6-well zebrafish injection molds, Adaptive Science Tools).

Microinjection day:

1. Collect embryos at or just before 1-cell stage.

2. Prepare injection mix. For a concentration series of RNA, dilute desired concentration in 0.1 M KCl and 0.5% phenol red. For MO, dilute a 4× Danieau Solution (232 mM NaCl, 2.8 mM KCl, 1.6 mM MgSO$_4$, 2.4 mM Ca(NO$_3$)$_2$, 20 mM HEPES pH 7.6) to 1× using desired amount of MO, water, and 0.5% phenol red.

3. Load injection mix into finely pulled glass needles (1-mm capillary tubes with filaments; World Precision Instruments, TW100F-4).

4. Break the needle tip using forceps and calibrate the needle to estimate the amount of liquid injected (typically 2 nL) using a 1 × 0.01 mm stage micrometer for droplet calibration (Fisher, 12-561-SM1).

5. Load eggs at the 1 or 2-cell stage into wells.

6. Inject into cytoplasmic streaming of the yolk (MO, mRNA) or the single cell (mRNA). See *The Zebrafish Book* (Chapter 5) [17] for an illustration of injection.

7. Use forceps to remove embryos from wells and put in egg water at 28.5°C to develop to desired stage.

Whole mount immunofluorescence of zebrafish embryos

We describe a standard protocol for the detection of protein expression throughout embryogenesis by immunofluorescence, which allows high-resolution two-dimensional and three-dimensional (3D) evaluations after confocal z-stack rendering. This protocol is convenient and reproducible for heart-specific markers such as the myocardial or atrial proteins detected by MF-20 and S46 antibodies, respectively. Specific antibodies may require treatment modifications, and suggestions for alternative procedures are included. Whole mount immunofluorescence is usually compared between wild-type and mutant lines or embryos after experimental protein knockdown or overexpression.

Prior to day 1

Prepare:

1. 0.3g/L 1-phenyl 2-thiourea (PTU) with egg water.
2. 0.4% (w/v) Zebrafish Tricaine Stock. Make small quantity, adjust to pH 7 using 1 M Tris (pH 9), and store in freezer.
3. 4% Paraformaldehyde (PFA), pH 7.4. Caution: toxic, use in hood. Prepare 200 mL in sterile 1× phosphate buffered saline (PBS). To get PFA into solution add a few droplets of 10 N NaOH. Cool to room temperature and adjust pH to ~7.4. Store aliquots at −20°C. Thaw aliquots at 65°C and cool on ice before use.

Zebrafish embryo preparation and fixation:

1. Dechorionate embryos at approximately 24 hours post fertilization (hpf).
2. Incubate dechorionated embryos in 0.3g/L PTU made with egg water at 28.5°C to inhibit melanogenesis and generate transparent embryos [21]. Place embryos back into incubator and allow embryos to develop to desired stage.
3. If embryos are older than 24 hpf, anesthetize them with 0.015% tricaine.
4. Fix zebrafish embryos in 4% PFA for 1.5 hours rocking at room temperature (RT) or overnight (O/N) at 4°C. Some antibodies may require fixation in 1–2% PFA for 30–60 minutes at RT. Other antibodies work better with Dent's fixation (80% EtOH, 20% dimethyl sulfoxide (DMSO)) O/N at −20°C.
5. Remove fixative and dispose of waste appropriately. Wash once with 100% MeOH 1×. Replace with fresh 100% MeOH and store embryos at −20°C. (Some antibodies may require skipping the MeOH step and proceed directly into PBS + 0.1% Tween (PBST) and antibody staining.)

Day 1

Prepare:

1. Blocking Solution: We prefer to use saponin during the blocking as this depletes the yolk contents, allowing for easier visualization of the heart. Make fresh 2% (w/v) saponin with sterile H₂O, vortex vigorously to get into solution. Dilute concentrated saponin 10-fold with the other block solutions. Final solution is PBS with 10% (v/v) serum (e.g. goat serum, chosen based on animal in which the secondary antibody was produced), 2 mg/mL BSA, and 0.2% saponin (w/v). Store O/N at 4°C for use the next day. Alternative block: 1% DMSO, 5 mg/mL BSA, 5% serum in PBST.

Primary antibody:

1. If embryos are stored in 100% MeOH, gradually change the solution to PBST through 5 to 10-minute incubations. (e.g. 75% MeOH: 25% PBST, 50:50, 25:75, 0:100). Keep in microfuge tubes or transfer to small dish.
2. Optional antigen retrieval step by enzymatic digestion: Digest embryos with 50–100 μL of 0.05% trypsin: 1 minute, late somitogenesis; 5 minutes, 24-hour embryos; 10 minutes, 48-hour embryos; 15 minutes, 72-hour embryos. Remove trypsin and wash 3 × 5 minutes in PBST.
3. Remove PBST and add 1 mL of blocking solution. Rock for 1 hour at RT (or O/N at 4°C).
4. Remove blocking solution. Add 200–500 μL of primary antibody diluted to appropriate concentration in blocking solution. A dilution of 1:250 for MF20 and S46 (Table 49.1) works well in our hands, but dilutions should be empirically determined for each antibody. Leave rocking O/N at 4°C (or 1–4 hour at RT).

Day 2

Secondary antibody:

1. Remove primary antibody. Wash 3 × 5 minutes in blocking solution (or PBST).
2. Add 200–500 μL secondary antibody diluted to appropriate concentration in blocking solution and incubate rocking for 1 hour at RT. We typically use a dilution of 1:1000 (Alexa Fluor 546 goat anti-mouse IgG2b for MF20 and Alexa Fluor 488 goat anti-mouse IgG1 for S46), but dilutions for each antibody should be empirically determined. Choose the secondary antibody based on the animal in which the primary antibody was produced and the class or subclass of the primary antibody. For example, if the primary antibody is a mouse monoclonal of the subclass IgM, a secondary antibody that reacts with IgM should be used goat anti-mouse IgM).

Table 49.1 Cardiac-specific antibodies and dyes

Antibody or dye	Name	Tissue specificity	Reference	Location
MF20 (Antibody)	Anti-meromyosin	Heart myocardium; slow and fast muscle fibers	[18, 22]	Developmental studies Hybridoma bank
S46 (Antibody)	Anti-myosin heavy polypeptide 6 (Previously known as *amhc*)	Atrium	[23]	Developmental studies Hybridoma bank
DAF-2 DA (Dye); DAR-4M AM (Dye)	4,5-Diaminofluorescein diacetate solution; Diaminorhodamine-4M AM	Outflow tract	[3]	Calbiochem, Cell Technology, Inc.

3. Wash 3 × 5 minutes in blocking solution (or PBST).

4. Add 200 ng/mL 4′,6-diamidino-2-pheylindole (DAPI) in PBS for 5 minutes.

5. Remove DAPI and wash 3 × 5 minutes with blocking solution (or PBST).

6. Mount zebrafish for microscopy. Zebrafish can be transferred to 3% methylcellulose or glycerol for imaging in a depression slide; alternatively they can be mounted in 1% low-melting agarose (see section Zebrafish live embryo cell tracking for preparation) or on a tape-bridged slide. To prepare tape-bridged slides, put zebrafish (heart side up for cardiac imaging, removing the tail helps to keep the zebrafish properly positioned) in a drop of glycerol with three stacked pieces of scotch tape on either side. Put a drop of stop-cock grease on each tape stack. Gently place a 22 mm × 22 mm coverslip over the zebrafish resting on the tape stack.

7. Image on fluorescent or confocal microscope. If a 3D reconstruction is desired, collect confocal z-stacks through the heart or vessels. Assemble stacks using available software (e.g. Zeiss Zen, Image J, ImagePro, Amira).

Zebrafish live embryo cell tracking

We describe a basic protocol that allows the capture of dynamic processes by imaging zebrafish embryos over a time course to track individual cells throughout early embryogenesis. This technique can be performed with a multitude of transgenic zebrafish lines (Table 49.2) and is successfully used in our laboratory employing the Hand2:eGPFxH2AF: mCherry reporter zebrafish line (Robert K. Ho, PhD, University of Chicago; Brian A. Link, PhD, Medical College of Wisconsin).

Prepare:

1. 0.4% Zebrafish Tricaine Stock, as described earlier.

2. 0.7% Low melting-point (LMP) agarose diluted in egg water.

Mount zebrafish:

1. Melt LMP agarose to 65°C in a water bath. Once liquid, add Zebrafish Tricaine Stock to agarose with a final concentration of 0.16% in order to immobilize the embryos.

2. In the meantime, screen embryos under a dissecting microscope for fluorescence, and separate embryos with the strongest signal.

3. Dechorionate zebrafish of interest.

4. Place embryos back in the incubator and allow the zebrafish to develop to desired stage. For example, we use 15 somite stage embryos to track cell migration from the heart–limb field to the site of heart development.

5. Once the agarose is fully melted, allow it to come to body temperature. Test temperature by holding tube against the inside of your wrist.

6. Using a transfer pipette, move embryos to clean glass-bottom culture dish (MatTek). Remove excess water using a micropipette with great care, avoiding any damage to the embryo.

7. Once the agarose is cooled to body temperature, cover embryo with a drop of agarose.

8. Before the agarose sets, properly position embryo depending on which structure you want to image using a fine-tipped dissecting probe. Mount fish at the bottom of the dish, as this helps to create clearer and crisper images.

9. Once agarose sets, cover fish with an extra layer of body temperature agarose.

Table 49.2 Transgenic (Tg) zebrafish lines labeling cardiovascular structures

Genotype	Phenotype	Reference
Tg(myl7: nRFP) Previously Tg(cmlc2: nRFP)	Cardiomyocyte nuclei labeled with RFP	[24]
Tg(myl7: egfp) Previously Tg(cmlc2: EGFP)	Myocardium labeled with GFP (Figure 49.1B)	[25]
Tg(Kdrl: EGFP) (Previously Tg(flk1: EGFP)	Endothelial cells including vasculature labeled with GFP	[26]
Tg(kdrl: mCherry) Previously Tg(flk1: mCherry)	Endothelial cells including vasculature labeled with mCherry (Figure 49.1C)	[27]
Tg(kdrl: nlsmCherry) Previously Tg(flk1: nlsmCherry)	Nuclei of endothelial cells including vasculature labeled with mCherry	[27]
Tg(fli1a: EGFP)	Endothelial cells including vasculature labeled with GFP	[28]
Tg(Tie2: EGFP)	Endothelial cells including vasculature labeled with GFP	[29]
Tg(gata1: DsRed)	Erythrocytes labeled with DsRed	[30]
casper; Tg(myl7: nuDsRed)	Formation of melanocytes and iridophores inhibited; cardiomyocyte nuclei labeled with DsRed	[16]

Image zebrafish:

1. Image zebrafish using appropriate confocal microscope (e.g. Zeiss LSM700 with heated stage and/or incubator set at 28.5°C).

    a. Place glass-bottom dish with mounted embryo onto the stage.

    b. Ensure that all cells of interest are in focus using a z-stack. Use the fastest scan possible while still being able to discern individual cells. Faster scans will prevent the laser from melting the agarose.

    c. Set up a time-lapse experiment. Ten minutes between stacks is sufficient to track cells individually.

2. After images are collected, assemble the maximum intensity projections of the z-stack into a movie using available software (e.g. Zeiss Zen, Image J, ImagePro, Amira).

Alternative approaches

If whole mount immunofluorescence cannot be utilized, then standard colorimetric immunohistochemistry techniques may be an option to visualize protein expression, although typically only one to two colors can be detected in colorimetric assays, which limits detection of multiple epitopes.

Alternatively, western blots can be performed to demonstrate the presence or absence of a protein. While protein blots do not provide information on protein localization, they may indicate potential post-translational protein modifications. If antibodies are not available for a particular gene product, then in situ hybridization (ISH) is the next universal choice to determine the localization of the respective mRNA in the developing heart or vasculature. If live embryo cell tracking cannot be utilized, standard staining techniques (e.g. whole mount immunofluorescence, in situ hybridization) at multiple time points should be considered. By examining a developmental sequence, first indications of cell migration patterns can be gained.

Weaknesses and strengths

There are numerous advantages when using whole mount immunofluorescence and live cell tracking of zebrafish embryos. Multiple proteins can be detected simultaneously and their localization within a tissue and cell can be determined in relation to the others. Fluorescent antibody staining can be combined with fluorescent transgenic lines to determine localization of a protein in a wild-type or mutant background.

Furthermore, fluorescent detection allows multiple proteins to be detected in space using 3D-rendered confocal z-stacks. In the case of live cell imaging, it is possible to track the migration of individual cells in space and time, which cannot be accomplished with any other methodology. The main weakness of these methods is the limited availability of antibodies for whole mount immunofluorescence or limited transgenic reporter lines for live embryo cell tracking (Table 49.2). Beyond the basic protocols described here, special microscopes and high-speed cameras may be needed to detect and capture particular developmental processes and such a set up could become prohibitive due to cost if it is not shared as part of a dedicated facility.

Conclusion

Whole mount immunofluorescence protein detection at high spatial resolution and dynamic live embryo fluorescent cell tracking throughout zebrafish development provide unique insight into tissue morphogenesis that cannot be achieved in other organisms. These techniques, in combination with transgenic and/or mutant zebrafish, MO knockdown, or mRNA overexpression, hold the potential for exciting new discoveries in cardiovascular research.

References

1 Pelster B, Burggren WW. Disruption of hemoglobin oxygen transport does not impact oxygen-dependent physiological processes in developing embryos of zebra fish (Danio rerio). *Circ Res* 1996; **79**: 358–362.

2 Stainier DY. Zebrafish genetics and vertebrate heart formation. *Nat Rev Genet* 2001; **2**: 39–48.

3 Grimes AC, Stadt HA, Shepherd IT, Kirby ML. Solving an enigma: arterial pole development in the zebrafish heart. *Dev Biol* 2006; **290**: 265–276.

4 Bill BR, Petzold AM, Clark KJ, Schimmenti LA, Ekker SC. A primer for morpholino use in zebrafish. *Zebrafish* 2009; **6**: 69–77.

5 Eisen JS, Smith JC. Controlling morpholino experiments: don't stop making antisense. *Development* 2008; **135**: 1735–1743.

6 Alexander J, Stainier DY, Yelon D. Screening mosaic F1 females for mutations affecting zebrafish heart induction and patterning. *Dev Genet* 1998; **22**: 288–299.

7 Chen JN, Haffter P, Odenthal J, Vogelsang E, Brand M, van Eeden FJ, *et al.* Mutations affecting the cardiovascular system and other internal organs in zebrafish. *Development* 1996; **123**: 293–302.

8 Stainier DY, Fouquet B, Chen JN, Warren KS, Weinstein BM, Meiler SE, *et al.* Mutations affecting the formation and function of the cardiovascular system in the zebrafish embryo. *Development* 1996; **123**: 285–292.

9 Warren KS, Wu JC, Pinet F, Fishman MC. The genetic basis of cardiac function: dissection by zebrafish (Danio rerio) screens. *Philos Trans R Soc Lond B Biol Sci* 2000; **355**: 939–944.

10 Arnaout R, Ferrer T, Huisken J, Spitzer K, Stainier DY, Tristani-Firouzi M, *et al.* Zebrafish model for human long QT syndrome. *Proc Natl Acad Sci U S A* 2007; **104**: 11316–11321.

11 Garrity DM, Childs S, Fishman MC. The heartstrings mutation in zebrafish causes heart/fin Tbx5 deficiency syndrome. *Development* 2002; **129**: 4635–4645.

12 Hassel D, Scholz EP, Trano N, Friedrich O, Just S, Meder B, *et al.* Deficient zebrafish ether-a-go-go-related gene channel gating causes short-QT syndrome in zebrafish reggae mutants. *Circulation* 2008; **117**: 866–875.

13 Peterson RT, Shaw SY, Peterson TA, Milan DJ, Zhong TP, Schreiber SL, *et al.* Chemical suppression of a genetic mutation in a zebrafish model of aortic coarctation. *Nat Biotechnol* 2004; **22**: 595–599.

14 Xu X, Meiler SE, Zhong TP, Mohideen M, Crossley DA, Burggren WW, *et al.* Cardiomyopathy in zebrafish due to mutation in an alternatively spliced exon of titin. *Nat Genet* 2002; **30**: 205–209.

15 Sun L, Lien CL, Xu X, Shung KK. In vivo cardiac imaging of adult zebrafish using high frequency ultrasound (45–75 MHz). *Ultrasound Med Biol* 2008; **34**: 31–39.

16 Hoage T, Ding Y, Xu X. Quantifying cardiac functions in embryonic and adult zebrafish. *Methods Mol Biol* 2012; **843**: 11–20.

17 Westerfield M. *The Zebrafish Book. A Guide for the Laboratory Use of Zebrafish (Danio rerio)*. Eugene: University of Oregon Press, 2000.

18 Miura GI, Yelon D. A guide to analysis of cardiac phenotypes in the zebrafish embryo. *Methods Cell Biol* 2011; **101**: 161–180.

19 Chico TJ, Ingham PW, Crossman DC. Modeling cardiovascular disease in the zebrafish. *Trends Cardiovasc Med* 2008; **18**: 150–155.

20 Mullins M. Microinjection Techniques: Injecting through the Chorion. Zebrafish Course 2010. Available at http://courses.mbl.edu/zebrafish/faculty/mullins/pdf/Mullins_InjectionhandoutZfishCourse2011.pdf

21 Karlsson J, von Hofsten J, Olsson PE. Generating transparent zebrafish: a refined method to improve detection of gene expression during embryonic development. *Mar Biotechnol (NY)* 2001; **3**: 522–527.

22 Han Y, Dennis JE, Cohen-Gould L, Bader DM, Fischman DA. Expression of sarcomeric myosin in the presumptive myocardium of chicken embryos occurs within six hours of myocyte commitment. *Dev Dyn* 1992; **193**: 257–265.

23 Yelon D, Horne SA, Stainier DY. Restricted expression of cardiac myosin genes reveals regulated aspects of heart tube assembly in zebrafish. *Dev Biol* 1999; **214**: 23–37.

24 Mably JD, Mohideen MA, Burns CG, Chen JN, Fishman MC. Heart of glass regulates the concentric growth of the heart in zebrafish. *Curr Biol* 2003; **13**: 2138–2147.

25 Burns CG, Milan DJ, Grande EJ, Rottbauer W, MacRae CA, Fishman MC, *et al*. High-throughput assay for small molecules that modulate zebrafish embryonic heart rate. *Nat Chem Biol* 2005; **1**: 263–264.

26 Jin SW, Beis D, Mitchell T, Chen JN, Stainier DY. Cellular and molecular analyses of vascular tube and lumen formation in zebrafish. *Development* 2005; **132**: 5199–5209.

27 Wang Y, Kaiser MS, Larson JD, Nasevicius A, Clark KJ, Wadman SA, *et al*. Moesin1 and Ve-cadherin are required in endothelial cells during in vivo tubulogenesis. *Development* 2010; **137**: 3119–3128.

28 Lawson ND, Weinstein BM. In vivo imaging of embryonic vascular development using transgenic zebrafish. *Dev Biol* 2002; **248**: 307–318.

29 Motoike T, Loughna S, Perens E, Roman BL, Liao W, Chau TC, *et al*. Universal GFP reporter for the study of vascular development. *Genesis* 2000; **28**: 75–81.

30 Traver D, Paw BH, Poss KD, Penberthy WT, Lin S, Zon LI, *et al*. Transplantation and in vivo imaging of multilineage engraftment in zebrafish bloodless mutants. *Nat Immunol* 2003; **4**: 1238–1246.

Vascular and cardiac studies in *Drosophila*

Lin Yu, Joseph P. Daniels, and Matthew J. Wolf

Duke University, Durham, NC, USA

Introduction

Traditionally, transgenic mouse models provide important insights into specific genes in the development of cardiovascular disease; however, mouse models are not readily amenable to large-scale genetic or pharmacologic drug screens. The limitations include the difficulty mapping phenotypes to genotypes for candidate gene identification, the costs associated with the maintenance of animal colonies, and the time required for the manifestation of phenotypes. To complement conventional mouse models, and circumvent some associated limitations, approaches using the unique genetic resources of the fruit fly, *Drosophila melanogaster*, to model human cardiomyopathies have been developed [1–3].

During the past several decades, intensive investigations based on lineage tracing and morphology of the embryonic fly heart have shown that the fly circulatory system develops from an orchestrated set of fundamental, evolutionarily conserved signals that occur in the mesoderm [4,5]. As the fly develops during the late larval and pupal stages, the circulatory system undergoes significant morphological changes to become the adult heart. The *Drosophila* heart is a linear tube composed of a single layer of cardiomyocytes that share similar signaling pathways and genes compared to mammalian hearts [3]. Although undoubtedly simpler than a mammalian heart, the fly cardiovascular system provides unique opportunities to precisely examine how genetic mutations cause abnormalities in cardiac myocyte function.

A variety of cardiomyopathies have been modeled using *Drosophila*. In general, dilated cardiomyopathies are the most well-characterized model and are based on measurements of systolic and diastolic chamber dimensions in partially dissected flies or *in vivo*. Changes in cardiac function based on measurements of cardiac chamber dimensions *in vivo* in the fly closely resemble assessments using echocardiography in mammals, including humans [2]. Additionally, mechanisms underlying myocardial calcium handling are conserved between flies and mammals, although the mammalian heart has a much more complex conduction system [6]. Furthermore, mutations in genes associated with human cardiovascular diseases recapitulate abnormalities in *Drosophila*. For example, mutations in structural proteins including troponin I (*hdp²* mutant) [2], tropomyosin (*TM2³* mutant) [2], dystrophin (*dysExel6184/dyskx43* mutant) [7], and delta-sarcoglycan (*Scgd⁸⁴⁰* mutant) [8] cause dilated cardiomyopathies in adult flies. Additionally, mutations in signaling molecules, ion channels, mitochondrial function, and metabolic enzymes, including epidermal growth factor receptor [9], Notch receptor ligand [10], potassium channels (KCNQ) [11], sestrin [12], CCR4-Not3 complex [1], Rho-GTPase Cdc42 [13], sterol regulatory element-binding protein (dSREBP) [14], and mitochondrial assembly regulatory factor (MARF) and optic atrophy (Opa)-1 [15], have been shown to cause

Manual of Research Techniques in Cardiovascular Medicine, First Edition. Edited by Hossein Ardehali, Roberto Bolli, and Douglas W. Losordo.

cardiac abnormalities in *Drosophila*. The modeling of cardiac hypertrophy in *Drosophila* is less well established compared to dilated cardiomyopathies; however, alterations in receptor tyrosine kinase signaling cause increased cardiomyocyte size consistent with cardiac hypertrophy (Wolf, *et al.* unpublished data).

The fly heart has also been used to investigate changes in diastolic function as related to aging and to model the effects of high-fat diets on cardiac function and lipotoxicity [16,17]. Furthermore, elegant studies demonstrate a high degree of conservation between the *Drosophila* and mammalian heart proteomes [18]. This suggests that the fly heart may provide a robust experimental platform to investigate changes in metabolic enzymes and proteins under conditions of cardiomyopathy. These observations, in conjunction with the tremendous resources that are available to researchers using *Drosophila*, also suggest that studies of fly mutants in the context of changes in diet may provide new insight into environmental exposures that impact cardiovascular diseases.

Of course, there are significant limitations to the use of *Drosophilas* as model of cardiovascular diseases [3]. First, the fly has an open circulatory system, a single cardiomyocyte cell layer, and a single heart chamber. Second, there is no coronary circulation, and oxygen transport occurs via diffusion. Therefore, ischemia–reperfusion studies that are amenable in mice cannot be conducted in the fly. However, cardiac function can be measured under conditions in which the entire fly is subjected to hypoxic conditions [19]. Third, although channels and calcium-handling mechanisms are conserved between flies and mammals, the conduction system is significantly less complex in *Drosophila* [6].

Several experimental methods have been developed to characterize cardiac function and structure in adult *Drosophila* [3]. Adult heart rate responses to externally applied electrical pacing can be monitored to characterize the effects of aging on cardiac parameters in adult flies [20]. Methods based on dissection of the surrounding tissues from the fly heart and perfusion in artificial hemolymph provide strategies to directly record cardiac chamber dimensions [20], measure calcium handling using genetically encoded calcium-dependent fluorescent indicators [6], or prepare specimens for immuno-histochemistry to visualize cardiac structures [21]. Optical coherence tomography (OCT), as described below, has been adapted to examine cardiac chamber size and function in awake, adult *Drosophila* [2]. Histological techniques have been developed to characterize heart wall thicknesses [9]. This chapter describes practical approaches to phenotype cardiac function and morphology in adult *Drosophila*, thereby providing opportunities to identify genes that affect heart function.

Protocols

Measurement of *in vivo* cardiac chamber dimension by optical coherence tomography (OCT)

The ability to measure cardiac chamber dimensions in whole animals has been a major advance in cardiovascular research. OCT is a noninvasive, nondestructive *in vivo* imaging technique that provides microscopic tomographic sectioning of biologic tissues and can produce images similar to echocardiography in mice and humans [2,22]. By measuring reflected light in the near-infra red range, OCT provides subsurface imaging with a spatial resolution of 2–8 microns without requiring direct contact between the probe and the tissue. Thus, strategies based on OCT can be used to screen for abnormalities in cardiac chamber size in intact adult flies. The following protocol is designed to obtain cardiac chamber measurements in live, adult flies using a Bioptigen OCT system (Bioptigen, Inc., Durham, NC); however, other OCT systems can be used.

Immobilizing adult flies:

1. Collect adult females that are between 2 and 14 days old, ideally 1 week old. Bodies should be of consistent size.

2. Anesthetize flies using standard CO_2 permeable flypad (Genesee Scientific, Inc.). Flies are then individually placed into 2 mm deep slits made with a standard razor blade using Petri dishes containing GelWax (Yaley Enterprises, Redding, CA). Flies should not be exposed to CO_2 for longer than ~10 minutes. Ensure that each fly is embedded evenly in the anterior–posterior orientation and in the lateral orientation. Do not embed the animal too deep into the gel since this can deform the cuticle, rendering the fly unusable for imaging. The fly should be embedded so that one-half to two-thirds of the body is below the surface of the gel (Figure 50.1A). Correctly immobilized flies will have the dorsal aspect facing the OCT source.

3. Allow 10 minutes for flies to recover, as ascertained by movement of the head, body, and extremities. Scan flies within 30 minutes of embedding. All imaging is conducted at room temperature (25°C) unless otherwise dictated by the experimental design.

Obtaining OCT images:

All OCT images are obtained using an ordered set of imaging parameters.

4. A 1 mm wide 2D B-mode OCT transverse image is obtained to ensure that the fly is oriented evenly along the anterior–posterior and the lateral axes.

5. 2D B-mode OCT longitudinal and transverse scanning is performed along the anterior–posterior direction to position the imaging plane in the first abdominal (A1) segment.

6. The cross-sectional image of the heart is centered in the middle of the imaging plane and the width of the 2D B-mode OCT transverse image is changed from 1 mm to 0.2 mm. Then the cross-sectional image of the heart is again centered in the middle of the imaging plane.

7. M-mode imaging of the cardiac chamber is obtained by stopping the scanning mirror in the midline and collecting continuous image data as a function of time. A series of M-mode images represents the dorsal/ ventral diameter of the heart tube at the A1 segment over a set period of time. Typically, >1000 axial lines are collected per cardiac cycle over several seconds. This provides sufficient temporal resolution to accurately define end-diastolic and end-systolic parameters. Several M-modes are acquired for each fly (Figure 50.1B).

8. After obtaining M-mode OCT images, return to 2D B-mode OCT longitudinal and transverse scanning once more to ensure proper anatomical localization throughout image acquisition. If the fly has moved during the acquisition of the M-mode then repeat Steps 4 through 7.

Processing OCT images and measuring cardiac parameters:

Imaging processing may differ according to the manufacturer of the OCT instrument. For our Bioptigen OCT system, each image file is recoded in ".OCT" format. The ".OCT" files are converted to JPG formats using ImageJ software and graphical user interface plugins. These plugins were developed to create M-mode images from .OCT files and can be obtained from Bioptigen, Inc., Durham, NC (http://www.bioptigen.com/index.html).

9. The cardiac chamber dimensions are measured from M-mode images. Measure the distance between the edge of the superior and inferior walls during mid-diastole: these measures are end diastolic dimension, or EDD, and the end systolic dimension, or ESD, respectively. Fractional shortening, or FS, is calculated as $[(EDD - ESD)/ EDD] \times 100$ and represents the extent of cardiac chamber area change during systole. Average measures from a minimum of three consecutive cardiac cycles during normal regular rhythm. All OCT measurements are calibrated to a reference standard. We use a 125 micron standard cover slip. Typically, control flies that have "normal" cardiac chamber dimensions (i.e. w^{1118}) have an EDD of ~76 ± 3 µm, an ESD of ~8 ± 2 µm, and a FS of ~90 ± 2% (Figure 50.1C). Flies that have dilated cardiomyopathy have increased ESD and EDD measurements (Figure 50.1D). For example, the hdp^2 mutant is used as a positive control ("dilated heart") in our studies and typically has an EDD of ~120 µm, an ESD of ~40–50 µm, and a FS of ~60–65%.

Cautions

1. Be careful to avoid motion artifacts. This is particularly important since the animals are awake and occasionally move.

2. Both the dorsal and the ventral walls of the heart tube must be visible during OCT imaging to accurately calculate cardiac dimensions. Additionally, flies that are placed too deep into the gel may develop deformation of the cuticle and adversely affect imaging of the heart.

3. Avoid imaging animals with unusually slow heart rates (<300 bpm).

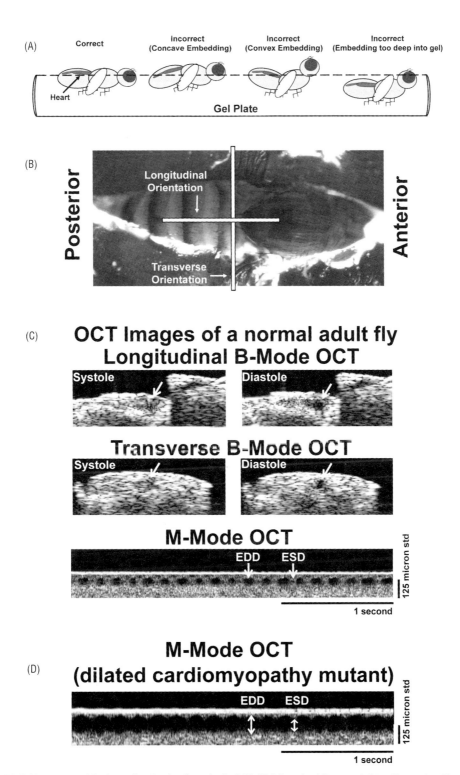

Figure 50.1 Measurement of *in vivo* cardiac chamber dimension by OCT. (A) Schematic of flies on gel plate with correct and incorrect immobilization. (B) Example of correctly immobilized fly showing longitudinal and transverse image planes. (C) Representative longitudinal and transverse B-mode images during systole and diastole in normal adult fly. A representative M-mode OCT image with EDD and ESD is shown. (D) Representative M-mode from a fly with dilated cardiomyopathy for comparison.

Limitations

OCT imaging provides excellent spatial and temporal resolution to accurately measure *in vivo* cardiac dimensions in intact animals. Current OCT instruments can achieve axial (spatial) resolution on the order of 2 to 8 microns, more than sufficient to measure cardiac chamber dimensions. The weaknesses of OCT are similar to those associated with echocardiography. Because images are obtained from reflected light, any dense material within the lumen of the heart or surrounding the heart can potentially interfere with image quality.

Other alternative methods routinely used rely on partially dissected preparations of adult fly hearts [20,23]. Typically, the tissues surrounding the heart are dissected away to provide a preparation that contains the heart and adherent noncardiac cells attached to the dorsal cuticle. This preparation is bathed in artificial hemolymph and can be thought of as analogous to a Langendorff preparation of isolated, perfused mammalian hearts. We find that approaches using both OCT and dissected specimens provide a more thorough assessment of cardiac chamber dimensions.

Characterization of heart wall thickness by histology

The ability to accurately assess changes in cardiac morphology and heart wall thickness is necessary to identify the effects of specific genetic mutations. Methods based on immunofluorescent labeling of dissected heart preparations have been developed and previously described [21]. We will describe methods to accurately measure heart wall thickness in adult *Drosophila* using serial transverse histological sections.

Fixation, dehydration, and equilibration in liquid paraffin

1. Fix 20 female flies into 10 mL Telly's fixation buffer (60% ethanol, 3.33% formalin, 4% glacial acetic acid) for at least 1 week at 4°C.

2. Dehydrate flies with serial ethanol washes in sealed glass vials: two 30 minute washes in 70% ethanol; two 30 minute washes in 80% ethanol; one 30 minute wash in 90% ethanol; one 30 minute wash in 95% ethanol; and two 30 minute washes in 100% ethanol containing 5% glycerol. Gentle rotation is used for each step.

3. Place flies in histology cassette (Gray Biopsy Cassette; Tissue-Tek, Sakura Finetek, USA, Inc.) and soak into 100% ethanol for 5 minutes. Then, wash the cassettes two times for 15 to 20 minutes in xylene.

4. Place the cassette in a suitable jar that contains liquid paraffin (Polyfin Paraffin, VWR) prewarmed to 56°C and tap the cassette to clear out any air bubbles. Next, place the jar into a 56°C vacuum oven for 20 minutes.

5. Next, remove the jar from the vacuum oven, tap out any bubbles again, and place the jar back in the vacuum oven for 40 minutes.

6. Remove the jar from the oven, exchange with fresh paraffin and place the jar back in the vacuum oven for 20 minutes.

7. Remove the jar from the vacuum oven, tap out bubbles again, and then place the jar back in the oven for overnight or up to 3 days.

Embedding specimens in paraffin blocks and sectioning

8. Embed one fly into one mold (Peel-A-Way disposable embedding T-8 molds, Polysciences, Inc.) with the fly positioned head up and posterior down in the paraffin. Allow paraffin to cool until solid.

9. Serial 8 μm thick sections are cut using a microtome (Leica #RM2135) and sectioned strips are briefly immersed in 40°C deionized water to expand the wax strip. Then, the sections are placed onto microscope slides and allowed to dry overnight at 37°C.

Hematoxylin and eosin staining:

10. Place slides into a slide holder and warm the slides to 55°C for 1 hour before staining.

11. Place the slides for two 15 minute incubations in xylene.

12. Rehydrate slides with serial ethanol gradient: two 2 minute washes in 100% ethanol; two 2 minute washes in 95% ethanol; one 2 minute wash in 80% ethanol; and one 2 minute wash in 70% ethanol.

13. Rinse the slides in 1 × PBS (phosphate buffered saline) and then soak the slides in tap water for 5 minutes.

14. Place slides in hematoxylin for 1.5 minutes followed by four changes in tap water.

15. Place slides in acid alcohol (500 mL volume: 350 mL 100% ethanol, 150 mL dH$_2$O, 5 mL 37%

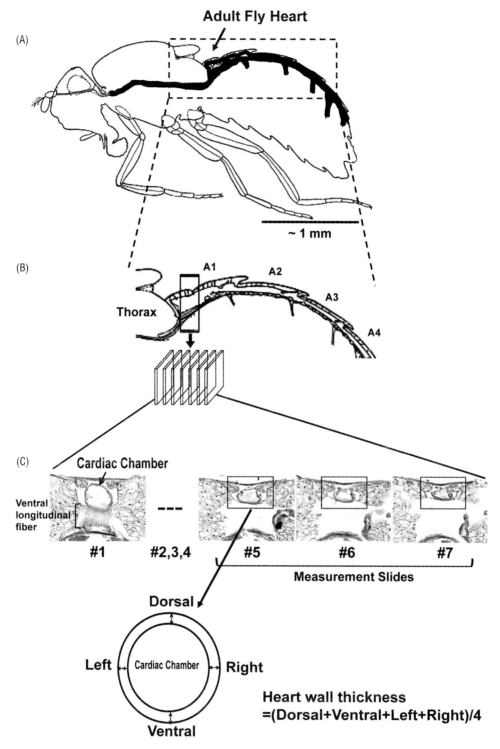

Figure 50.2 Characterization of heart wall thickness by histology. (A) Schematic of the adult fly circulatory system. (B) Region of the adult fly heart that is evaluated by serial histological sectioning. (C) Representative serial H&E stained sections through the fly heart and general method used to calculate wall thicknesses.

HCl) for 5 seconds followed by four changes in tap water.

16. Place slides in Scott's solution (24 mM sodium bicarbonate and 80 mM magnesium sulfate; we use Scott's solution from Electron Microscopy Sciences, Inc.) for 20 seconds followed by four changes in tap water.

17. Place the slides in 80% ethanol for 2 minutes.

18. Place the slides in Eosin for 40 seconds followed by four changes in tap water.

19. Perform two 2 minute washes in 95% ethanol and then two 2 minute washes in 100% ethanol.

20. Incubate the slides twice in xylene for 15 minutes.

21. Add three drops of Cytoseal-XYL (Thermo Scientific Inc.) onto slide and lay cover slip flat onto the slide. Incubate the slides at 37°C overnight to cure.

Heart wall thickness measurement:

22. Examine serial sections for each fly and photograph serial images from the first appearance of the heart in the thorax (Figure 50.2).

23. The landmark section is the section with the last *en face* appearance of the ventral longitudinal fiber, also called the dorsal diaphragm. Typically, we designate this landmark section as number 1 and photograph serial sections towards the abdomen. Heart wall thickness is measured in sections number 5–7 (Figure 50.2). These regions are analogous to the positions of the heart measured by OCT.

24. Use ImageJ to measure the width of heart wall on dorsal, ventral, left, and right side of the heart tube.

Limitations

This method is used to measure the heart wall thickness. Heart lumen dimensions are not generally measured using this method. Instead, we rely on OCT measurements as described earlier.

Conclusions

Drosophila-based research offers powerful resources to address questions pertaining to human cardiovascular diseases. Mutations identified in human genetic studies can be validated using the fruit fly model. Additionally, studies using the adult fly have the potential to identify genes that cause or modify cardiomyopathies. Ultimately, translating the results of genetic screens conducted in *Drosophila* to humans has the potential to identify new therapies to treat cardiomyopathies.

References

1 Neely GG, Kuba K, Cammarato A, Isobe K, Amann S, Zhang L, *et al.* A global in vivo Drosophila RNAi screen identifies NOT3 as a conserved regulator of heart function. *Cell* 2010; **141**: 142–153.

2 Wolf MJ, Amrein H, Izatt JA, Choma MA, Reedy MC, Rockman HA, *et al.* Drosophila as a model for the identification of genes causing adult human heart disease. *Proc Natl Acad Sci U S A* 2006; **103**: 1394–1399.

3 Wolf MJ, Rockman HA. Drosophila, genetic screens, and cardiac function. *Circ Res* 2011; **109**: 794–806.

4 Bodmer R, Venkatesh TV. Heart development in Drosophila and vertebrates: conservation of molecular mechanisms. *Dev Genet* 1998; **22**: 181–186.

5 Reim I, Frasch M. Genetic and genomic dissection of cardiogenesis in the Drosophila model. *Pediatr Cardiol* 2010; **31**: 325–334.

6 Lin N, Badie N, Yu L, Abraham D, Cheng H, Bursac N, *et al.* A method to measure myocardial calcium handling in adult Drosophila. *Circ Res* 2011; **108**: 1306–1315.

7 Taghli-Lamallem O, Akasaka T, Hogg G, Nudel U, Yaffe D, Chamberlain JS, *et al.* Dystrophin deficiency in Drosophila reduces lifespan and causes a dilated cardiomyopathy phenotype. *Aging Cell* 2008; **7**: 237–249.

8 Allikian MJ, Bhabha G, Dospoy P, Heydemann A, Ryder P, Earley JU, *et al.* Reduced life span with heart and muscle dysfunction in Drosophila sarcoglycan mutants. *Hum Mol Genet* 2007; **16**: 2933–2943.

9 Yu L, Lee T, Lin N, Wolf MJ. Affecting Rhomboid-3 function causes a dilated heart in adult Drosophila. *PLoS Genet* 2010; **6**: e1000969.

10 Kim IM, Wolf MJ, Rockman HA. Gene deletion screen for cardiomyopathy in adult Drosophila identifies a new notch ligand. *Circ Res* 2010; **106**: 1233–1243.

11 Ocorr K, Reeves NL, Wessells RJ, Fink M, Chen HS, Akasaka T, *et al.* KCNQ potassium channel mutations cause cardiac arrhythmias in Drosophila that mimic the effects of aging. *Proc Natl Acad Sci U S A* 2007; **104**: 3943–3948.

12 Lee JH, Budanov AV, Park EJ, Birse R, Kim TE, Perkins GA, *et al.* Sestrin as a feedback inhibitor of TOR that prevents age-related pathologies. *Science* 2010; **327**: 1223–1228.

13 Qian L, Wythe JD, Liu J, Cartry J, Vogler G, Mohapatra B, *et al.* Tinman/Nkx2-5 acts via miR-1 and upstream of Cdc42 to regulate heart function across species. *J Cell Biol* 2011; **193**: 1181–1196.

14 Lim HY, Wang W, Wessells RJ, Ocorr K, Bodmer R. Phospholipid homeostasis regulates lipid metabolism and cardiac function through SREBP signaling in Drosophila. *Genes Dev* 2011; **25**: 189–200.

15 Dorn GW, 2nd, Clark CF, Eschenbacher WH, Kang MY, Engelhard JT, Warner SJ, *et al.* MARF and Opa1 control mitochondrial and cardiac function in Drosophila. *Circ Res* 2011; **108**: 12–17.

16 Luong N, Davies CR, Wessells RJ, Graham SM, King MT, Veech R, *et al.* Activated FOXO-mediated insulin resistance is blocked by reduction of TOR activity. *Cell Metab* 2006; **4**: 133–142.

17 Wessells R, Fitzgerald E, Piazza N, Ocorr K, Morley S, Davies C, *et al.* d4eBP acts downstream of both dTOR and dFoxo to modulate cardiac functional aging in Drosophila. *Aging Cell* 2009; **8**: 542–552.

18 Cammarato A, Ahrens CH, Alayari NN, Qeli E, Rucker J, Reedy MC, *et al.* A mighty small heart: the cardiac proteome of adult Drosophila melanogaster. *PLoS One* 2011; **6**: e18497.

19 Coquin L, Feala JD, McCulloch AD, Paternostro G. Metabolomic and flux-balance analysis of age-related decline of hypoxia tolerance in Drosophila muscle tissue. *Mol Syst Biol* 2008; **4**: 233.

20 Ocorr K, Fink M, Cammarato A, Bernstein S, Bodmer R. Semi-automated optical heartbeat analysis of small hearts. *J Vis Exp* 2009; (**31**) pii: 1435.

21 Alayari NN, Vogler G, Taghli-Lamallem O, Ocorr K, Bodmer R, Cammarato A, *et al.* Fluorescent labeling of Drosophila heart structures. *J Vis Exp* 2009; (**32**) pii: 1423.

22 Huang D, Swanson EA, Lin CP, Schuman JS, Stinson WG, Chang W, *et al.* Optical coherence tomography. *Science* 1991; **254**: 1178–1181.

23 Wessells RJ, Fitzgerald E, Cypser JR, Tatar M, Bodmer R. Insulin regulation of heart function in aging fruit flies. *Nat Genet* 2004; **36**: 1275–1281.

Index

Note: Page references in *italics* refer to Figures; those in **bold** refer to Tables

---

Manual of Research Techniques in Cardiovascular Medicine, First Edition. Edited by Hossein Ardehali, Roberto Bolli, and
Douglas W. Losordo.
© 2014 John Wiley & Sons, Ltd. Published 2014 by John Wiley & Sons, Ltd.